Personalized Precision Medicine: Role of Epigenetic Biomarkers

Personalized Precision Medicine: Role of Epigenetic Biomarkers

Editor: Tommy Royal

AMERICAN
MEDICAL PUBLISHERS
www.americanmedicalpublishers.com

AMERICAN
MEDICAL PUBLISHERS
www.americanmedicalpublishers.com

Cataloging-in-Publication Data

Personalized precision medicine : role of epigenetic biomarkers / edited by Tommy Royal.
p. cm.
Includes bibliographical references and index.
ISBN 979-8-88740-371-7
1. Epigenetics. 2. Genetics. 3. Biochemical markers. 4. Personalized medicine.
5. Medical genetics. I. Royal, Tommy.
QH450 .P47 2023
572.865--dc23

American Medical Publishers,
41 Flatbush Avenue,
1st Floor, New York,
NY 11217, USA

ISBN 979-8-88740-371-7 (Hardback)

Contents

Preface

The purpose of the book is to provide a glimpse into the dynamics and to present opinions and studies of some of the scientists engaged in the development of new ideas in the field from very different standpoints. This book will prove useful to students and researchers owing to its high content quality.

Epigenetics is the study of heritable phenotype changes that do not entail changes in the DNA sequence. Epigenetic abnormalities have emerged as the most promising biomarkers for diagnosis and prognosis in the early stage of illnesses, such as cancer, autoimmune diseases and psychological disorders. A medical model in which people are divided into groups with medical decisions, practices, interventions and products being tailored to the individual patient based on their predicted response or risk of disease is referred as personalized medicine. The terms precision medicine and personalized medicine are utilized interchangeably for describing the concept. Diagnostic testing is used often in personalized medicine to determine suitable and optimal therapies based on a patient's genetic content, or other molecular or cellular analysis. Certain aspects of personalized medicine utilize genetic information, such as pharmacogenomics. With the help of genomics, proteomics and imaging techniques, molecular scale data of the patients is obtained easily. These molecular biomarkers are then used in determining the prognosis of diseases such as cancer. The readers would gain knowledge that would broaden their perspective about personalized precision medicine through this book. Also included herein is a detailed explanation of the role of epigenetic biomarkers. This book will help the readers in keeping pace with the rapid changes in this field of study.

At the end, I would like to appreciate all the efforts made by the authors in completing their chapters professionally. I express my deepest gratitude to all of them for contributing to this book by sharing their valuable works. A special thanks to my family and friends for their constant support in this journey.

Editor

1

Epigenetic Biomarkers in the Management of Ovarian Cancer: Current Perspectives

Alka Singh[1]*, Sameer Gupta*[2] *and Manisha Sachan*[1*]

[1] *Department of Biotechnology, Motilal Nehru National Institute of Technology, Allahabad, India,* [2] *Department of Surgical Oncology, King George Medical University, Lucknow, India*

***Correspondence:**
Manisha Sachan
manishas@mnnit.ac.in;
manishas77@rediffmail.com

Ovarian cancer (OC) causes significant morbidity and mortality as neither detection nor screening of OC is currently feasible at an early stage. Difficulty to promptly diagnose OC in its early stage remains challenging due to non-specific symptoms in the early-stage of the disease, their presentation at an advanced stage and poor survival. Therefore, improved detection methods are urgently needed. In this article, we summarize the potential clinical utility of epigenetic signatures like DNA methylation, histone modifications, and microRNA dysregulation, which play important role in ovarian carcinogenesis and discuss its application in development of diagnostic, prognostic, and predictive biomarkers. Molecular characterization of epigenetic modification (methylation) in circulating cell free tumor DNA in body fluids offers novel, non-invasive approach for identification of potential promising cancer biomarkers, which can be performed at multiple time points and probably better reflects the prevailing molecular profile of cancer. Current status of epigenetic research in diagnosis of early OC and its management are discussed here with main focus on potential diagnostic biomarkers in tissue and body fluids. Rapid and point of care diagnostic applications of DNA methylation in liquid biopsy has been precluded as a result of cumbersome sample preparation with complicated conventional methods of isolation. New technologies which allow rapid identification of methylation signatures directly from blood will facilitate sample-to answer solutions thereby enabling next-generation point of care molecular diagnostics. To date, not a single epigenetic biomarker which could accurately detect ovarian cancer at an early stage in either tissue or body fluid has been reported. Taken together, the methodological drawbacks, heterogeneity associated with ovarian cancer and non-validation of the clinical utility of reported potential biomarkers in larger ovarian cancer populations has impeded the transition of epigenetic biomarkers from lab to clinical settings. Until addressed, clinical implementation as a diagnostic measure is a far way to go.

Keywords: biomarker, cell free DNA, diagnosis, DNA methylation, epigenetics, epithelial ovarian cancer

KEYPOINTS

- Prompt diagnosis remains challenging due to non-specific symptoms in the early-stage of the disease, their presentation at an advanced stage and poor survival.
- DNA methylation occurs very early in malignant transformation and their utility as biomarker holds great promise to overcome the false positive detection of ovarian cancer using current standard serum marker CA125.
- Not even a single report has suggested or demonstrated a good epigenetic marker for early and accurate detection of OC in either tissue or fluid. Thus, early detection still remains a huge unmet need. However, analysis of a panel of aberrant methylation based epigenetic markers in blood-based non-invasive assay could pave its way into clinical implementation.

INTRODUCTION

Ovarian cancer, a molecularly heterogeneous disease, remains the most lethal disease among gynecological malignancies. Representing as the third most frequent cancer among female gynecological system carcinoma, ovarian cancer is associated with the highest mortality rates. Despite constituting only 3% of all female cancer, the annual incidence of ovarian cancer worldwide is 220,000 with 21,290 estimated numbers of new cases and 14,600 estimated deaths annually (Siegel et al., 2015). Typical diagnosis of more than 70% of OC cases, at an advanced disease stage is one of the potent reasons for high fatality rate and carries poor prognosis with current therapies. The median age of disease presentation in ovarian cancer is 60 years and its lifetime risk is one in seventy with an overall lifetime mortality of one in ninety five (Cannistra, 2004; Howe et al., 2006).

Epithelial ovarian cancer (E0C) comprises 90% of all forms of OC cases and is characterized by heterogeneity at histopathological, clinical and molecular level. The exact cause for the ovarian malignancy still remains unknown. A strong familiar history either of ovarian or breast cancer has been described as important risk factors associated with OC. More than one-fifth of ovarian carcinomas (about 23%) have hereditary susceptibility and germline mutations of BRCA1 and BRCA2 tumor suppressor genes; in particular contribute to 65–85% of these cases (Ramus et al., 2007). An association of hormonal risk in postmenopausal women is suggested by over 50% of deaths. In addition, parity, pregnancy, lactation, tubal ligation, and oral contraceptive use are associated with reduced risk and have been found to be protective factors against disease development.

Rapid growth, non-specific clinical symptoms at early stage of the disease and lack of early diagnostic methods make prompt diagnosis challenging. As a result, EOC is typically diagnosed at an advanced stage (FIGO III/IV), when the tumor has spread beyond the pelvis and even unlikely to be completely removed by surgery. The long term survival rates for women with disseminated malignancies are low (10–30%). However, diagnosis of ovarian cancer at the localized stage (confinement of lesion still to the ovaries) is highly curable (over 95% 5 year survival rate; Siegel et al., 2011). To improve the overall survival of women diagnosed with EOC and to overcome the non-specific clinical manifestation of EOC, identification of molecular biomarkers of preclinical or early stage EOC tumors is critically needed. A better understanding of EOC genome portrait will help in the identification of promising biomarkers of clinical utility for early diagnosis of OC.

MOLECULAR CLASSIFICATION

The primary OC were classified into epithelial (60%), germ cell (30%), and sex-cord stromal tumors (8%), by the World Health Organization (WHO) classification and tumor morphology system (2014). A large majority of OC, almost 80–85%, are of epithelial origin. However, a small proportion accounting approximately 10% of all OC falls into germ cell and sex-cord stromal tumor categories (Devouassoux-Shisheboran and Genestie, 2015). Further on the basis of disease dissemination, the American Joint committee on Cancer/Tumor Node Metastasis (AJCC/TNM) and International Federation of Gynecology and Obstetrics (FIGO) staging systems, classified ovarian cancer into various stages. The confinement of tumors to the ovaries is represented by stage I and II whereas stage III is associated with local metastasis (usually lymph) and stage IV with distal organ metastases (Yarbro et al., 1999).

EOCs have been further sub-categorized based on following two criteria: (a) firstly, on the degree of proliferation, grade and extent of invasion into Benign (adenoma and cystadenoma), low malignant potential (LMP) and malignant (b) and secondly based on tumor histopathological grade and molecular characteristics, EOC malignant tumors are classified into serous (70%, most common), endometrioid (10–20%), clear cell (12%), mucinous (3%) and less commonly, transitional (6%), squamous, mixed, and undifferentiated (<1%) subtypes (Bowtell, 2010; Devouassoux-Shisheboran and Genestie, 2015; Earp and Cunningham, 2015; **Figure 1**) On the basis of histological type and grade, these tumors exhibit different genetic and epidemiological risk factors, pattern of spread, molecular abnormalities, response to targeted therapies and disease prognosis (Devouassoux-Shisheboran and Genestie, 2015; Earp and Cunningham, 2015).

Almost a decade ago, a dualistic classification system recognized Type I and Type II EOC tumors (Shih and Kurman, 2004; Vang et al., 2009). Type I EOCs are generally low grade serous carcinomas but also include mucinous, endometrioid, and clear cell subtype tumors. They are thought to arise from a low malignant potential precursor, are characterized as slow growing with low levels of chromosomal instability, intact DNA repair machinery and harbor mutations in KRAS, BRAF, and ERBB2 at a high frequency. Type II EOCs arise *de novo* and are comprised of high-grade serous carcinoma. These aggressive tumors also include malignant mixed mesodermal and undifferentiated carcinomas, are characterized by rapid growth with no identified precursor lesions, high levels of chromosomal aberrations along with high frequency of TP53,

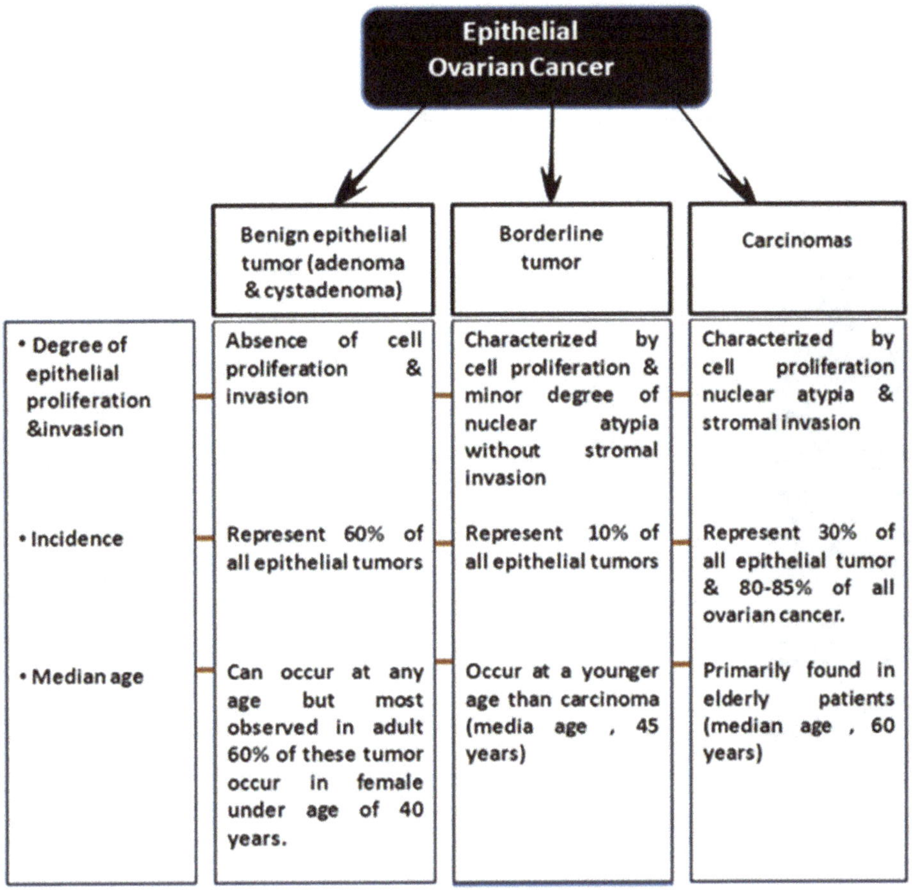

FIGURE 1 | Sub-classification of epithelial ovarian tumors.

BRCA1/2 mutations. They constitute 70% of EOC cases (Jayson et al., 2014; **Figure 2**).

The cells of origin of ovarian cancer are still debated. Two models with respect to the origin of ovarian cancer have been proposed: (1) origin from ovarian surface epithelium (OSE), (2) from the fallopian tube. Taken together, the pro-inflammatory environment due to ovulation events, expression pattern of ovarian inclusion cysts and biomarkers which are shared by OSE and malignant growth, form the basis of first model. On contrary, tubal precursor lesions, genetic evidence of BRCA1/2 mutation carriers and recent studies strongly implicate a non-ovarian origin and form the basis of the later model. To date, neither model has evidently revealed superiority over the other. Thus, it is speculated that the HGSOC could have arisen from two different sites which undergo similar changes and could be a possible reason for tumor heterogeneity (Klotz and Wimberger, 2017). It has also been postulated that aberrantly methylated Mullerian duct cells migrate into ovarian stroma where they are supported by the epigenetically/ genetically altered stromal environment, facilitating a cascade of events which culminate in ovarian carcinogenesis. Epigenetic profiling of endocervical glandular cells would facilitate in prediction of risk or early detection of ovarian cancer (Jones et al., 2010).

SCREENING AND EARLY DETECTION

OC is generally characterized by few non-specific early symptoms, presentation of the disease at a late stage and poor survival. Difficulty to diagnose it in its early stages still remains challenging. Early diagnosis, screening and personalized treatment is still the biggest unmet need to combat this devastating disease. Unavailability of early cancer-specific diagnostic markers and ubiquitous acquisition of drug resistance to targeted therapies are the most striking obstacles for the effective OC treatment.

Clinically, serum antigen-125 (CA125) is the most extensively studied, established and utilized diagnostic marker of EOC, despite its elevation marked by only 47% of early-stage EOC (Woolas et al., 1993). Additionally, aberrantly elevated serum CA125 have been reported in several benign conditions of endometriosis, pregnancy, peritonitis, pelvic inflammatory disease, uterine fibroids, menstrual cycle, liver cirrhosis. Its elevation is also associated with several malignancies such as lung and colorectal cancer (Jacobs and Bast, 1989). Moreover, poor specificity, high false positive rate, and low positive prediction value make CA125 alone unsuitable as an EOC diagnostic marker.

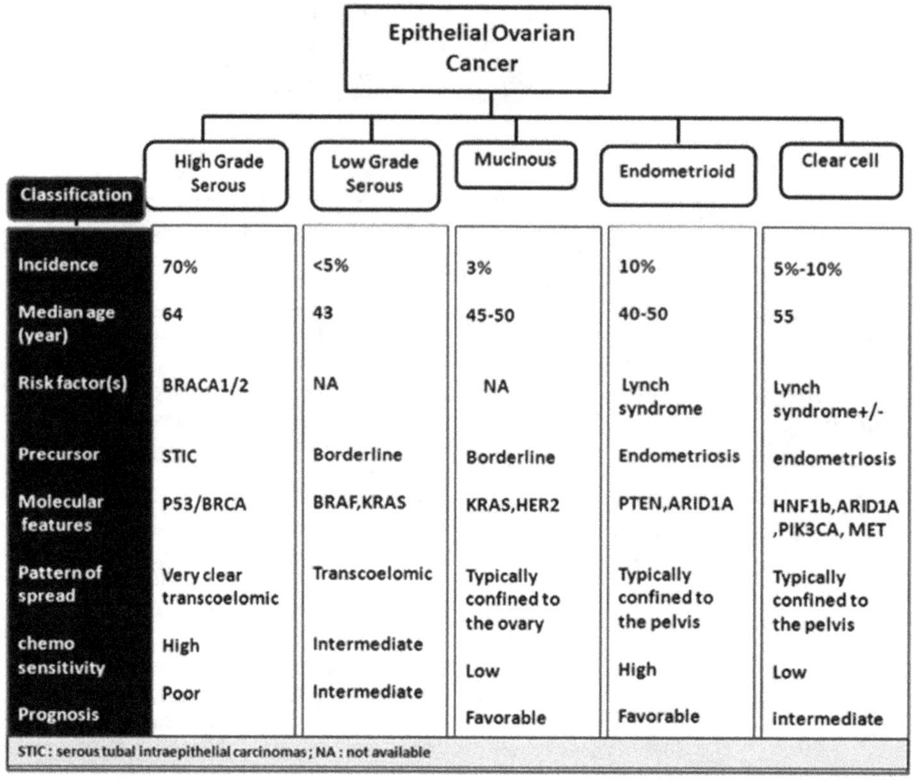

FIGURE 2 | Phenotypic- genotypic classification of epithelial ovarian cancer subtypes.

However, CA125 is more suitable markers for tumor recurrence (Clarke-Pearson, 2009).

For clinical needs to diagnose OC at an early stage, the conventional screening methods such as serum cancer antigen 125 (CA125) concentrations, transvaginal ultrasound probe and magnetic resonance imaging have not shown reliability in reducing population mortality or morbidity due to high false-negatives rates and lower sensitivity and specificity (Menon and Jacobs, 2000; Jacobs and Menon, 2004; Munkarah et al., 2007). Therefore, methods for early detection are critically required. Owing to the low incidence rate of OC amongst postmenopausal women, a logistic diagnostic screening test warrants the need of high sensitivity (>75%) and specificity (>99.6%) to attain a positive prediction value (PPV) of 10%. Novel biomarkers for early-stage diagnosis are being explored and it is more likely that a combination of biomarkers could achieve these required diagnostic criteria (Moore et al., 2010).

To determine the effect of screening on OC mortality, several randomized controlled trial in general population had been undertaken. Recently, both CA125 and transvaginal sonography (TVS) was evaluated in the Prostate, Lung, Colorectal, and Ovarian (PLCO) cancer screening trial, however no significant difference was observed in OC mortality between screening and conventional care arms (Buys et al., 2011). The United Kingdom Collaborative Trial of Ovarian Cancer Screening (UKCTOCS), being considered as the largest prospective randomized trial, comprised of over 200,000 asymptomatic postmenopausal women who were screened with TVS alone and combined TVS and CA125. Although improvement in specificity of detection was achieved on combining CA125 with TVS, however these trials failed to attain the requisite diagnostic accuracy of 99.6% specificity (Menon et al., 2009). CA125 together with HE4 has somewhat improved sensitivity and specificity of detection which correctly identified 76.4% of cancer samples and 95% of cancer negative samples. This accuracy was notably higher than either marker alone. However further validation is still required (Moore et al., 2010). According to the Guide to Clinical Preventive Services 2010–2011, it has been mentioned that neither of any screening test [serum antigen-125 (CA-125), ultrasound imaging, pelvic examination or any earlier diagnosis methods] was able to improve OC survival rates U. S. Preventive Services Task Force (2010).

The Risk of Malignancy Index, widely used at present, particularly UK, is a score based on ultrasound variables, menopausal status and CA125 (Jacobs et al., 1990). Its sensitivity is the determining criteria for a patient to be sent to experts by referring gynecologist provided objective assessment score is lower (78%) (Geomini et al., 2009). Transvaginal sonography (TVS) is based on a formal scoring model system. Though highly sensitive and being considered as an ideal method for second stage diagnosis, the major limitation associated with this method is its high dependency on individual expertise (Yazbek et al., 2008). Therefore, in clinical practice to discriminate benign and malignant ovarian tumors is still a significant challenge. The availability of biomarker or their combination which can potentially detect ovarian cancer at its earliest stage with required sensitivity and specificity would help in improving clinical outcomes.

MARKERS FOR OVARIAN CANCER DIAGNOSIS AND MANAGEMENT

Protein Markers

As discussed before, a suitable screening test for OC early stage diagnosis will require high sensitivity and high specificity. Current practices for screening of OC include transvaginal ultrasonography, biomarker analysis, or a combination of both. To date, a number of potential biomarkers for early diagnosis of OC have been identified through intense research in proteomic and genomic. Here, we summarize a comprehensive account of recent researches on explored novel and robust serum based biomarkers for the non-invasive early stage screening of ovarian cancer (**Table 1**).

Although being considered as the "gold standard" biomarker for detection of OC, its clinical relevance mainly falls in evaluating disease recurrence. Other biochemical markers such as lysophosphatidic acid, human epididymis protein 4 (HE4), inhibins (which are members of TGF-β subfamily), Mesothelin (associated with migration and metastasis) (Huang et al., 2006), Osteopontin, and YKL-40 have been reported to be elevated in sera of patients with OC amongst various studies, which could be of diagnostic significance for improved cancer detection, most likely in various combination with one another and /or with CA125 (Rosenthal et al., 2006; Moore et al., 2010). The most promising molecular biomarker of all these, to date are HE4 and Mesothelin. So far, US FDA has only approved CA125 and HE4 for monitoring disease progression/recurrence, but not for screening purpose (Rosenthal et al., 2006).

For the triage of pelvic mass, the multivariate index assay OVA1, constituting measurements of 5-proteins: CA125-II, apolipoprotein A1, transthyretin, beta 2 microglobulin, and transferrin, has been approved by FDA since 2009. Although, the test had improved sensitivity but compromised in revealing diagnostic potential with its low specificity upon replacement of CA125 with the multivariate index assay (Nguyen et al., 2013). Elevated levels of Kallikrein 6 and 7 (KLK6 and KLK7) was reported in sera of ovarian carcinoma subtypes, depicting their potential to improve early detection of OC. Other biomarkers with potential clinical significance for early diagnosis in women with EOC include GSTT1, Prostasin (PRSS8), KLK6, KLK7, FOLR1, and ALDH1, which are currently under research and clinical trials (Sarojini et al., 2012).

Evaluation of several prediagnostic multimarker panels along with PLCO screening trial has identified promising biomarkers which are able to distinguish ovarian cancer cases from normal control groups; for instance, a four biomarker panel consisting of CA-125, HE4, CEA, and VCAM-1 effectively discriminated early stage OC from healthy controls with sensitivity of 86% at 98% specificity (Lin et al., 2009). Another panel constituting of CA-125, ApoA1, TTR, and H418, was able to differentiate OC patients at early stage of disease from cancer-free healthy control samples with 74% sensitivity at 97% specificity (Zhang et al., 2004). Still to date, no panel of biomarkers that has been examined amongst numerous studies could outperform CA125 alone, in distinguishing between the two groups. The sensitivity and specificity of serum based non-invasive biomarkers for improved ovarian cancer detection from various studies as well as the currently active/completed clinical trials evaluating potent biochemical markers of clinical significance for early diagnosis of EOC are summarized in **Tables 2, 3** respectively.

Genetic Marker

About 23% of ovarian tumors have been associated with hereditary conditions and the genetic abnormalities in about 65–85% of hereditary ovarian carcinomas is the germline mutation in BRCA (breast cancer early onset genes BRCA1 and BRCA2) genes which are essential for DNA repair as well as in maintaining genomic stability and integrity. The cumulative lifetime risk of EOC for a woman with BRCA1 and BRCA2 mutation is 39–46% and 12–20%, respectively (Ramus et al., 2007). Lifetime risk to develop breast cancer and ovarian cancer is enhanced up to 85% and up to 54% respectively in the carriers of BRCA1 and BRCA2 mutations. Association of several tumor suppressor genes and oncogenes (tumor suppressor gene TP53 in Li- Fraumeni syndrome, mismatch repair genes (MMR) in Lynch syndrome, genes involved with double strand break repair system: BARD1, CHEK2, RAD51, and PALB2) with hereditary ovarian cancer has been reported. Till date, around 16 genes have been reported to be associated with hereditary ovarian carcinogenesis while several other mutations are yet unknown and need to be further explored (Toss et al., 2015).

Epigenetic Marker

Epigenetics is the mechanism for the regulation of gene expression without any alternation in the primary DNA sequence (Jones and Laird, 1999; Jones and Baylin, 2002; Feinberg and Tycko, 2004). DNA methylation, modification of histone proteins and miRNAs are the key modulator in regulating several cellular processes such as cell differentiation, embryogenesis, inactivation of X chromosome, genome imprinting, and many others (Jones, 2001; Reik and Lewis, 2005; Kacem and Feil, 2009; Portela and Esteller, 2010). The epigenetic alternations involve interplay between DNA methylation, histone modification and micro RNA expression to modulate gene expression during development and cancer progression. (1) The global hypomethylation, largely of repetitive DNA which results in demethylation of several oncogenes and (2) localized hypermethylation at promoters of various tumor suppressor genes leading to their transcriptional silencing, are two opposite epigenetic phenomenon involved in tumorigenesis (Sharma et al., 2010). DNA methyltransferase (DNMT) mediated methylation of deoxycytosine located within the CpG dinucleotides is the best known and widely studied epigenetic mechanism leading to transcription repression in cancer (Bird and Wolffe, 1999; Hendrich and Bird, 2000; Bird,

TABLE 1 | Novel tumor biochemical markers for early detection of ovarian cancer.

Biochemical marker	Nature	Origin/function	Status	Source	Clinical utility	References
CA125	Glycoprotein antigen	Expressed by fetal amniotic epithelium and coelomic epithelium	Elevated Early stage: 47% Advanced stage: >90%	Serum	Valuable marker for tumor recurrence Limitations: Unsuitable for early detection due to insufficient sensitivity and being elevated in other conditions	Clarke-Pearson, 2009; Moore et al., 2010
HE4	Protease	Serum maturation	Elevated Serous: 93% Endometrioid: 100%	Serum	Histotype differentiation and screening	Hough et al., 2000; Lu et al., 2004; Moore et al., 2008
Mesothelin	Glycosylphosphatidylinositol-linked cell surface molecule	*Expressed by mesothelial cells *Involved in metastasis	Elevated Early stage: 60%	Urine	Early screening	McIntosh et al., 2004; Tang et al., 2013
Transthyretin	An acute phase reactant and major carrier of serum thyroxine	Tumor development	Downregulated in EOC patients	Serum	Early stage screening	Mählck and Grankvist, 1994; Schweigert and Sehouli, 2005; Nosov et al., 2009
ApoA1	Constituent of high density lipoproteins	Prevents tumor development	Downregulated in ovarian cancer patients	Serum	Early stage screening	Gadomska et al., 2005; Kim et al., 2012
Kallikrein	Family of Serine proteases *Human KLK family: 15 members *Chromosome position: 19q13.3–4	Regulates proteolytic cascades	Elevated: 12KLK/15	Serum	Elevated KLK-6 and−10 in OC cases with low level of CA125. Useful marker for OC detection	Borgoño and Diamandis, 2004; Rosen et al., 2005
Osteopontin	An adhesive glycoprotein	*Synthesized by osteoblasts and vascular endothelial cells *Associated with bone remodeling and immune function	Elevated in invasive and borderline ovarian cancer tumors	Plasma	Early stage screening	Kim et al., 2002

2002). DNA methylation is known to be the earliest event during carcinogenesis and plays a crucial role in silencing of tumor suppressor genes (Sharma et al., 2010; Teschendorff and Widschwendter, 2012; Teschendorff et al., 2012, 2016; Bartlett et al., 2016). Promoter methylation mediated epigenetic silencing of gene is regulated by the recruitment of MBD (methyl CpG binding proteins such as MeCP2, MBD1, MBD2, and MBD4) which in turn regulates chromatin state by recruiting histone modifying and chromatin-remodeling complexes (repressors) at the site of methylation, which subsequently generates condensed chromatin structure and results in transcriptional repression (Esteller, 2007; Lopez-Serra and Esteller, 2008). On contrary, epigenetic activation of gene is regulated by recruitment of Cfp1 and histone methyltransferase Setd1 which aids in generating an open chromatin structure by creating domains which are enriched with active histone marks (acetylation and H3K4 trimethylation) (Thomson et al., 2010, p. 1; Jones and Baylin, 2007; **Supplementary Figure 1**). Increasing evidences has revealed the significant role of DNA methylation in cancer development and progression, right from transcriptional silencing of tumor suppressor genes to the activation of oncogenes and consequently promoting metastasis (Costello and Plass, 2001; Herman and Baylin, 2003; Wilting and Dannenberg, 2012). Apparently, it is quite evident now that DNA methylation plays an equal or possibly even greater role than the genetic lesion such as mutations, deletion and translocations which have been associated for long, with malignant transformations and carcinogenesis (Chan T. A. et al., 2008). For instance, though the familial breast cancer susceptibility gene 1 (BRCA1) mutations contributes to 5–10% of EOC, promoter hypermethylation of non-mutated BRCA1 allele is the second disruptive event to the development of this cancer (Barton et al., 2008).

Tissue Biomarkers

Diagnosis

So far, several methylation based signatures have been reported in EOC. Here, we summarize an overview of some of the extensively studied potential biomarkers of diagnostic utility in ovarian cancer (**Table 6**). In ovarian cancer, a large number of tumor suppressor genes have been identified to be silenced by promoter hypermethylation and downregulated includes DAPK, LOT1, TMS1/ASC, and PAR4 (pro-apoptotic function and cell cycle regulation), p16, SPARC, ANGPTL2, and CTGF (tumor suppressor activity), ICAM-1 and CDH1 (cell adhesion), PEG31 (role in imprinting) and many others (**Tables 4, 5**). In

TABLE 2 | Specificity and sensitivity of early detection biomarkers for ovarian cancer from various studies.

Biochemical biomarker	Source	Population tested	Clinical prediction		References
			Sensitivity	Specificity	
HE4	Serum	147 Cancer (111 ovarian cancer cases), 285 Benign, 66 controls	79.3%	98.9%	Molina et al., 2011
HE4 + CA125	Serum	383 Benign and 89 Cancer	100% 92.30%	74.20% 76.0 %	Moore et al., 2011
Osteopontin	Plasma	46 Benign, 47 cancer, 51 ovarian cancer, 107 controls	-	-	Kim et al., 2002
Prostasin + CA125	Serum	64 cancer, 137 control	92%	94%	Mok et al., 2001
KLK6	Serum	141 Benign, 146 ovarian cancer, 97 controls	21–26%	95%	Diamandis et al., 2003
KLK6+ CA125	Serum	141 Benign, 146 ovarian cancer, 97 controls	42%	90%	Diamandis et al., 2003
B7-H4	Serum	1,023 cancer, 997 Benign (236 ovarian cancer cases, 260 controls)	45%	97%	Simon et al., 2006
B7-H4 + CA125	Serum	1,023 cancer, 997 Benign (236 ovarian cancer cases, 260 controls)	65%	97%	Simon et al., 2007
CA125/IL-6/IL-8/VEGF/EGF	Serum	44 Early-stage cancers 37 Benign, 45 controls	84%	95%	Gorelik, 2005
CA125/IL-6/G-CSF/VEGF/EGF	Serum	44 Early-stage cancers 37 Benign, 45 controls	86.5%	93%	Gorelik, 2005
CA125/HE4/Glycodelin/ PLAUR/MUC1/PAI-1	Serum	200 Cancers (133 stage I/II), 396 Healthy controls	80.5%	96.5%	Havrilesky et al., 2008
Leptin/Prolactin/ Osteopontin/IGF2	Serum	100 Cancers, 106 controls	95%	94%	Mor et al., 2005
CA125 HE4 Mesothelin	Serum	143 Cancers, 124 benign, 344 controls	78% 68–82% 31–44%	98% 98% 98%	Shah et al., 2009
Leptin/Prolactin/ Osteopontin/IGF2/MIF/ CA125	Serum	Training: 113 cancers, 181 controls Test: 43 cancers, 181 Controls	95.3%	99.4%	Visintin et al., 2008
CA125/ CA19- 9 /EGFR /CRP/ Myoglobin/APOA1/ APOC3/MIP1A/ IL-6/IL-18/ Tenascin C	Serum	115 Cancers, 93 benign 24 Controls, 13 non-ovarian cancers	91.3%	88.5%	Amonkar et al., 2009
CA-125, HE4, SI	Serum	74 cancer, 137 controls	84%	98.5%	Andersen et al., 2010
RIM, ROMA, CA-125, HE4,	Serum	445 Benign, 31 borderline, and 162 malignant tumors	Postmenopausal 89, 91, 92, and 72% Premenopausal 87, 87, 96, and 83%	Postmenopausal 80, 77, 80, and 92% Premenopausal 90, 81, 60, 91%	Lycke et al., 2018
CA-125 HE4 TTR	Serum	130 Benign, 126 ovarian cancer, 400 controls	64.29% 46.4% 78.6%	53.57% 43.3% 68.8%	Zheng et al., 2018
CA-125, HE4, TK1	Serum	75 ovarian cancer, 40 Benign, 35 controls	94.18%	79.53%	Xi et al., 2017
CA-125+HE4, HE4+FOLR1	Serum	150 benign controls, 216 ovarian cancer, 20 controls	67% 65%	95% 95%	Leung et al., 2016
CA-125, ApoA1, TTR	Serum	200 cancer, 142 controls	74%	97%	Zhang et al., 2004
CA125, HE4, MMP-7, CA72-4	Serum	142 stage I cancer, 217 controls	83.2%	98%	Simmons et al., 2016
CA-125, CA 72–4, MCSF	Plasma	123 cancer, 224 controls	70%	98%	Edgell et al., 2010
CA-125, TTR, ApoA1	Serum	20 cancer, 82 controls	89%	92%	Su et al., 2007
CA-125, HE4, CEA, VCAM-1	Serum	456 cancer, 2,000 controls	86–93%	98%	Lin et al., 2009
CA-125, CRP, SAA, IL-6, IL-8	Plasma	150 cancer, 212 controls	94.1%	91.3%	Edgell et al., 2010
S100A4	Serum	160 cancer, 52 Benign, 52 controls	78%	92%	Lv et al., 2018
KPNA2	Serum	162 cancer, 48 controls	71.4%	81.2%	Huang et al., 2017
Septin-9 Clusterin	Plasma	137 EOC, 12 borderline,51 benign, 58 controls	82.5% 71.5%	50.0% 41.4%	Lyu et al., 2018

TABLE 3 | Clinical trials (currently active or completed) for evaluating novel biomarkers of ovarian cancer.

Biochemical marker	Setting	Phase	Samples (*n*)	Status	Clinical trial no.	Primary clinical outcome	References
All biomarkers	Adnexal mass	1	500 (E)	Completed	NCT01466049	Screening	NA
HE4 + CA125	Pelvic mass	0	566	Completed	NCT00315692	Cancer vs. benign disease	Moore et al., 2009
CA125	Low risk women	1	9500 (E)	Recruiting	NCT00539162	Rate of increase in CA125 over time	NA
HE4 + CA125	Adnexal mass	1	512	Completed	NCT00987649	Initial cancer risk assessment	NA
CA125+ HE4	High risk women	1	1208 (E)	Active, not recruiting	NCT01121640	PPV of screening protocol	NA
CA125	High risk women	2	2400 (E)	Withdrawn	NCT00080639	Screening	NA
Mesothelin	Low risk women	0	250 (E)	Unknown	NCT000155740	Screening	NA
FOLR1	Stage I ovarian cancer	2	50 (E)	Terminated	NCT01511055	Sensitivity and specificity of Intraoperative imaging (IOI) with folate	NA
CA125 + TVU	Ovarian disease	0	750 (E)	Terminated	NCT01292733	CA125 measurement in blood over time	NA
CA125± TVU	Postmenopausal	0	48230	Completed	NCT00058032	Screening post menopausal women	Menon et al., 2009; Jacobs et al., 2011
CA125	High risk women	0	2430	Unknown	NCT00039559	Sensitivity and specificity of early detection for ovarian cancer	NA
CA125+ TVU	High genetic risk women	0	5000 (E)	Completed	NCT00033488	Screening women at high genetic risk for ovarian cancer	NA
CA125	High risk women	0	6000 (E)	Recruiting	NCT00005095	Screening	NA
Combined methods	Ovarian neoplasms	0	36000	Unknown	NCT01178736	Low- cost screening	NA
Interventional	High risk women	0	1500	Recruiting	NCT00849199	Genetic testing, screening	NA
All biomarkers	High risk women	0	250 (E)	Unknown	NCT00854399	Overall survival	NA
Tumor markers	High risk women	0	5000	Completed	NCT00267072	Early stage detection	NA
DNA markers	Ovarian cancer	0	118 (E)	Active, not recruiting	NCT00879840	Assessment of screening modalities	NA
BRCA1/2 Mutation	Ovarian neoplasms	0	1500	Completed	NCT00001468	Identifying BRCA1/2 mutation	NA
BRCA	Epithelial ovarian cancer	0	600 (E)	Completed	NCT03229122	Genetic Testing of BRCA	NA
All biomarkers	High risk women	0	500(E)	Recruiting	NCT03150121	Identification of uterine lavage-based biomarkers for early detection	NA
All biomarkers	High risk women	0	6000	Recruiting	NCT00005095	Early stage detection and prevention	NA
CA125	High genetic risk women	0	40	Completed	NCT00043472	Screening	NA
DNA markers	Women with serous epithelial ovarian cancer	0	250	Not yet recruiting	NCT03622385	Early detection of high grade serous epithelial ovarian cancer	NA

TVU, transvaginal ultrasonography; (w), women; (E), estimated enrollment; IOI, intraoperative imaging. Source: http://clinicaltrials.gov/.

ovarian cancer, some of the most frequently methylated genes include OPCML (tumor suppressor activity), TES (involved in regulation of cell motility) and RASSF1A (tumor suppressor activity as well as an inhibitor of the anaphase-promoting complex) (Barton et al., 2008). Promoter methylation of HOXA10 and HOXA11, which are involved in very early ovarian tumor initiation effectively distinguished normal and malignant ovaries (Fiegl et al., 2008; Widschwendter et al., 2009). Methylation induced silencing of PTEN has also been frequently observed in primary epithelial ovarian carcinomas (Kurose et al., 2001). CTGF (encodes the connective tissue growth factor) (Kikuchi et al., 2007; Barbolina et al., 2009), CCBE1 (hypothesized to be involved in regulation of cell motility) (Barton et al., 2010), HIC1 (a p53 target gene) (Rathi et al., 2002), CDH13 (Makarla et al., 2005), and CDH1 (the loss of which correlates with the upregulation of matrix metalloproteinases and metastasis- promoting protein a 5-integrin) (Sawada et al., 2008) act as metastasis suppressors.

TABLE 4 | List of most frequently epigenetically dysregulated genes in ovarian cancer.

S. No	Gene	Function	Epigenetic event	References
1.	Survivin	Apoptotic inhibitor	Downregulated	Mirza et al., 2002
2.	GATA 4	Transcription factor	Downregulated	Caslini et al., 2006; Cai et al., 2009
3.	APC	Regulation of cell adhesion	Downregulated	Tam et al., 2007
4.	ARHI	Ras homolog, maternally imprinted putative tumor suppressor. Negative regulator of cancer growth and progression	Downregulated	Yu et al., 2003; Fu et al., 2015
5.	BRCA 1	DNA damage response	Downregulated	Baldwin et al., 2000; Wilcox et al., 2005; Press et al., 2008
6.	DAPK	Apoptosis	Downregulated	Bai et al., 2004
7.	Estrogen receptor β	Transcriptional activator	Downregulated	Suzuki et al., 2008
8.	hMLH 1	DNA mismatch repair	Downregulated	Meng et al., 2008; Zhang H. et al., 2008
9.	hMSH 2	DNA mismatch repair	Downregulated	Zhang H. et al., 2008
10.	ICAM 1	Cell/matrix adhesion	Downregulated	Arnold et al., 2001
11.	LOT1	Apoptosis	Downregulated	Abdollahi et al., 2003; Kamikihara et al., 2005
12.	OPCML	Cell adhesion	Downregulated	Sellar et al., 2003; Teodoridis et al., 2005; Zhang J. et al., 2006
13.	PACE-4	Serine protease	Downregulated	Fu et al., 2003
14.	RASSFIA	Microtubule stability	Downregulated	Agathanggelou et al., 2001; Yoon et al., 2001
15.	PEG 3	Apoptosis	Downregulated	Feng W. et al., 2008
16.	DLEC 1	Unknown	Downregulated	Kwong et al., 2006
17.	ARLTS 1	Premature termination of translation	Downregulated	Petrocca et al., 2006
18.	TCEAL 7	Cell death regulation	Downregulated	Chien et al., 2005
19.	P16	Cell cycle control	Downregulated	Milde-Langosch et al., 1998; Katsaros et al., 2004
20.	TMS1	Apoptosis	Downregulated	Akahira et al., 2004a
21.	WT1	Transcription factor	Downregulated	Kaneuchi et al., 2005
22.	14-3-3 SIGMA	Regulation of cell growth and differentiation	Downregulated	Kaneuchi et al., 2004
23.	DR 4	Apoptosis	Downregulated	Horak et al., 2005
24.	FBXO 32	Apoptosis (?)	Downregulated	Chou et al., 2010
25.	IGFBP-3	Antiproliferative, pro-apoptosis, and invasion suppressor	Downregulated	Torng et al., 2009
26.	SFRP5	Modulator of Wnt signaling	Downregulated	Su et al., 2010
27.	CCBE 1	Migration and cell survival	Downregulated	Barton et al., 2010
28.	RUNX3	Transcription factor	Downregulated	Zhang et al., 2009
29.	CHFR	Cell cycle control	Downregulated	Gao et al., 2009
30.	Maspin(SERPINBS)	Protease inhibitor	Expressed	Rose et al., 2006
31.	FANCF	DNA repair(?)	Up regulated	Taniguchi et al., 2003
32.	Synuclein gamma	Unknown	Up regulated	Gupta et al., 2003
33.	TUBB3	Formation of microtubules	Up regulated	Izutsu et al., 2008
34.	CLDN3	Tight junction protein	Up regulated	Honda et al., 2007
35.	HOXA10	Transcription factor	Up regulated	Cheng et al., 2010
36.	FBXW7	Ubiquitin ligase mediates ubiquitylation of oncoproteins	Downregulated	Kitade et al., 2016
37.	SPARC	Membrane-associated glycoprotein, normal development, anti-proliferative, and de-adhesive properties angiogenesis, ECM production	Downregulated	Socha et al., 2009
38.	HIC1	Transcriptional repressor	Downregulated	Pieretti et al., 1995; Rathi et al., 2002; Teodoridis et al., 2005; Tam et al., 2007
39.	Rarβ	Transcriptional regulator of cell growth	Downregulated	Makarla et al., 2005; Tam et al., 2007
40.	GSTP1	Intra cellular detoxification	Downregulated	Makarla et al., 2005; Bol et al., 2010

(Continued)

TABLE 4 | Continued

S. No	Gene	Function	Epigenetic event	References
41.	TBX15	Development of mesodermal derivative	Downregulated	Gozzi et al., 2016
42.	HUSIF 1	Modulate heparin binding growth factor signaling promote Wnt signaling pathway	Downregulated	Staub et al., 2007
43.	SFRP1	Inhibitor of Wnt/β-catenin signaling pathway	Downregulated	Su et al., 2009; Kardum et al., 2017
44.	RunX1T1	Putative SMAD4 target/TGFβ/SMAD4 signaling	Downregulated	Yeh et al., 2011
45.	ANGPTL2	Secreted glycoprotein involved in angiogenesis	Downregulated	Kikuchi et al., 2008
46.	CTGF	Adhesion molecule, motility modulator	Downregulated	Kikuchi et al., 2007
47.	FOXD3	Transcriptional regulator of development, cell maintenance, and lineage specification	Downregulated	Luo et al., 2019
48.	NISCH	Encodes imidazoline receptor Nischarin, regulates cellular migration, and invasion upon interacting with PAK1, LIMK, Rac1, and LKB1	Downregulated	Li J. et al., 2015
49.	ABCA1	A TGF-β target, regulator of cholesterol efflux and metabolism	Downregulated	Chou et al., 2015, p. 1
50.	TIMP2	A EZH2 target, endogenous regulator of matrix metalloproteinases, repressor of metastasis	Downregulated	Yi et al., 2017
51.	PCDH17	Transmembrane protein belonging to cadherin superfamily, potential calcium-dependent cell-adhesion protein	Downregulated	Baranova et al., 2018
52.	LDOC1	A nuclear transcription factor, regulator of NFκB Signaling	Downregulated	Buchholtz et al., 2014
53.	RGS2	Regulator of GTPase activity of G protein subunits. Negative regulator of angiotensin-activated signaling pathway	Downregulated	Cacan, 2017
54.	PRTFDC1	Unknown	Downregulated	Cai et al., 2007
55.	DDR	Subclass of RTKs, associated with cell differentiation, proliferation, adhesion, migration, and invasion	Downregulated	Chung et al., 2017
56.	ARNTL	Circadian gene	Downregulated	Yeh et al., 2014
57.	GULP1	Apoptosis, lipid homeostasis, regulator of Arf6-mediated signaling	Downregulated	Maldonado et al., 2018, p. 1
58.	TGFB1	Adhesion, essential for function of microfibrils and interacts with fibronectin and integrins	Downregulated	Kang et al., 2010
59.	SALL2	Cellular quiescence factor, neural development	Downregulated	Sung et al., 2013
60.	PDZ-LIM	Ubiquitination of nuclear p65, inflammation	Downregulated	Zhao et al., 2016
61.	KLF11	Inhibitory regulator of TGFβ signaling, promotes apoptosis	Downregulated	Wang et al., 2015
62.	GBGT1	Encodes glycosyltransferase which plays role in synthesis of Forssman glycolipid	Downregulated	Jacob et al., 2014

Methylation induced repression of these suppressors correlates with invasive EOC.

Several studies have identified the association of tumor-specific gene methylation with molecular, clinical, and pathological characteristics of epithelial ovarian carcinomas. For instance, highest degree of promoter methylation of SFN (an inhibitor of cell cycle progression), TMS1 and WT1 has been demonstrated in clear-cell ovarian tumors than in other histological types (Kaneuchi et al., 2004, p. 14; Terasawa et al., 2004; Kaneuchi et al., 2005; Teodoridis et al., 2005). Another finding suggests that promoter methylation of RASSF1A, APC, GSTP1, and MGMT correlates with the presence of invasive ovarian carcinomas (Makarla et al., 2005). Hypermethylation of FOXD3 correlated with tumor suppressive role (inhibition of proliferation, migration and promotion of apoptosis) in ovarian cancer cells and thus could serve as a potential therapeutic target for diagnosis of ovarian cancer (Luo et al., 2019).

Using a high-throughput approach to screen genes that showed highest differential methylation between ovarian cancer and normal tissue, Melnikov et al. identified 10 genes to be informative in tissue samples which include: BRCA1, EP300, NR3C1, MLH1, DNAJC15, CDKN1C, TP73, PGR, THBS1, and TMS1. A maximum sensitivity of 69% with 70% specificity was attained on testing the potential of several combinations of these genes to discriminate normal from cancer tissue. Since, all tumors analyzed were of advanced stage (either stage IIIA or higher), therefore, the potential of this panel to diagnose EOC at an early stage is unknown (Melnikov et al., 2009). Ibanez de Caceres et al. demonstrated that hypermethylation of atleast one of the six genes in panel (BRCA1, RASSF1A, APC, $p14^{arf}$, $p16^{ink4a}$, and DAPK) could be detected in 70/ 71 (99%) of EOCs using methylation specific PCR. Furthermore, none of the normal non-neoplastic tissue showed methylation, revealing a specificity of 100%. Additionally, across all histological subtypes, grades, stages as well as age, hypermethylation of TSGs was observed (Ibanez de Caceres et al., 2004). Taken together, these results support hypermethylation of these tumor suppressor genes as a relatively early event in ovarian carcinogenesis and could serve as

TABLE 5 | List of hypermethylated genes in ovarian cancer.

Gene	Frequency of hypermethylation in ovarian cancer	Ovarian cancer subtype	Frequency of hypermethylation in normal tissue	Method	References
RASSF1A	15.6–50%	S, M, E, CC	0–13%	MSP	Yoon et al., 2001; Makarla et al., 2005; Choi et al., 2006; Bol et al., 2010
DAPK	50–67% (full)	S, CC, E, M, CS, PDA	50% (Partial)	MSP	Collins et al., 2006; Häfner et al., 2011
p16(CDKN2A)	16.9–42%	S, M, E	0–25%	MSP	Strathdee et al., 2001; Rathi et al., 2002; Tam et al., 2007
HIC1	15.9–51.7%	Not specific	12.5–19%; 11.1%	MSP	Strathdee et al., 2001; Ongenaert et al., 2008
OPCML	46.5–83.3%	Not specific	0%	Restriction enzyme cut analysis, MSP	Czekierdowski et al., 2006a; Zhang J. et al., 2006
MLH1	10%	S, E, M, CC, MIX	0% ADJ NLS	MSP	Strathdee et al., 2001
TERT	29.8%	S, M, E, CC	30%	qMSP	Widschwendter A. et al., 2004
PTEN	16.9%	E, S, M, CC	0%	MSP	Ongenaert et al., 2008
ING1	24%	S, M, E, CC, PDA	0%	MSP	Shen et al., 2005
ITGA8	13.3%	S, E, M, CC, SCC	0% END cyst	MSP	Cai et al., 2007
MGMT	9%	S, M, CC, E, UN	16%	MSP	Makarla et al., 2005
MINT25	16%	S, E, M, CC, MIX	0% ADJ NLS	MSP	Strathdee et al., 2001
APC	18–47.2%	S, M, CC, E, UN	0–25%	MSP	Rathi et al., 2002; Makarla et al., 2005; Ongenaert et al., 2008
BRCA1	10–24%	S, E, M, CC, MIX	0–5.5% ADJ NLS	MSP	Strathdee et al., 2001; Rathi et al., 2002; Ibanez de Caceres et al., 2004
CASP8	3%	S, E, M, CC, MIX	0% ADJ NLS	MSP	Strathdee et al., 2001
CDH1 (E-cadherin)	26–29%	S, M, CC, E, UN	6%	MSP	Rathi et al., 2002; Makarla et al., 2005
CDH13 (H-cadherin)	18–22%	S,M, CC, E, UN	8–13%	MSP	Rathi et al., 2002; Makarla et al., 2005
DCR1	43%	NS	0%	MSP	Shivapurkar et al., 2004
GPR150	26.6%	S, E, M, CC, SCC	0% END cyst	MSP	Cai et al., 2007
Htr (TERC)	24%	S, E, M, CC, MIX	0% ADJ NLS	MSP	Strathdee et al., 2001

ADJ NLS, Adjacent normals; CC, Clear cell; CS, Carcinosarcoma; E, Endometroid; END, Endometrial; M, Mucinous; MIX, Mixed; MSP, Methylation-specific PCR; NS, Not specified; PDA, Poorly differentiated adenocarcinoma; QMSP, Quantitative methylation-specific PCR; S, Serous; SCC, Squamous cell carcinoma; UN, Undifferentiated.

a potential biomarker for detection and accurate discrimination of EOC at early stage.

Using 7- genes panel [secreted frizzled receptor proteins 1, 2 4, 5 (SFRP1, 2, 4, 5), SRY box1 (SOX1), paired box gene 1(PAX1), and LIM homeobox transcription factor 1, alpha (LMX1A)], Sui et al. investigated methylation in 126 primary ovarian tumors, 75 benign ovarian tumors and 14 borderline ovarian tumors and in 26 OC serum samples. Their findings indicated that promoter methylation of any one of SOX1, PAX1, and SFRP1 could distinguish EOC patients from normal control with a sensitivity of 73.08% and a specificity of 75%. Though these test scores are higher than those of CA125 alone, however it is probably not high enough to warrant its implementation as a diagnostic test for individual patients. Moreover, as no specification of tumor stage within the studied group was provided, the performance of this panel in detection of EOC at an early stage therefore remains unclear (Su et al., 2009).

Hypomethylation induced abnormal expression of several oncogenes such as CLDN4 (encodes an integral component of tight junctions) (Honda et al., 2006; Litkouhi et al., 2007), MAL (mal, T-cell differentiation protein) (Lee et al., 2010), BORIS (a cancer testis antigen family candidate oncogenes) (Woloszynska-Read et al., 2007), and IGF2 (an imprinted gene involved in other malignancies) (Murphy et al., 2006) has been demonstrated in ovarian carcinomas. Promoter hypomethylation induced upregulation of other cancer-associated genes in ovarian cancer includes maspin (SERPINB5) (Rose et al., 2006), MCJ (Strathdee et al., 2004, 2005), and SNCG (synucelin-γ) (Gupta et al., 2003; Czekierdowski et al., 2006b), which encodes an activator of the MAPK and Elk-1 signaling cascades. Hypomethylation of SNCG, MASPIN, and CLDN4 correlates with advanced-stage and metastasis while that of BORIS is linked with disease presence.

Hypomethylation of Sat2 (satellite 2) DNA in the juxtacentromeric region of chromosome 1 and 16 has been

TABLE 6 | Epigenetic biomarkers for ovarian cancer detection.

Epigenetic marker	Source	Sensitivity /specificity	Technique	References
GTF2A1 and HAAO	Tumor tissue	Presence of malignancy 95/88%; 89/82%	qMSP	Huang et al., 2009
HOXA9 and SCGB3A1	Tumor tissue	Early stage carcinoma (18/24, $p = 0.002$) (5/25, $p = 0.020$)	MSP	Wu et al., 2007
RASSF1A and HIC1	Tumor tissue	Early stage ovarian carcinomas 34/100, 2/68, OR = 0.3 34/100, 10/68, OR = 0.4	MSP	Feng Q. et al., 2008
RASSF1A, GSTP1, MGMT, APC	Tumor tissue	Presence of invasive tumors RASSF1A: 30% vs. 0%; GSTP1: 9% vs. 0%; MGMT: 9% vs. 0%; APC:22% vs. 0%;	MSP	Barton et al., 2008
SPARC	Tumor tissue	Association with tumor grade Methylation frequency: 68%	MSP	Socha et al., 2009
CDH13, CRABP1, HOXA9, and SCGB3A1	Tumor tissue	Histological subtype differentiation CDH13, CRABP1, HOXA9 and SCGB3A1 ($P = 0.041$, $P < 0.001$, $P = 0.007$, $P < 0.001$)	MSP	Wu et al., 2007
CTGF	Tumor tissue	Inversely correlated with invasive disease	cDNA microarray analysis	Barbolina et al., 2009
CCBE1	Tumor tissue	Inversely correlated with metastasis 6/11 (55%) in OC cell lines 38/81 (41%) OC tumors.	Small-interfering RNA (siRNA)-mediated knockdown	Barton et al., 2010
HIC1	Tumor tissue	Presence of malignancy Methylation frequency: 35%	MSP	Rathi et al., 2002
CDH1	Tumor tissue	Inversely correlated with metastasis	Small-interfering RNA (siRNA)-mediated knockdown	Sawada et al., 2008
SFN, TMS1, and WTI	Tumor tissue	Methylation exclusive for Clear cell subtype	MSP	Barton et al., 2008
hMLH1, CDKN2A, and MGMT	Matched tumors	Associated with development of Synchronous endometrial and ovarian cancer Methylation frequency: 39, 41, and 48%	MSP	Furlan, 2006
14-3-3s	Tumor tissue	Advanced stage ovarian carcinomas	MSP, quantitative reverse transcription-PCR	Akahira et al., 2004b
HOXA11	Tumor tissue	Presence of malignancy, Suboptimal tumor debulking and poor outcome (relative risk for death = 3.4)	MethyLight assay	Fiegl et al., 2008
10 gene panel	Tumor tissue	Presence of serous adenocarcinoma (69.4% sensitivity and 70.2% specificity)	Microarray Mediated Methylation Assay (MethDet test)	Melnikov et al., 2009
Polycomb group target genes in particular HOXA9	Normal endometrium	Hoxa9 hypermethylation association with increased risk (12.3 fold) of ovarian cancer	MethyLight assay	Widschwendter et al., 2009
SNCG, MASPIN, and CLDN4	Tumor tissue	Advanced stage ovarian carcinomas	Small-interfering RNA (siRNA)-mediated knockdown, qRT-PCR	Gupta et al., 2003; Rose et al., 2006; Choi et al., 2007; Honda et al., 2007
PCDH17	Tumor tissue	Presence of malignancy	Next-generation sequencing, Methylation-sensitive high-resolution melting Analysis	Baranova et al., 2018
EGFL7 and RASSF1	Tumor tissue	Early stage disease detection and progression	DNA methylation microarray assay, Bisulfite pyrosequencing	Rattanapan et al., 2018
LDOC1	Ovarian cancer cell line	Early stage disease detection	RT-PCR and real-time PCR	Buchholtz et al., 2014
GPR150, ITGA8, and HOXD11	Ovarian cancer cell line	Tumor marker	Methylation-sensitive-representational difference analysis (MS-RDA) and MSP	Cai et al., 2007

(Continued)

TABLE 6 | Continued

Epigenetic marker	Source	Sensitivity /specificity	Technique	References
TGFBI	Tumor tissue and ovarian cancer cell line	Presence of malignancy	Real-time RT-PCR, MS-PCR, and bisulfite sequencing	Kang et al., 2010
DAPK1 and SOX1	Tumor tissue	Early stage disease	MethyLight	Kaur et al., 2016
BORIS	Tumor tissue	Presence of malignancy	qRT-PCR	Woloszynska-Read et al., 2007
long-intergenic non-coding RNA (lincRNA) gene (LOC134466)	Tumor tissue and ovarian cancer cell line	Potential novel diagnostic biomarker for high grade (Type II) serous ovarian carcinoma (HGSOC)	MeDIP-Chip and Sequenom massARRAY methylation analysis	Gloss et al., 2012

reported in ovarian cancer (Qu et al., 1999). A significant increase in hypomethylation of chromosome 1 Sat2 and chromosome 1 satellite α from non-neoplastic tissue toward ovarian cancer tissue was observed. Higher hypomethylation levels were observed in serous and endometrioid tumors in comparison to mucinous. Moreover, extensive hypomethylation was prevalent in high grade or advanced stage tumors (Widschwendter M. et al., 2004). Taken together, consistent higher expression levels along with hypomethylation of L1 and human endogenous retrovirus-W retrotransposons (repetitive sequences widely distributed throughout the genome) has been reported in malignant ovarian tumors against normal control samples (Menendez et al., 2004). It has been hypothesized that promotion in homologous recombination as a result of increased hypomethylation, leads to chromosomal aberrations associated with carcinogenesis (Kolomietz et al., 2002; Symer et al., 2002).

Prognosis

Potential prognostic biomarker includes FBXO32, which correlates with advanced stage and shorter disease free survival (Chou et al., 2010), Ribosomal DNA (18S and 28S) linked with prolonged disease free survival (Chan, 2005), IGFBP-3, correlates with disease progression and death in early stage EOC (Wiley et al., 2006b) and HOXA11, association with postsurgical residual tumor and poor outcome (Fiegl et al., 2008). Methylation of ≥ 1 gene of SFRP1, SFRP2, and SOX1 correlated with short disease free survival while SOX1, LMX1A, and SFRP1 methylation was associated with recurrence and short overall survival (Su et al., 2009). A progression-free survival prediction accuracy of 95% is reported by Wei et al. with hMLH1, IGFP3, and NEUROD1 among a panel of 112 highly discriminatory loci (Wei, 2006). Furthermore, detection of prognostic epigenetic biomarker has also been described in plasma as well as peritoneal fluid. Methylation of hMLH1, analyzed in 138 plasma samples predicted poor survival (hazard ratio: 1.99) (Gifford, 2004) while CDH1, CDH13, and APC (out of a 15 gene panel) analyzed in peritoneal fluid from 57 ovarian cancer patients could predict overall survival (Suehiro et al., 2008). Huang et al. recently reported that the epigenetic loss of heparin sulfate 3-O-sulfation makes ovarian cancer cells sensitive to oncogenic signals and could predict prognosis, thereby reflecting the utility of HS3ST2 for targeted therapy (Huang et al., 2018).

Recently using genome-wide methylation data analysis, five-methylation signature (SLC39A14, PREX2, KCNIP2, CORO6, and EFNB1) were reported as novel independent prognostic biomarker for patients with ovarian serous cystadenocarcinoma, which significantly associated with OS of patients. Moreover, these signatures exhibited higher sensitivity and specificity to predict OSC prognosis (AUC = 0.715), which reflects their clinical significance in improving outcome prediction. Furthermore, these 5- methylation signatures were more accurate over known biomarkers in predicting prognostic survival of OSC patients (Guo T. Y. et al., 2018). Promoter methylation of BRCA1 has been reported to be associated significantly with increased PFS of patients with OC undergoing adjuvant platinum–taxane-based chemotherapy ($P = 0.008$) as well for the patients with disease recurrence (PFS = 18.5 months over 12.8 months for patients without BRCA1 promoter methylation), thereby reflecting that promoter methylation of BRCA1 could be a better predictive marker of response to platinum–taxane-based chemotherapy in sporadic Epithelial ovarian carcinoma (Ignatov et al., 2014).

Another study highlights the potential of CDH1, DLEC1, and SFRP5 gene methylation panel as a prognostic biomarker in advanced stage OC patients. Presence of two or more methylated genes in patients significantly correlated with disease recurrence (hazard ratio: 1.91; $p = 0.002$) and shorter overall survival and disease free survival (hazard ratio: 1.96; $p = 0.006$) (Lin et al., 2018). Liu et al. reported the prognostic potential of C/EBPβ (a transcription factor) which augments chemoresistance of ovarian cancer cells by maintaining an open chromatin state via reprogramming H3K79 methylation of multiple drug-resistance genes upon direct interaction with DOT1L (DNA methyltransferase), thus provides a new insight for more precise therapeutics options in OC by identifying and targeting the key regulators of epigenetics (Liu et al., 2018).

Several recent researches have suggested the hypermethylation and reduced expression is prognostic for shorter progression free survival. For instance, using genome wide array analyses, Hafner et al. reported 220 differentially methylated region with short and long PFS. Validation experiments on a large cohort of type II EOC revealed the association of RUNX3/CAMK2N1 with poor clinical outcome (Lower PFS), indicating the prognostic potential of these genes (Häfner et al., 2016). Few studies have highlighted the tight link between promoter methylation and metastasis. For instance, stimulation of ovarian cancer cell lines by TGFβ, which is a key player in metastasis, extensively change promoter methylation of genes that are associated with

EMT (Epithelial-mesenchymal transition) and progression of cancer (Cardenas et al., 2014). Deng et al. reported the tumor suppressive role of IQGAP2 which suppresses the ovarian cancer progression via suppressing Epithelial-mesenchymal transition by regulating Wnt/β signaling, thereby providing a potential biomarker and therapeutic strategy to combat ovarian cancer diagnosis (Deng et al., 2016).

Brachova et al. studied the association of oncomorphic TP53 mutation on patient outcome diagnosed with advanced EOC. Oncomorphic TP53 mutation correlated with worse progression free survival, higher risk of recurrence and higher rate of platinum resistance (Brachova et al., 2015). Dai et al. explored the association of methylation-based prognostic biomarkers within key ovarian cancer-related pathways with progression free survival to platinum based chemotherapy in HGSOC. NKD1, VEGFB, and PRDX2 were identified as the best predictors of progression free survival (PFS: HR $= 2.3$ $p = 3.3 \times 10{-}5$; Overall Survival: HR $= 1.9$, $p = 0.007$). Further validation using independent TCGA data set revealed the significant association of VEGFA, VEGFB, and VEGFC promoter methylation with progression free survival (Dai et al., 2013).

Promoter hypomethylation and expression of PRAME correlates with increased survival in high grade serous ovarian carcinoma (Zhang et al., 2016). Promoter hypomethylation and increased expression of proto-oncogenes is predictive for more aggressiveness and metastasis of disease and thereby lower survival, which is evident from recent studies on GABRP, SLC6A12, MGAT3, CT45, CA9, MUC13, and AGR2 (Sung et al., 2014a,b,c, 2017a,b; Zhang et al., 2015; Kohler et al., 2016). Hypomethylation of Sat2 DNA (Chr 1) was associated relapse and poor prognosis (Widschwendter M. et al., 2004), and LINE1 was linked with poorer overall survival and lower progression free survival (Pattamadilok et al., 2008; **Table 7**).

Another important study by Wei et al. reported 112 methylated loci which were prognostic for reduced PFS and could predict PFS with an accuracy of 95% using Significance Analysis of Microarray and Prediction Analysis of Microarray algorithm (Wei, 2006). Twenty-two hypermethylated loci were identified by global methylation profiling of 485 tumor samples of clear-cell ovarian cancer in a recent study. These hypermethylated loci were associated with 9 genes (VWA1, FOXP1, FGFRL1, LINC00340, KCNH2, ANK1, ATXN2, NDRG21, and SLC16A11). Further, methylation induced silencing of KCNH2 (HERG, a potassium channel) could be a better prognostic factor for poor survival provided increased proliferation was mediated by overexpression of Eag family members. However, further validation on larger cohort is still warranted (Cicek et al., 2013). Huang et al. identified 63 differentially methylated regions of prognostic relevance which significantly correlated with poor PFS. Further, epigenetic silencing of regulators of hedgehog signaling pathway ZIC1 and ZIC4 was associated with increased proliferation, migration, and invasion. Additionally, promoter hypermethylation of ZIC1 significantly correlated with poor survival and thus could serve as prognostic determinant for patient outcome (Huang et al., 2013).

Another study describes that the global methylome status of HGSOC PDX (patient-derived xenografts) resembled with global methylation in corresponding patient tumor over several generations and could be efficiently modulated by demethylating agents. C-terminal Src kinase (CSK), a novel epigenetically regulated gene and associated pathways were also identified. Low CSK methylation significantly correlated with improved PFS and OS in HGSOC patients (Tomar et al., 2016). Koestler et al. using integrative global methylation and single nucleotide polymorphisms analysis identified DNA methylation marks (13 unique CpGs and 17 unique SNPs) which could mediate EOC genetic risk (Koestler et al., 2014).

Recently, Sharma et al. investigated epigenetic regulation of POTE gene family, which is localized to autosomal pericentromeric region. POTE gene family is over-expressed in HGSOC. Epigenetic silencing of POTE gene was functionally verified by experiments involving treatment with Decitabine and DNMT knockout cell lines. In addition expression of individual gene in POTE gene family correlated with chemoresistance and poor clinical outcome in HGSOC patients. Furthermore, several epigenetic alternations (pericentromeric activation, global and locus-specific L1 hypomethylation, and locus-specific 5' CpG hypomethylation) served as a determinant for regulation of epigenetic activation of POTE gene (Sharma et al., 2019).

In conclusion, these studies provides insight to the association of several potential methylation based prognostic biomarkers with clinical outcome in ovarian carcinoma and further suggest that these reports on epigenome wide interrogation of DNA methylation warrants detailed functional analysis of loci sufficiently discriminating OC with normal state. New targets identified through comprehensive methylome analysis in OC have significant translational potential to pave the design of future clinical investigations and therapeutics.

Predictive

Methylation mediated transcriptional repression of specific drug-response genes results in acquisition of drug resistance and significantly extends its impact on different facets of chemotherapeutic actions: membrane entry/exit, drug metabolism, response to cellular injury, DNA repair, apoptosis etc., in cancer cells. Hypermethylated genes such as hMLH1, ASS1 (arginine biosynthesis-related gene), ESR2 (encoding ER-β), and SFRP5 (encodes an inhibitor of oncogenic WNT signaling pathway) have been implicated in platinum resistance. Three studies well defined in ovarian cancer includes: Methylation of either BRCA1, GSTP1, or MGMT significantly correlates with improved response to chemotherapy ($p = 0.013$) (Teodoridis et al., 2005). Hypermethylation of RASSF1A and CABIN1 have been reported to correlate with response to adjuvant therapy. Patients who responded to therapy had moderately higher frequencies of RASSF1A hypermethylation (OR $= 0.4$) and significantly higher frequencies of CABIN1 hypermethylation (OR $= 0.1$) (Feng Q. et al., 2008). Strathdee et al. demonstrated that high levels of MCJ methylation significantly correlated with poor response to therapy ($p = 0.027$) and poor overall survival ($p = 0.023$; HR $= 2.9$) (Strathdee et al., 2005). Hypomethylation induced upregulation of ABCG2 (multidrug transporter) MAL (determinant of platinum resistance) and TUBB3 (determinant of taxane resistance) genes have been described in advanced

TABLE 7 | Epigenetic biomarkers for ovarian cancer prognostication.

Epigenetic marker	Source	Clinical prediction	References
182-gene panel	Tumor tissue	HR 2.5 for PFS	Wei et al., 2002
112-gene panel	Tumor tissue	Prediction accuracy of 95% for shorter Disease free survival	Wei, 2006
SFRP1, *SFRP2*, and *SOX1*	Tumor tissue	Correlates with shorter Disease free survival	Su et al., 2009
SOX1, *LMX1A*, and *SFRP1*	Tumor tissue	Correlates with shorter overall survival	Su et al., 2009
hMLH1	Plasma	If hypermethylated HR:1.99 for OS	Gifford, 2004
HOXA10, HOXA11	Tumor tissue	RR for death:3.4, if HOXA11 methylated	Fiegl et al., 2008, p. 11
18S and 28S rDNA	Tumor tissue	Prolonged DFS	Chan, 2005
EN2	Tumor tissue	Short progression free survival	McGrath et al., 2018
MYLK3	Tumor tissue	Higher methylation level significantly predicted better overall survival with least residual disease	Phelps et al., 2017
FBXO32	Tumor tissue	Advanced stage and short DFS	Chou et al., 2010
Panel of IGFFBP3, p16, BRCA1, GSTP1, ER-α, hMLH1	Tumor tissue	Seven fold increased risk of short DFS HR: 6.53 for disease progression	Wiley et al., 2006a
RUNX3, CAMK2N1	Tumor tissue and ovarian cancer cell line	Short overall survival	Häfner et al., 2016
ABCA1	Tumor tissue and ovarian cancer cell line	Shorter overall survival	Chou et al., 2015
GULP1	ovarian cancer cell line	Residual disease, worse overall survival, and disease specific survival	Maldonado et al., 2018, p. 1
FZD4, DVL1, and ROCK1	Tumor tissue	Correlated with early disease relapse	Dai et al., 2011
DNA hypomethylated genes			
15 gene panel	Peritoneal fluid	Short overall survival	Muller, 2004
Sat 2 DNA (Chr1)	Tumor tissue	RR for relapse:4.1, RR for death:9.4 if region methylated	Widschwendter M. et al., 2004
LINE1	Tumor tissue	Lower methylation level significantly predicted poor OS and PFS	Pattamadilok et al., 2008
ATG4A, HIST1H2BN	Tumor tissue	Poor progression free survival	Liao et al., 2014

ovarian carcinoma cases with drug-acquired chemoresistance (Izutsu et al., 2008; Balch et al., 2010; Lee et al., 2010; **Table 8**).

Recently Pulliam et al. demonstrated the combinatorial effect of DNA methyltransferase inhibitor (DNMTi) guadecitabine and the Poly (ADP-ribose) polymerase (PARP) inhibitors (PARPi) talazoparib in resensitizing PARPi resistant breast and ovarian cancer irrespective of BRCA status. Synergistic effect of guadecitabine and talazoparib increased ROS accumulation, and further sensitized the breast and ovarian cancer cells toward PARPi sensitivity by subsequent activation of cAMP/PKA signaling which in turn promoted PARP activation. Furthermore, DNMTi augmented PARP "trapping" by talazoparib. The finding of this complementary model supports further clinical exploration of this combination therapy in PARPi-resistant cancers (Pulliam et al., 2018). Another study using integrated global methylation analysis on extreme chemoresponsive HGSOC patients identified four genes of clinical relevance (FZD10, FAM83A, MYO18B, and MKX) as epigenetic marker of platinum based chemoresponse, of which, FZD10 was reported as functionally validated marker of platinum sensitivity (Tomar et al., 2017). Promoter methylation of OPCML was significantly associated with poor overall survival of OC patients and thus could be of use in predicting disease prognosis (Zhou et al., 2014).

A recent study has described induction of hypomethylation in resistant ovarian cancer patients upon treatment with cisplatin, though, in the intergenic regions, the loss of methylation was primarily observed (Lund et al., 2017). Hypomethylation of developmental genes MSX1 and TMEM88 correlated with platinum resistance in patients with ovarian cancer (Bonito et al., 2016; de Leon et al., 2016). Stimulation of EMT by non-coding RNA HOTAIR has been reported to be regulated by DNA methylation and is indicative of resistance to carboplatin (Teschendorff et al., 2015). Likewise, another study highlights promotion of platinum resistance by TET. Induction of EMT by TET is mediated by demethylation of Vimentin promoter in ovarian carcinoma (Han et al., 2017).

A recent study has described how methylome-targeting strategies could bring forth anti-tumor effect. Guadecitabine-mediated induction of global hypomethylation not only affects metabolic and immune responses but also activates tumor suppressor genes which eventually contribute to platinum drug re-sensitization in ovarian cancer. This might offer utility in improving survival outcomes of patients with ovarian cancer

TABLE 8 | Epigenetic biomarkers for ovarian cancer prediction.

Epigenetic marker	Source	Clinical prediction	References
Methylation of >1 of BRCA1, GSTP1, and MGMT	Tumor tissue	Association with improved response to chemotherapy	Teodoridis et al., 2005
RASSF1A, CABIN1	Tumor tissue	Association with response to chemotherapy	Feng Q. et al., 2008
ASS1	Tumor tissue	Determinant of Platinum resistance	Nicholson et al., 2009
HSulf1	Tumor tissue	Determinant of Platinum resistance	Staub et al., 2007
SFRP5	Tumor tissue	Determinant of Platinum resistance	Su et al., 2010
hMLH1	Plasma	Relapse of Chemoresistant tumor	Gifford, 2004
ESR2	Tumor tissue	Determinant of Platinum resistance	Yap et al., 2009
MCJ	Tumor tissue	Association with response to chemotherapy and overall survival	Strathdee et al., 2005
TUBB3	Tumor tissue	Taxane resistance	Izutsu et al., 2008
MSX1	Ovarian cancer cell line	Sensitivity to platinum drug	Bonito et al., 2016
TBX2	Tumor tissue	Sensitivity to platinum drug	Tasaka et al., 2017
MAL	Tumor tissue	Platinum resistance	Lee et al., 2010

(Fang et al., 2018). Another recent study has highlighted the tumor suppressor role of ZNF671 and its methylation could act as a predictor for early recurrence of serous ovarian carcinoma (Mase et al., 2019). Another important study by M. Keita et al. has for the first time reported the exclusive association of massive DNA hypomethylation with poorly differentiated tumors, which correlates with disease aggressiveness and progression. This report also raises concern over the adverse effect of use of demethylating agents which probably aid the activation of oncogenes and prometastatic genes (Keita et al., 2013).

In conclusion, it is speculated that the combinatorial therapies utilizing epigenetic inhibitors holds promise and would be most effective for chemo-resensitization of resistant tumors, possibly by restoration of pathways associated with drug response, and thus would subsequently implicate improved survival outcomes as well as personalized treatment for this devastating disease.

Histone Modifications in Ovarian Cancer

Compared with DNA methylation, the evidence on chromatin modification in development of ovarian cancer is limited. Histone modification mediated regulation of cell cycle regulatory proteins such as cyclin B1 (Valls et al., 2005), p21 (Richon et al., 2000), and ADAM19 (Chan M. W. et al., 2008) have been described in various reports. Association of histone modifications with aberrant class III β tubulin protein expression (Izutsu et al., 2008), reduction of PACE3 expression (Fu et al., 2003) and silencing of survivin (Mirza et al., 2002) has been reported in ovarian tumorigenesis. Upregulation of tumor suppressor Rb and CDKN1 (cyclin-dependent kinase inhibitor) by histone acetylation was described by Strait et al. (2002). Moreover, the overexpression of HDACs 1–3 in ovarian cancer has been reported to be associated with high grade tumors and resulting poor prognosis (Weichert et al., 2008). On the other note, the derepression of claudin-3 and claudin-4 was found to be associated with loss of trimethylated histone 3 lysine 27 (H3K27me3) (Kwon et al., 2010). The transcriptional repression of osteoprotegerin (OPG) has been reported to be mediated by reduced histone 3 lysine 4 trimethylation (H3K4me3) and increased H3K27me3 (Lu et al., 2009). Similarly, the association of transcriptional silencing of GATA4 and GATA6 with hypoacetylation of histones H3 and H4 and loss of trimethylated histone 3l ysine 4 (H3K4me3) has been described by Caslini et al. (2006).

A very recent report has provided insight into the mechanism associated with development and progression of OC. Early Loss of E3 ubiquitin ligase RNF20 and histone H2B monoubiquitylation (H2Bub1) has been reported to drive ovarian tumorigenesis by altering chromatin accessibility and thereby activating immune signaling pathways (IL6), and this loss has been defined by majority of high grade serous ovarian carcinomas tumors (Hooda et al., 2019). Cacan et al. reported that the loss of FAS expression which contributes to drug resistance is mediated by histone deacetylase 1 (HDAC1) in chemoresistant OC cells (Cacan, 2016). Recently Tang et al. highlighted the repression of histone H3 lysine 27 trimethylation (H3K27me3) which was mitigated by AMP-activated protein kinase (AMPK) phosphorylation upon treatment with metformin thus implicated the antitumor effect of metformin and suggested its utility in the treatment of EOC patients who are not diabetic (Tang et al., 2018).

In another study, the mechanism associated with upregulation of ABCB1 was conferred to chromatin remodeling (via p300 mediated H3K9ac and AR complex binding to ARE4) which in turn leads to the development of taxol resistant phenotype. It was shown that the upregulation of p300 and GCN5 (HATs) was associated with overexpression of ABCB1 and resistance to taxol and PI3K/AKT pathway which is activated by taxol, mediates the regulation of the expression of p300 and AR. These results further reveal the significance of AKT/p300/AR axis as a novel treatment strategy in combating taxol resistance (Sun et al., 2019). Using ChIP-seq approach, Curry et al. identified genome-wide bivalent domains (H3K27me3 and H3K4me3) at gene promoter in tumor samples which were collected pre and post platinum resistance acquisition, and showed that these representative poised gene sets are pre-disposed to hypermethylation induced epigenetic silencing during acquisition of drug resistance, thus provides novel insights to prevent emergence of drug resistance (Curry et al., 2018).

Yi et al. reported that Enhancer of zeste homolog 2 (EZH2) mediates repression of tissue inhibitor of metalloproteinases

2(TIMP2) by H3K27me3 and DNA methylation thereby facilitating ovarian cancer metastasis (Yi et al., 2017). In similar context, another study highlighted silencing of ARHI in ovarian cancer which was synergistically mediated by Enhancer of zeste homolog 2 (EZH2) induced H3K27me3 and DNA methylation. Furthermore increased EZH2 expression correlated with worse overall survival rates, implicating prognostic potential of EZH2 in EOC (Fu et al., 2015). Repression of Regulator of G-protein signaling 2 (RGS2) via histone deacetylases (HDACs) and DNA methyltransferase I in chemoresistant OC cells has been reported recently by Cacan et al., and utility of their inhibitors might serve as a novel approach to overcome chemoresistance in ovarian cancer (Cacan, 2017).

Clinical Application of Epigenetic Biomarker in Liquid Biopsies for Ovarian Cancer Management

Cell Free DNA Biology

Advancement in the understanding underlying molecular pathogenesis of cancer, along with advancements in molecular techniques has facilitated the study of molecular alternations associated with cancer development at an early stage in body fluids. Circulating cell free DNA which are believed to have derived from tumor cells, reflect specific genetic and epigenetic alternations, and thus may offer potential non-invasive viable biomarkers for several cancer, capable of providing valuable information regarding disease progression and response to therapy in real time.

In 1948, the existence of cell free DNA was first described by Mandel and Métais. Cell free DNA are derived from necrotic and apoptotic cells, commonly released by all cell types. Further, numerous subsequent studies confirmed that the tumor-specific pattern of alterations, such as chromosomal abnormality, somatic mutations, resistance mutation, aberrant methylation and copy number variations could be found in cfDNA, which can serve as potential target for diagnosis of cancer through non-invasive approach (Leon et al., 1977; Polivka et al., 2015; **Figure 3**).

Numerous studies support the detection of methylation signature in almost any body fluid (such as serum, plasma, smears, nipple fluid aspirate, and vaginal fluid etc.). As sampling of blood can be considered as minimal invasive process, thus serves as an ideal substrate for methylation analysis. The average concentrations of circulating cell free DNA in healthy subjects is 30 ng/ml. However, in cancer patients, the average concentration of cell free serum DNA is higher, approximately 180 ng/ml as dying cancer cells release tumor DNA into the blood (Gormally et al., 2007). The average length of circulating cfDNA, which are usually fragmented, is 140 to 170 bp and of which, only a fraction of few thousand amplifiable copies of cfDNA /ml of blood, might be of diagnostic relevance (Gormally et al., 2007; Polivka et al., 2015). The levels of circulating cell free DNA in serum is abnormally high in early as well as advanced-stage tumors (Perlin and Moquin, 1972; Leon et al., 1977). For this phenomenon, the proposed two primary mechanisms includes: either cells in cancer tissue undergoes *in situ* apoptosis and/or necrosis or cells might detach from tumors and extravasate into bloodstream where they undergo lysis (**Figure 4**).

Since its first validation, the potential application of circulating DNA in research settings and for non-invasive management of cancer as "liquid biopsy" is expanding with improvement in molecular and genomic techniques. Numerous studies have demonstrated that tumor specific aberrant methylation can also be detected in cfDNA of patients with different tumor types such as lung, prostate, breast and colorectal cancer and further confirmed altered methylation as an independent diagnostic/ prognostic marker (Board et al., 2008; Brock et al., 2008; Lofton-Day et al., 2008; Vlassov et al., 2010). Warren et al. developed a highly sensitive non-invasive test for screening of colorectal cancer based on methylation of SEPT9 in plasma which could specifically detect all stages and locations of colorectal cancers (Warren et al., 2011). Hypermethylation of Vim gene is strongly correlated with the occurrence of colorectal cancer. Similarly hypermethylation of SHOX2 in sputum has been used as biomarker for distinguishing malignant and benign lung diseases (Kneip et al., 2011). Gstp1 methylation status in urine is strongly correlated with early onset of prostate cancer (Belinsky, 2004).

Numerous reports have highlighted the potential of DNA methylation based biomarkers for non-invasive detection of cancer utilizing cell free DNA. Recently, using integrated methylome analysis Wei et al. reported hypermethylation of SPG20, a putative STAT3 target, for non-invasive detection of gastric cancer at an early stage (Wei et al., 2019). Yang et al. explored the potential of eight gene panel for non-invasive detection of lung cancer using qMSP and revealed that the promoter methylation of any of the eight gene could detect the disease with a sensitivity of 72% with 91% specificity, reflecting the utility of plasma DNA methylation as a novel approach for detection of lung cancer at early stage (Yang et al., 2018).

Similarly, promoter methylation of OPCML and HOXD9 assessed in serum cell free DNA using methylation-sensitive high-resolution melting, was detected with a sensitivity of 62.50% with specificity of 100%, thus could serve as a non-invasive differential biomarker to prevent misdiagnosis of cholangiocarcinoma (CCA) and other biliary diseases (Wasenang et al., 2019). Further, for the management of pancreatic cancer and its early detection Eissa et al. analyzed the methylation of ADAMTS1 and BNC1 in cfDNA using qMSP, which exhibited a sensitivity of 94.8% and specificity of 91.6% with a AUC of 0.95 reflecting diagnostic potential of this blood based two-gene panel in detection of pancreatic cancer at an early stage (Eissa et al., 2019). Methylation of APC, FOXA1, and RASSF1A in cell free DNA served as a best performing cassette in terms of diagnostic and prognostic value, revealing a sensitivity, specificity and accuracy over 70% suggesting its putative utility in management of breast cancer (Salta et al., 2018).

Other studies using genome-wide methylation profiling of serum/plasma cell-free DNA have identified potential biomarkers for clinical utility. For instance, Xu et al. using MeDIP-seq approach reported 10 significant differentially methylated genes as potent biomarker for lung cancer clinical application (Xu et al., 2019). Similarly, using genome-wide methylome profiling and

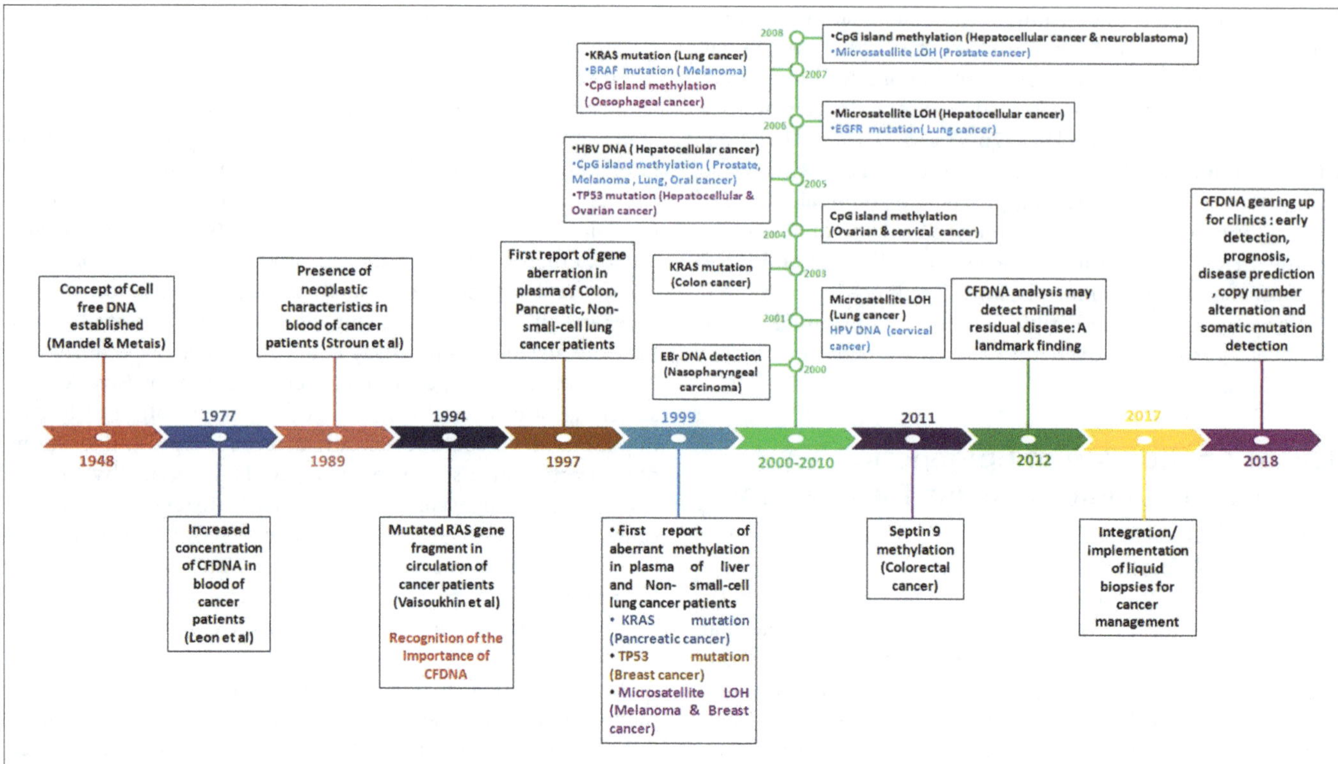

FIGURE 3 | Timeline reflecting the detection of genetic and epigenetic alternations in Cell-free DNA in blood of patients with different cancer type.

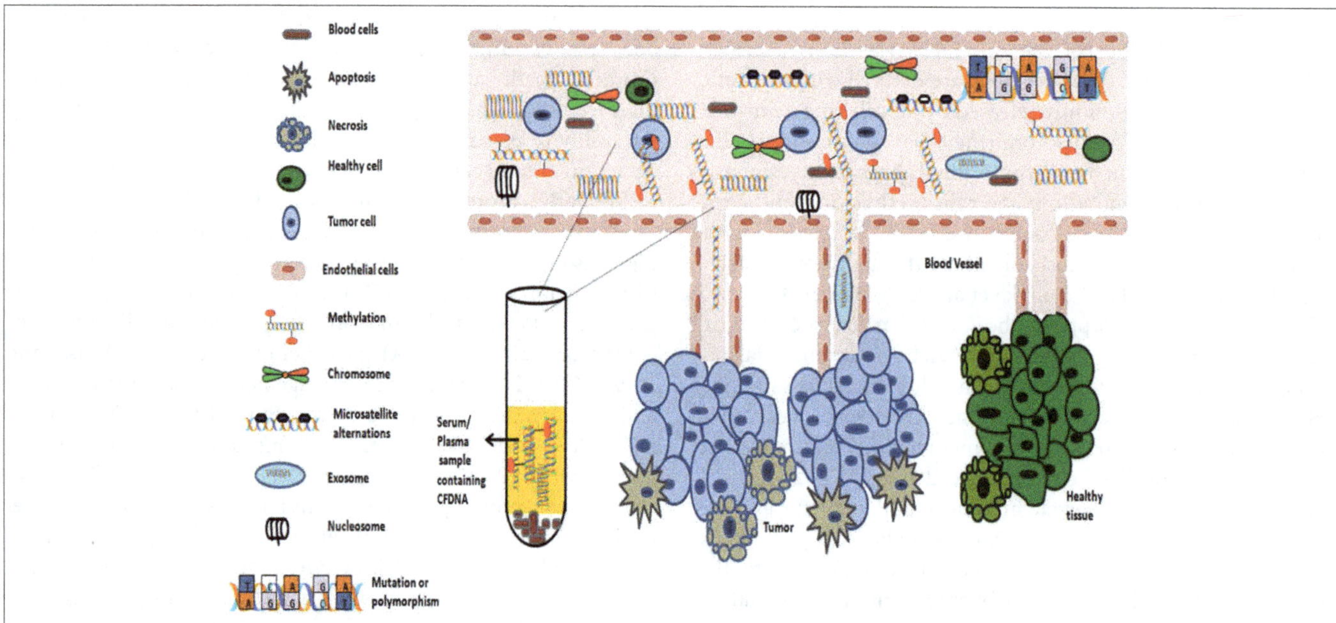

FIGURE 4 | Origin of Cell-free DNA in blood.

Sequenom MassARRAY approach, it was reported that promoter methylation of CASZ1, CDH13, and ING2 could serve as a potent noninvasive biomarker for detection of esophageal cancer at early stage (Wang H.Q. et al., 2018).

Challenges

The analysis of blood borne cell-free DNA has tremendous potential to enable rapid, non-invasive molecular diagnosis of cancer. They are of great clinical relevance as they provide specific targets for initial diagnosis, permit monitoring of treatment efficacy as well as information about tumor profile and its dynamics which are critical for treatment decisions (De Mattos-Arruda et al., 2014; Lewis et al., 2015).

The advantages of analyzing tumor specific DNA methylation in cell free serum DNA includes, improved sensitivity as cfDNA can be easily amplified by PCR, fewer false positive rate as methylation pattern is generally conserved throughout the progression of disease, stability during sample collection as abnormal DNA methylation is chemically as well as biologically stable and remains relatively unaffected by physiological condition at the time of sample collection, increased technical sensitivity and specificity for gene specific assays as well as offers assay design advantages over genetic alternation that might be interspersed throughout a given gene. Furthermore, DNA methylation is a positively detectable signal, unlike a loss of signal as in chromosomal deletions (Wittenberger et al., 2014).

Several limitations in the methylation detection of cell free serum DNA includes extremely low amount of available cfDNA, missing bisulfite conversions as they are usually fragmented, low sensitivity demonstrated by a single marker and time-consuming, complicated and expensive conventional techniques for cfDNA isolation. The most commonly used technique for methylation detection is MSP PCR (methylation specific PCR) which is a bisulfite-conversion- based method. The limitation of bisulfite conversion of cfDNA is the missing DNA. Because of the technical difficulties of DNA methylation analysis, only few DNA methylation based markers has been identified to date, which apply only to a fraction of gynecological cancers including breast, ovarian and endometrial cancers (Wittenberger et al., 2014; Lewis et al., 2015).

The two technological challenges to be addressed include (1) the detection of low abundant tumor-specific DNA methylation patterns through methylation specific PCR priming or probing with high signal-to-noise ratio (2) the determination of methylation status of consecutive sites in individual DNA molecules with single base-pair resolution. This requires methylation-independent priming and sequence analysis of combined PCR product. Clinically the major problem associated with DNA methylation assays is to detect scarcely abundant alleles within high background levels of non-target molecules. However, with the advent of digital MethyLight assay together with rapid advances in next generation sequencing based technologies, these issues can be overcome. One example of this novel approach is the development of the PraenaTest™ (LifeCodexx, Germany) (Weisenberger et al., 2008).

Serum Based Epigenetic Biomarker

Tumor-specific methylation-based biomarkers might possibly prove valuable for monitoring disease prognosis and different pathological determinants; however, non-invasive analysis and characterization of biomarkers in body fluids offers more feasibility in early screening and detection of the disease as well in monitoring the response to therapy. Numerous studies have reported aberrant methylation in ovarian cancer as discussed earlier; there are relatively few reports of serum/plasma methylation biomarkers for earlier detection of OC. Various studies that demonstrated striking detection sensitivities and specificities in non-invasive assays, thereby supporting the promising utility of these biomarkers for early screening and detection of OC has been summarized in **Table 9.**

MicroRNAs in Ovarian Cancer

Aberrant expression of microRNAs has been confirmed in ovarian carcinogenesis. A decrease in mRNA levels of the miR-processing enzymes in OC malignant cases against normal controls, strongly implicates an overall tumor suppressive role of miRs in ovarian tumorigenesis (Merritt et al., 2008; Pampalakis et al., 2010). Overexpression of Drosha and Dicer was significantly associated with better survival, while low expression of Drosha was associated with suboptimal surgical cytoreduction and low expression of Dicer with advanced tumor stage, thereby further implicating the tumor suppressive role of microRNAs in OC (Merritt et al., 2008; Faggad et al., 2010). With respect to ovarian cancer, the potential targets for several upregulated miRs includes pro-apoptotic, metastasis-suppressing or antiproliferation gene products while those for the downregulated miRs includes growth signaling, prometastatic- or anti-apoptosis-associated proteins. A list of upregulated/downregulated miRs involved in ovarian cancer development is shown in **Table 10**. A list of aberrantly expressed miRs which could serve as a promising biomarker for detection of ovarian cancer has been summarized in **Table 11**. Chao et al. reported that in advanced stage cancer, miR-187 regulates carcinogenesis through Dab2 dependent EMT (epithelial-to-mesenchymal transition) (Chao et al., 2012, p. 2). Furthermore, other studies have described miR-199a, miR-200a, miR-200b, miR-200c, and miR-214 as significantly overexpressed and miR-100 and miRNAlet-7i as significantly downregulated in ovarian tumors (Iorio et al., 2007; Yang H. et al., 2008; Yang N. et al., 2008). Several miRNA signatures that could distinguish ovarian tumors based on histological subtypes has been studied such as miR-200b and miR-141 was observed to be overexpressed in serous and endometrioid subtypes; upregulated of miR-21, miR-203, and miR-205 correlated with endometrioid histotype; downregulated miR-145 correlated with serous and clear cell subtype, while downregulated miR 222 was associated with endometrioid and clear cell subtype (Iorio et al., 2007).

Recently, Braga et al. described methylation of miR-9-1, miR-9-3, and miR-130b which strongly correlated with progression of OC (Braga et al., 2018a). Different histotype of ovarian carcinomas reflect differential expression of specific miRNAs which might serve as a valid biomarker. Agostini et al. reported significant overexpression of miR-192, miR-194, and miR-215 in mucinous subtype of ovarian carcinomas. However their expression was downregulated in other subtypes and sex cord-stromal tumors (Agostini et al., 2018).

A list of promising aberrantly expressed miRs which could be of prognostic and predictive relevance in ovarian cancer has been summarized in **Table 11**. A lower ratio of miR-221 to miR-222 significantly correlated with worse overall survival in predominantly high grade, advanced stage sporadic ovarian carcinomas (Wurz et al., 2010). Downregulation of miR-141,

TABLE 9 | Non-invasive epigenetic DNA methylation biomarkers for ovarian cancer.

Epigenetic marker(s)	Source	Patient/sample	Clinical prediction	Technology	References
Methylation of ≥1 gene of BRCA1, RASSF1A, APC, p14ARF, p16INK4A, or DAPK	Serum and cytologically negative peritoneal fluid	50 serum, 40 peritoneal fluid from EOC patients along with 40 control serum and peritoneal fluid samples	Presence of malignancy Sensitivity: 41/50 (82% for serum) 28/30 (93% for peritoneal fluid), Specificity: 100% (all tumor stages).	Methylation-specific-PCR (MSP)	Ibanez de Caceres et al., 2004
DAPK	Whole peripheral blood DNA	26 peripheral blood samples	Sensitivity: 14/16 (54%) for DAPK-methylation-positive samples: Specificity: 10/10 (100%) for DAPK methylation negative	Methylation-specific PCR (MSP)	Collins et al., 2006
Methylation of ≥1 gene of SOX1, PAX1 or SFRP1	Serum	46 (26 ovarian cancer cases and 20 patients with a benign condition	Sensitivity: 73.08% Specificity: 75%	Methylation-specific PCR (MSP)	Su et al., 2009
Methylation of 7-gene panel (APC, RASSF1A, CDH1, RUNX3, TFPI2, SFRP5, and OPCML	Serum	202 patients (87 EOC cases, 53 benign cases and 62 controls)	Sensitivity of 7-gene panel: 85.3% Specificity of 7-gene panel: 90.5% in stage I EOC Sensitivity of CA125: 56.1% Specificity of CA125: 64.15%	Multiplex methylation-specific PCR (MSP)	Zhang et al., 2013
10-gene panel (Combination of BRCA1, HIC1,PAX5,PGR, THBS1)	Plasma	66 (33 cancer cases and 33 control)	Presence of malignancy Sensitivity: 61% Specificity: 85%	Microarray based multiplex assay(MethDet56 technique)	Melnikov et al., 2009
Several gene panel (RASSF1A and PGR-PROX) (RASSF1A, CALCA and EP300)	Serum	90 (30 EOC cases, 30 cases with Benign disease along with 30 controls non neoplastic samples)	Methylation of RASSF1A and PGR-PROX Sensitivity: 80.0% Specificity:73.3% Methylation of RASSF1A, CALCA and EP300 Sensitivity: 90.0% Specificity: 86.7%.	Microarray based Assay(MethDet 56)	Liggett et al., 2011
OPCML	Serum	194 (71 EOC, 43 benign and 80 controls non neoplastic samples)	Sensitivity: 87.18% Specificity: 93.75% Accuracy: 90.14%	Nested Methylation -specific PCR (MSP)	Wang et al., 2017
RASSF1A	Plasma	53 samples including OC tumors, adjacent tumor cell free tissues and paired plasma circulating tumor DNA	Sensitivity: 33/53 (62.3%), RASSF1A methylation of paired plasma CtDNA showed slight concordant with primary tumor samples ($P = 0.227$, 2-sided Pearson $\chi 2$ test, $k = 0.156$). Significantly correlates with overall survival	Real-time methylation specific-PCR (real-time MSP) and methylation-sensitive high-resolution melting analysis (MS-HRMA)	Giannopoulou et al., 2017
ESR1	Plasma	Group A: 66 OC cases Group B: 53 OC case along with 50 paired plasma samples	Sensitivity of detection: 38%. ESR1 methylation predicted better clinical outcomes: overall survival ($P = 0.027$), progression-free survival ($P = 0.041$)	Real-time methylation-specific PCR (real-time MSP) assay	Giannopoulou et al., 2018
3-gene panel	Serum	For assay development: 151 cases and for validation study 250 cases with different conditions in 3 sets	Pre-chemotherapy Sensitivity: 41.4% Specificity: 90.7% Post chemotherapy Responders: 78% non-responders: 86%	Targeted ultra-high coverage bisulfite sequencing	Widschwendter et al., 2017

miR−200a, miR-200b, miR-200c, and miR-429 correlated with poor progression free survival. Moreover, multivariate analysis of relevant clinicopathological variables such as debulking status, stage and grade of tumor revealed the correlation of miR-429 expression with recurrence-free survival (Leskela et al., 2010). Downregulated miR-422b and miR-34c correlated with decreased disease-specific survival in HGSOC patients with BRCA1/2 abnormalities (Lee et al., 2009).

In ovarian cancer, overexpression of miR-214 has been specifically associated with the degradation of PTEN mRNA which further leads to the activation of Akt pathway and has been correlated with platinum resistance (Yang H. et al., 2008). Downregulation of miR-Let7i has been reported in platinum-resistance ovarian tumors; however its gain of function resulted in restoration of drug sensitivity of chemoresistance OC cells (Yang N. et al., 2008).

TABLE 10 | List of dysregulated miRNAs in ovarian cancer.

	Mechanism(s)	miR(s)	Targets	Consequence(s) leading to tumorigenesis	References
Upregulated	c-myc activation	130a	MCSF, GAX and HOXA5	Chemotherapy resistance, angiogenesis, and dedifferentiation	Taylor and Gercel-Taylor, 2008; Eitan et al., 2009
	Copy gain	27a and 451	ZBTB10, Myt-1, HMGB2, HOXA2, and CYP1B1	Multidrug export, oncogenic signaling and reduced apoptotic potential	Shibata et al., 2006; Zhang L. et al., 2006
		213	APP and SATB2	Chemoresistance	Boren et al., 2009
		199a, 200a, b, c and 335	TGFβ, ZEB1, ZEB2, BAP1, GATA4, GATA6, TNC, FN1, EXOC5, and TUBB3	Mesenchymal–epithelial transition	Weisenberger et al., 2008; Su et al., 2009; Liggett et al., 2011; Giannopoulou et al., 2017; Wang et al., 2017
	Hypomethylation	203	p63, SOCS-3, ABL1, MCEF, and ADAMTS6	Unknown	Iorio et al., 2007; Lee et al., 2009
		205	ZEB1, ZEB2, E2F1, ERBB3, PKCe, and SHIP2	Mesenchymal–epithelial transition, oncogenic signal transduction	Iorio et al., 2007; Yu et al., 2008; Lee et al., 2009
		21	PDCD4[†], RPS7[†], NCAPG[†], TPM1, and PTEN	Reduced apoptotic potential and anchorage independence	Iorio et al., 2007; Laios et al., 2008; Sorrentino et al., 2008; Eitan et al., 2009; Lee et al., 2009; Resnick et al., 2009; Yang et al., 2009
	Unknown	340	PAM, RTN3, PPL, RNF34, and ZNF513	Chemoresistance	Boren et al., 2009
		221/222	KIT, AIP1, p21, p57, TCF12, RIMS3, and ARNT	Cell cycle progression and angiogenesis	Merritt et al., 2008; Vlassov et al., 2010; Kneip et al., 2011
Downregulated	C/EBPα Downregulation	1	FOXP1, HDAC4 c-Met, Pim1 and HAND2	Tumor growth, cell motility and proliferation	Iorio et al., 2007
	DNA methylation and copy loss	137	CDK6, MITF, KLF12, and PDLIM3	Cell cycle progression and dedifferentiation	Iorio et al., 2007; Zhang L. et al., 2008
		140	c-SRK, MMP13 and FGF2	Oncogenic signaling	Iorio et al., 2007; Zhang L. et al., 2008
		150	c-Myb, MAK9, Akt3, and MAP2K4	Oncogenic signaling	Zhang L. et al., 2008
		551a	LPHN1, ERBB4, and ZFP36	Oncogenic signaling	Dahiya et al., 2008
		9	NF-kB[†], Bcl2[†], Bcl6, FGF[†], and b-Raf	Oncogenic signaling	Leon et al., 1977; Weisenberger et al., 2008; Faggad et al., 2010; Kneip et al., 2011
		184	TTK69, K10, and Sax(A)	Dedifferentiation	Zhang L. et al., 2008
	Unknown	30b and d	CTGF	Invasion/metastasis	Laios et al., 2008
		98	HMGA2, LIN28B, and HIC2	Oncogenic signaling and cancer stemness	Dahiya et al., 2008
		517a and b	CREAP-1, MAPKAPK5, NFKBIE, and PTK2B	Chemoresistance and oncogenic signaling	Lee et al., 2009
		Let-7i	HMGA2, LIN28Bm TRIM71, and IGF2BP1	Chemoresistance	Yang N. et al., 2008
		662	NEGR1, MKX, and CSF3	Unknown	Dahiya et al., 2008

Several studies have recently highlighted the diagnostic and prognostic relevance of several miRNAs, their association with overall survival of patients and have shown that they could serve as putative biomarker as well as therapeutic target for ovarian cancer management. For instance, Li et al. have reported tumor suppressive role of miR-542-3p, which directly targets CDK14 and was observed significantly downregulated in EOC tissue and OC cell lines (Li et al., 2019).

Si et al. highlighting the therapeutic significance of miR-27a in OC, reported miR-27a mediated regulation of proliferation, chemosensitivity and invasion of OC by targeting Cullin 5 (CUL5) (Si et al., 2019, p. 5). Another study by Jia et al. reported the tumor suppressive role of miR-34 in regulation of tumor proliferation via inducting autophagy and apoptosis and suppression of cell invasion by targeting Notch 1 (Jia et al., 2019, p. 1). Wang et al. utilizing integrated meta-analysis approach

TABLE 11 | List of misexpressed miRNAs in ovarian cancer.

Epigenetic marker	Alternations in miRNAs	Source	Methodology	Clinical prediction	References
Dicer, Drosha mRNA	Downregulated	Tumor tissue and ovarian cancer cell lines	Quantitative RT-PCR, gene expression array	Advanced tumor stage and Suboptimal tumor debulking	Merritt et al., 2008; Faggad et al., 2010; Pampalakis et al., 2010
let-7i, miR-221,−30c,−152 and−193 miR-185,−106a,−181a, −210,−423,−103,−107 and let-7c	Downregulated Upregulated	Tumor tissue from Endometrial cancer, normal endometrial and atypical hyperplasia	Quantitative RT-PCR, microarray analysis	Association with Endometrial cancer development	Boren et al., 2008
miR-124-1,−124-2,−124-3,−127,−132,−137,−193A, 375 and−339	Downregulated	Tumor tissue	Quantitative RT-PCR, MSP, direct Sanger sequencing	EOC metastasis (including peritoneal macro-metastases)	Loginov et al., 2018
let-7i	Downregulated	Tumor tissue and ovarian cancer cell lines	miRNA Microarray, Stem-loop real-time RT-PCR (TaqMan miRNA assay)	Associated with increased resistance to chemotherapy drugs, cis-platinum, and short progression-free survival	Yang N. et al., 2008
miR-30c,−130a, and−335	Downregulated	Paclitaxel and cisplatin resistant cancer cell lines	miRNA Microarray, qPCR, Northern blots	Association with development of chemoresistance	Sorrentino et al., 2008
miR- 199b-5p	Downregulated	Cisplatin-sensitive and -resistant ovarian cancer cell lines	miRCURY LNA^{TM} microRNA array and Q-PCR	Development of acquired chemoresistance through the activation of JAG1-Notch1 signaling cascade	Liu et al., 2014
miR-34a, miR-34b*/c	Downregulated	Tumor tissue	Quantitative RT-PCR, *in- situ* hybridization	Associated with motility and invasion by regulation of MET, progression of disease to advanced stages	Corney et al., 2010
miR−34a,−200a,−200b, −449b,−509-3p,−509-3-5p, −513a-5p and −574-5p	Upregulated	Tumor tissue	MicroRNA microarray	Differentially expressed in Stage I disease	Eitan et al., 2009
miR-302b,−22, and−373 miR-148b and−211	Upregulated Downregulated	Tumor tissue and ovarian cancer cell lines	MicroRNA microarray, Quantitative Real time PCR (Taqman based)	Discriminates serous vs. non-serous disease	Iorio et al., 2007
miR-7, 34c-5p, 146b-5p and 449a	Upregulated	Tumor tissue	Massively parallel pyrosequencing, TaqMan qRT-PCR assays	Serous adenocarcinoma	Wyman et al., 2009
miR-23p,−125a-3p,−125a-5p,−130a,−146b-5p,−193a-3p,−193a-5p,−423-5p,−451 and−491-5p	Upregulated	Tumor tissue	MicroRNA microarray	Differentially expressed in Stage III disease	Eitan et al., 2009
miRs 100, 199a, 200a, and 214	Upregulated	Tumor tissue and ovarian cancer cell line	miRNA array and Northern blot analysis, quantitative reverse transcription-PCR.	Late clinical stage and high-grade tumors, negative regulation of PTEN by miR-214 thereby inducing cell survival and cisplatin resistance	Yang H. et al., 2008
miR-302b,−325,−299-5p,−222, and−324-3p miR-212 and−150	Upregulated Downregulated	Tumor tissue and ovarian cancer cell lines	MicroRNA microarray, Quantitative Real time PCR (Taqman based)	Differentiates Serous vs. endometrioid disease	Iorio et al., 2007
miR-325,−22,−302c,−299-5p,−373, and−196b miR-9 and−18	Upregulated Downregulated	Tumor tissue and ovarian cancer cell lines	MicroRNA microarray, Quantitative Real time PCR (Taqman based)	Associated with Poor differentiation	Iorio et al., 2007
miR-30a,−30a*, and−486-5p	Upregulated	Tumor tissue and ovarian cancer cell lines	MicroRNA microarray, Quantitative Real time PCR (Taqman based)	Clear cell disease	Iorio et al., 2007

(Continued)

TABLE 11 | Continued

Epigenetic marker	Alternations in miRNAs	Source	Methodology	Clinical prediction	References
Methylation of let-7a-3	Downregulated	Tumor tissue	Real-time methylation-specific PCR and real-time reverse Transcription-PCR, direct Sanger sequencing	Favorable prognosis	Lu et al., 2007, p. 3
miR-449b	Upregulated	Tumor tissue	MicroRNA microarray	Good prognosis	Eitan et al., 2009
let-7e	Upregulated	Paclitaxel and cisplatin resistant cancer cell lines	miRNA Microarray, qPCR, Northern blots	Associated with resistance to Paclitaxel	Sorrentino et al., 2008
miR-200a,−200b, and−429	Upregulated	Primary tumor and ovarian cancer cell line	Real-time reverse transcription-PCR	Long disease free survival and delayed recurrence, prognostic marker in advanced ovarian cancer	Cochrane et al., 2009; Hu et al., 2009
miRs 100, 199a, 200a, and 214	Upregulated	Tumor tissue and ovarian cancer cell line	miRNA array and Northern blot analysis, quantitative reverse transcription-PCR.	Late clinical stage and high-grade tumors	Yang H. et al., 2008
Methylation of miR-34a	Downregulated	Tumor tissue	Quantitative reverse transcription-PCR, MethyLight assay	Inversely associated with grade, p53 mutation, and dualistic tumor type. Reduced progression free survival and worsen overall survival.	Schmid et al., 2016
Methylation of miR-199a-3p	Downregulated	Tumor tissue and ovarian cancer cell line	Methylation-specific PCR and bisulphite sequencing	Tumor aggressiveness and enhanced cisplatin resistance through promoting DDR1 expression	Deng et al., 2017
Methylation of 10 miRNA genes (miR-124-2,−124-3,−125B-1,−127,−129-2,−137, −193A,−203A,−339,−375)	Downregulated	Tumors tissue and matched peritoneal metastases	Methylation-specific PCR	Involved in metastasis	Loginov et al., 2018
(miR-34b/c, miR-9-1, miR-124-3, miR-129-2, and miR-107)	Downregulated	Tumor tissue	Methylation-specific PCR	Associated with clinical grade and metastasis. High sensitivity and specificity reveals its diagnostic potential (87–94%, AUC = 0.92).	Braga et al., 2018b
miR-150	Downregulated	Tumor tissue	Real time PCR	Correlated with shorter progression free survival	Wilczynski et al., 2018
miR-4443 and miR-5195-3p	Downregulated	Tumor tissue	Real time PCR	Correlates with metastasis and tumor progression	Ebrahimi and Reiisi, 2019
miR-148a	Downregulated	Plasma samples and ovarian cancer cell line	Real time PCR	Associated with poor prognosis, tumor growth and metastasis	Gong et al., 2016
(hsa-miR-135, 150,−340, 625, 1908, 3187,−96,−196b,−449c, and−1275)	Downregulated	Tumor tissue	Small RNA sequencing, quantitative RT-PCR	Associated with survival	Chen et al., 2018
miR-595	Downregulated	Tumor tissue	qRT-PCR	Correlated with shorter overall survival	Zhou et al., 2017
miR-498	Downregulated	Tumor tissue	qPCR	Correlated with shorter overall survival and progression free survival	Cong et al., 2015

(Continued)

TABLE 11 | Continued

Epigenetic marker	Alternations in miRNAs	Source	Methodology	Clinical prediction	References
miR-9	Downregulated	Tumor tissue and ovarian cancer cell line	Real time PCR, luciferase reporter assay, Western Blot, Methylation study, RNAi technique, and cytotoxicity Assay	Resistance to paclitaxel by targeting CCNG1.	Li X. et al., 2015
miR-508-3p	Downregulated	Tumor tissue and ovarian cancer cell line	System biology approach, qRT-PCR, methylation PCR, RNA sequencing, immuno blot	Predictor for mesenchymal subtype and metastasis	Zhao et al., 2019
hsa-miR-1273g-3p	Downregulated	Serum samples of recurrent epithelial ovarian cancer patients	Microarray and qRT-PCR	Prognostic biomarker for recurrence	Günel et al., 2018

have shown the oncogenic role of miRNA-27a by mediating FOXO1 and its inhibition could serve as a new strategy in combating ovarian cancer (Wang Z. et al., 2018, p. 1). Hu et al. identified miR-934 as an oncogene in OC by directly targeting BRMS1L, and thus could serve as a therapeutic marker (Hu et al., 2019). It has been reported that miR-1294 was identified to be downregulated in EOC and correlated with tumor progression and shorter overall survival, thereby could serve as an independent prognostic indicator (Guo W. et al., 2018).

Liu et al. provided insights into the oncogenic role of microRNA-96 (miR-96-5p) in ovarian cancer. Its significant overexpression was found in tissue as well as serum samples. Overexpression of miR-96-5p was correlated with increased proliferation and migration by suppressing Caveolae1 (CAV1) and inhibiting AKT signaling pathway and its downstream proteins (Cyclin D1 and P70), thus implying that miR-96-5p could serve as a promising therapeutic target for ovarian cancer (Liu et al., 2019, p. 1). Similarly, Chaluvally-Raghavan et al. reported that miR551b-3p which is an oncogenic microRNA, directly upregulates STAT3 expression and further deregulates proliferation and metastasis *in vivo* and *in vitro*. Reduced expression of STAT3 in OC cells *in vitro* and *in vivo* via anti-miR551b-3p leads to reduction in growth of ovarian tumor *in vivo*, thereby implying that it could serve as promising therapeutic target in future for ovarian cancer (Chaluvally-Raghavan et al., 2016).

In another study, miR-152 mediated suppression of tumor proliferation along with promotion of apoptosis via repression of ERBB3 was reported, thus demonstrating miR-152 as a potential therapeutic target (Li et al., 2017, p. 3). Liu et al. reported association of miR-506 with better response to therapy as well as long PFS and overall survival in OC patients. Further, it sensitized cancer cells to chemotherapy by directly targeting RAD51 and thus could be of therapeutic importance (Liu et al., 2015).

10 miRs which were identified using genome wide MicroRNA expression profiling were capable to discriminate malignant tissue samples from normal with a sensitivity of 97% and specificity of 92% (Wang et al., 2014). Biamonte et al. have reported tumor suppressive role of miR-let-7g and significant association of its reduced expression in both tissue as well as serum with chemoresistance in advanced stage EOC patient which reflects its potential as a predictive biomarker to monitor response to chemotherapy (Biamonte et al., 2019). Kobayashi et al. have shown significant overexpression of serum miR-1290 in advance stage HGSOC in comparison to early stage. Moreover, it was capable to discriminate patients with HGSOC from patients with malignancies of other histological subtypes with a sensitivity of 47% and specificity of 85% (AUC = 0.76), thus reflecting diagnostic potential of miR-1290 for HGSOC (Kobayashi et al., 2018).

Mahmoud et al. examined the diagnostic significance of serum miR-21 and reported that its upregulation was significantly negatively correlated with Programmed Cell Death-4 (PDCD4) expression in EOC patients (Mahmoud et al., 2018). Another study highlighted significantly elevated expression of serum exosomal miR-93, miR-145, and miR-200c in OC. Moreover, the sensitivity for miR-145 and miR-200c was 91.6 and 90.0% which was far superior in comparison with CA125, thus these serum exosomal microRNAs could be of diagnostic relevance for preoperative diagnosis of OC (Kim et al., 2019). miR-21 was observed significantly overexpressed in the sera of EOC patients and its elevated expression correlated with shorter overall survival (Xu et al., 2013). Further, downregulation of serum miR-25 and miR-93 and upregulation of miR-7 and miR-429 have been reported in OC patients. In addition, the sensitivity and specificity achieved by these four serum miRs were 93 and 92% to discriminate cancer patients from non-neoplastic control samples, deciphering their diagnostic significance in EOC. Moreover serum miR-429 correlated with overall survival and could serve as an independent prognostic indicator (Meng et al., 2015). Findings from another study reveal the relevance of serum miR-141 and miR-200c in OC diagnosis and prognosis. Both of these miRs were identified to be overexpressed in serum of EOC patients; however miR-200c displayed a descending expression trend across tumor stage (early to advance) while an escalating expression trend was observed in case of miR-141. Moreover, the sensitivity for miR-141 and miR-200c were 0.69 and 0.72 with a specificity of 0.72 and 0.70, respectively, to discriminate cancerous samples from normal control [AUC = 0.75 and 0.79, respectively]. Furthermore, high serum miR-200c correlated with higher survival rate. On contrary, low serum miR-141 correlated with higher survival rate (Gao and Wu, 2015).

Langhe et al. using Exiqon platform explored a 4-miR panel in serum of EOC patients for their diagnostic utility and found that these miRs were significantly downregulated in EOC patients. Furthermore these miRs target WNT signaling, AKT/mTOR signaling and TLR-4/MyD88 to regulate ovarian cancer progression and resistance (Langhe et al., 2015). Overexpression of serum miR-200a, miR-200b, and miR-200c which have been observed in EOC patients, correlates with aggressive disease progression and could be indicative of disease prognosis and patient survival (Zuberi et al., 2015). Higher serum concentration of exosomal miR-200b and miR-200c correlated with shorter overall survival, which suggests its prognostic relevance. (Meng et al., 2016b) Serum miR-200a, miR-200b, and miR-200c differentiated cancerous and benign tumors with 83% sensitivity and 100% specificity, which reflect that these miRs could be of diagnostic utility (Meng et al., 2016a).

These miRs though hold great potential for their utility in ovarian cancer management; however its therapeutical implementation still remains a challenge. To address this, well-designed clinical study as well as validated methodologies is essentially warranted.

Expert Commentary

It is now well-established that DNA methylation occurs very early in malignant transformation and their utility as biomarker holds great promise to overcome the false positive detection of ovarian cancer using current standard serum marker CA125. In this review, we highlight the recent epigenetic biomarkers analyzed in tissue and body fluids for early detection of OC. Strikingly; to date no single epigenetic biomarker facilitating early diagnosis of OC has made transition to the clinics. The probable reasons for this could be: the heterogeneous nature of EOC, difference in sample processing, assay design, technique used and approach could explain the variations observed in methylation frequencies amongst various studies for individual genes. Most of the studies for methylation analysis of genes were conducted on small sample size and in particular the normal control samples were insufficient to conclude the specificity of the assay. Therefore, further studies on larger sample size are necessary to be conducted to determine the potential of methylation if it could serve as biomarker for early EOC screening or not. Another limitation is the absence of standardized reference value for methylation analysis when trying to analyze if a particular locus is hyper or hypomethylated. To overcome this, currently, methylation cut off points which are based on already published reports or consensus are used.

The majority of the reports highlight the methylation status of gene or genes in a panel. No epigenetic biomarker screening study has been performed till date. However, for the detection figures approaching current screening modalities (89.5% sensitivity and 99.8% specificity) has been achieved by Ibanez de Caceres et al. (2004) with 82% sensitivity and 100% specificity (Ibanez de Caceres et al., 2004). All 30 control cases showed 0 false positive rate and further replication of the study on the basis of this sample size would give a false positive rate between 0 and 11.4% (95% confidence interval), thereby indicating that perfect specificity would unlikely hold up in the follow-up studies. In view of these considerations regarding the study of Ibanez de Caceres et al. are left to follow-up studies to shed light on. However, none of the report has been further validated undertaking follow up studies on a larger cohort and prospective study design thereby limiting the utility of the reported findings.

Molecular analysis of epigenetic modification (methylation) in circulating cell free tumor DNA in fluids serves as a novel, non-invasive approach for identification of potential promising cancer biomarkers, which can be performed at multiple time points and probably better reflects the prevailing molecular profile of cancer. Very few studies analyzing the methylation status of genes in blood-based assay for ovarian cancer diagnosis has been reported. Careful precision handling and processing of liquid biopsy for cell free DNA extraction is critically needed.

Future Prospects

Over the last decade, an exponential progress in DNA methylation based biomarker development has been witnessed. Owing to the stability of DNA and methylation pattern, a number of cfDNA as well as tissue based screening assay has paved its way into clinics. The commercial success of several tests based on DNA methylation biomarkers for early detection of colon, lung and prostate cancer and prediction of bladder cancer along with various markers under validation study shows that the time for transition into clinics can be relatively rapid. New technologies which allow rapid identification of methylation signatures directly from blood will facilitate sample-to answer solutions thereby enabling next-generation point of care molecular diagnostics. Moreover, ongoing work on liquid biopsies together with the recent advanced technologies such as digital PCR, bisulfite sequencing, methyl immune-precipitation coupled with next-generation sequencing, and methylation arrays along with advanced statistical data analysis may mitigate the problematic issues for the development of non-invasive method thereby overcoming the existing challenges to personalized medicine.

AUTHOR CONTRIBUTIONS

AS wrote the manuscript. SG and MS edited the final version of the manuscript.

REFERENCES

Abdollahi, A., Pisarcik, D., Roberts, D., Weinstein, J., Cairns, P., and Hamilton, T. C. (2003). LOT1 (PLAGL1/ZAC1), the candidate tumor suppressor gene at chromosome 6q24-25, is epigenetically regulated in cancer. *J. Biol. Chem.* 278, 6041–6049. doi: 10.1074/jbc.M210361200

Agathanggelou, A., Honorio, S., Macartney, D. P., Martinez, A., Dallol, A., Rader, J., et al. (2001). Methylation associated inactivation of RASSF1A from region 3p21.3 in lung, breast and ovarian tumours. *Oncogene* 20, 1509–1518. doi: 10.1038/sj.onc.1204175

Agostini, A., Brunetti, M., Davidson, B., Trop,é, C. G., Eriksson, A. G. Z., Heim, S., et al. (2018). The microRNA miR-192/215 family is upregulated in mucinous ovarian carcinomas. *Sci. Rep.* 8:11069. doi: 10.1038/s41598-018-29332-7

Akahira, J., Sugihashi, Y., Ito, K., Niikura, H., Okamura, K., and Yaegashi, N. (2004a). Promoter methylation status and expression of TMS1 gene in human epithelial ovarian cancer. *Cancer Sci.* 95, 40–43. doi: 10.1111/j.1349-7006.2004.tb03168.x

Akahira, J., Sugihashi, Y., Suzuki, T., Ito, K., Niikura, H., Moriya, T., et al. (2004b). Decreased expression of 14-3-3 sigma is associated with advanced disease in human epithelial ovarian cancer: its correlation with aberrant DNA methylation. *Clin. Cancer Res. Off. J. Am. Assoc. Cancer Res.* 10, 2687–2693. doi: 10.1158/1078-0432.CCR-03-0510

Amonkar, S. D., Bertenshaw, G. P., Chen, T.-H., Bergstrom, K. J., Zhao, J., Seshaiah, P., et al. (2009). Development and preliminary evaluation of a multivariate index assay for ovarian cancer. *PLoS ONE* 4:e4599. doi: 10.1371/journal.pone.0004599

Andersen, M. R., Goff, B. A., Lowe, K. A., Scholler, N., Bergan, L., Drescher, C. W., et al. (2010). Use of a symptom index, CA125, and HE4 to predict ovarian cancer. *Gynecol. Oncol.* 116, 378–383. doi: 10.1016/j.ygyno.2009.10.087

Arnold, J. M., Cummings, M., Purdie, D., and Chenevix-Trench, G. (2001). Reduced expression of intercellular adhesion molecule-1 in ovarian adenocarcinomas. *Br. J. Cancer* 85, 1351–1358. doi: 10.1054/bjoc.2001.2075

Bai, T., Tanaka, T., Yukawa, K., Maeda, M., and Umesaki, N. (2004). Reduced expression of death-associated protein kinase in human uterine and ovarian carcinoma cells. *Oncol. Rep.* 11, 661–665. doi: 10.3892/or.11.3.661

Balch, C., Matei, D. E., Huang, T. H.-M., and Nephew, K. P. (2010). Role of epigenomics in ovarian and endometrial cancers. *Epigenomics* 2, 419–447. doi: 10.2217/epi.10.19

Baldwin, R. L., Nemeth, E., Tran, H., Shvartsman, H., Cass, I., Narod, S., et al. (2000). BRCA1 promoter region hypermethylation in ovarian carcinoma: a population-based study. *Cancer Res.* 60, 5329–5333.

Baranova, I., Kovarikova, H., Laco, J., Dvorak, O., Sedlakova, I., Palicka, V., et al. (2018). Aberrant methylation of PCDH17 gene in high-grade serous ovarian carcinoma. *Cancer Biomark.* 23, 125–133. doi: 10.3233/CBM-181493

Barbolina, M. V., Adley, B. P., Kelly, D. L., Shepard, J., Fought, A. J., Scholtens, D., et al. (2009). Downregulation of connective tissue growth factor by three-dimensional matrix enhances ovarian carcinoma cell invasion. *Int. J. Cancer* 125, 816–825. doi: 10.1002/ijc.24347

Bartlett, T. E., Chindera, K., McDermott, J., Breeze, C. E., Cooke, W. R., Jones, A., et al. (2016). Epigenetic reprogramming of fallopian tube fimbriae in BRCA mutation carriers defines early ovarian cancer evolution. *Nat. Commun.* 7:11620. doi: 10.1038/ncomms11620

Barton, C. A., Gloss, B. S., Qu, W., Statham, A. L., Hacker, N. F., Sutherland, R. L., et al. (2010). Collagen and calcium-binding EGF domains 1 is frequently inactivated in ovarian cancer by aberrant promoter hypermethylation and modulates cell migration and survival. *Br. J. Cancer* 102, 87–96. doi: 10.1038/sj.bjc.6605429

Barton, C. A., Hacker, N. F., Clark, S. J., and O'Brien, P. M. (2008). DNA methylation changes in ovarian cancer: implications for early diagnosis, prognosis and treatment. *Gynecol. Oncol.* 109, 129–139. doi: 10.1016/j.ygyno.2007.12.017

Belinsky, S. A. (2004). Gene-promoter hypermethylation as a biomarker in lung cancer. *Nat. Rev. Cancer* 4, 707–717. doi: 10.1038/nrc1432

Biamonte, F., Santamaria, G., Sacco, A., Perrone, F. M., Di Cello, A., Battaglia, A. M., et al. (2019). MicroRNA let-7g acts as tumor suppressor and predictive biomarker for chemoresistance in human epithelial ovarian cancer. *Sci. Rep.* 9:5668. doi: 10.1038/s41598-019-42221-x

Bird, A. (2002). DNA methylation patterns and epigenetic memory. *Genes Dev.* 16, 6–21. doi: 10.1101/gad.947102

Bird, A. P., and Wolffe, A. P. (1999). Methylation-induced repression–belts, braces, and chromatin. *Cell* 99, 451–454. doi: 10.1016/S0092-8674(00)81532-9

Board, R. E., Knight, L., Greystoke, A., Blackhall, F. H., Hughes, A., Dive, C., et al. (2008). DNA methylation in circulating tumour DNA as a biomarker for cancer. *Biomark. Insights* 2, 307–319. doi: 10.1177/117727190700200003

Bol, G. M., Suijkerbuijk, K. P. M., Bart, J., Vooijs, M., van der Wall, E., and van Diest, P. J. (2010). Methylation profiles of hereditary and sporadic ovarian cancer. *Histopathology* 57, 363–370. doi: 10.1111/j.1365-2559.2010.03642.x

Bonito, N. A., Borley, J., Wilhelm-Benartzi, C. S., Ghaem-Maghami, S., and Brown, R. (2016). Epigenetic regulation of the homeobox gene MSX1 associates with platinum-resistant disease in high-grade serous epithelial ovarian cancer. *Clin. Cancer Res.* 22, 3097–3104. doi: 10.1158/1078-0432.CCR-15-1669

Boren, T., Xiong, Y., Hakam, A., Wenham, R., Apte, S., Chan, G., et al. (2009). MicroRNAs and their target messenger RNAs associated with ovarian cancer response to chemotherapy. *Gynecol. Oncol.* 113, 249–255. doi: 10.1016/j.ygyno.2009.01.014

Boren, T., Xiong, Y., Hakam, A., Wenham, R., Apte, S., Wei, Z., et al. (2008). MicroRNAs and their target messenger RNAs associated with endometrial carcinogenesis. *Gynecol. Oncol.* 110, 206–215. doi: 10.1016/j.ygyno.2008.03.023

Borgoño, C. A., and Diamandis, E. P. (2004). The emerging roles of human tissue kallikreins in cancer. *Nat. Rev. Cancer* 4, 876–890. doi: 10.1038/nrc1474

Bowtell, D. D. L. (2010). The genesis and evolution of high-grade serous ovarian cancer. *Nat. Rev. Cancer* 10, 803–808. doi: 10.1038/nrc2946

Brachova, P., Mueting, S. R., Carlson, M. J., Goodheart, M. J., Button, A. M., Mott, S. L., et al. (2015). TP53 oncomorphic mutations predict resistance to platinum- and taxane-based standard chemotherapy in patients diagnosed with advanced serous ovarian carcinoma. *Int. J. Oncol.* 46, 607–618. doi: 10.3892/ijo.2014.2747

Braga, E. A., Loginov, V. I., Burdennyi, A. M., Filippova, E. A., Pronina, I. V., Kurevlev, S. V., et al. (2018a). Five Hypermethylated MicroRNA genes as potential markers of ovarian cancer. *Bull. Exp. Biol. Med.* 164, 351–355. doi: 10.1007/s10517-018-3988-y

Braga, E. A., Loginov, V. I., Filippova, E. A., Burdennyi, A. M., Pronina, I. V., Kazubskaya, T. P., et al. (2018b). Diagnostic value of a group of MicroRNA genes hypermethylated in ovarian carcinoma. *Bull. Exp. Biol. Med.* 166, 253–256. doi: 10.1007/s10517-018-4326-0

Brock, M. V., Hooker, C. M., Ota-Machida, E., Han, Y., Guo, M., Ames, S., et al. (2008). DNA methylation markers and early recurrence in stage I lung cancer. *N. Engl. J. Med.* 358, 1118–1128. doi: 10.1056/NEJMoa0706550

Buchholtz, M.-L., Brüning, A., Mylonas, I., and Jückstock, J. (2014). Epigenetic silencing of the LDOC1 tumor suppressor gene in ovarian cancer cells. *Arch. Gynecol. Obstet.* 290, 149–154. doi: 10.1007/s00404-014-3177-9

Buys, S. S., Partridge, E., Black, A., Johnson, C. C., Lamerato, L., Isaacs, C., et al. (2011). Effect of screening on ovarian cancer mortalitys (PLCO) cancer screening randomized controlled trial. *JAMA* 305, 2295–2303. doi: 10.1001/jama.2011.766

Cacan, E. (2016). Histone deacetylase-1-mediated suppression of FAS in chemoresistant ovarian cancer cells. *Anticancer Res.* 36, 2819–2826.

Cacan, E. (2017). Epigenetic regulation of RGS2 (Regulator of G-protein signaling 2) in chemoresistant ovarian cancer cells. *J. Chemother.* 29, 173–178. doi: 10.1080/1120009X.2016.1277007

Cai, K. Q., Caslini, C., Capo-chichi, C. D., Slater, C., Smith, E. R., Wu, H., et al. (2009). Loss of GATA4 and GATA6 expression specifies ovarian cancer histological subtypes and precedes neoplastic transformation of ovarian surface epithelia. *PLoS ONE* 4:e6454. doi: 10.1371/journal.pone.0006454

Cai, L., Abe, M., Izumi, S., Imura, M., Yasugi, T., and Ushijima, T. (2007). Identification of PRTFDC1 silencing and aberrant promoter methylation of GPR150, ITGA8 and HOXD11 in ovarian cancers. *Life Sci.* 80, 1458–1465. doi: 10.1016/j.lfs.2007.01.015

Cannistra, S. A. (2004). Cancer of the ovary. *N. Engl. J. Med.* 351, 2519–2529. doi: 10.1056/NEJMra041842

Cardenas, H., Vieth, E., Lee, J., Segar, M., Liu, Y., Nephew, K. P., et al. (2014). TGF-β induces global changes in DNA methylation during the epithelial-to-mesenchymal transition in ovarian cancer cells. *Epigenetics* 9, 1461–1472. doi: 10.4161/15592294.2014.971608

Caslini, C., Capo-Chichi, C. D., Roland, I. H., Nicolas, E., Yeung, A. T., and Xu, X. X. (2006). Histone modifications silence the GATA transcription factor genes in ovarian cancer. *Oncogene* 25:5446. doi: 10.1038/sj.onc.1209533

Chaluvally-Raghavan, P., Jeong, K. J., Pradeep, S., Silva, A. M., Yu, S., Liu, W., et al. (2016). Direct upregulation of STAT3 by MicroRNA-551b-3p deregulates growth and metastasis of ovarian cancer. *Cell Rep.* 15, 1493–1504. doi: 10.1016/j.celrep.2016.04.034

Chan, M. W., Huang, Y.-W., Hartman-Frey, C., Kuo, C.-T., Deatherage, D., Qin, H., et al. (2008). Aberrant transforming growth factor beta1 signaling and SMAD4 nuclear translocation confer epigenetic repression of ADAM19 in ovarian cancer. *Neoplasia* 10, 908–919. doi: 10.1593/neo.08540

Chan, M. W. Y. (2005). Hypermethylation of 18S and 28S Ribosomal DNAs predicts progression-free survival in patients with ovarian cancer. *Clin. Cancer Res.* 11, 7376–7383. doi: 10.1158/1078-0432.CCR-05-1100

Chan, T. A., Glockner, S., Yi, J. M., Chen, W., Van Neste, L., Cope, L., et al. (2008). Convergence of mutation and epigenetic alterations identifies common genes in cancer that predict for poor prognosis. *PLoS Med.* 5:e114. doi: 10.1371/journal.pmed.0050114

Chao, A., Lin, C.-Y., Lee, Y.-S., Tsai, C.-L., Wei, P.-C., Hsueh, S., et al. (2012). Regulation of ovarian cancer progression by microRNA-187 through targeting disabled homolog-2. *Oncogene* 31, 764–775. doi: 10.1038/onc.2011.269

Chen, S. F., Liu, Z., Chaurasiya, S., Dellinger, T. H., Lu, J., Wu, X., et al. (2018). Identification of core aberrantly expressed microRNAs in serous ovarian carcinoma. *Oncotarget* 9, 20451–20466. doi: 10.18632/oncotarget.24942

Cheng, W., Jiang, Y., Liu, C., Shen, O., Tang, W., and Wang, X. (2010). Identification of aberrant promoter hypomethylation of HOXA10 in ovarian cancer. *J. Cancer Res. Clin. Oncol.* 136, 1221–1227. doi: 10.1007/s00432-010-0772-4

Chien, J., Staub, J., Avula, R., Zhang, H., Liu, W., Hartmann, L. C., et al. (2005). Epigenetic silencing of TCEAL7 (Bex4) in ovarian cancer. *Oncogene* 24, 5089–5100. doi: 10.1038/sj.onc.1208700

Choi, Y.-L., Kang, S. Y., Shin, Y. K., Choi, J. S., Kim, S. H., Lee, S.-J., et al. (2006). Aberrant hypermethylation of RASSF1A promoter in ovarian borderline tumors and carcinomas. *Virchows Arch. Int. J. Pathol.* 448, 331–336. doi: 10.1007/s00428-005-0091-3

Choi, Y.-L., Kim, J., Kwon, M. J., Choi, J. S., Kim, T.-J., Bae, D.-S., et al. (2007). Expression profile of tight junction protein claudin 3 and claudin 4 in ovarian serous adenocarcinoma with prognostic correlation. *Histol. Histopathol.* 22, 1185–1195. doi: 10.14670/HH-22.1185

Chou, J.-L., Huang, R.-L., Shay, J., Chen, L.-Y., Lin, S.-J., Yan, P. S., et al. (2015). Hypermethylation of the TGF-β target, ABCA1 is associated with poor prognosis in ovarian cancer patients. *Clin. Epigenetics* 7:1. doi: 10.1186/s13148-014-0036-2

Chou, J.-L., Su, H.-Y., Chen, L.-Y., Liao, Y.-P., Hartman-Frey, C., Lai, Y.-H., et al. (2010). Promoter hypermethylation of FBXO32, a novel TGF-beta/SMAD4 target gene and tumor suppressor, is associated with poor prognosis in human ovarian cancer. *Lab. Investig. J. Tech. Methods Pathol.* 90, 414–425. doi: 10.1038/labinvest.2009.138

Chung, V. Y., Tan, T. Z., Huang, R.-L., Lai, H.-C., and Huang, R. Y.-J. (2017). Loss of discoidin domain receptor 1 (DDR1) via CpG methylation during EMT in epithelial ovarian cancer. *Gene* 635, 9–15. doi: 10.1016/j.gene.2017.09.001

Cicek, M. S., Koestler, D. C., Fridley, B. L., Kalli, K. R., Armasu, S. M., Larson, M. C., et al. (2013). Epigenome-wide ovarian cancer analysis identifies a methylation profile differentiating clear-cell histology with epigenetic silencing of the HERG K+ channel. *Hum. Mol. Genet.* 22, 3038–3047. doi: 10.1093/hmg/ddt160

Clarke-Pearson, D. L. (2009). Clinical practice. Screening for ovarian cancer. *N. Engl. J. Med.* 361, 170–177. doi: 10.1056/NEJMcp0901926

Cochrane, D. R., Spoelstra, N. S., Howe, E. N., Nordeen, S. K., and Richer, J. K. (2009). MicroRNA-200c mitigates invasiveness and restores sensitivity to microtubule-targeting chemotherapeutic agents. *Mol. Cancer Ther.* 8, 1055–1066. doi: 10.1158/1535-7163.MCT-08-1046

Collins, Y., Dicioccio, R., Keitz, B., Lele, S., and Odunsi, K. (2006). Methylation of death-associated protein kinase in ovarian carcinomas. *Int. J. Gynecol. Cancer Off. J. Int. Gynecol. Cancer Soc.* 16 (Suppl. 1), 195–199. doi: 10.1136/ijgc-00009577-200602001-00031

Cong, J., Liu, R., Wang, X., Wang, J., Wang, H., and Hou, J. (2015). Low miR-498 expression levels are associated with poor prognosis in ovarian cancer. *Eur. Rev. Med. Pharmacol. Sci.* 19, 4762–4765.

Corney, D. C., Hwang, C.-I., Matoso, A., Vogt, M., Flesken-Nikitin, A., Godwin, A. K., et al. (2010). Frequent downregulation of miR-34 family in human ovarian cancers. *Clin. Cancer Res.* 16, 1119–1128. doi: 10.1158/1078-0432.CCR-09-2642

Costello, J. F., and Plass, C. (2001). Methylation matters. *J. Med. Genet.* 38, 285–303. doi: 10.1136/jmg.38.5.285

Curry, E., Zeller, C., Masrour, N., Patten, D. K., Gallon, J., Wilhelm-Benartzi, C. S., et al. (2018). Genes predisposed to DNA hypermethylation during acquired resistance to chemotherapy are identified in ovarian tumors by bivalent chromatin domains at initial diagnosis. *Cancer Res.* 78, 1383–1391. doi: 10.1158/0008-5472.CAN-17-1650

Czekierdowski, A., Czekierdowska, S., Szymanski, M., Wielgos, M., Kaminski, P., and Kotarski, J. (2006a). Opioid-binding protein/cell adhesion molecule-like (OPCML) gene and promoter methylation status in women with ovarian cancer. *Neuro Endocrinol. Lett.* 27, 609–613.

Czekierdowski, A., Czekierdowska, S., Wielgos, M., Smolen, A., Kaminski, P., and Kotarski, J. (2006b). The role of CpG islands hypomethylation and abnormal expression of neuronal protein synuclein-gamma (SNCG) in ovarian cancer. *Neuro Endocrinol. Lett.* 27, 381–386.

Dahiya, N., Sherman-Baust, C. A., Wang, T.-L., Davidson, B., Shih, I.-M., Zhang, Y., et al. (2008). MicroRNA expression and identification of putative miRNA targets in ovarian cancer. *PLoS ONE* 3:e2436. doi: 10.1371/journal.pone.0002436

Dai, W., Teodoridis, J. M., Zeller, C., Graham, J., Hersey, J., Flanagan, J. M., et al. (2011). Systematic CpG Islands methylation profiling of genes in the Wnt pathway in epithelial ovarian cancer identifies biomarkers of progression-free survival. *Clin. Cancer Res.* 17, 4052–4062. doi: 10.1158/1078-0432.CCR-10-3021

Dai, W., Zeller, C., Masrour, N., Siddiqui, N., Paul, J., and Brown, R. (2013). Promoter CpG Island methylation of genes in key cancer pathways associates with clinical outcome in high-grade serous ovarian cancer. *Clin. Cancer Res.* 19, 5788–5797. doi: 10.1158/1078-0432.CCR-13-1217

de Leon, M., Cardenas, H., Vieth, E., Emerson, R., Segar, M., Liu, Y., et al. (2016). Transmembrane protein 88 (TMEM88) promoter hypomethylation is associated with platinum resistance in ovarian cancer. *Gynecol. Oncol.* 142, 539–547. doi: 10.1016/j.ygyno.2016.06.017

De Mattos-Arruda, L., Weigelt, B., Cortes, J., Won, H. H., Ng, C. K. Y., Nuciforo, P., et al. (2014). Capturing intra-tumor genetic heterogeneity by *de novo* mutation profiling of circulating cell-free tumor DNA: a proof-of-principle. *Ann. Oncol. Off. J. Eur. Soc. Med. Oncol.* 25, 1729–1735. doi: 10.1093/annonc/mdu239

Deng, Y., Zhao, F., Hui, L., Li, X., Zhang, D., Lin, W., et al. (2017). Suppressing miR-199a-3p by promoter methylation contributes to tumor aggressiveness and cisplatin resistance of ovarian cancer through promoting DDR1 expression. *J. Ovarian Res.* 10. doi: 10.1186/s13048-017-0333-4

Deng, Z., Wang, L., Hou, H., Zhou, J., and Li, X. (2016). Epigenetic regulation of IQGAP2 promotes ovarian cancer progression via activating Wnt/β-catenin signaling. *Int. J. Oncol.* 48, 153–160. doi: 10.3892/ijo.2015.3228

Devouassoux-Shisheboran, M., and Genestie, C. (2015). Pathobiology of ovarian carcinomas. *Chin. J. Cancer* 34, 50–55. doi: 10.5732/cjc.014.10273

Diamandis, E. P., Scorilas, A., Fracchioli, S., Van Gramberen, M., De Bruijn, H., Henrik, A., et al. (2003). Human kallikrein 6 (hK6): a new potential serum biomarker for diagnosis and prognosis of ovarian carcinoma. *J. Clin. Oncol. Off. J. Am. Soc. Clin. Oncol.* 21, 1035–1043. doi: 10.1200/JCO.2003.02.022

Earp, M. A., and Cunningham, J. M. (2015). DNA methylation changes in epithelial ovarian cancer histotypes. *Genomics* 106, 311–321. doi: 10.1016/j.ygeno.2015.09.001

Ebrahimi, S. O., and Reiisi, S. (2019). Downregulation of miR-4443 and miR-5195-3p in ovarian cancer tissue contributes to metastasis and tumorigenesis. *Arch. Gynecol. Obstet.* 299, 1453–1458. doi: 10.1007/s00404-019-05107-x

Edgell, T., Martin-Roussety, G., Barker, G., Autelitano, D. J., Allen, D., Grant, P., et al. (2010). Phase II biomarker trial of a multimarker diagnostic for ovarian cancer. *J. Cancer Res. Clin. Oncol.* 136, 1079–1088. doi: 10.1007/s00432-009-0755-5

Eissa, M. A. L., Lerner, L., Abdelfatah, E., Shankar, N., Canner, J. K., Hasan, N. M., et al. (2019). Promoter methylation of ADAMTS1 and BNC1 as potential biomarkers for early detection of pancreatic cancer in blood. *Clin. Epigenetics* 11:59. doi: 10.1186/s13148-019-0650-0

Eitan, R., Kushnir, M., Lithwick-Yanai, G., David, M. B., Hoshen, M., Glezerman, M., et al. (2009). Tumor microRNA expression patterns associated with resistance to platinum based chemotherapy and survival in ovarian cancer patients. *Gynecol. Oncol.* 114, 253–259. doi: 10.1016/j.ygyno.2009.04.024

Esteller, M. (2007). Epigenetic gene silencing in cancer: the DNA hypermethylome. *Hum. Mol. Genet.* 16, R50–R59. doi: 10.1093/hmg/ddm018

Faggad, A., Budczies, J., Tchernitsa, O., Darb-Esfahani, S., Sehouli, J., Müller, B. M., et al. (2010). Prognostic significance of Dicer expression in ovarian cancer-link to global microRNA changes and oestrogen receptor expression. *J. Pathol.* 220, 382–391. doi: 10.1002/path.2658

Fang, F., Cardenas, H., Huang, H., Jiang, G., Perkins, S. M., Zhang, C., et al. (2018). Genomic and epigenomic signatures in ovarian cancer associated with resensitization to platinum drugs. *Cancer Res.* 78, 631–644. doi: 10.1158/0008-5472.CAN-17-1492

Feinberg, A. P., and Tycko, B. (2004). The history of cancer epigenetics. *Nat. Rev. Cancer* 4, 143–153. doi: 10.1038/nrc1279

Feng, Q., Deftereos, G., Hawes, S. E., Stern, J. E., Willner, J. B., Swisher, E. M., et al. (2008). DNA hypermethylation, Her-2/neu overexpression and p53 mutations in ovarian carcinoma. *Gynecol. Oncol.* 111, 320–329. doi: 10.1016/j.ygyno.2008.07.036

Feng, W., Marquez, R. T., Lu, Z., Liu, J., Lu, K. H., Issa, J.-P. J., et al. (2008). Imprinted tumor suppressor genes ARHI and PEG3 are the most frequently down-regulated in human ovarian cancers by loss of heterozygosity and promoter methylation. *Cancer* 112, 1489–1502. doi: 10.1002/cncr.23323

Fiegl, H., Windbichler, G., Mueller-Holzner, E., Goebel, G., Lechner, M., Jacobs, I. J., et al. (2008). HOXA11 DNA methylation–a novel prognostic biomarker in ovarian cancer. *Int. J. Cancer* 123, 725–729. doi: 10.1002/ijc.23563

Fu, Y., Campbell, E. J., Shepherd, T. G., and Nachtigal, M. W. (2003). Epigenetic regulation of proprotein convertase PACE4 gene expression in human ovarian cancer cells. *Mol. Cancer Res.* 1, 569–576.

Fu, Y., Chen, J., Pang, B., Li, C., Zhao, J., and Shen, K. (2015). EZH2-Induced H3K27me3 is Associated with epigenetic repression of the ARHI tumor-suppressor gene in ovarian cancer. *Cell Biochem. Biophys.* 71, 105–112. doi: 10.1007/s12013-014-0168-1

Furlan, D. (2006). The high frequency of *de novo* promoter methylation in synchronous primary endometrial and ovarian carcinomas. *Clin. Cancer Res.* 12, 3329–3336. doi: 10.1158/1078-0432.CCR-05-2679

Gadomska, H., Grzechocinska, B., Janecki, J., Nowicka, G., Powolny, M., and Marianowski, L. (2005). Serum lipids concentration in women with benign and malignant ovarian tumours. *Eur. J. Obstet. Gynecol. Reprod. Biol.* 120, 87–90. doi: 10.1016/j.ejogrb.2004.02.045

Gao, Y., Lou, G., Zhang, G.-M., Sun, X.-W., Ma, Y.-Y., Yang, Y.-M., et al. (2009). CHFR promoter hypermethylation and reduced CHFR mRNA expression in ovarian cancer. *Int. J. Biol. Markers* 24, 83–89. doi: 10.1177/172460080902400204

Gao, Y., and Wu, J. (2015). MicroRNA-200c and microRNA-141 as potential diagnostic and prognostic biomarkers for ovarian cancer. *Tumor Biol.* 36, 4843–4850. doi: 10.1007/s13277-015-3138-3

Geomini, P., Kruitwagen, R., Bremer, G. L., Cnossen, J., and Mol, B. W. J. (2009). The accuracy of risk scores in predicting ovarian malignancy: a systematic review. *Obstet. Gynecol.* 113, 384–394. doi: 10.1097/AOG.0b013e318195ad17

Giannopoulou, L., Chebouti, I., Pavlakis, K., Kasimir-Bauer, S., and Lianidou, E. S. (2017). RASSF1A promoter methylation in high-grade serous ovarian cancer: a direct comparison study in primary tumors, adjacent morphologically tumor cell-free tissues and paired circulating tumor DNA. *Oncotarget* 8:21429. doi: 10.18632/oncotarget.15249

Giannopoulou, L., Mastoraki, S., Buderath, P., Strati, A., Pavlakis, K., Kasimir-Bauer, S., et al. (2018). ESR1 methylation in primary tumors and paired circulating tumor DNA of patients with high-grade serous ovarian cancer. *Gynecol. Oncol.* 150, 355–360. doi: 10.1016/j.ygyno.2018.05.026

Gifford, G. (2004). The Acquisition of hMLH1 Methylation in Plasma DNA after chemotherapy predicts poor survival for ovarian cancer patients. *Clin. Cancer Res.* 10, 4420–4426. doi: 10.1158/1078-0432.CCR-03-0732

Gloss, B. S., Patterson, K. I., Barton, C. A., Gonzalez, M., Scurry, J. P., Hacker, N. F., et al. (2012). Integrative genome-wide expression and promoter DNA methylation profiling identifies a potential novel panel of ovarian cancer epigenetic biomarkers. *Cancer Lett.* 318, 76–85. doi: 10.1016/j.canlet.2011.12.003

Gong, L., Wang, C., Gao, Y., and Wang, J. (2016). Decreased expression of microRNA-148a predicts poor prognosis in ovarian cancer and associates with tumor growth and metastasis. *Biomed. Pharmacother.* 83, 58–63. doi: 10.1016/j.biopha.2016.05.049

Gorelik, E. (2005). Multiplexed immunobead-based cytokine profiling for early detection of ovarian cancer. *Cancer Epidemiol. Biomarkers Prev.* 14, 981–987. doi: 10.1158/1055-9965.EPI-04-0404

Gormally, E., Caboux, E., Vineis, P., and Hainaut, P. (2007). Circulating free DNA in plasma or serum as biomarker of carcinogenesis: practical aspects and biological significance. *Mutat. Res. Mutat. Res.* 635, 105–117. doi: 10.1016/j.mrrev.2006.11.002

Gozzi, G., Chelbi, S. T., Manni, P., Alberti, L., Fonda, S., Saponaro, S., et al. (2016). Promoter methylation and downregulated expression of the TBX15 gene in ovarian carcinoma. *Oncol. Lett.* 12, 2811–2819. doi: 10.3892/ol.2016.5019

Günel, T., Gumusoglu, E., Dogan, B., Ertem, F. B., Hosseini, M. K., Cevik, N., et al. (2018). Potential biomarker of circulating hsa-miR-1273g-3p level for detection of recurrent epithelial ovarian cancer. *Arch. Gynecol. Obstet.* 298, 1173–1180. doi: 10.1007/s00404-018-4913-3

Guo, T. Y., Xu, H.-Y., Chen, W. J., Wu, M.-X., and Dai, X. (2018). Downregulation of miR-1294 associates with prognosis and tumor progression in epithelial ovarian cancer. *Eur. Rev. Med. Pharmacol. Sci.* 22, 7646–7652.

Guo, W., Zhu, L., Yu, M., Zhu, R., Chen, Q., and Wang, Q. (2018). A five-DNA methylation signature act as a novel prognostic biomarker in patients with ovarian serous cystadenocarcinoma. *Clin. Epigenetics* 10:142. doi: 10.1186/s13148-018-0574-0

Gupta, A., Godwin, A. K., Vanderveer, L., Lu, A., and Liu, J. (2003). Hypomethylation of the synuclein gamma gene CpG island promotes its aberrant expression in breast carcinoma and ovarian carcinoma. *Cancer Res.* 63, 664–673.

Häfner, N., Diebolder, H., Jansen, L., Hoppe, I., Dürst, M., and Runnebaum, I. B. (2011). Hypermethylated DAPK in serum DNA of women with uterine leiomyoma is a biomarker not restricted to cancer. *Gynecol. Oncol.* 121, 224–229. doi: 10.1016/j.ygyno.2010.11.018

Häfner, N., Steinbach, D., Jansen, L., Diebolder, H., Dürst, M., and Runnebaum, I. B. (2016). RUNX3 and CAMK2N1 hypermethylation as prognostic marker for epithelial ovarian cancer: prognostic methylation markers for EOC. *Int. J. Cancer* 138, 217–228. doi: 10.1002/ijc.29690

Han, X., Zhou, Y., You, Y., Lu, J., Wang, L., Hou, H., et al. (2017). TET1 promotes cisplatin-resistance via demethylating the vimentin promoter in ovarian cancer: TET1 in ovarian cancer. *Cell Biol. Int.* 41, 405–414. doi: 10.1002/cbin.10734

Havrilesky, L. J., Whitehead, C. M., Rubatt, J. M., Cheek, R. L., Groelke, J., He, Q., et al. (2008). Evaluation of biomarker panels for early stage ovarian cancer detection and monitoring for disease recurrence. *Gynecol. Oncol.* 110, 374–382. doi: 10.1016/j.ygyno.2008.04.041

Hendrich, B., and Bird, A. (2000). Mammalian methyltransferases and methyl-CpG-binding domains: proteins involved in DNA methylation. *Curr. Top. Microbiol. Immunol.* 249, 55–74. doi: 10.1007/978-3-642-59696-4_4

Herman, J. G., and Baylin, S. B. (2003). Gene silencing in cancer in association with promoter hypermethylation. *N. Engl. J. Med.* 349, 2042–2054. doi: 10.1056/NEJMra023075

Honda, H., Pazin, M. J., D'Souza, T., Ji, H., and Morin, P. J. (2007). Regulation of the CLDN3 gene in ovarian cancer cells. *Cancer Biol. Ther.* 6, 1733–1742. doi: 10.4161/cbt.6.11.4832

Honda, H., Pazin, M. J., Ji, H., Wernyj, R. P., and Morin, P. J. (2006). Crucial roles of Sp1 and epigenetic modifications in the regulation of the CLDN4 promoter in ovarian cancer cells. *J. Biol. Chem.* 281, 21433–21444. doi: 10.1074/jbc.M603767200

Hooda, J., Novak, M., Salomon, M. P., Matsuba, C., Ramos, R. I., MacDuffie, E., et al. (2019). Early loss of histone H2B monoubiquitylation alters chromatin accessibility and activates key immune pathways that facilitate progression of ovarian cancer. *Cancer Res.* 79, 760–772. doi: 10.1158/0008-5472.CAN-18-2297

Horak, P., Pils, D., Haller, G., Pribill, I., Roessler, M., Tomek, S., et al. (2005). Contribution of epigenetic silencing of tumor necrosis factor-related apoptosis inducing ligand receptor 1 (DR4) to TRAIL resistance and ovarian cancer. *Mol. Cancer Res.* 3, 335–343. doi: 10.1158/1541-7786.MCR-04-0136

Hough, C. D., Sherman-Baust, C. A., Pizer, E. S., Montz, F. J., Im, D. D., Rosenshein, N. B., et al. (2000). Large-scale serial analysis of gene expression reveals genes differentially expressed in ovarian cancer. *Cancer Res.* 60, 6281–6287.

Howe, H. L., Wu, X., Ries, L. A. G., Cokkinides, V., Ahmed, F., Jemal, A., et al. (2006). Annual report to the nation on the status of cancer, 1975–2003, featuring cancer among U.S. Hispanic/Latino populations. *Cancer* 107, 1711–1742. doi: 10.1002/cncr.22193

Hu, X., Macdonald, D. M., Huettner, P. C., Feng, Z., El Naqa, I. M., Schwarz, J. K., et al. (2009). A miR-200 microRNA cluster as prognostic marker in advanced ovarian cancer. *Gynecol. Oncol.* 114, 457–464. doi: 10.1016/j.ygyno.2009.05.022

Hu, Y., Zhang, Q., Cui, J., Liao, Z.-J., Jiao, M., Zhang, Y.-B., et al. (2019). Oncogene miR-934 promotes ovarian cancer cell proliferation and inhibits cell apoptosis through targeting BRMS1L. *Eur. Rev. Med. Pharmacol. Sci.* 23, 5595–5602. doi: 10.26355/eurrev_201907_18293

Huang, C.-Y., Cheng, W.-F., Lee, C.-N., Su, Y.-N., Chien, S.-C., Tzeng, Y.-L., et al. (2006). Serum mesothelin in epithelial ovarian carcinoma: a new screening marker and prognostic factor. *Anticancer Res.* 26, 4721–4728.

Huang, L., Zhou, Y., Cao, X.-P., Lin, J.-X., Zhang, L., Huang, S.-T., et al. (2017). KPNA2 is a potential diagnostic serum biomarker for epithelial ovarian cancer and correlates with poor prognosis. *Tumor Biol.* 39:101042831770628. doi: 10.1177/1010428317706289

Huang, R.-L., Chen, H.-J., Chen, L.-Y., Chao, T.-K., Lin, W.-Y., Liew, P.-L., et al. (2018). Epigenetic loss of heparan sulfate 3-O-sulfation sensitizes ovarian carcinoma to oncogenic signals and predicts prognosis: less 3-O-sulfated HS sensitizes prognostic signals. *Int. J. Cancer* 143, 1943–1953. doi: 10.1002/ijc.31580

Huang, R.-L., Gu, F., Kirma, N. B., Ruan, J., Chen, C.-L., Wang, H.-C., et al. (2013). Comprehensive methylome analysis of ovarian tumors reveals hedgehog signaling pathway regulators as prognostic DNA methylation biomarkers. *Epigenetics* 8, 624–634. doi: 10.4161/epi.24816

Huang, Y.-W., Jansen, R. A., Fabbri, E., Potter, D., Liyanarachchi, S., Chan, M. W. Y., et al. (2009). Identification of candidate epigenetic biomarkers for ovarian cancer detection. *Oncol. Rep.* 22, 853–861. doi: 10.3892/or_00000509

Ibanez de Caceres, I., Battagli, C., Esteller, M., Herman, J. G., Dulaimi, E., Edelson, M. I., et al. (2004). Tumor cell-specific BRCA1 and RASSF1A hypermethylation in serum, plasma, and peritoneal fluid from ovarian cancer patients. *Cancer Res.* 64, 6476–6481. doi: 10.1158/0008-5472.CAN-04-1529

Ignatov, T., Eggemann, H., Costa, S. D., Roessner, A., Kalinski, T., and Ignatov, A. (2014). BRCA1 promoter methylation is a marker of better response to platinum–taxane-based therapy in sporadic epithelial ovarian cancer. *J. Cancer Res. Clin. Oncol.* 140, 1457–1463. doi: 10.1007/s00432-014-1704-5

Iorio, M. V., Visone, R., Di Leva, G., Donati, V., Petrocca, F., Casalini, P., et al. (2007). MicroRNA signatures in human ovarian cancer. *Cancer Res.* 67, 8699–8707. doi: 10.1158/0008-5472.CAN-07-1936

Izutsu, N., Maesawa, C., Shibazaki, M., Oikawa, H., Shoji, T., Sugiyama, T., et al. (2008). Epigenetic modification is involved in aberrant expression of class III beta-tubulin, TUBB3, in ovarian cancer cells. *Int. J. Oncol.* 32, 1227–1235. doi: 10.3892/ijo_32_6_1227

Jacob, F., Hitchins, M. P., Fedier, A., Brennan, K., Nixdorf, S., Hacker, N. F., et al. (2014). Expression of GBGT1 is epigenetically regulated by DNA methylation in ovarian cancer cells. *BMC Mol. Biol.* 15:24. doi: 10.1186/1471-2199-15-24

Jacobs, I., and Bast, R. C. (1989). The CA 125 tumour-associated antigen: a review of the literature. *Hum. Reprod. Oxf. Engl.* 4, 1–12. doi: 10.1093/oxfordjournals.humrep.a136832

Jacobs, I., Gentry-Maharaj, A., Burnell, M., Manchanda, R., Singh, N., Sharma, A., et al. (2011). Sensitivity of transvaginal ultrasound screening for endometrial cancer in postmenopausal women: a case-control study within the UKCTOCS cohort. *Lancet Oncol.* 12, 38–48. doi: 10.1016/S1470-2045(10)70268-0

Jacobs, I., Oram, D., Fairbanks, J., Turner, J., Frost, C., and Grudzinskas, J. G. (1990). A risk of malignancy index incorporating CA 125, ultrasound and menopausal status for the accurate preoperative diagnosis of ovarian cancer. *Br. J. Obstet. Gynaecol.* 97, 922–929. doi: 10.1111/j.1471-0528.1990.tb02448.x

Jacobs, I. J., and Menon, U. (2004). Progress and challenges in screening for early detection of ovarian cancer. *Mol. Cell. Proteomics* 3, 355–366. doi: 10.1074/mcp.R400006-MCP200

Jayson, G. C., Kohn, E. C., Kitchener, H. C., and Ledermann, J. A. (2014). Ovarian cancer. *Lancet* 384, 1376–1388. doi: 10.1016/S0140-6736(13)62146-7

Jia, Y., Lin, R., Jin, H., Si, L., Jian, W., Yu, Q., et al. (2019). MicroRNA-34 suppresses proliferation of human ovarian cancer cells by triggering autophagy and apoptosis and inhibits cell invasion by targeting Notch 1. *Biochimie* 160, 193–199. doi: 10.1016/j.biochi.2019.03.011

Jones, A., Lechner, M., Fourkala, E.-O., Kristeleit, R., and Widschwendter, M. (2010). Emerging promise of epigenetics and DNA methylation for the diagnosis and management of women's cancers. *Epigenomics* 2, 9–38. doi: 10.2217/epi.09.47

Jones, P. A. (2001). The role of DNA methylation in mammalian epigenetics. *Science* 293, 1068–1070. doi: 10.1126/science.1063852

Jones, P. A., and Baylin, S. B. (2002). The fundamental role of epigenetic events in cancer. *Nat. Rev. Genet.* 3:415. doi: 10.1038/nrg816

Jones, P. A., and Baylin, S. B. (2007). The epigenomics of cancer. *Cell* 128, 683–692. doi: 10.1016/j.cell.2007.01.029

Jones, P. A., and Laird, P. W. (1999). Cancer-epigenetics comes of age. *Nat. Genet.* 21, 163–167. doi: 10.1038/5947

Kacem, S., and Feil, R. (2009). Chromatin mechanisms in genomic imprinting. *Mamm. Genome* 20, 544–556. doi: 10.1007/s00335-009-9223-4

Kamikihara, T., Arima, T., Kato, K., Matsuda, T., Kato, H., Douchi, T., et al. (2005). Epigenetic silencing of the imprinted geneZAC by DNA methylation is an early event in the progression of human ovarian cancer. *Int. J. Cancer* 115, 690–700. doi: 10.1002/ijc.20971

Kaneuchi, M., Sasaki, M., Tanaka, Y., Shiina, H., Verma, M., Ebina, Y., et al. (2004). Expression and methylation status of 14-3-3 sigma gene can characterize the different histological features of ovarian cancer. *Biochem. Biophys. Res. Commun.* 316, 1156–1162. doi: 10.1016/j.bbrc.2004.02.171

Kaneuchi, M., Sasaki, M., Tanaka, Y., Shiina, H., Yamada, H., Yamamoto, R., et al. (2005). WT1 and WT1-AS genes are inactivated by promoter methylation in ovarian clear cell adenocarcinoma. *Cancer* 104, 1924–1930. doi: 10.1002/cncr.21397

Kang, S., Dong, S. M., and Park, N.-H. (2010). Frequent promoter hypermethylation of TGFBI in epithelial ovarian cancer. *Gynecol. Oncol.* 118, 58–63. doi: 10.1016/j.ygyno.2010.03.025

Kardum, V., Karin, V., Glibo, M., Skrtic, A., Martic, T. N., Ibisevic, N., et al. (2017). Methylation-associated silencing of SFRP1 gene in high-grade serous ovarian carcinomas. *Ann. Diagn. Pathol.* 31, 45–49. doi: 10.1016/j.anndiagpath.2017.07.002

Katsaros, D., Cho, W., Singal, R., Fracchioli, S., Rigault De La Longrais, I. A., Arisio, R., et al. (2004). Methylation of tumor suppressor gene p16 and prognosis of epithelial ovarian cancer. *Gynecol. Oncol.* 94, 685–692. doi: 10.1016/j.ygyno.2004.06.018

Kaur, M., Singh, A., Singh, K., Gupta, S., and Sachan, M. (2016). Development of a multiplex MethyLight assay for the detection of DAPK1 and SOX1 methylation in epithelial ovarian cancer in a north Indian population. *Genes Genet. Syst.* 91, 175–181. doi: 10.1266/ggs.15-00051

Keita, M., Wang, Z.-Q., Pelletier, J.-F., Bachvarova, M., Plante, M., Gregoire, J., et al. (2013). Global methylation profiling in serous ovarian cancer is indicative for distinct aberrant DNA methylation signatures associated with tumor aggressiveness and disease progression. *Gynecol. Oncol.* 128, 356–363. doi: 10.1016/j.ygyno.2012.11.036

Kikuchi, R., Tsuda, H., Kanai, Y., Kasamatsu, T., Sengoku, K., Hirohashi, S., et al. (2007). Promoter hypermethylation contributes to frequent inactivation of a putative conditional tumor suppressor gene connective tissue growth factor in ovarian cancer. *Cancer Res.* 67, 7095–7105. doi: 10.1158/0008-5472.CAN-06-4567

Kikuchi, R., Tsuda, H., Kozaki, K., Kanai, Y., Kasamatsu, T., Sengoku, K., et al. (2008). Frequent inactivation of a putative tumor suppressor, angiopoietin-like protein 2, in ovarian cancer. *Cancer Res.* 68, 5067–5075. doi: 10.1158/0008-5472.CAN-08-0062

Kim, J.-H., Skates, S. J., Uede, T., Wong, K., Schorge, J. O., Feltmate, C. M., et al. (2002). Osteopontin as a potential diagnostic biomarker for ovarian cancer. *JAMA* 287, 1671–1679. doi: 10.1001/jama.287.13.1671

Kim, S., Choi, M. C., Jeong, J.-Y., Hwang, S., Jung, S. G., Joo, W. D., et al. (2019). Serum exosomal miRNA-145 and miRNA-200c as promising biomarkers for preoperative diagnosis of ovarian carcinomas. *J. Cancer* 10, 1958–1967. doi: 10.7150/jca.30231

Kim, Y.-W., Bae, S. M., Lim, H., Kim, Y. J., and Ahn, W. S. (2012). Development of multiplexed bead-based immunoassays for the detection of early stage ovarian cancer using a combination of serum biomarkers. *PLoS ONE* 7:e44960. doi: 10.1371/journal.pone.0044960

Kitade, S., Onoyama, I., Kobayashi, H., Yagi, H., Yoshida, S., Kato, M., et al. (2016). FBXW7 is involved in the acquisition of the malignant phenotype in epithelial ovarian tumors. *Cancer Sci.* 107, 1399–1405. doi: 10.1111/cas.13026

Klotz, D. M., and Wimberger, P. (2017). Cells of origin of ovarian cancer: ovarian surface epithelium or fallopian tube? *Arch. Gynecol. Obstet.* 296, 1055–1062. doi: 10.1007/s00404-017-4529-z

Kneip, C., Schmidt, B., Seegebarth, A., Weickmann, S., Fleischhacker, M., Liebenberg, V., et al. (2011). SHOX2 DNA methylation is a biomarker for the diagnosis of lung cancer in plasma. *J. Thorac. Oncol.* 6, 1632–1638. doi: 10.1097/JTO.0b013e318220ef9a

Kobayashi, M., Sawada, K., Nakamura, K., Yoshimura, A., Miyamoto, M., Shimizu, A., et al. (2018). Exosomal miR-1290 is a potential biomarker of high-grade serous ovarian carcinoma and can discriminate patients from those with malignancies of other histological types. *J. Ovarian Res.* 11:81. doi: 10.1186/s13048-018-0458-0

Koestler, D. C., Chalise, P., Cicek, M. S., Cunningham, J. M., Armasu, S., Larson, M. C., et al. (2014). Integrative genomic analysis identifies epigenetic marks that mediate genetic risk for epithelial ovarian cancer. *BMC Med. Genomics* 7:260. doi: 10.1158/1538-7445.AM2014-260

Kohler, R. S., Anugraham, M., López, M. N., Xiao, C., Schoetzau, A., Hettich, T., et al. (2016). Epigenetic activation of *MGAT3* and corresponding bisecting GlcNAc shortens the survival of cancer patients. *Oncotarget* 7:51674–51686. doi: 10.18632/oncotarget.10543

Kolomietz, E., Meyn, M. S., Pandita, A., and Squire, J. A. (2002). The role of Alu repeat clusters as mediators of recurrent chromosomal aberrations in tumors. *Genes. Chromosomes Cancer* 35, 97–112. doi: 10.1002/gcc.10111

Kurose, K., Zhou, X.-P., Araki, T., Cannistra, S. A., Maher, E. R., and Eng, C. (2001). Frequent loss of PTEN Expression Is Linked to Elevated Phosphorylated Akt levels, but not associated with p27 and Cyclin D1 expression, in primary epithelial ovarian carcinomas. *Am. J. Pathol.* 158, 2097–2106. doi: 10.1016/S0002-9440(10)64681-0

Kwon, M. J., Kim, S.-S., Choi, Y.-L., Jung, H. S., Balch, C., Kim, S.-H., et al. (2010). Derepression of CLDN3 and CLDN4 during ovarian tumorigenesis is associated with loss of repressive histone modifications. *Carcinogenesis* 31, 974–983. doi: 10.1093/carcin/bgp336

Kwong, J., Lee, J.-Y., Wong, K.-K., Zhou, X., Wong, D. T. W., Lo, K.-W., et al. (2006). Candidate tumor-suppressor gene DLEC1 is frequently downregulated by promoter hypermethylation and histone hypoacetylation in human epithelial ovarian cancer. *Neoplasia* 8, 268–278. doi: 10.1593/neo.05502

Laios, A., O'Toole, S., Flavin, R., Martin, C., Kelly, L., Ring, M., et al. (2008). Potential role of miR-9 and miR-223 in recurrent ovarian cancer. *Mol. Cancer* 7:35. doi: 10.1186/1476-4598-7-35

Langhe, R., Norris, L., Saadeh, F. A., Blackshields, G., Varley, R., Harrison, A., et al. (2015). A novel serum microRNA panel to discriminate benign from malignant ovarian disease. *Cancer Lett.* 356, 628–636. doi: 10.1016/j.canlet.2014.10.010

Lee, C.-H., Subramanian, S., Beck, A. H., Espinosa, I., Senz, J., Zhu, S. X., et al. (2009). MicroRNA profiling of BRCA1/2 mutation-carrying and non-mutation-carrying high-grade serous carcinomas of ovary. *PLoS ONE* 4:e7314. doi: 10.1371/journal.pone.0007314

Lee, P. S., Teaberry, V. S., Bland, A. E., Huang, Z., Whitaker, R. S., Baba, T., et al. (2010). Elevated MAL expression is accompanied by promoter hypomethylation and platinum resistance in epithelial ovarian cancer. *Int. J. Cancer* 126, 1378–1389. doi: 10.1002/ijc.24797

Leon, S. A., Shapiro, B., Sklaroff, D. M., and Yaros, M. J. (1977). Free DNA in the serum of cancer patients and the effect of therapy. *Cancer Res.* 37, 646–650.

Leskela, S., Leandro-Garcia, L. J., Mendiola, M., Barriuso, J., Inglada-Perez, L., Munoz, I., et al. (2010). The miR-200 family controls -tubulin III expression and is associated with paclitaxel-based treatment response and progression-free survival in ovarian cancer patients. *Endocr. Relat. Cancer* 18, 85–95. doi: 10.1677/ERC-10-0148

Leung, F., Bernardini, M. Q., Brown, M. D., Zheng, Y., Molina, R., Bast, R. C., et al. (2016). Validation of a novel biomarker panel for the detection of ovarian cancer. *Cancer Epidemiol. Biomarkers Prev.* 25, 1333–1340. doi: 10.1158/1055-9965.EPI-15-1299

Lewis, J. M., Heineck, D. P., and Heller, M. J. (2015). Detecting cancer biomarkers in blood: challenges for new molecular diagnostic and point-of-care tests using cell-free nucleic acids. *Expert Rev. Mol. Diagn.* 15, 1187–1200. doi: 10.1586/14737159.2015.1069709

Li, J., He, X., Dong, R., Wang, Y., Yu, J., and Qiu, H. (2015). Frequent loss of NISCH promotes tumor proliferation and invasion in ovarian cancer via inhibiting the FAK signal pathway. *Mol. Cancer Ther.* 14, 1202–1212. doi: 10.1158/1535-7163.MCT-14-0911

Li, J., Shao, W., and Feng, H. (2019). MiR-542-3p, a microRNA targeting CDK14, suppresses cell proliferation, invasiveness, and tumorigenesis of epithelial ovarian cancer. *Biomed. Pharmacother.* 110, 850–856. doi: 10.1016/j.biopha.2018.11.104

Li, L.-W., Xiao, H.-Q., Ma, R., Yang, M., Li, W., and Lou, G. (2017). miR-152 is involved in the proliferation and metastasis of ovarian cancer through repression of ERBB3. *Int. J. Mol. Med.* 41, 1529–1535. doi: 10.3892/ijmm.2017.3324

Li, X., Pan, Q., Wan, X., Mao, Y., Lu, W., Xie, X., et al. (2015). Methylation-associated Has-miR-9 deregulation in paclitaxel- resistant epithelial ovarian carcinoma. *BMC Cancer* 15:1. doi: 10.1186/s12885-015-1509-1

Liao, Y.-P., Chen, L.-Y., Huang, R.-L., Su, P.-H., Chan, M. W. Y., Chang, C.-C., et al. (2014). Hypomethylation signature of tumor-initiating cells predicts poor prognosis of ovarian cancer patients. *Hum. Mol. Genet.* 23, 1894–1906. doi: 10.1093/hmg/ddt583

Liggett, T. E., Melnikov, A., Yi, Q., Replogle, C., Hu, W., Rotmensch, J., et al. (2011). Distinctive DNA methylation patterns of cell-free plasma DNA in women with malignant ovarian tumors. *Gynecol. Oncol.* 120, 113–120. doi: 10.1016/j.ygyno.2010.09.019

Lin, B., White, J. T., Wu, J., Lele, S., Old, L. J., Hood, L., et al. (2009). Deep depletion of abundant serum proteins reveals low-abundant proteins as potential biomarkers for human ovarian cancer. *Proteomics Clin. Appl.* 3, 853–861. doi: 10.1002/prca.200800141

Lin, H.-W., Fu, C.-F., Chang, M.-C., Lu, T.-P., Lin, H.-P., Chiang, Y.-C., et al. (2018). *CDH1*, *DLEC1* and *SFRP5* methylation panel as a prognostic marker for advanced epithelial ovarian cancer. *Epigenomics* 10, 1397–1413. doi: 10.2217/epi-2018-0035

Litkouhi, B., Kwong, J., Lo, C.-M., Smedley, J. G., McClane, B. A., Aponte, M., et al. (2007). Claudin-4 overexpression in epithelial ovarian cancer is associated with hypomethylation and is a potential target for modulation of tight junction barrier function using a C-terminal fragment of *Clostridium perfringens* enterotoxin. *Neoplasia* 9, 304–314. doi: 10.1593/neo.07118

Liu, B., Zhang, J., and Yang, D. (2019). miR-96-5p promotes the proliferation and migration of ovarian cancer cells by suppressing Caveolae1. *J. Ovarian Res.* 12:57. doi: 10.1186/s13048-019-0533-1

Liu, D., Zhang, X.-X., Li, M.-C., Cao, C.-H., Wan, D.-Y., Xi, B.-X., et al. (2018). C/EBPβ enhances platinum resistance of ovarian cancer cells by reprogramming H3K79 methylation. *Nat. Commun.* 9:1739. doi: 10.1038/s41467-018-03590-5

Liu, G., Yang, D., Rupaimoole, R., Pecot, C. V., Sun, Y., Mangala, L. S., et al. (2015). Augmentation of response to chemotherapy by microRNA-506 through regulation of RAD51 in serous ovarian cancers. *J. Natl. Cancer Inst.* 107:djv108. doi: 10.1093/jnci/djv108

Liu, M. X., Siu, M. K. Y., Liu, S. S., Yam, J. W. P., Ngan, H. Y. S., and Chan, D. W. (2014). Epigenetic silencing of microRNA-199b-5p is associated with acquired chemoresistance via activation of JAG1-Notch1 signaling in ovarian cancer. *Oncotarget* 5, 944–958. doi: 10.18632/oncotarget.1458

Lofton-Day, C., Model, F., Devos, T., Tetzner, R., Distler, J., Schuster, M., et al. (2008). DNA methylation biomarkers for blood-based colorectal cancer screening. *Clin. Chem.* 54, 414–423. doi: 10.1373/clinchem.2007.095992

Loginov, V. I., Pronina, I. V., Burdennyy, A. M., Filippova, E. A., Kazubskaya, T. P., Kushlinsky, D. N., et al. (2018). Novel miRNA genes deregulated by aberrant methylation in ovarian carcinoma are involved in metastasis. *Gene* 662, 28–36. doi: 10.1016/j.gene.2018.04.005

Lopez-Serra, L., and Esteller, M. (2008). Proteins that bind methylated DNA and human cancer: reading the wrong words. *Br. J. Cancer* 98, 1881–1885. doi: 10.1038/sj.bjc.6604374

Lu, K. H., Patterson, A. P., Wang, L., Marquez, R. T., Atkinson, E. N., Baggerly, K. A., et al. (2004). Selection of potential markers for epithelial ovarian cancer with gene expression arrays and recursive descent partition analysis. *Clin. Cancer Res. Off. J. Am. Assoc. Cancer Res.* 10, 3291–3300. doi: 10.1158/1078-0432.CCR-03-0409

Lu, L., Katsaros, D., Rigault de la Longrais, I. A., Sochirca, O., and Yu, H. (2007). Hypermethylation of let-7a-3 in Epithelial Ovarian Cancer Is Associated with

Low Insulin-like Growth Factor-II Expression and Favorable Prognosis. *Cancer Res.* 67, 10117–10122. doi: 10.1158/0008-5472.CAN-07-2544

Lu, T.-Y., Kao, C.-F., Lin, C.-T., Huang, D.-Y., Chiu, C.-Y., Huang, Y.-S., et al. (2009). DNA methylation and histone modification regulate silencing of OPG during tumor progression. *J. Cell. Biochem.* 108, 315–325. doi: 10.1002/jcb.22256

Lund, R. J., Huhtinen, K., Salmi, J., Rantala, J., Nguyen, E. V., Moulder, R., et al. (2017). DNA methylation and transcriptome changes associated with cisplatin resistance in ovarian cancer. *Sci. Rep.* 7:1469. doi: 10.1038/s41598-017-01624-4

Luo, G., Chen, C., Wang, J., Yue, H., Tian, Y., Yang, P., et al. (2019). FOXD3 may be a new cellular target biomarker as a hypermethylation gene in human ovarian cancer. *Cancer Cell Int.* 19:44. doi: 10.1186/s12935-019-0755-8

Lv, Y., Niu, Z., Guo, X., Yuan, F., and Liu, Y. (2018). Serum S100 calcium binding protein A4 (S100A4, metatasin) as a diagnostic and prognostic biomarker in epithelial ovarian cancer. *Br. J. Biomed. Sci.* 75, 88–91. doi: 10.1080/09674845.2017.1394052

Lycke, M., Kristjansdottir, B., and Sundfeldt, K. (2018). A multicenter clinical trial validating the performance of HE4, CA125, risk of ovarian malignancy algorithm and risk of malignancy index. *Gynecol. Oncol.* 151, 159–165. doi: 10.1016/j.ygyno.2018.08.025

Lyu, N., Wang, Y., Wang, J., Zhang, Z., and Kong, W. (2018). Study on early diagnosis of epithelial ovarian cancer by analysis of plasma septin-9 and clusterin level. *J. Cancer Res. Ther.* 14:444. doi: 10.4103/0973-1482.181178

Mählck, C. G., and Grankvist, K. (1994). Plasma prealbumin in women with epithelial ovarian carcinoma. *Gynecol. Obstet. Invest.* 37, 135–140. doi: 10.1159/000292542

Mahmoud, E. H., Fawzy, A., and, A., Elshimy, R. A. (2018). Serum MicroRNA-21 negatively relates to expression of programmed cell death-4 in patients with epithelial ovarian cancer. *Asian Pac. J. Cancer Prev.* 19, 33–38.

Makarla, P. B., Saboorian, M. H., Ashfaq, R., Toyooka, K. O., Toyooka, S., Minna, J. D., et al. (2005). Promoter hypermethylation profile of ovarian epithelial neoplasms. *Clin. Cancer Res.* 11, 5365–5369. doi: 10.1158/1078-0432.CCR-04-2455

Maldonado, L., Brait, M., Izumchenko, E., Begum, S., Chatterjee, A., Sen, T., et al. (2018). Integrated transcriptomic and epigenomic analysis of ovarian cancer reveals epigenetically silenced GULP1. *Cancer Lett.* 433, 242–251. doi: 10.1016/j.canlet.2018.06.030

Mase, S., Shinjo, K., Totani, H., Katsushima, K., Arakawa, A., Takahashi, S., et al. (2019). *ZNF671* DNA methylation as a molecular predictor for the early recurrence of serous ovarian cancer. *Cancer Sci.* 110, 1105–1116. doi: 10.1111/cas.13936

McGrath, S. E., Annels, N., Madhuri, T. K., Tailor, A., Butler-Manuel, S. A., Morgan, R., et al. (2018). Engrailed-2 (EN2) – a novel biomarker in epithelial ovarian cancer. *BMC Cancer* 18:943. doi: 10.1186/s12885-018-4816-5

McIntosh, M. W., Drescher, C., Karlan, B., Scholler, N., Urban, N., Hellstrom, K. E., et al. (2004). Combining CA 125 and SMR serum markers for diagnosis and early detection of ovarian carcinoma. *Gynecol. Oncol.* 95, 9–15. doi: 10.1016/j.ygyno.2004.07.039

Melnikov, A., Scholtens, D., Godwin, A., and Levenson, V. (2009). Differential methylation profile of ovarian cancer in tissues and plasma. *J. Mol. Diagn.* 11, 60–65. doi: 10.2353/jmoldx.2009.080072

Menendez, L., Benigno, B. B., and McDonald, J. F. (2004). L1 and HERV-W retrotransposons are hypomethylated in human ovarian carcinomas. *Mol. Cancer* 3:12. doi: 10.1186/1476-4598-3-12

Meng, C.-F., Dai, D.-Q., and Guo, K.-J. (2008). [Effects of 5-Aza-2′-deoxycytidine and trichostatin A on DNA methylation and expression of hMLH1 in ovariancancer cell line COC1/DDP]. *Ai Zheng* 27, 1251–1255.

Meng, X., Joosse, S. A., Müller, V., Trillsch, F., Milde-Langosch, K., Mahner, S., et al. (2015). Diagnostic and prognostic potential of serum miR-7, miR-16, miR-25, miR-93, miR-182, miR-376a and miR-429 in ovarian cancer patients. *Br. J. Cancer* 113, 1358–1366. doi: 10.1038/bjc.2015.340

Meng, X., Müller, V., Milde-Langosch, K., Trillsch, F., Pantel, K., and Schwarzenbach, H. (2016a). "Circulating Cell-Free miR-373, miR-200a, miR-200b and miR-200c in Patients with Epithelial Ovarian Cancer," in *Circulating Nucleic Acids in Serum and Plasma – CNAPS IX*, eds P. B. Gahan, M. Fleischhacker, and B. Schmidt (Cham: Springer International Publishing), 3–8. doi: 10.1007/978-3-319-42044-8_1

Meng, X., Müller, V., Milde-Langosch, K., Trillsch, F., Pantel, K., and Schwarzenbach, H. (2016b). Diagnostic and prognostic relevance of circulating exosomal miR-373, miR-200a, miR-200b and miR-200c in patients with epithelial ovarian cancer. *Oncotarget* 7. doi: 10.18632/oncotarget.7850

Menon, U., Gentry-Maharaj, A., Hallett, R., Ryan, A., Burnell, M., Sharma, A., et al. (2009). Sensitivity and specificity of multimodal and ultrasound screening for ovarian cancer, and stage distribution of detected cancers: results of the prevalence screen of the UK Collaborative Trial of Ovarian Cancer Screening (UKCTOCS). *Lancet Oncol.* 10, 327–340. doi: 10.1016/S1470-2045(09)70026-9

Menon, U., and Jacobs, I. J. (2000). Recent developments in ovarian cancer screening. *Curr. Opin. Obstet. Gynecol.* 12, 39–42. doi: 10.1097/00001703-200002000-00007

Merritt, W. M., Lin, Y. G., Han, L. Y., Kamat, A. A., Spannuth, W. A., Schmandt, R., et al. (2008). Dicer, Drosha, and outcomes in patients with ovarian cancer. *N. Engl. J. Med.* 359, 2641–2650. doi: 10.1056/NEJMoa0803785

Milde-Langosch, K., Ocon, E., Becker, G., and Löning, T. (1998). p16/MTS1 inactivation in ovarian carcinomas: high frequency of reduced protein expression associated with hyper-methylation or mutation in endometrioid and mucinous tumors. *Int. J. Cancer* 79, 61–65.

Mirza, A., McGuirk, M., Hockenberry, T. N., Wu, Q., Ashar, H., Black, S., et al. (2002). Human survivin is negatively regulated by wild-type p53 and participates in p53-dependent apoptotic pathway. *Oncogene* 21, 2613–2622. doi: 10.1038/sj.onc.1205353

Mok, S. C., Chao, J., Skates, S., Wong, K., Yiu, G. K., Muto, M. G., et al. (2001). Prostasin, a potential serum marker for ovarian cancer: identification through microarray technology. *J. Natl. Cancer Inst.* 93, 1458–1464. doi: 10.1093/jnci/93.19.1458

Molina, R., Escudero, J. M., Aug,é, J. M., Filella, X., Foj, L., Torn,é, A., et al. (2011). HE4 a novel tumour marker for ovarian cancer: comparison with CA 125 and ROMA algorithm in patients with gynaecological diseases. *Tumour Biol. J. Int. Soc. Oncodevelopmental Biol. Med.* 32, 1087–1095. doi: 10.1007/s13277-011-0204-3

Moore, R. G., Brown, A. K., Miller, M. C., Skates, S., Allard, W. J., Verch, T., et al. (2008). The use of multiple novel tumor biomarkers for the detection of ovarian carcinoma in patients with a pelvic mass. *Gynecol. Oncol.* 108, 402–408. doi: 10.1016/j.ygyno.2007.10.017

Moore, R. G., MacLaughlan, S., and Bast, R. C. (2010). Current state of biomarker development for clinical application in epithelial ovarian cancer. *Gynecol. Oncol.* 116, 240–245. doi: 10.1016/j.ygyno.2009.09.041

Moore, R. G., McMeekin, D. S., Brown, A. K., DiSilvestro, P., Miller, M. C., Allard, W. J., et al. (2009). A novel multiple marker bioassay utilizing HE4 and CA125 for the prediction of ovarian cancer in patients with a pelvic mass. *Gynecol. Oncol.* 112, 40–46. doi: 10.1016/j.ygyno.2008.08.031

Moore, R. G., Miller, M. C., Disilvestro, P., Landrum, L. M., Gajewski, W., Ball, J. J., et al. (2011). Evaluation of the diagnostic accuracy of the risk of ovarian malignancy algorithm in women with a pelvic mass. *Obstet. Gynecol.* 118, 280–288. doi: 10.1097/AOG.0b013e318224fce2

Mor, G., Visintin, I., Lai, Y., Zhao, H., Schwartz, P., Rutherford, T., et al. (2005). Serum protein markers for early detection of ovarian cancer. *Proc. Natl. Acad. Sci. U.S.A.* 102, 7677–7682. doi: 10.1073/pnas.0502178102

Muller, H. M. (2004). Analysis of methylated genes in peritoneal fluids of ovarian cancer patients: a new prognostic tool. *Clin. Chem.* 50, 2171–2173. doi: 10.1373/clinchem.2004.034090

Munkarah, A., Chatterjee, M., and Tainsky, M. A. (2007). Update on ovarian cancer screening: *Curr. Opin. Obstet. Gynecol.* 19, 22–26. doi: 10.1097/GCO.0b013e328011ec99

Murphy, S. K., Huang, Z., Wen, Y., Spillman, M. A., Whitaker, R. S., Simel, L. R., et al. (2006). Frequent IGF2/H19 domain epigenetic alterations and elevated IGF2 expression in epithelial ovarian cancer. *Mol. Cancer Res.* 4, 283–292. doi: 10.1158/1541-7786.MCR-05-0138

Nguyen, L., Cardenas-Goicoechea, S. J., Gordon, P., Curtin, C., Momeni, M., Chuang, L., et al. (2013). Biomarkers for early detection of ovarian cancer. *Womens Health* 9, 171–187. doi: 10.2217/WHE.13.2

Nicholson, L. J., Smith, P. R., Hiller, L., Szlosarek, P. W., Kimberley, C., Sehouli, J., et al. (2009). Epigenetic silencing of argininosuccinate synthetase confers resistance to platinum-induced cell death but collateral sensitivity to arginine auxotrophy in ovarian cancer. *Int. J. Cancer* 125, 1454–1463. doi: 10.1002/ijc.24546

Nosov, V., Su, F., Amneus, M., Birrer, M., Robins, T., Kotlerman, J., et al. (2009). Validation of serum biomarkers for detection of early-stage ovarian cancer. *Am. J. Obstet. Gynecol.* 200, 639.e1–5. doi: 10.1016/j.ajog.2008.12.042

Ongenaert, M., Van Neste, L., De Meyer, T., Menschaert, G., Bekaert, S., and Van Criekinge, W. (2008). PubMeth: a cancer methylation database combining text-mining and expert annotation. *Nucl. Acids Res.* 36, D842–D846. doi: 10.1093/nar/gkm788

Pampalakis, G., Diamandis, E. P., Katsaros, D., and Sotiropoulou, G. (2010). Down-regulation of dicer expression in ovarian cancer tissues. *Clin. Biochem.* 43, 324–327. doi: 10.1016/j.clinbiochem.2009.09.014

Pattamadilok, J., Huapai, N., Rattanatanyong, P., Vasurattana, A., Triratanachat, S., Tresukosol, D., et al. (2008). LINE-1 hypomethylation level as a potential prognostic factor for epithelial ovarian cancer. *Int. J. Gynecol. Cancer* 18, 711–717. doi: 10.1111/j.1525-1438.2007.01117.x

Perlin, E., and Moquin, R. B. (1972). Serum DNA levels in patients with malignant disease. *Am. J. Clin. Pathol.* 58, 601–602. doi: 10.1093/ajcp/58.5.601

Petrocca, F., Iliopoulos, D., Qin, H. R., Nicoloso, M. S., Yendamuri, S., Wojcik, S. E., et al. (2006). Alterations of the tumor suppressor gene ARLTS1 in ovarian cancer. *Cancer Res.* 66, 10287–10291. doi: 10.1158/0008-5472.CAN-06-2289

Phelps, D. L., Borley, J. V., Flower, K. J., Dina, R., Darb-Esfahani, S., Braicu, I., et al. (2017). Methylation of MYLK3 gene promoter region: a biomarker to stratify surgical care in ovarian cancer in a multicentre study. *Br. J. Cancer* 116, 1287–1293. doi: 10.1038/bjc.2017.83

Pieretti, M., Cavalieri, C., Conway, P. S., Gallion, H. H., Powell, D. E., and Turker, M. S. (1995). Genetic alterations distinguish different types of ovarian tumors. *Int. J. Cancer* 64, 434–440. doi: 10.1002/ijc.2910640614

Polivka, J., Pesta, M., and Janku, F. (2015). Testing for oncogenic molecular aberrations in cell-free DNA-based liquid biopsies in the clinic: are we there yet? *Expert Rev. Mol. Diagn.* 15, 1631–1644. doi: 10.1586/14737159.2015.1110021

Portela, A., and Esteller, M. (2010). Epigenetic modifications and human disease. *Nat. Biotechnol.* 28, 1057–1068. doi: 10.1038/nbt.1685

Press, J. Z., De Luca, A., Boyd, N., Young, S., Troussard, A., Ridge, Y., et al. (2008). Ovarian carcinomas with genetic and epigenetic BRCA1 loss have distinct molecular abnormalities. *BMC Cancer* 8:17. doi: 10.1186/1471-2407-8-17

Pulliam, N., Fang, F., Ozes, A. R., Tang, J., Adewuyi, A., Keer, H., et al. (2018). An effective epigenetic-PARP inhibitor combination therapy for breast and ovarian cancers independent of BRCA mutations. *Clin. Cancer Res.* 24, 3163–3175. doi: 10.1158/1078-0432.CCR-18-0204

Qu, G., Dubeau, L., Narayan, A., Yu, M. C., and Ehrlich, M. (1999). Satellite DNA hypomethylation vs. overall genomic hypomethylation in ovarian epithelial tumors of different malignant potential. *Mutat. Res.* 423, 91–101. doi: 10.1016/S0027-5107(98)00229-2

Ramus, S. J., Harrington, P. A., Pye, C., DiCioccio, R. A., Cox, M. J., Garlinghouse-Jones, K., et al. (2007). Contribution of *BRCA1* and *BRCA2* mutations to inherited ovarian cancer. *Hum. Mutat.* 28, 1207–1215. doi: 10.1002/humu.20599

Rathi, A., Virmani, A. K., Schorge, J. O., Elias, K. J., Maruyama, R., Minna, J. D., et al. (2002). Methylation profiles of sporadic ovarian tumors and nonmalignant ovaries from high-risk women. *Clin. Cancer Res.* 8, 3324–3331.

Rattanapan, Y., Korkiatsakul, V., Kongruang, A., Chareonsirisuthigul, T., Rerkamnuaychoke, B., Wongkularb, A., et al. (2018). EGFL7 and RASSF1 promoter hypermethylation in epithelial ovarian cancer. *Cancer Genet.* 224–225, 37–40. doi: 10.1016/j.cancergen.2018.04.117

Reik, W., and Lewis, A. (2005). Co-evolution of X-chromosome inactivation and imprinting in mammals. *Nat. Rev. Genet.* 6, 403–410. doi: 10.1038/nrg1602

Resnick, K. E., Alder, H., Hagan, J. P., Richardson, D. L., Croce, C. M., and Cohn, D. E. (2009). The detection of differentially expressed microRNAs from the serum of ovarian cancer patients using a novel real-time PCR platform. *Gynecol. Oncol.* 112, 55–59. doi: 10.1016/j.ygyno.2008.08.036

Richon, V. M., Sandhoff, T. W., Rifkind, R. A., and Marks, P. A. (2000). Histone deacetylase inhibitor selectively induces p21WAF1 expression and gene-associated histone acetylation. *Proc. Natl. Acad. Sci. U.S.A.* 97, 10014–10019. doi: 10.1073/pnas.180316197

Rose, S. L., Fitzgerald, M. P., White, N. O., Hitchler, M. J., Futscher, B. W., De Geest, K., et al. (2006). Epigenetic regulation of maspin expression in human ovarian carcinoma cells. *Gynecol. Oncol.* 102, 319–324. doi: 10.1016/j.ygyno.2005.12.025

Rosen, D. G., Wang, L., Atkinson, J. N., Yu, Y., Lu, K. H., Diamandis, E. P., et al. (2005). Potential markers that complement expression of CA125 in epithelial ovarian cancer. *Gynecol. Oncol.* 99, 267–277. doi: 10.1016/j.ygyno.2005.06.040

Rosenthal, A. N., Menon, U., and Jacobs, I. J. (2006). Screening for ovarian cancer. *Clin. Obstet. Gynecol.* 49, 433–447. doi: 10.1097/00003081-200609000-00004

Salta, S., P., Nunes, S., Fontes-Sousa, M., Lopes, P., Freitas, M., et al. (2018). A DNA methylation-based test for breast cancer detection in circulating cell-free DNA. *J. Clin. Med.* 7:420. doi: 10.3390/jcm7110420

Sarojini, S., Tamir, A., Lim, H., Li, S., Zhang, S., Goy, A., et al. (2012). Early detection biomarkers for ovarian cancer. *J. Oncol.* 2012, 1–15. doi: 10.1155/2012/709049

Sawada, K., Mitra, A. K., Radjabi, A. R., Bhaskar, V., Kistner, E. O., Tretiakova, M., et al. (2008). Loss of E-cadherin promotes ovarian cancer metastasis via alpha 5-integrin, which is a therapeutic target. *Cancer Res.* 68, 2329–2339. doi: 10.1158/0008-5472.CAN-07-5167

Schmid, G., Notaro, S., Reimer, D., Abdel-Azim, S., Duggan-Peer, M., Holly, J., et al. (2016). Expression and promotor hypermethylation of miR-34a in the various histological subtypes of ovarian cancer. *BMC Cancer* 16:102. doi: 10.1186/s12885-016-2135-2

Schweigert, F. J., and Sehouli, J. (2005). Transthyretin, a biomarker for nutritional status and ovarian cancer. *Cancer Res.* 65:1114; author reply 1114.

Sellar, G. C., Watt, K. P., Rabiasz, G. J., Stronach, E. A., Li, L., Miller, E. P., et al. (2003). OPCML at 11q25 is epigenetically inactivated and has tumor-suppressor function in epithelial ovarian cancer. *Nat. Genet.* 34, 337–343. doi: 10.1038/ng1183

Shah, C. A., Lowe, K. A., Paley, P., Wallace, E., Anderson, G. L., McIntosh, M. W., et al. (2009). Influence of ovarian cancer risk status on the diagnostic performance of the serum biomarkers mesothelin, HE4, and CA125. *Cancer Epidemiol. Biomarkers Prev.* 18, 1365–1372. doi: 10.1158/1055-9965.EPI-08-1034

Sharma, A., Albahrani, M., Zhang, W., Kufel, C. N., James, S. R., Odunsi, K., et al. (2019). Epigenetic activation of POTE genes in ovarian cancer. *Epigenetics* 14, 185–197. doi: 10.1080/15592294.2019.1581590

Sharma, S., Kelly, T. K., and Jones, P. A. (2010). Epigenetics in cancer. *Carcinogenesis* 31, 27–36. doi: 10.1093/carcin/bgp220

Shen, D.-H., Chan, K. Y.-K., Khoo, U.-S., Ngan, H. Y.-S., Xue, W.-C., Chiu, P.-M., et al. (2005). Epigenetic and genetic alterations of p33ING1b in ovarian cancer. *Carcinogenesis* 26, 855–863. doi: 10.1093/carcin/bgi011

Shibata, D., Mori, Y., Cai, K., Zhang, L., Yin, J., Elahi, A., et al. (2006). RAB32 hypermethylation and microsatellite instability in gastric and endometrial adenocarcinomas. *Int. J. Cancer* 119, 801–806. doi: 10.1002/ijc.21912

Shih, I.-M., and Kurman, R. J. (2004). Ovarian tumorigenesis: a proposed model based on morphological and molecular genetic analysis. *Am. J. Pathol.* 164, 1511–1518. doi: 10.1016/S0002-9440(10)63708-X

Shivapurkar, N., Toyooka, S., Toyooka, K. O., Reddy, J., Miyajima, K., Suzuki, M., et al. (2004). Aberrant methylation of trail decoy receptor genes is frequent in multiple tumor types. *Int. J. Cancer* 109, 786–792. doi: 10.1002/ijc.20041

Si, L., Jia, Y., Lin, R., Jian, W., Yu, Q., and Yang, S. (2019). 10.1016/j.biochi.2019.03.011. *Arch. Biochem. Biophys.* 668, 9–15. doi: 10.1016/j.abb.2019.04.009

Siegel, R., Ward, E., Brawley, O., and Jemal, A. (2011). Cancer statistics, 2011: The impact of eliminating socioeconomic and racial disparities on premature cancer deaths. *CA Cancer J. Clin.* 61, 212–236. doi: 10.3322/caac.20121

Siegel, R. L., Miller, K. D., and Jemal, A. (2015). Cancer Statistics, 2015. *CA Cancer J. Clin.* 65, 5–29. doi: 10.3322/caac.21254

Simmons, A. R., Clarke, C. H., Badgwell, D. B., Lu, Z., Sokoll, L. J., Lu, K. H., et al. (2016). Validation of a biomarker panel and longitudinal biomarker performance for early detection of ovarian cancer. *Int. J. Gynecol. Cancer* 26, 1070–1077. doi: 10.1097/IGC.0000000000000737

Simon, I., Katsaros, D., Rigault de la Longrais, I., Massobrio, M., Scorilas, A., Kim, N. W., et al. (2007). B7-H4 is over-expressed in early-stage ovarian cancer and is independent of CA125 expression. *Gynecol. Oncol.* 106, 334–341. doi: 10.1016/j.ygyno.2007.03.035

Simon, I., Zhuo, S., Corral, L., Diamandis, E. P., Sarno, M. J., Wolfert, R. L., et al. (2006). B7-h4 is a novel membrane-bound protein and a candidate serum and tissue biomarker for ovarian cancer. *Cancer Res.* 66, 1570–1575. doi: 10.1158/0008-5472.CAN-04-3550

Socha, M. J., Said, N., Dai, Y., Kwong, J., Ramalingam, P., Trieu, V., et al. (2009). Aberrant Promoter Methylation of Sparc in Ovarian Cancer. *Neoplasia* 11, 126–135. doi: 10.1593/neo.81146

Sorrentino, A., Liu, C.-G., Addario, A., Peschle, C., Scambia, G., and Ferlini, C. (2008). Role of microRNAs in drug-resistant ovarian cancer cells. *Gynecol. Oncol.* 111, 478–486. doi: 10.1016/j.ygyno.2008.08.017

Staub, J., Chien, J., Pan, Y., Qian, X., Narita, K., Aletti, G., et al. (2007). Epigenetic silencing of HSulf-1 in ovarian cancer:implications in chemoresistance. *Oncogene* 26, 4969–4978. doi: 10.1038/sj.onc.1210300

Strait, K. A., Dabbas, B., Hammond, E. H., Warnick, C. T., Iistrup, S. J., and Ford, C. D. (2002). Cell cycle blockade and differentiation of ovarian cancer cells by the histone deacetylase inhibitor trichostatin A are associated with changes in p21, Rb, and Id proteins. *Mol. Cancer Ther.* 1, 1181–1190.

Strathdee, G., Appleton, K., Illand, M., Millan, D. W., Sargent, J., Paul, J., et al. (2001). Primary ovarian carcinomas display multiple methylator phenotypes involving known tumor suppressor genes. *Am. J. Pathol.* 158, 1121–1127. doi: 10.1016/S0002-9440(10)64059-X

Strathdee, G., Davies, B. R., Vass, J. K., Siddiqui, N., and Brown, R. (2004). Cell type-specific methylation of an intronic CpG island controls expression of the MCJ gene. *Carcinogenesis* 25, 693–701. doi: 10.1093/carcin/bgh066

Strathdee, G., Vass, J. K., Oien, K. A., Siddiqui, N., Curto-Garcia, J., and Brown, R. (2005). Demethylation of the MCJ gene in stage III/IV epithelial ovarian cancer and response to chemotherapy. *Gynecol. Oncol.* 97, 898–903. doi: 10.1016/j.ygyno.2005.03.023

Su, F., Lang, J., Kumar, A., Ng, C., Hsieh, B., Suchard, M. A., et al. (2007). Validation of candidate serum ovarian cancer biomarkers for early detection. *Biomark. Insights* 2, 369–375. doi: 10.1177/117727190700200011

Su, H.-Y., Lai, H.-C., Lin, Y.-W., Chou, Y.-C., Liu, C.-Y., and Yu, M.-H. (2009). An epigenetic marker panel for screening and prognostic prediction of ovarian cancer. *Int. J. Cancer* 124, 387–393. doi: 10.1002/ijc.23957

Su, H.-Y., Lai, H.-C., Lin, Y.-W., Liu, C.-Y., Chen, C.-K., Chou, Y.-C., et al. (2010). Epigenetic silencing of SFRP5 is related to malignant phenotype and chemoresistance of ovarian cancer through Wnt signaling pathway. *Int. J. Cancer* 127, 555–567. doi: 10.1002/ijc.25083

Suehiro, Y., Okada, T., Okada, T., Anno, K., Okayama, N., Ueno, K., et al. (2008). Aneuploidy predicts outcome in patients with endometrial carcinoma and is related to lack of CDH13 hypermethylation. *Clin. Cancer Res.* 14, 3354–3361. doi: 10.1158/1078-0432.CCR-07-4609

Sun, N., Kohli, A., Huang, S., Chang, T., and Chao, C. C. -K. (2019). Androgen receptor transcriptional activity and chromatin modifications on the *ABCB1/MDR* gene are critical for taxol resistance in ovarian cancer cells. *J. Cell. Physiol.* 234, 8760–8775. doi: 10.1002/jcp.27535

Sung, C. K., Li, D., Andrews, E., Drapkin, R., and Benjamin, T. (2013). Promoter methylation of the SALL2 tumor suppressor gene in ovarian cancers. *Mol. Oncol.* 7, 419–427. doi: 10.1016/j.molonc.2012.11.005

Sung, H. Y., Choi, E. N., Lyu, D., Park, A. K., Ju, W., and Ahn, J.-H. (2014a). Aberrant hypomethylation-mediated AGR2 overexpression induces an aggressive phenotype in ovarian cancer cells. *Oncol. Rep.* 32, 815–820. doi: 10.3892/or.2014.3243

Sung, H. Y., Ju, W., and Ahn, J.-H. (2014b). DNA hypomethylation-mediated overexpression of carbonic anhydrase 9 induces an aggressive phenotype in ovarian cancer cells. *Yonsei Med. J.* 55:1656. doi: 10.3349/ymj.2014.55.6.1656

Sung, H. Y., Park, A. K., Ju, W., and Ahn, J.-H. (2014c). overexpression of mucin 13 due to promoter methylation promotes aggressive behavior in ovarian cancer cells. *Yonsei Med. J.* 55:1206. doi: 10.3349/ymj.2014.55.5.1206

Sung, H. Y., Yang, S.-D., Ju, W., and Ahn, J.-H. (2017a). Aberrant epigenetic regulation of GABRP associates with aggressive phenotype of ovarian cancer. *Exp. Mol. Med.* 49:e335. doi: 10.1038/emm.2017.62

Sung, H. Y., Yang, S.-D., Park, A. K., Ju, W., and Ahn, J.-H. (2017b). Aberrant hypomethylation of *solute carrier family 6 member 12* promoter induces metastasis of ovarian cancer. *Yonsei Med. J.* 58:27. doi: 10.3349/ymj.2017.58.1.27

Suzuki, F., Akahira, J.-I., Miura, I., Suzuki, T., Ito, K., Hayashi, S.-I., et al. (2008). Loss of estrogen receptor beta isoform expression and its correlation with aberrant DNA methylation of the 5'-untranslated region in human epithelial ovarian carcinoma. *Cancer Sci.* 99, 2365–2372. doi: 10.1111/j.1349-7006.2008.00988.x

Symer, D. E., Connelly, C., Szak, S. T., Caputo, E. M., Cost, G. J., Parmigiani, G., et al. (2002). Human l1 retrotransposition is associated with genetic instability *in vivo*. *Cell* 110, 327–338. doi: 10.1016/S0092-8674(02)00839-5

Tam, K. F., Liu, V. W. S., Liu, S. S., Tsang, P. C. K., Cheung, A. N. Y., Yip, A. M. W., et al. (2007). Methylation profile in benign, borderline and malignant ovarian tumors. *J. Cancer Res. Clin. Oncol.* 133, 331–341. doi: 10.1007/s00432-006-0178-5

Tang, G., Guo, J., Zhu, Y., Huang, Z., Liu, T., Cai, J., et al. (2018). Metformin inhibits ovarian cancer via decreasing H3K27 trimethylation. *Int. J. Oncol.* 52, 1899–1911. doi: 10.3892/ijo.2018.4343

Tang, Z., Qian, M., and Ho, M. (2013). The role of mesothelin in tumor progression and targeted therapy. *Anticancer Agents Med. Chem.* 13, 276–280. doi: 10.2174/1871520611313020014

Taniguchi, T., Tischkowitz, M., Ameziane, N., Hodgson, S. V., Mathew, C. G., Joenje, H., et al. (2003). Disruption of the Fanconi anemia-BRCA pathway in cisplatin-sensitive ovarian tumors. *Nat. Med.* 9, 568–574. doi: 10.1038/nm852

Tasaka, R., Fukuda, T., Shimomura, M., Inoue, Y., Wada, T., Kawanishi, M., et al. (2017). TBX2 expression is associated with platinum-sensitivity of ovarian serous carcinoma. *Oncol. Lett.* 15, 3085–3090. doi: 10.3892/ol.2017.7719

Taylor, D. D., and Gercel-Taylor, C. (2008). MicroRNA signatures of tumor-derived exosomes as diagnostic biomarkers of ovarian cancer. *Gynecol. Oncol.* 110, 13–21. doi: 10.1016/j.ygyno.2008.04.033

Teodoridis, J. M., Hall, J., Marsh, S., Kannall, H. D., Smyth, C., Curto, J., et al. (2005). CpG island methylation of DNA damage response genes in advanced ovarian cancer. *Cancer Res.* 65, 8961–8967. doi: 10.1158/0008-5472.CAN-05-1187

Terasawa, K., Sagae, S., Toyota, M., Tsukada, K., Ogi, K., Satoh, A., et al. (2004). Epigenetic inactivation of TMS1/ASC in ovarian cancer. *Clin. Cancer Res. Off. J. Am. Assoc. Cancer Res.* 10, 2000–2006. doi: 10.1158/1078-0432.CCR-0932-03

Teschendorff, A. E., Gao, Y., Jones, A., Ruebner, M., Beckmann, M. W., Wachter, D. L., et al. (2016). DNA methylation outliers in normal breast tissue identify field defects that are enriched in cancer. *Nat. Commun.* 7:10478. doi: 10.1038/ncomms10478

Teschendorff, A. E., Jones, A., Fiegl, H., Sargent, A., Zhuang, J. J., Kitchener, H. C., et al. (2012). Epigenetic variability in cells of normal cytology is associated with the risk of future morphological transformation. *Genome Med.* 4:24. doi: 10.1186/gm323

Teschendorff, A. E., Lee, S.-H., Jones, A., Fiegl, H., Kalwa, M., Wagner, W., et al. (2015). HOTAIR and its surrogate DNA methylation signature indicate carboplatin resistance in ovarian cancer. *Genome Med.* 7:108. doi: 10.1186/s13073-015-0233-4

Teschendorff, A. E., and Widschwendter, M. (2012). Differential variability improves the identification of cancer risk markers in DNA methylation studies profiling precursor cancer lesions. *Bioinformatics* 28, 1487–1494. doi: 10.1093/bioinformatics/bts170

Thomson, J. P., Skene, P. J., Selfridge, J., Clouaire, T., Guy, J., Webb, S., et al. (2010). CpG islands influence chromatin structure via the CpG-binding protein Cfp1. *Nature* 464, 1082–1086. doi: 10.1038/nature08924

Tomar, T., Alkema, N. G., Schreuder, L., Meersma, G. J., de Meyer, T., van Criekinge, W., et al. (2017). Methylome analysis of extreme chemoresponsive patients identifies novel markers of platinum sensitivity in high-grade serous ovarian cancer. *BMC Med.* 15:116. doi: 10.1186/s12916-017-0870-0

Tomar, T., de Jong, S., Alkema, N. G., Hoekman, R. L., Meersma, G. J., Klip, H. G., et al. (2016). Genome-wide methylation profiling of ovarian cancer patient-derived xenografts treated with the demethylating agent decitabine identifies novel epigenetically regulated genes and pathways. *Genome Med.* 8:107. doi: 10.1186/s13073-016-0361-5

Torng, P.-L., Lin, C.-W., Chan, M. W., Yang, H.-W., Huang, S.-C., and Lin, C.-T. (2009). Promoter methylation of IGFBP-3 and p53 expression in ovarian endometrioid carcinoma. *Mol. Cancer* 8:120. doi: 10.1186/1476-4598-8-120

Toss, A., Tomasello, C., Razzaboni, E., Contu, G., Grandi, G., Cagnacci, A., et al. (2015). Hereditary ovarian cancer: not only *BRCA* 1 and 2 genes. *BioMed Res. Int.* 2015, 1–11. doi: 10.1155/2015/341723

U. S. Preventive Services Task Force (2010). *The Guide to Clinical Preventive Services 2010 - 2011: Recommendations of the U.S. Preventive Services Task Force.* Rockville, MD: Agency for Healthcare Research and Quality (US) Available online at: http://www.ncbi.nlm.nih.gov/books/NBK56707/ (accessed December 19, 2017).

Valls, E., Sánchez-Molina, S., and Martínez-Balbás, M. A. (2005). Role of histone modifications in marking and activating genes through mitosis. *J. Biol. Chem.* 280, 42592–42600. doi: 10.1074/jbc.M507407200

Vang, R., Shih, I.-M., and Kurman, R. J. (2009). Ovarian low-grade and high-grade serous carcinoma: pathogenesis, clinicopathologic and molecular biologic features, and diagnostic problems. *Adv. Anat. Pathol.* 16, 267–282. doi: 10.1097/PAP.0b013e3181b4fffa

Visintin, I., Feng, Z., Longton, G., Ward, D. C., Alvero, A. B., Lai, Y., et al. (2008). Diagnostic markers for early detection of ovarian cancer. *Clin. Cancer Res.* 14, 1065–1072. doi: 10.1158/1078-0432.CCR-07-1569

Vlassov, V. V., Laktionov, P. P., and Rykova, E. Y. (2010). Circulating nucleic acids as a potential source for cancer biomarkers. *Curr. Mol. Med.* 10, 142–165. doi: 10.2174/156652410790963295

Wang, B., Yu, L., Luo, X., Huang, L., Li, Q., Shao, X., et al. (2017). Detection of OPCML methylation, a possible epigenetic marker, from free serum circulating DNA to improve the diagnosis of early-stage ovarian epithelial cancer. *Oncol. Lett.* 14, 217–223. doi: 10.3892/ol.2017.6111

Wang, G., Li, X., Tian, W., Wang, Y., Wu, D., Sun, Z., et al. (2015). Promoter DNA methylation is associated with *KLF11* expression in epithelial ovarian cancer: promoter Dna Methylation Is Associated With *KLF11* Expression. *Genes. Chromosomes Cancer* 54, 453–462. doi: 10.1002/gcc.22257

Wang, H.-Q., Yang, C.-Y., Wang, S.-Y., Wang, T., Han, J.-L., Wei, K., et al. (2018). Cell-free plasma hypermethylated CASZ1, CDH13 and ING2 are promising biomarkers of esophageal cancer. *J. Biomed. Res.* 32, 424–433. doi: 10.7555/JBR.32.20170065

Wang, L., Zhu, M.-J., Ren, A.-M., Wu, H.-F., Han, W.-M., Tan, R.-Y., et al. (2014). A Ten-MicroRNA signature identified from a genome-wide MicroRNA expression profiling in human epithelial ovarian cancer. *PLoS ONE* 9:e96472. doi: 10.1371/journal.pone.0096472

Wang, Z., Ji, G., Wu, Q., Feng, S., Zhao, Y., Cao, Z., et al. (2018). Integrated microarray meta-analysis identifies miRNA-27a as an oncogene in ovarian cancer by inhibiting FOXO1. *Life Sci.* 210, 263–270. doi: 10.1016/j.lfs.2018.08.043

Warren, J. D., Xiong, W., Bunker, A. M., Vaughn, C. P., Furtado, L. V., Roberts, W. L., et al. (2011). Septin 9 methylated DNA is a sensitive and specific blood test for colorectal cancer. *BMC Med.* 9:133. doi: 10.1186/1741-7015-9-133

Wasenang, W., Chaiyarit, P., Proungvitaya, S., and Limpaiboon, T. (2019). Serum cell-free DNA methylation of OPCML and HOXD9 as a biomarker that may aid in differential diagnosis between cholangiocarcinoma and other biliary diseases. *Clin. Epigenetics* 11:39. doi: 10.1186/s13148-019-0634-0

Wei, K.-L., Chou, J.-L., Chen, Y.-C., Jin, H., Chuang, Y.-M., Wu, C.-S., et al. (2019). Methylomics analysis identifies a putative STAT3 target, SPG20, as a noninvasive epigenetic biomarker for early detection of gastric cancer. *PLoS ONE* 14:e0218338. doi: 10.1371/journal.pone.0218338

Wei, S. H. (2006). Prognostic DNA methylation biomarkers in ovarian cancer. *Clin. Cancer Res.* 12, 2788–2794. doi: 10.1158/1078-0432.CCR-05-1551

Wei, S. H., Chen, C.-M., Strathdee, G., Harnsomburana, J., Shyu, C.-R., Rahmatpanah, F., et al. (2002). Methylation microarray analysis of late-stage ovarian carcinomas distinguishes progression-free survival in patients and identifies candidate epigenetic markers. *Clin. Cancer Res.* 8, 2246–2252.

Weichert, W., Denkert, C., Noske, A., Darb-Esfahani, S., Dietel, M., Kalloger, S. E., et al. (2008). Expression of class I histone deacetylases indicates poor prognosis in endometrioid subtypes of ovarian and endometrial carcinomas. *Neoplasia* 10, 1021–1027. doi: 10.1593/neo.08474

Weisenberger, D. J., Trinh, B. N., Campan, M., Sharma, S., Long, T. I., Ananthnarayan, S., et al. (2008). DNA methylation analysis by digital bisulfite genomic sequencing and digital MethyLight. *Nucleic Acids Res.* 36, 4689–4698. doi: 10.1093/nar/gkn455

Widschwendter, A., Müller, H. M., Hubalek, M. M., Wiedemair, A., Fiegl, H., Goebel, G., et al. (2004). Methylation status and expression of human telomerase reverse transcriptase in ovarian and cervical cancer. *Gynecol. Oncol.* 93, 407–416. doi: 10.1016/j.ygyno.2004.01.036

Widschwendter, M., Apostolidou, S., Jones, A. A., Fourkala, E. O., Arora, R., Pearce, C. L., et al. (2009). HOXA methylation in normal endometrium from premenopausal women is associated with the presence of ovarian cancer: a proof of principle study. *Int. J. Cancer* 125, 2214–2218. doi: 10.1002/ijc.24599

Widschwendter, M., Jiang, G., Woods, C., Müller, H. M., Fiegl, H., Goebel, G., et al. (2004). DNA hypomethylation and ovarian cancer biology. *Cancer Res.* 64, 4472–4480. doi: 10.1158/0008-5472.CAN-04-0238

Widschwendter, M., Zikan, M., Wahl, B., Lempiäinen, H., Paprotka, T., Evans, I., et al. (2017). The potential of circulating tumor DNA methylation analysis for the early detection and management of ovarian cancer. *Genome Med.* 9:116. doi: 10.1186/s13073-017-0500-7

Wilcox, C. B., Baysal, B. E., Gallion, H. H., Strange, M. A., and DeLoia, J. A. (2005). High-resolution methylation analysis of the BRCA1 promoter in ovarian tumors. *Cancer Genet. Cytogenet.* 159, 114–122. doi: 10.1016/j.cancergencyto.2004.12.017

Wilczynski, M., Zytko, E., Danielska, J., Szymanska, B., and Dzieniecka, M., Nowak, M., et al. (2018). Clinical significance of miRNA-21,−103,−129,−150 in serous ovarian cancer. *Arch. Gynecol. Obstet.* 297, 741–748. doi: 10.1007/s00404-018-4660-5

Wiley, A., Katsaros, D., Chen, H., Rigault de la Longrais, I. A., Beeghly, A., Puopolo, M., et al. (2006a). Aberrant promoter methylation of multiple genes in malignant ovarian tumors and in ovarian tumors with low malignant potential. *Cancer* 107, 299–308. doi: 10.1002/cncr.21992

Wiley, A., Katsaros, D., Fracchioli, S., and Yu, H. (2006b). Methylation of the insulin-like growth factor binding protein-3 gene and prognosis of epithelial ovarian cancer. *Int. J. Gynecol. Cancer* 16, 210–218. doi: 10.1111/j.1525-1438.2006.00299.x

Wilting, R. H., and Dannenberg, J.-H. (2012). Epigenetic mechanisms in tumorigenesis, tumor cell heterogeneity and drug resistance. *Drug Resist. Updat.* 15, 21–38. doi: 10.1016/j.drup.2012.01.008

Wittenberger, T., Sleigh, S., Reisel, D., Zikan, M., Wahl, B., Alunni-Fabbroni, M., et al. (2014). DNA methylation markers for early detection of women's cancer: promise and challenges. *Epigenomics* 6, 311–327. doi: 10.2217/epi.14.20

Woloszynska-Read, A., James, S. R., Link, P. A., Yu, J., Odunsi, K., and Karpf, A. R. (2007). DNA methylation-dependent regulation of BORIS/CTCFL expression in ovarian cancer. *Cancer Immun.* 7, 21.

Woolas, R. P., Xu, F. J., Jacobs, I. J., Yu, Y. H., Daly, L., Berchuck, A., et al. (1993). Elevation of multiple serum markers in patients with stage I ovarian cancer. *J. Natl. Cancer Inst.* 85, 1748–1751. doi: 10.1093/jnci/85.21.1748

Wu, Q., Lothe, R. A., Ahlquist, T., Silins, I., Tropé, C. G., Micci, F., et al. (2007). DNA methylation profiling of ovarian carcinomas and their *in vitro* models identifies HOXA9, HOXB5, SCGB3A1, and CRABP1 as novel targets. *Mol. Cancer* 6:45. doi: 10.1186/1476-4598-6-45

Wurz, K., Garcia, R. L., Goff, B. A., Mitchell, P. S., Lee, J. H., Tewari, M., et al. (2010). MiR-221 and MiR-222 alterations in sporadic ovarian carcinoma: relationship to CDKN1B, CDKNIC and overall survival. *Genes. Chromosomes Cancer.* 49, 577–584. doi: 10.1002/gcc.20768

Wyman, S. K., Parkin, R. K., Mitchell, P. S., Fritz, B. R., O'Briant, K., Godwin, A. K., et al. (2009). Repertoire of microRNAs in epithelial ovarian cancer as determined by next generation sequencing of small RNA cDNA Libraries. *PLoS ONE* 4:e5311. doi: 10.1371/journal.pone.0005311

Xi, Q.-P., Pu, D.-H., and Lu, W.-N. (2017). Research on application value of combined detection of serum CA125, HE4 and TK1 in the diagnosis of ovarian cancer. *Eur. Rev. Med. Pharmacol. Sci.* 21, 4536–4541.

Xu, W., Lu, J., Zhao, Q., Wu, J., Sun, J., Han, B., et al. (2019). Genome-wide plasma cell-free DNA methylation profiling identifies potential biomarkers for lung cancer. *Dis. Markers* 2019, 1–7. doi: 10.1155/2019/4108474

Xu, Y.-Z., Xi, Q.-H., Ge, W.-L., and Zhang, X.-Q. (2013). Identification of serum MicroRNA-21 as a biomarker for early detection and prognosis in human epithelial ovarian cancer. *Asian Pac. J. Cancer Prev.* 14, 1057–1060. doi: 10.7314/APJCP.2013.14.2.1057

Yang, H., Kong, W., He, L., Zhao, J.-J., O'Donnell, J. D., Wang, J., et al. (2008). MicroRNA expression profiling in human ovarian cancer: miR-214 induces cell survival and cisplatin resistance by targeting PTEN. *Cancer Res.* 68, 425–433. doi: 10.1158/0008-5472.CAN-07-2488

Yang, N., Kaur, S., Volinia, S., Greshock, J., Lassus, H., Hasegawa, K., et al. (2008). MicroRNA microarray identifies Let-7i as a novel biomarker and therapeutic target in human epithelial ovarian cancer. *Cancer Res.* 68, 10307–10314. doi: 10.1158/0008-5472.CAN-08-1954

Yang, Y., Chaerkady, R., Beer, M. A., Mendell, J. T., and Pandey, A. (2009). Identification of miR-21 targets in breast cancer cells using a quantitative proteomic approach. *Proteomics* 9, 1374–1384. doi: 10.1002/pmic.200800551

Yang, Z., Qi, W., Sun, L., Zhou, H., Zhou, B., and Hu, Y. (2018). 10.1186/s13148-019-0634-0. *Adv. Clin. Exp. Med.* 28, 361–366. doi: 10.17219/acem/84935

Yap, O. W. S., Bhat, G., Liu, L., and Tollefsbol, T. O. (2009). Epigenetic modifications of the Estrogen receptor beta gene in epithelial ovarian cancer cells. *Anticancer Res.* 29, 139–144.

Yarbro, J. W., Page, D. L., Fielding, L. P., Partridge, E. E., and Murphy, G. P. (1999). American Joint Committee on Cancer prognostic factors consensus conference. *Cancer* 86, 2436–2446.

Yazbek, J., Raju, S. K., Ben-Nagi, J., Holland, T. K., Hillaby, K., and Jurkovic, D. (2008). Effect of quality of gynaecological ultrasonography on management of patients with suspected ovarian cancer: a randomised controlled trial. *Lancet Oncol.* 9, 124–131. doi: 10.1016/S1470-2045(08)70005-6

Yeh, C.-M., Shay, J., Zeng, T.-C., Chou, J.-L., Huang, T. H.-M., Lai, H.-C., et al. (2014). Epigenetic silencing of ARNTL, a circadian gene and potential tumor suppressor in ovarian cancer. *Int. J. Oncol.* 45, 2101–2107. doi: 10.3892/ijo.2014.2627

Yeh, K.-T., Chen, T.-H., Yang, H.-W., Chou, J.-L., Chen, L.-Y., Yeh, C.-M., et al. (2011). Aberrant TGFβ/SMAD4 signaling contributes to epigenetic silencing of a putative tumor suppressor, RunX1T1 in ovarian cancer. *Epigenetics* 6, 727–739. doi: 10.4161/epi.6.6.15856

Yi, X., Guo, J., Guo, J., Sun, S., Yang, P., Wang, J., et al. (2017). EZH2-mediated epigenetic silencing of TIMP2 promotes ovarian cancer migration and invasion. *Sci. Rep.* 7:3568. doi: 10.1038/s41598-017-03362-z

Yoon, J. H., Dammann, R., and Pfeifer, G. P. (2001). Hypermethylation of the CpG island of the RASSF1A gene in ovarian and renal cell carcinomas. *Int. J. Cancer* 94, 212–217. doi: 10.1002/ijc.1466

Yu, J., Ryan, D. G., Getsios, S., Oliveira-Fernandes, M., Fatima, A., and Lavker, R. M. (2008). MicroRNA-184 antagonizes microRNA-205 to maintain SHIP2 levels in epithelia. *Proc. Natl. Acad. Sci. U.S.A.* 105, 19300–19305. doi: 10.1073/pnas.0803992105

Yu, Y., Fujii, S., Yuan, J., Luo, R. Z., Wang, L., Bao, J., et al. (2003). Epigenetic regulation of ARHI in breast and ovarian cancer cells. *Ann. N. Y. Acad. Sci.* 983, 268–277. doi: 10.1111/j.1749-6632.2003.tb05981.x

Zhang, H., Zhang, S., Cui, J., Zhang, A., Shen, L., and Yu, H. (2008). Expression and promoter methylation status of mismatch repair gene hMLH1 and hMSH2 in epithelial ovarian cancer. *Aust. N. Z. J. Obstet. Gynaecol.* 48, 505–509. doi: 10.1111/j.1479-828X.2008.00892.x

Zhang, J., Ye, F., Chen, H., Ye, D., Lu, W., and Xie, X. (2006). [Deletion of OPCML gene and promoter methylation in ovarian epithelial carcinoma]. *Zhongguo Yi Xue Ke Xue Yuan Xue Bao* 28, 173–177.

Zhang, L., Huang, J., Yang, N., Greshock, J., Megraw, M. S., Giannakakis, A., et al. (2006). microRNAs exhibit high frequency genomic alterations in human cancer. *Proc. Natl. Acad. Sci. U.S.A.* 103, 9136–9141. doi: 10.1073/pnas.0508889103

Zhang, L., Volinia, S., Bonome, T., Calin, G. A., Greshock, J., Yang, N., et al. (2008). Genomic and epigenetic alterations deregulate microRNA expression in human epithelial ovarian cancer. *Proc. Natl. Acad. Sci. U.S.A.* 105, 7004–7009. doi: 10.1073/pnas.0801615105

Zhang, Q., Hu, G., Yang, Q., Dong, R., Xie, X., Ma, D., et al. (2013). A multiplex methylation-specific PCR assay for the detection of early-stage ovarian cancer using cell-free serum DNA. *Gynecol. Oncol.* 130, 132–139. doi: 10.1016/j.ygyno.2013.04.048

Zhang, S., Wei, L., Zhang, A., Zhang, L., and Yu, H. (2009). RUNX3 gene methylation in epithelial ovarian cancer tissues and ovarian cancer cell lines. *Omics J. Integr. Biol.* 13, 307–311. doi: 10.1089/omi.2009.0030

Zhang, W., Barger, C. J., Eng, K. H., Klinkebiel, D., Link, P. A., Omilian, A., et al. (2016). PRAME expression and promoter hypomethylation in epithelial ovarian cancer. *Oncotarget* 7, 45352–45369. doi: 10.18632/oncotarget.9977

Zhang, W., Barger, C. J., Link, P. A., Mhawech-Fauceglia, P., Miller, A., Akers, S. N., et al. (2015). DNA hypomethylation-mediated activation of *Cancer/Testis Antigen 45* (*CT45*) genes is associated with disease progression and reduced survival in epithelial ovarian cancer. *Epigenetics* 10, 736–748. doi: 10.1080/15592294.2015.1062206

Zhang, Z., Bast, R. C., Yu, Y., Li, J., Sokoll, L. J., Rai, A. J., et al. (2004). Three biomarkers identified from serum proteomic analysis for the detection of early stage ovarian cancer. *Cancer Res.* 64, 5882–5890. doi: 10.1158/0008-5472.CAN-04-0746

Zhao, L., Wang, W., Xu, L., Yi, T., Zhao, X., Wei, Y., et al. (2019). Integrative network biology analysis identifies miR-508-3p as the determinant for the mesenchymal identity and a strong prognostic biomarker of ovarian cancer. *Oncogene* 38, 2305–2319. doi: 10.1038/s41388-018-0577-5

Zhao, L., Yu, C., Zhou, S., Lau, W. B., Lau, B., Luo, Z., et al. (2016). Epigenetic repression of PDZ-LIM domain-containing protein 2 promotes ovarian cancer via NOS2-derived nitric oxide signaling. *Oncotarget* 7, 1408–1420. doi: 10.18632/oncotarget.6368

Zheng, X., Chen, S., Li, L., Liu, X., Liu, X., Dai, S., et al. (2018). Evaluation of HE4 and TTR for diagnosis of ovarian cancer: comparison with CA-125. *J. Gynecol. Obstet. Hum. Reprod.* 47, 227–230. doi: 10.1016/j.jogoh.2018.03.010

Zhou, F., Tao, G., Chen, X., Xie, W., Liu, M., and Cao, X. (2014). Methylation of OPCML promoter in ovarian cancer tissues predicts poor patient survival. *Clin. Chem. Lab. Med.* 52, 735–742. doi: 10.1515/cclm-2013-0736

Zhou, Q.-H., Zhao, Y.-M., Jia, L.-L., and Zhang, Y. (2017). Mir-595 is a significant indicator of poor patient prognosis in epithelial ovarian cancer. *Eur. Rev. Med. Pharmacol. Sci.* 21, 4278–4282.

Zuberi, M., Mir, R., Das, J., Ahmad, I., Javid, J., Yadav, P., et al. (2015). Expression of serum miR-200a, miR-200b, and miR-200c as candidate biomarkers in epithelial ovarian cancer and their association with clinicopathological features. *Clin. Transl. Oncol.* 17, 779–787. doi: 10.1007/s12094-015-1303-1

2

Essential Role of Histone Replacement and Modifications in Male Fertility

Tong Wang[1†], Hui Gao[1†], Wei Li[1,2] and Chao Liu[1,2*]*

[1] State Key Laboratory of Stem Cell and Reproductive Biology, Institute of Zoology, Chinese Academy of Sciences, Beijing, China, [2] College of Life Sciences, University of Chinese Academy of Sciences, Beijing, China

***Correspondence:**
Wei Li
leways@ioz.ac.cn
Chao Liu
liuchao@ioz.ac.cn

†These authors have contributed equally to this work

Spermiogenesis is a complex cellular differentiation process that the germ cells undergo a distinct morphological change, and the protamines replace the core histones to facilitate chromatin compaction in the sperm head. Recent studies show the essential roles of epigenetic events during the histone-to-protamine transition. Defects in either the replacement or the modification of histones might cause male infertility with azoospermia, oligospermia or teratozoospermia. Here, we summarize recent advances in our knowledge of how epigenetic regulators, such as histone variants, histone modification and their related chromatin remodelers, facilitate the histone-to-protamine transition during spermiogenesis. Understanding the molecular mechanism underlying the modification and replacement of histones during spermiogenesis will enable the identification of epigenetic biomarkers of male infertility, and shed light on potential therapies for these patients in the future.

Keywords: spermiogenesis, histone-to-protamine transition, histone variants, histone modification, male infertility

INTRODUCTION

Spermatogenesis is the process of male gamete production with successive cellular differentiation, which can be subdivided into spermatogonial mitosis, spermatocytic meiosis and spermiogenesis (Roosen-Runge, 1962; Hess and Renato De Franca, 2008). During spermatogenesis, SSC (spermatogonial stem cells) undergo self-renewal and differentiate into spermatogonia that perform meiosis to generate haploid germ cells and ensure the genetic diversity through meiotic recombination (Rathke et al., 2014; Bao and Bedford, 2016). Then, the haploid germ cells undergo spermiogenesis with a distinct morphological change and chromatin compaction in the sperm nuclei to prevent the paternal genome from mutagenesis and damage (Govin et al., 2004; Bao and Bedford, 2016). During the nuclear chromatin re-organization in spermiogenesis, the majority of the somatic histones are firstly replaced by testis-specific histone variants, and transition proteins (TPs) are subsequently incorporated in the nuclei of spermatids, protamines (PRMs) further replace TPs in the late spermatids to pack the genome into the highly condensed sperm nucleus (Rathke et al., 2014; Bao and Bedford, 2016). During the histone-to-protamine transition, the histone variants and specific histone modifications play essential roles by modulating the chromatin compaction and higher-order chromatin structure (**Table 1**) (Boskovic and Torres-Padilla, 2013; Bao and Bedford, 2016; Hada et al., 2017; Hao et al., 2019). Defects in either the replacement or the modification of histones might result in azoospermia, oligospermia or teratozoospermia, which leads to male infertility (**Table 2**). The focus of this review is on recent advances in our knowledge of how epigenetic regulators, such as histone variants, histone modification and their

TABLE 1 | The main histone variants and modifications during the histone-to-protamine transition.

Type	Histone	Name	Period	Function	Reference
Histone variants	H1	H1T	Spermatocytes to elongating spermatids	Maintain open chromatin configuration and no detectable phenotype in H1t-null testis	Delucia et al., 1994; Khadake and Rao, 1995; Drabent et al., 2000; Fantz et al., 2001
		H1T2	Round spermatids and elongating spermatids	Indispensable for the replacement of histones with protamines and chromatin condensation	Martianov et al., 2005; Tanaka et al., 2005
		HILS1	Elongating and elongated spermatids	Contribute to the open chromatin structure	Yan et al., 2003; Mishra et al., 2018
	H2A	TH2A	Spermatocytes to elongated spermatids	Contribute to the open chromatin structure and cooperate with TH2B to regulate TP2 incorporation	Padavattan et al., 2015; Shinagawa et al., 2015; Padavattan et al., 2017
		H2AL2	Elongating and elongated spermatids	Assemble open nucleosomes and allow TPs incorporation	Govin et al., 2007; Barral et al., 2017
		H2A.B	Spermatocytes to round spermatids	Destabilize chromatin and modulate the dynamics of H2AL2 removal and TP1 incorporation and	Soboleva et al., 2012; Soboleva et al., 2017; Anuar et al., 2019
	H2B	Th2B	Spermatocytes, round spermatids and elongating spermatids	Destabilize chromatin and regulate the TPs and PRMs incorporation	Meistrich et al., 1985; Montellier et al., 2013
	H3	H3.3	All types of germ cell	Contribute to the open chromatin structure, modulate TP1 removal and PRM1 incorporation	Bramlage et al., 1997; Couldrey et al., 1999; Van Der Heijden et al., 2007; Thakar et al., 2009; Chen et al., 2013; Tang et al., 2015
		H3T	Spermatocytes, round spermatids and elongating spermatids	Contribute to the open chromatin and required for spermatogonial differentiation and ensures entry into meiosis	Tachiwana et al., 2010; Ueda et al., 2017
Histone modifications	Acetylation	H4K5/8/12ac	Spermatogonia, spermatocytes and elongating spermatids	Essential for destabilization and remodeling of nucleosomes, TPs incorporation	Hazzouri et al., 2000;Gaucher et al., 2012; Qian et al., 2013; Bell et al., 2014; Dong et al., 2017; Ketchum et al., 2018
		H4K16ac	Elongating spermatids		
	Ubiquitination	UbH2A	Spermatocytes and elongating spermatids	Essential for the recruitment of the MOF acetyltransferase complex to modulate H4K16ac and histone removal	Chen et al., 1998; Baarends et al., 1999; Lu et al., 2010; Gou et al., 2017; Meng et al., 2019; Wang et al., 2019
		UbH2B	Spermatocytes and elongating spermatids		
	Methylation	H3K4me3	Spermatogonia, spermatocytes, round spermatids and elongating spermatids	Essential for the recruitment of PYGO2 to recognize HAT to facilitate H3 acetylation; recruit PHF7 to catalyze H2A ubiquitination to facilitate the histone removal	Godmann et al., 2007; Song et al., 2011; Nair et al., 2008; Wang et al., 2019
		H3K9me1/2/3	Spermatogonia, Round spermatids and elongating spermatids	Regulate the *Tnps* and *Prms* genes expression	Okada et al., 2007
		H3K36me3	Spermatocytes and round spermatids	Regulate the *Tnps* and *Prms* genes expression	Zuo et al., 2018
		H3K79me3	Elongating spermatids	Correlate with histone H4 hyperacetylation to regulate histone-to-protamine transition	Dottermusch-Heidel et al., 2014
	Phosphorylation	γH2AX	Spermatocytes elongating spermatids	Require for the normal quantities of H3, H4 and PRM2 precursor and intermediate	Li et al., 2005; Spiridonov et al., 2005; Jha et al., 2017
		H4S1	Spermatocyte, round spermatids and elongating spermatids	Essential for chromatin compaction and concomitantly histone accessibility	Krishnamoorthy et al., 2006; Zhang et al., 2016
	Other	Crotonylation	Elongating spermatids	Facilitate TP1 and PRM2 incorporation	Liu et al., 2017b
		PARsylation	Elongating spermatids	Require for histone removal and TP1 incorporation	Meyer-Ficca et al., 2009; Meyer-Ficca et al., 2011; Meyer-Ficca et al., 2015

TABLE 2 | Mouse models related with the histone-to-protamine transition.

Gene	Phenotype	Function	Reference
H1t	Fertility and no spermatogenesis abnormalities	Dispensable for histone-to-protamine transition	Drabent et al., 2000; Fantz et al., 2001
H1t2	Reduced fertility with delayed nuclear condensation and aberrant elongation of spermatids	Indispensable for the incorporation of PRMs and proper chromatin condensation	Martianov et al., 2005; Tanaka et al., 2005
Th2b	Fertility with normal spermatogenesis in *Th2b*-null mice Infertility with abnormal spermatozoa in TH2B C-terminus modified mice	Destabilize chromatin and regulate TPs and PRMs incorporation	Montellier et al., 2013
Th2a/Th2b	Infertility with accumulated spermatocytes at interkinesis and abnormal spermatozoa	Indispensable for cohesin release and TP2 incorporation	Shinagawa et al., 2015
H2al2	Infertility and the sperm chromatin show a compaction defects	Assemble open nucleosomes and allow TPs incorporation	Barral et al., 2017
H2a.b	Reduced fertility with abnormal spermatozoa	Destabilize chromatin and modulate the dynamics of H2AL2 removal and TP1 incorporation	Anuar et al., 2019
H3f3a	Reduced fertility with dysmorphic spermatozoa	Require for normal development of some spermatids	Tang et al., 2015
H3f3b	Infertility with abnormal spermatozoa and reduced sperm count	Indispensable for spermatogenesis related genes expression, TP1 removal and PRM1 incorporation	Yuen et al., 2014
H3t	Infertility with azoospermia	Require for spermatogonial differentiation and ensures entry into meiosis	Ueda et al., 2017
Epc1	Infertility with abnormal round spermatids to elongating spermatids transition	Require for round spermatids maturation by regulating histone acetylation and TP2 incorporation	Dong et al., 2017
Tip60	The germ cell is arrested at the RS stage	Contribute to round spermatids maturation by regulating histone acetylation and TP2 incorporation	Dong et al., 2017
Sirt1	Reduced fertility with abnormal spermatozoa and decreased sperm count	Require for acetylation of H4K5, H4K8 and H4K12 histone, and TP2 incorporation	Bell et al., 2014
Brdt	Infertility with complete absence of post-meiotic cells in *Brdt*-null mice Infertility with abnormal spermatids in *Brdt*$^{\Delta BD1/\Delta BD1}$ mice	Control the chromatin organization and meiotic sex chromosome inactivation; the first bromodomain of BRDT is essential to link histone removal and TPs, PRMs incorporation	Shang et al., 2007; Dhar et al., 2012; Gaucher et al., 2012; Manterola et al., 2018
Pa200	Reduced fertility with abnormal spermatozoa and decreased sperm count	Recognize acetylated histones and mediate the core histones for acetylation dependent degradation through proteasomes	Khor et al., 2006; Qian et al., 2013
Rnf8	Infertility with abnormal spermatozoa and reduced sperm count	Require for histone ubiquitination and modulate H4K16ac to facilitate histone removal and TPs, PRMs incorporation	Lu et al., 2010
Miwi	Infertility with abnormal spermatozoa and reduced sperm count in *Miwi* D-box mutations mice	Essential for nuclear translocation of RNF8 and facilitates the histone ubiquitination and further histone removal	Gou et al., 2017
L3mbtl2	Reduced fertility with abnormal spermatozoa and decreased sperm count	Require for the RNF8-UbH2A pathway and further PRM1 incorporation	Meng et al., 2019
Phf7	Infertility with abnormal spermatozoa and decreased sperm count	Recognize the H3K4me3/me2 and catalyze H2A ubiquitination to facilitate the histone removal	Wang et al., 2019
Pygo2	Infertile with abnormal spermatozoa and decreased sperm count in *Pygo2* reduced mice	Recognize H3K4me3 and recruit HAT to facilitate H3 acetylation and expression of *Prms*, *Tnp2*, and *H1fnt*.	Nair et al., 2008
Jhdm2a	Infertile with abnormal spermatozoa and decreased sperm count	Control H3K9 methylation at the promoter of *Tnp1* and *Prm1* genes and regulate their expression	Okada et al., 2007
Setd2	Infertility with round spermatid arrest	Catalyze H3K36me3 and facilitate the activation of *Tnps* and *Prms* genes	Zuo et al., 2018
Tssk6	Infertility with abnormal spermatozoa	Mediate γH2AX to possess normal quantities of histone H3, H4 and PRM2 precursor and intermediate	Spiridonov et al., 2005; Jha et al., 2017
Cdyl	Reduced fertility with decreased sperm count and motility	Regulate histone crotonylation to facilitate TP1 and PRM2 incorporation	Liu et al., 2017b
Parp11	Infertility with teratozoospermia	Modulate PARsylation to facilitate chromatin condensation	Meyer-Ficca et al., 2015
Parg110	Reduced fertility with poor sperm chromatin quality	Dispensable for histone removal and TP1 incorporation	Meyer-Ficca et al., 2009; Meyer-Ficca et al., 2011
Tnp1	Reduced fertility with subtle abnormal spermatozoa and decreased spermatozoa	Dispensable for histone displacement as the compensation by TP2 and PRM2 precursor	Yu et al., 2000
Tnp2	Reduced fertility with abnormal spermatozoa	Dispensable for histone displacement but necessary for maintaining the normal processing of PRM2 and the completion of chromatin condensation	Zhao et al., 2001

(Continued)

TABLE 2 | Continued

Gene	Phenotype	Function	Reference
Tnp1/Tnp2	Infertile with abnormal spermatozoa and decreased sperm count	Indispensable for PRM2 incorporation and chromatin condensation	Shirley et al., 2004
Prm1	Infertile with abnormal spermatozoa and decreased sperm count	Indispensable for spermiogenesis and chromatin condensation	Cho et al., 2001
Prm2	Infertile with abnormal spermatozoa and decreased sperm count		
Camk4	Infertile with abnormal spermatozoa and decreased sperm count	Mediate the phosphorylation of PRM2 and facilitate basic nuclear proteins removal	Wu et al., 2000

related chromatin remodelers, regulate the highly orchestrated chromatin re-organization and facilitate the histone-to-protamine transition during spermiogenesis.

HISTONE VARIANTS

In eukaryotes, nucleosomes are the packing units of DNA, which contain four types of canonical histones (H2A, H2B, H3, and H4) and the linker histone H1 (Talbert and Henikoff, 2010; Kowalski and Palyga, 2012). While canonical histone expression is typically coupled to DNA replication, some non-canonical histones (histone variants) that are distinct form their canonical paralogues in amino acid sequence, are constitutively expressed and have roles in a wide range of processes (Talbert and Henikoff, 2010). Many histones variants are expressed during spermiogenesis and modulate the chromatin structure to facilitate the histone-to-protamine replacement (Mccarrey et al., 2005; Govin et al., 2007). Here, we summarize the recent advances in our understanding of the role of histone variants during the histone-to-protamine transition.

H1 VARIANTS

Linker histones contribute to form and stabilize the higher-order chromatin structure (Bednar et al., 1998). In mammals, there are about 11 different subtypes of histone H1 (Happel and Doenecke, 2009). Among these, H1T, H1T2, and HILS1 are testis-specific H1 variants (**Figure 1**) (Happel and Doenecke, 2009).

H1T is exclusively detected as early as mid- to late pachytene spermatocytes, and maintains high expression levels in the elongating spermatids (**Figure 1**) (Drabent et al., 1996; Drabent et al., 2003). Biochemical and biophysical studies found that, distinct from other somatic H1 variants, H1T binds less tightly to H1-depleted nucleosomes, suggesting it may maintain a relatively open chromatin configuration to facilitate histone replacement during spermiogenesis (Delucia et al., 1994; Khadake and Rao, 1995). Unexpectedly, *H1t*-null mice are fertile and exhibit no spermatogenesis abnormalities, and the histone-to-protamine transition in *H1t*-deficient testis is normal (Drabent et al., 2000; Fantz et al., 2001). Although the expression of some canonical subtypes, including H1.1, H1.2, and H1.4, is enhanced in *H1t*-null mice, elevated levels of H1.1 or H1.2 could not be observed in the *H1t*-deficient spermatids (Drabent et al., 2003), indicating some other types of H1 variants may play redundant roles in the histone-to-protamine transition.

H1T2 selectively localizes at the apical pole in the nucleus of round and elongating spermatids but not in mature spermatozoa (**Figure 1**) (Martianov et al., 2005). Distinct from H1T, H1T2 is critical for spermiogenesis, as homozygous *H1t2*-mutant males are infertile due to delayed nuclear condensation and aberrant elongation of spermatids. Further analysis shows the protamine levels are substantially reduced in *H1t2*-null spermatozoa (Martianov et al., 2005; Tanaka et al., 2005), indicating H1T2 is necessary for the incorporation of protamines, and proper chromitin condensation during the histone-to-protamine transition.

HILS1 is strongly expressed in the nuclei of elongating and elongated spermatids (**Figure 1**) (Yan et al., 2003). HILS1 is the least conserved H1 variant, and a poor condenser of chromatin compared with somatic H1, demonstrating the idea that HILS1 may have a distinct role in the histone-to-protamine transition (Yan et al., 2003; Mishra et al., 2018). In *Drosophila*, *Mst77F* encodes a linker histone-like protein that is similar with the mammalian HILS1 protein and expressed in elongating spermatids (Raja and Renkawitz-Pohl, 2005). The disruption of *Mst77F* cause male sterile as producing spermatozoa with malformed heads. Although the histone-to-protamine transition occurs independently of *Mst77F*, the nuclei of spermatid fail to properly condense after the histone-to-protamine replacement in *Mst77F* mutant male (Kimura and Loppin, 2016). However, the functional roles of HILS1 in mammalian spermiogenesis need further investigation.

H2A VARIANTS

Multiple testis-specific H2A variants have been identified in mammals, including TH2A, H2AL1, H2AL2, H2AL3 and H2A.B (Trostleweige et al., 1982; Govin et al., 2007; Soboleva et al., 2012).

TH2A is present and actively synthesized in early primary spermatocytes and gradually disappears during condensation of spermatid nuclei (**Figure 1**) (Shires et al., 1976; Trostleweige et al., 1982). TH2A could contribute to the open chromatin structure, as crystal structures of nucleosome core particles (NCPs) with TH2A show the H-bonding interactions between the TH2A/TH2A′ L1 loops are lost and the histone dimer-DNA contacts are dramatically decreased (Padavattan et al., 2015; Padavattan et al., 2017). Although a *Th2a*-knockout mouse model has yet

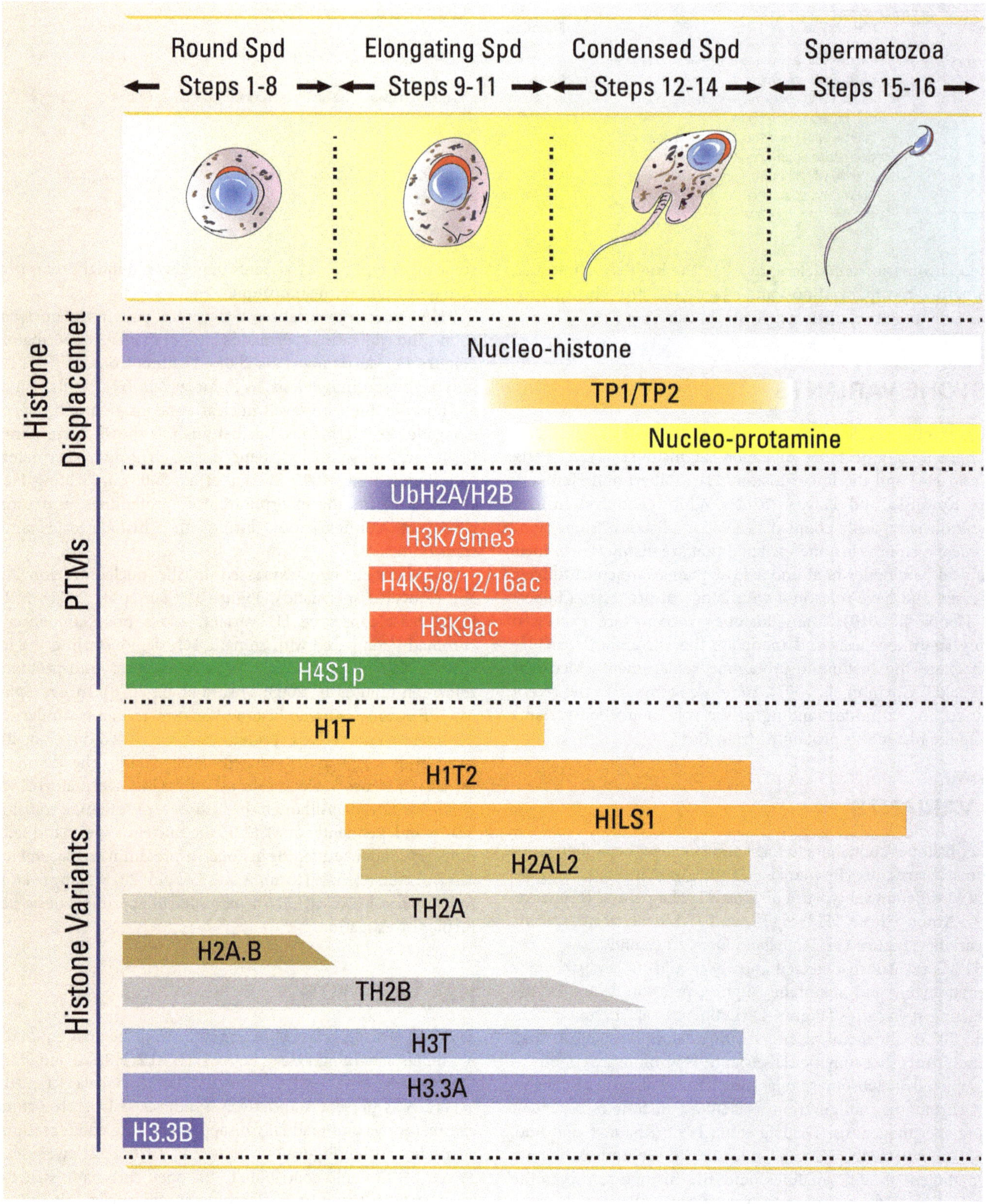

FIGURE 1 | Summary of critical time points and epigenetic events during the histone-to-protamine transition. The haploid germ cells undergo a dramatic morphological change, and nuclear chromatin re-organization starts from round spermatid (Spd) to mature spermatozoa. Detailed studies of the indicated histone variants and histone modification might establish the precise epigenetic events of spermiogenesis.

to be established, mice with knockouts of the testis-specific H2B variants *Th2a* and *Th2b* exhibit male infertility with few sperm in the epididymis (Shinagawa et al., 2015). In this double-knockout mouse, impaired chromatin incorporation of transition protein 2 (TP2) and elevated H2B could be observed in the mutant testis, suggesting the TH2A and TH2B may regulate the function in chromatin dynamics or the total histone levels to facilitate the histone replacement during spermatogenesis (Shinagawa et al., 2015). As the *Th2b*-null male mice show normal spermatogenesis and fertility (Montellier et al., 2013), the histone replacement defect in *Th2a*/*Th2b* double-knockout male mice is probably caused by the depletion of *Th2a* or their synergistic effect.

In late-developing post-meiotic male germ cells, H2AL2 is specifically expressed in condensing spermatids that correlates with the expression of TPs (**Figure 1**) (Govin et al., 2007). By comparing *H2al2*-null mice to wild-type mice, H2AL2 was demonstrated to be required to load TPs onto the nucleosome and for efficient PRMs assembly during the histone-to-protamine transition. Additionally, the nucleosome reconstitution assays revealed that the incorporation of H2A.L.2 can drastically modulate the nucleosome structure to facilitate TPs invading the nucleosomes and further transformation (Barral et al., 2017). Thus, H2AL2 could assemble open nucleosomes and allow TPs invading, which further promotes protamine processing and sperm genome compaction.

H2A.B is spatially and temporally regulated during spermatogenesis and detectable from the pachytene stage to the round spermatids (**Figure 1**) (Soboleva et al., 2012; Soboleva et al., 2017). *In vitro* studies show that H2A.B is able to destabilize chromatin and has unfolding properties to chromatin (Soboleva et al., 2012), indicating H2A.B might promote chromatin reorganization and further histones displacement by TPs. Male *H2a.b*-null male mice are subfertile due to the production of abnormal spermatozoa and clogged seminiferous tubules (Anuar et al., 2019). In *H2a.b*-null elongating spermatids, H2AL2 could not be detected in pericentric heterochromatin, and the replacement of TP1 by protamines appears to be delayed (Anuar et al., 2019). These results indicate H2A.B might modulate the dynamics of H2AL2 and TP1 chromatin incorporation and removal to participate in the histone-to-protamine transition.

H2B VARIANTS

The testis-specific histone variant TH2B is one of the earliest histone variants identified in testis (Shires et al., 1975). TH2B massively replaces somatic H2B during meiosis and remains the main type of H2B in round and elongating spermatids (Meistrich et al., 1985; Montellier et al., 2013), suggesting TH2B might be indispensable for meiotic and post-meiotic germ cells. The crystal structure analysis shows the TH2B could not form the water-mediated hydrogen bonds with H4R78 (Urahama et al., 2014), which may affect the stability of the TH2B nucleosome and facilitate histone replacement during spermiogenesis. In a *Th2b* mutant mouse, which contains modified C-terminus of the TH2B protein and causes a dominant-negative effect, males were infertile and severe abnormalities were seen in the elongating spermatids, which affected subnucleosomal transitional states during histone replacement (Boskovic and Torres-Padilla, 2013; Montellier et al., 2013). In contrast, *Th2b*-null mice are fertile and show normal spermatogenesis process, indicating a compensatory mechanism that rescues deficiency of TH2B in the histone-to-protamine transition. Indeed, in *Th2b*-null testis, the expression of somatic H2B was significantly increased and elevated methylation of H4R35, H4R55, H4R67, and H2BR72 could be detected in *Th2b*-null spermatids. As H4R35, H4R55, H4R67, and H2BR72 participate in the interactions of histone–DNA and histone–histone, and their methylation may impair these intranucleosomal interactions (Hoghoughi et al., 2018). Thus, the elevated somatic H2B and histone modification in *Th2b*-null spermatids might rescue the *Th2b* deficiency in testis (Montellier et al., 2013; Bao and Bedford, 2016).

In humans, H2BFWT is a testis-specific histone, is synthesized and aggregated in testes, and single nucleotide polymorphisms (SNPs) in this gene is highly associated with male infertility (Churikov et al., 2004; Lee et al., 2009; Ying et al., 2012; Rafatmanesh et al., 2018; Teimouri et al., 2018). And spermatid-specific H2B (ssH2B) and H2BL1 have been identified and are strongly enriched in round or elongating spermatids, similar to that of TPs and protamines (Moss and Orth, 1993; Unni et al., 1995; Govin et al., 2007). However, the functional roles of these H2B variants in the histone-to-protamine transition still need to be further elucidated.

H3 VARIANTS

In addition to the two canonical histones H3.1 and H3.2, three additional H3 variants have been identified and expressed in mammal testes, including H3.3, H3T and H3.5 (Rathke et al., 2014; Bao and Bedford, 2016).

H3.3 differs from canonical H3.1 with five amino acids, is expressed throughout mouse seminiferous tubules, and accumulates in the XY body of spermatocytes (Bramlage et al., 1997; Van Der Heijden et al., 2007). Biochemical and biophysical studies show that H3.3 contributes to an open chromatin configuration and promotes transcription through disrupting the higher-order chromatin structure (Thakar et al., 2009; Chen et al., 2013). H3.3 could be encoded by two gene paralogs in mammal, *H3f3a* and *H3f3b*, and the depletion of either *H3f3a* or *H3f3b* causes male infertility. The disruption of *H3f3a* produces abnormal spermatozoa (Couldrey et al., 1999; Tang et al., 2015), and the loss of *H3f3b* leads to growth defects and death at birth, with surviving *H3f3b*-null males showing complete infertility (Yuen et al., 2014). In *H3f3b*-null germ cells, the TP1 is abnormally deposited in elongating spermatids while PRM1 could not be observed in in elongated spermatids and mature spermatozoa, indicating that *H3f3b* is required for chromatin reorganization and the histone-to-protamine transition (Yuen et al., 2014). H3T (H3.4) is exclusively expressed in the spermatocyte and diminishes in the elongating spermatids (Ueda et al., 2017). Biochemical studies clearly indicate that, in the H3T nucleosome, the DNA around the entry-exit regions shows more flexible than that of the H3.1-containing nucleosome, and that the H3T-containing polynucleosome could formed more open configuration than that of H3.1 (Tachiwana et al., 2010). However, the disruption of H3T leads to sterile males with azoospermia, as spermatocyte and spermatids are absent in the *H3t*-null testes (Ueda et al., 2017). Thus, the function of H3T in the later stage of spermatogenesis need further investigated by using spatially and temporally specific knockout mouse models.

H3.5 is highly expressed in human testis and specifically observed in spermatogonia and spermatocytes (Shiraishi et al., 2017). *In vitro* studies reveal that the H3.5-specific L103 residue, reduces the hydrophobic interaction with histone H4 in the H3.5-containing nucleosome, which corresponds to the H3.3 Phe104 residue (Urahama et al., 2016). H3.5 is significantly reduced in non-obstructive azoospermia (NOA) patients (Shiraishi et al., 2017), whereas the precise roles of H3.5 in spermatogenesis remain largely unknown.

HISTONE MODIFICATION

Covalent conjugation of different post-translational modification of histones has a dramatic effect on the chromatin conformation by affecting the stability of the nucleosome and the histone-DNA interaction (Bao and Bedford, 2016). Many types of histone modifications have been identified to facilitate the histone-to-protamine transition, including acetylation, ubiquitination, methylation, and phosphorylation (Luense et al., 2016).

ACETYLATION

Hyperacetylated histones could facilitate histone eviction, and the acetylation of H2A, H2B, H3, H4 and histone variants have been detected in mammal testis (Grimes and Henderson, 1984a; Grimes and Henderson, 1984b; Oliva and Mezquita, 1986; Oliva et al., 1987). In *Drosophila*, inactivation of histone acetyltransferases by anacardic acid prevents the histones degradation and further a protamine incorporation during spermiogenesis (Awe and Renkawitz-Pohl, 2010), suggesting that histone acetylation is essential for the histone-to-protamine replacement.

H4 acetylation (H4K5ac, H4K8ac, H4K12ac, and H4K16ac) shows a spatial distribution pattern during spermatogenesis and is indispensable for the histone-to-protamine transition (Bao and Bedford, 2016; Ketchum et al., 2018). H4K5ac, H4K8ac and H4K12ac are expressed in spermatogonia and pre-leptotene spermatocytes, disappear in leptotene to pachytene spermatocytes, reappeared in elongating spermatids, and finally disappeared in condensing spermatids (**Figure 1**) (Hazzouri et al., 2000; Ketchum et al., 2018). In contrast, H4K16ac could only be detected in elongating spermatids (**Figure 1**) (Ketchum et al., 2018). *In vitro* analysis shows that H4 acetylation is essential for destabilization and remodeling of nucleosomes, and the incorporation of H4K16ac into nucleosomes prevents the formation of compact chromatin fibers and influence chromatin forming cross-fiber interactions (Tse et al., 1998; Shogren-Knaak et al., 2006; Kan et al., 2009). These findings indicate that H4 acetylation modulates higher order chromatin structure to facilitate the histone-to-protamine transition. EPC1 (Enhancer Of Polycomb Homolog 1) and TIP60 (Tat-interactive protein, 60 kDa), which are two components for the mammalian NuA4 (nucleosome acetyltransferase of H4) complexes (**Figure 2**) (Doyon et al., 2004), are co-localized to the nuclear periphery near the acrosomes in both round spermatids and elongating spermatids (Dong et al., 2017). The depletion of either *Epc1* or *Tip60* perturbs histone hyperacetylation, especially H4 acetylation, and affects histone replacement during spermiogenesis (Dong et al., 2017). Another gene that may play a role in acetylation is SIRT1 (Sirtuin 1), a member of the NAD+-dependent deacetylase. Germ cell-specific *Sirt1* knockout mice display reduced male fertility due to decreased spermatozoa number and increased proportion of abnormal spermatozoa (Bell et al., 2014; Liu et al., 2017a). In *Sirt1*-null elongating and elongated spermatids, acetylation levels of H4K5, H4K8 and H4K12 are decreased and TP2 could not co-localize in the nucleus, leading to a chromatin condensation defect in *Sirt1*-null spermatozoa (Bell et al., 2014). Thus, SIRT1 may modulate other factors to promote H4 acetylation and the histone-to-protamine transition.

The histone acetylation might be recognized by some chromatin remodelers to confer downstream signaling, and the double bromodomain and extra-terminal domain (BET) proteins have been identified to be critical epigenetic readers binding to acetylated histones and modulating changes in chromatin structure and organization during spermiogenesis (Berkovits and Wolgemuth, 2013). BRDT is a testis-specific BET member protein, which is expressed specifically in spermatocytes and spermatids, and contains two bromodomains that specifically recognize acetylated lysine residues (Shang et al., 2007; Dhar et al., 2012; Manterola et al., 2018). BRDT binds the hyperacetylated histone H4 tail and co-localizes with acetylated H4 in elongating spermatids (Pivot-Pajot et al., 2003; Govin et al., 2006). Remodeling assays have shown BRDT regulated the chromatin reorganization dependent acetylation in round spermatids (Dhar et al., 2012). In mice, the disruption of the first bromodomain in BRDT resulted in male sterility by producing the morphologically abnormal spermatids (Shang et al., 2007). In elongating spermatids with BRDT containing a knockout of bromodomain 1 (BD1), TPs and protamines remained in the cytoplasm and histone replacement did not occur, suggesting BRDT is required for the histone-to-protamine transition by mediating the replacement of acetylated histones (**Figure 2**) (Gaucher et al., 2012). Furthermore, BRDT was found to bind with the N-terminus of SMARCE1 (SWI/SNF-related matrix-associated actin-dependent regulator of chromatin subfamily E member 1), a member of the SWI/SNF family of ATP-dependent chromatin remodeling complexes (Dhar et al., 2012), indicating BRDT may cooperate with SMARCE1 to facilitate the histone-to-protamine transition during spermiogenesis (**Figure 2**).

Proteasomes catalyze ATP- and polyubiquitin-dependent protein degradation, and they are made up of a 20S catalytic core particle (CP) and regulatory particle (RP). The 20S CP could be activated by cooperation with various RPs, such as PA700/19S, PA28α/β, PA28γ, and PA200 (Stadtmueller and Hill, 2011). PA200 is highly expressed in the testis, and the disruption of PA200

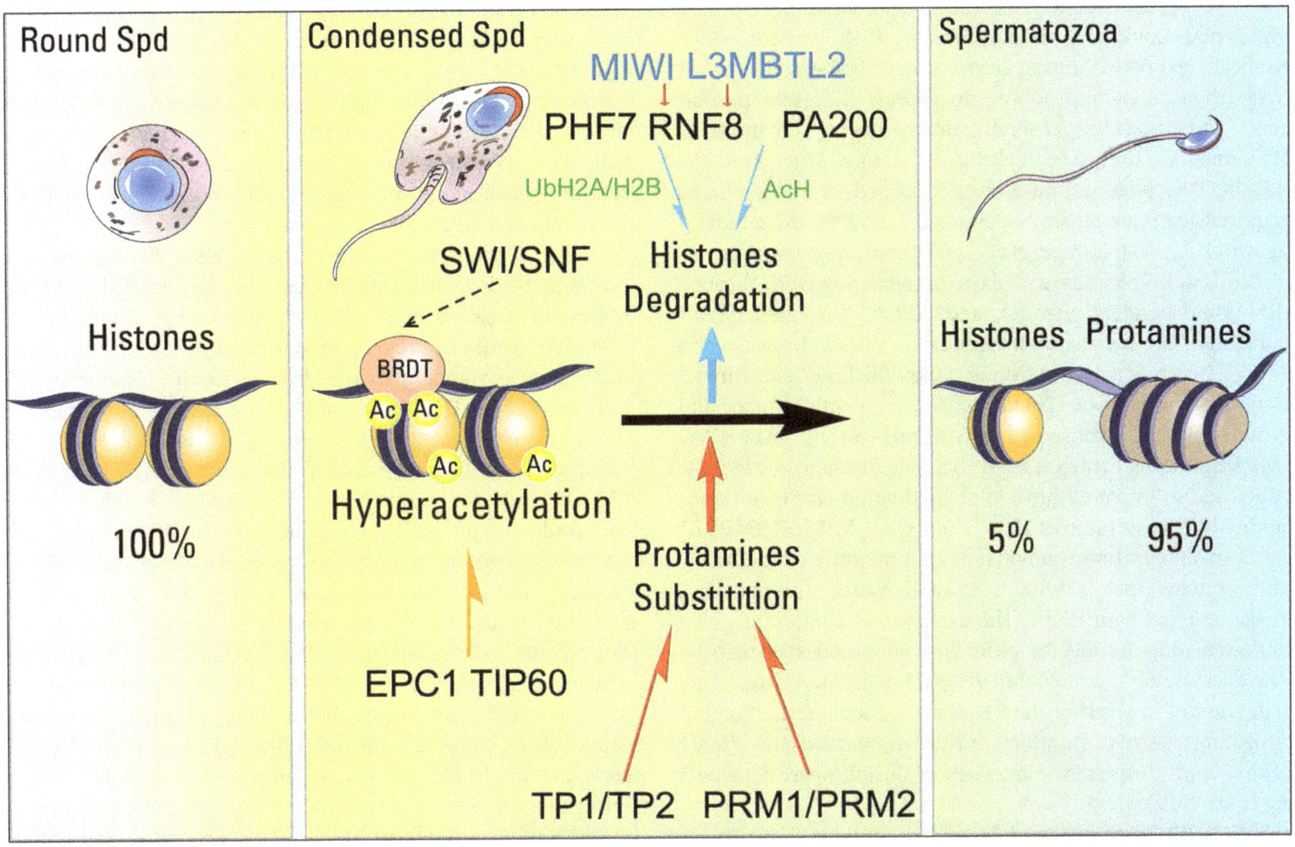

FIGURE 2 | The key factors related to the histone-to-protamine transition. Global incorporation of various H2A, H2B and H3 histone variants creates highly unstable nucleosomes, which then undergo histone hyperacetylation by EPC1/TIP60 or some other nucleosome acetyltransferase complexes. Acetylation at critical lysines further destabilizes the nucleosomes, while tail acetylation generates a platform for the recruitment of BRDT. BRDT interacts with the SWI/SNF family protein then starts the process of histone eviction and replacement by TPs. Evicted acetylated histones would then be recognized by PA200 and degraded by proteasomes during spermatogenesis. RNF8 could catalyze the ubiquitination of H2A. Ubiquitinated H2A and H2B control H4K16ac by regulating the association of MOF to the chromatin and facilitates histone removal in elongating spermatids. MIWI binds to RNF8 in the cytoplasm of early spermatids (Spd) through a Piwi-interacting RNA (piRNA)-independent manner, and promotes the nuclear translocation of RNF8 in late spermatids to catalyze histone ubiquitination and trigger histone removal. L3MBTL2 could interact with RNF8 and facilitate RNF8-dependent histone ubiquitination-related histone removal. PHF7 could recognize the H3K4me3/me2 and catalyze H2A ubiquitination to facilitate histone removal in elongating spermatids.

results in male infertility and severe defects in spermatogenesis (Ustrell et al., 2005; Khor et al., 2006). During spermiogenesis, PA200 regulatory could directly recognize acetylated histones through a bromodomain-like module and promote their ubiquitin-independent degradation. In *Pa200*-null spermatids, results showed that H2B, H3 and elevated H4K16ac could be detected at the end of the elongation stage (Qian et al., 2013). Thus, PA200 specifically recognizes acetylated histones and mediates the core histones for acetylation dependent degradation through proteasomes during spermatogenesis (**Figure 2**).

UBIQUITINATION

Ubiquitin is a 76 amino acid protein that is attached to target proteins to regulate several cellular processes, such as protein degradation, cell signaling, autophagy, DNA damage responses and so on (Hershko and Ciechanover, 1998; Pickart, 2001; Welchman et al., 2005; Komander and Rape, 2012). Ubiquitinated H2A and H2B are enriched in spermatocytes and elongating spermatids (Chen et al., 1998; Baarends et al., 1999). RNF8 is an ubiquitin E3 ligase that participates in DDR (DNA damage repair) by catalyzing the ubiquitination of H2A to promote the recruitment of some DNA damage response factors on the damage sites (Ma et al., 2011). The disruption of *Rnf8* causes significant late-stage developmental defects in spermatids due to problematic histone-to-protamine replacement, with the canonical histones being detectable in *Rnf8*-deficient mature spermatozoa (Lu et al., 2010). In *Rnf8*-null mice, both ubiquitinated H2A and H2B are decreased in the testes and H4K16ac is dramatically decreased as well (Lu et al., 2010). Further studies showed that ubiquitinated H2A and H2B were essential for the efficient recruitment of the MOF (males absent on the first) acetyltransferase complex, which is highly expressed in elongating spermatids and responsible for H4K16 acetylation in the chromatin (Akhtar and Becker, 2000; Lu et al., 2010). Thus, RNF8 catalyzed histone ubiquitination could modulate H4K16ac by regulating the localization of MOF on the chromatin and facilitate histone removal in the elongating spermatids.

The RNF8-dependent histone ubiquitination during spermiogenesis could also be modulated by PIWI protein, which is specifically expressed during germline development and enlists piRNAs (Piwi-interacting RNAs) to repress TE (transposable elements) and protect the germ cell genome integrity (Juliano et al., 2011; Siomi et al., 2011; Gou et al., 2017). In mice, *Miwi*, *Mili*, and *Miwi2*, the *Piwi* paralogs, have been identified in the testis and are required for male fertility (Deng and Lin, 2002; Kuramochi-Miyagawa et al., 2004; Carmell et al., 2007). During spermiogenesis, MIWI binds to RNF8 in the cytoplasm of early spermatids through a piRNAs-independent manner, and APC/C mediated MIWI degradation in late spermatids is essential for nuclear translocation of RNF8, which catalyzes histone ubiquitination and further facilitates histone removal (Gou et al., 2017). In both humans and mice, mutations in the conserved destruction box (D-box) of HIWI and MIWI proteins, which lead to their stabilization, cause male infertility due to impaired histone ubiquitination and histone-to-protamine transition (Gou et al., 2017). Except MIWI, L3MBTL2 (Lethal 3 malignant brain tumor like 2), a member of the MBT-domain proteins that is implicated in chromatin compaction, could also interact with RNF8. The depletion of *L3mbtl2* in germ cells affected male fertility by producing abnormal spermatozoa and the decrease of sperm counts. *L3mbtl2* deficiency also caused the reduction of in levels of the RNF8 and histone ubiquitination in elongating spermatids, which further influenced the PRM1 deposition and chromatin condensation during spermiogenesis (Meng et al., 2019).

PHF7 (PHD Finger Protein 7), which contains PHD (plant homeodomain) and RING finger domain, has been identified as a novel H2A ubiquitination E3 ligase in mouse testis (Hou et al., 2012; Wang et al., 2019). PHF7 is specifically located in the elongating spermatid nuclei, and the disruption of *Phf7* led to male mouse infertility as reduction of sperm count and the increased proportion of abnormal spermatozoa (Wang et al., 2019). PHF7 could recognize the H3K4me3/me2 through its PHD domain and catalyze H2A ubiquitination by its RING domain. In *Phf7*-null spermatids, the H2A ubiquitination was dramatically decreased that resulted in the histone retention and protamine replacement defect (**Figure 2**) (Wang et al., 2019). Therefore, PHF7 has dual roles during the histone-to-protamine transition that works as an epigenetic reader by recognizing H3K4me3/me2 and as an epigenetic writer through catalyzing H2A ubiquitination to promote histone removal.

METHYLATION

Multiple histone methylation have been identified in elongating spermatids, for instance H3K4me2, H3K4me3, H3K9me2, H3K9me3, H3K27me3, H3K79me2, and H3K79me3 (Godmann et al., 2007; Song et al., 2011; De Vries et al., 2012; Dottermusch-Heidel et al., 2014). Among them, the methylation of H3K4 and plus acetylation might help to achieve a more-open chromatin configuration, whereas H3K9 and H3K27 methylation are known to be associated with a more-repressed chromatin configuration (Rathke et al., 2014), indicating a balance of "opened" and "closed" chromatin regions during the histone-to-protamine transition. As some histone methyltransferases and demethylases are detectable during spermiogenesis (Godmann et al., 2007; Liu et al., 2010; Ushijima et al., 2012), the histone methylation may be dynamically regulated in testis. Although few mouse models exist that allow precise detection of methylation activity that directly regulates histone replacement during spermiogenesis, some studies have revealed that histone methylation may modulate the histone-to-protamine transition through some other ways. PYGO2 (Pygopus homolog 2) comprises a C-terminal PHD finger, which can recognize the H3K4me3 and is specifically located in the elongating spermatid nuclei. In mice, the reduction of *Pygo2* influenced the *Tnp*, *Prm* genes expression and caused the abnormal nuclear condensation, which further led to male sterility (Nair et al., 2008). Furthermore, PYGO2 associates with a histone acetyltransferase (HAT) activity, and the acetylation of H3 is disrupted in *Pygo2* reduced elongating spermatids (Nair et al., 2008), indicating PYGO2 may recognize H3K4me3 through its PHD domain and could recruit HAT to facilitate H3 acetylation and further histone-to-protamine transitions. As described before, PHF7 could recognize the H3K4me3/me2 and catalyze H2A ubiquitination to facilitate the histone-to-protamine transitions (Wang et al., 2019). The predominant histone methyltransferase SETD2 (SET domain–containing 2) catalyzes the H3K36me3, and knocking out *Setd2* in mouse germ cells causes aberrant spermiogenesis, resulting in complete male infertility. Moreover, the disruption of SETD2 causes complete loss of H3K36me3 and impaired activation of *Tnp* and *Prm* genes (Zuo et al., 2018), indicating H3K36me3 may regulate the histone-to-protamine transition by activating *Tnp* and *Prm* genes expression. Contrarily, JHDM2A (JmjC-domain-containing histone demethylase 2A) is an H3K9me2/1-specific demethylase. The loss of *Jhdm2a* in mice exhibits post-meiotic chromatin condensation defects and leads to male infertility. Although global H3K9 methylation has no effect in *Jhdm2a*-null testis, JHDM2A directly binds to and controls H3K9 methylation at the promoter of *Tnp1* and *Prm1* genes, which further regulates the sperm genome packaging and chromatin condensation (Okada et al., 2007).

PHOSPHORYLATION

Histone phosphorylation is involved in various cellular processes (Rossetto et al., 2012; Bao and Bedford, 2016), and dynamic histone phosphorylation have been observed during spermatogenesis (Govin et al., 2010; Bao and Bedford, 2016). The phosphorylation of histone H2AX at residue Ser139 (γH2AX) plays important roles in many biological processes, such as meiotic recombination and male sex chromosome inactivation in germ cells (Li et al., 2005). γH2AX is detectable in elongating spermatids, and TSSK6 has been identified to be responsible for the H2AX phosphorylation during spermiogenesis (Jha et al., 2017). In mice, targeted deletion of *Tssk6* leads to male sterility caused by the impairment in morphology and motility of spermatozoa (Spiridonov et al., 2005). In spermatozoa, the loss of TSSK6 blocks γH2AX formation, resulting in elevated H3, H4 and the precursor and intermediate of PRM2 (Jha et al., 2017). These results indicate that TSSK6 may mediate γH2AX to participate in the histone-to-protamine transition. H4S1 phosphorylation is highly expressed in mouse spermatocyte, round and elongating spermatids (Krishnamoorthy et al., 2006; Zhang et al., 2016). H4S1 phosphorylation has been found to be essential for chromatin compaction and concomitantly histone accessibility (Krishnamoorthy et al., 2006; Wendt and Shilatifard, 2006), suggesting that H4S1 phosphorylation is required for histone replacement during spermiogenesis. Outside the canonical histones, many phosphorylated residues have been identified, using mass spectrometry analyses, that exist on different testis-specific histone variants, such as H1T, HILS1, TH2A, TH2B (Sarg et al., 2009; Pentakota et al., 2014; Mishra et al., 2015; Luense et al., 2016; Hada et al., 2017). Although many core histones and histone variants phosphorylation have been identified in germ cells, their physiological roles need further investigation.

OTHER MODIFICATIONS

A variety of histone lysine modifications have been identified, including butyrylation, crotonylation, malonylation, propionylation, and succinylation (Tan et al., 2011; Sabari et al., 2017). Kcr (Lysine crotonylation) is a newly identified histone modification and is detectable in elongating spermatids, which regulated testis-specific genes activation in post-meiotic germ cells (Tan et al., 2011). The CDYL (chromodomain Y-like) protein, which contains a C-terminal CoAP domain that interacts with CoA to achieve its crotonyltransferase activity, may suppress the histone Kcr by converting crotonyl-CoA to β-hydroxybutyryl-CoA. Accordingly, *Cdyl*-deficient male mice show reduced fertility, decreased epididymal sperm count and sperm cell motility, and dysregulated histone Kcr (Liu et al., 2017b). In the *Cdyl*-deficient mouse testes, further analysis showed that the elevated TP1 and PRM2 were localized in a chromatin-free regions (Liu et al., 2017b), suggesting that histone crotonylation is essential for the histone-to-protamine transition during spermiogenesis.

Poly-ADP-ribosylation (PARsylation) is a common protein PTM (post-translational modification) observed in higher eukaryotes and involved in many different fundamental cellular functions. All of core histones and the linker histone H1 can be ADP-ribosylated (Gagne et al., 2006; Messner and Hottiger, 2011), which could be catalyzed by poly(ADP-ribose) polymerases, such as PARP1 and PARP2, and resolved by PARG (PAR glycohydrolase) (Gibson and Kraus, 2012). The PARP1, PARP2 and PARsylation proteins are specifically detected in elongating spermatids (Meyer-Ficca et al., 2005), and the perturbed PARsylation causes reduced male fertility with abnormal retention of core histones, H1T and HILS1 in mature spermatozoa (Meyer-Ficca et al., 2009; Meyer-Ficca et al., 2011; Meyer-Ficca et al., 2015). Thus, PARsylation is essential for the histone-to-protamine replacement, yet the precise PARsylation histone sites need further characterization.

TRANSITION PROTEINS

Between histone eviction and protamine incorporation in the nuclei of spermatids, about ninety percent of the chromatin components consist of TPs, which are arginine- and lysine-rich proteins encoded by *Tnp1* and *Tnp2* (Meistrich et al., 2003). However, the functional roles of each TP are still controversial (Rathke et al., 2014). TP1 could reduce the melting temperature of DNA and relax the DNA from core particles of nucleosome, whereas TP2 tends to compact the nucleosomal DNA by increasing its melting temperature, indicating TP2 may promote DNA condensation while TP1 facilitates the eviction of the histones (Singh and Rao, 1988; Akama et al., 1998; Kolthur-Seetharam et al., 2009; Rathke et al., 2014). However, a separate study that shown that neither TP1 nor TP2 leads to the conformation changes in supercoiled DNA (Levesque et al., 1998). These differences might reveal their unique roles during mammal spermiogenesis, as single knockout of either *Tnp1* or *Tnp2* leads to little morphological alteration of spermatozoa in mouse models. Elevated TP2 and TP1 proteins could be observed in *Tnp1*-null and *Tnp2*-null spermatids, respectively (Yu et al., 2000; Zhao et al., 2001). Thus, TP1 and TP2 may compensate for each other *in vivo*. Indeed, *Tnp1* and *Tnp2* double-knockout mice show severe abnormal spermiogenesis with a general decrease in sperm motility and abnormal sperm morphology (Shirley et al., 2004). The chromatin condensation is perturbed in the *Tnp1* and *Tnp2* double-knockout mice as severe histones retention is detectable, indicating TPs function redundantly yet have unique roles in the histone-to-protamine transition (Shirley et al., 2004; Zhao et al., 2004; Bao and Bedford, 2016).

PROTAMINES

Protamines are basic proteins that replace TPs in late spermatids (Rathke et al., 2014; Bao and Bedford, 2016). Two protamine genes (*Prm1* and *Prm2*) localize on the same chromosome in both humans and mice (Balhorn, 2007). Protamines tightly interact with DNA *via* a central arginine-rich DNA-binding domain (Balhorn, 2007). Unlike *Tnp* genes, the disruption of either *Prm1* or *Prm2* leads to the male infertility (Cho et al., 2001). Protamines have multiple PTM sites, and a total of 11 PTMs have been identified on the protamines of mouse spermatozoa, including acetylation, phosphorylation and methylation (Brunner et al., 2014). One site of interest is PRM2 S55, which is a candidate phosphorylated substrate residue of CAMK4 (Ca^{2+}/calmodulin-dependent protein kinase IV) (Wu et al., 2000). Targeted *Camk4* knockout male mice are infertile, and the transition protein displacement by PRM2 is perturbed as a specific loss of PRM2 and prolonged retention of TP2 in *Camk4*-null spermatids. *In vitro*, PRM2 could be phosphorylated by CAMK4, implicating CAMK4 mediated PRM2 phosphorylation is required for the protamine incorporation during spermiogenesis (Wu et al., 2000). Thus, the specific post-translational modifications on protamines may also be essential for the histone-to-protamine transition.

CONCLUSION AND FUTURE PERSPECTIVES

During the histone-to-protamine transition, many epigenetic regulators work together to facilitate paternal genome re-organization and packaging into the highly condensed nuclei of spermatozoa, through histone variation, specific histone modification and their related chromatin remodelers. Any defects during the histone-to-protamine transition would lead to male infertility (Bao and Bedford, 2016). While the morphological changes during spermiogenesis are well characterized, the precise molecular mechanisms underlying the chromatin re-organization, in particular the transition from histones to protamines, are still unclear. It's difficult to characterize the dynamic processes that occur during histone eviction, transition protein incorporation and protamine insertion. Moreover, 10% of the spermatozoa population in the epididymis has not yet completed the histone-to-protamine transition (Yoshida et al., 2018). These problems may be ascribed to a lack of experimental methods, which could fully recapitulate germ cell development *in vitro*. Further physiological insights may be gained by developing an *in vitro* germ-cell culture system that more accurately recapitulates the *in vivo* histone-to-protamine transition.

Many histone variants modulate histone replacement by regulating the chromatin structure; therefore, nucleosomes containing these histone variants often maintain a relatively decondensed and open chromatin configuration, facilitating histone replacement during spermiogenesis. The redundant function of histone variants in modulating chromatin configuration ensures that defects in some histone variants have a limited effect on spermatogenesis. Indeed, some mutant histone variants in mouse models are dispensable for male fertility, and mice may show elevated levels of compensatory histones or histone variants. However, the redundant function of histone variants makes it difficult to explore the precise role of each histone variant in histone replacement.

Although many histone modifications have been identified during the histone-to-protamine transition, many studies are descriptive and correlative. The direct manipulation of histone modification sites to reveal function is still urgently needed. With the development of gene editing tools, for example the CRISPR/Cas9 system, mouse models disrupting these histone modifications may be generated and used to elucidate function and *in vivo* relevance in the future. The following open-ended questions still need to be answered to provide in-depth investigation in the field.

(1) In addition to the histone variants and modifications mentioned above, what other novel histone variants and modifications participate in the histone-to-protamine transition? How can we identify them?
(2) How and where do histone variants replace canonical histones? What signal is needed to initiate replacement?
(3) As histone variants and modifications are identified that participate in the histone-to-protamine transition, how do we establish an epigenetic modulating network for this process? Which type of histone code is the initiating code?
(4) Histone hyperacetylation works as a determining event during the histone-to-protamine transition. Is this histone hyperacetylation an initial signal or an indirect consequence of prior events?
(5) What's the relationship between these histone variants and modifications? What's the mechanism underlying the cross talk between them?
(6) Chromatin assembly is modulated by histone chaperones or other chromatin remodelers. What's the functional role of histone chaperones during the histone-to-protamine transition? Which histone variants or modifications send a signal to the chaperones?
(7) How do the transition proteins replace the histone? How do protamines replace the transition proteins? What are the detailed functional roles of transition proteins?
(8) Are there still post-translational modifications that need to be discovered in order to more accurately describe how histone modification plays a role in spermatozoa maturation?

These questions and their underlying ideas need further investigation and refining to help us more thoroughly understand the complex molecular relationships and exact regulating mechanisms of the histone-to-protamine transition.

AUTHOR CONTRIBUTIONS

WT and HG wrote the manuscript and drew the figures; CL and WL proposed the idea and revised the manuscript. All authors listed have made a substantial, direct and intellectual contribution to the work and approved it for publication.

FUNDING

This work was supported by the Strategic Priority Research Program of the Chinese Academy of Sciences (Grant No. XDA16020701), the National Key R&D Program of China (grant 2016YFA0500901, 2018YFC1004202), the National Natural Science Foundation of China (grants 31771501, 91649202) and the Youth Innovation Promotion Association CAS (2018109).

ACKNOWLEDGMENTS

We thank Tracey Baas for critical reading of the manuscript.

REFERENCES

Akama, K., Sato, H., Hasegawa, S., Shimada, I., and Nakano, M. (1998). Transition protein 1 from boar late spermatid nuclei having DNA-melting activity is a dimeric protein. *Biochem. Mol. Biol. Int.* 44, 315–323. doi: 10.1080/15216549800201332

Akhtar, A., and Becker, P. B. (2000). Activation of transcription through histone H4 acetylation by MOF, an acetyltransferase essential for dosage compensation in *Drosophila*. *Mol. Cell* 5, 367–375. doi: 10.1016/S1097-2765(00)80431-1

Anuar, N. D., Kurscheid, S., Field, M., Zhang, L., Rebar, E., Gregory, P., et al. (2019). Gene editing of the multi-copy H2A.B gene and its importance for fertility. *Genome Biol.* 20, 23. doi: 10.1186/s13059-019-1633-3

Awe, S., and Renkawitz-Pohl, R. (2010). Histone H4 acetylation is essential to proceed from a histone- to a protamine-based chromatin structure in spermatid nuclei of *Drosophila melanogaster*. *Syst. Biol. in Reprod. Med.* 56, 44–61. doi: 10.3109/19396360903490790

Baarends, W. M., Hoogerbrugge, T. W., Roest, H. P., Ooms, M., Vreeburg, J., Hoeijmakers, J. H. J., et al. (1999). Histone ubiquitination and chromatin remodeling in mouse spermatogenesis. *Dev. Biol.* 207, 322–333. doi: 10.1006/dbio.1998.9155

Balhorn, R. (2007). The protamine family of sperm nuclear proteins. *Genome Biol.* 8, 1–8. doi: 10.1186/gb-2007-8-9-227

Bao, J., and Bedford, M. T. (2016). Epigenetic regulation of the histone-to-protamine transition during spermiogenesis. *Reproduction* 151, R55–R70. doi: 10.1530/REP-15-0562

Barral, S., Morozumi, Y., Tanaka, H., Montellier, E., Govin, J., De Dieuleveult, M., et al. (2017). Histone Variant H2A.L.2 Guides transition protein-dependent protamine assembly in male germ cells. *Mol. Cell* 66, 89–101 e108. doi: 10.1016/j.molcel.2017.02.025

Bednar, J., Horowitz, R. A., Grigoryev, S. A., Carruthers, L. M., Hansen, J. C., Koster, A. J., et al. (1998). Nucleosomes, linker DNA, and linker histone form a unique structural motif that directs the higher-order folding and compaction of chromatin. *Proc. Natl. Acad. Sci. U. S. A.* 95, 14173–14178. doi: 10.1073/pnas.95.24.14173

Bell, E. L., Nagamori, I., Williams, E. O., Del Rosario, A. M., Bryson, B. D., Watson, N., et al. (2014). SirT1 is required in the male germ cell for differentiation and fecundity in mice. *Development* 141, 3495–3504. doi: 10.1242/dev.110627

Berkovits, B. D., and Wolgemuth, D. J. (2013). The role of the double bromodomain-containing BET genes during mammalian spermatogenesis. *Gametogenesis* 102, 293–326. doi: 10.1016/B978-0-12-416024-8.00011-8

Boskovic, A., and Torres-Padilla, M. E. (2013). How mammals pack their sperm: a variant matter. *Genes Dev.* 27, 1635–1639. doi: 10.1101/gad.226167.113

Bramlage, B., Kosciessa, U., and Doenecke, D. (1997). Differential expression of the murine histone genes H3.3A and H3.3B. *Differentiation* 62, 13–20. doi: 10.1046/j.1432-0436.1997.6210013.x

Brunner, A. M., Nanni, P., and Mansuy, I. M. (2014). Epigenetic marking of sperm by post-translational modification of histones and protamines. *Epigenet. Chromatin* 7, 1–12. doi: 10.1186/1756-8935-7-2

Carmell, M. A., Girard, A., Van De Kant, H. J. G., Bourc'his, D., Bestor, T. H., De Rooij, D. G., et al. (2007). MIWI2 is essential for spermatogenesis and repression of transposons in the mouse male germline. *Dev. Cell* 12, 503–514. doi: 10.1016/j.devcel.2007.03.001

Chen, H. Y., Sun, J. M., Zhang, Y., Davie, J. R., and Meistrich, M. L. (1998). Ubiquitination of histone H3 in elongating spermatids of rat testes. *J. Biol. Chem.* 273, 13165–13169. doi: 10.1074/jbc.273.21.13165

Chen, P., Zhao, J. C., Wang, Y., Wang, M., Long, H. Z., Liang, D., et al. (2013). H3.3 actively marks enhancers and primes gene transcription via opening higher-ordered chromatin. *Genes Dev.* 27, 2109–2124. doi: 10.1101/gad.222174.113

Cho, C., Willis, W. D., Goulding, E. H., Haesook, J. H., Choi, Y. C., Hecht, N. B., and Eddy, E. M. (2001). Haploinsufficiency of protamine-1 or-2 causes infertility in mice. *Nat. Genet.* 28, 82–86. doi: 10.1038/ng0501-82

Churikov, D., Siino, J., Svetlova, M., Zhang, K. L., Gineitis, A., Bradbury, E. M., et al. (2004). Novel human testis-specific histone H2B encoded by the interrupted gene on the X chromosome. *Genomics* 84, 745–756. doi: 10.1016/j.ygeno.2004.06.001

Couldrey, C., Carlton, M. B. L., Nolan, P. M., Colledge, W. H., and Evans, M. J. (1999). A retroviral gene trap insertion into the histone 3.3A gene causes partial neonatal lethality, stunted growth, neuromuscular deficits and male sub-fertility in transgenic mice. *Hum. Mol. Genet.* 8, 2489–2495. doi: 10.1093/hmg/8.13.2489

De Vries, M., Ramos, L., Housein, Z., and De Boer, P. (2012). Chromatin remodelling initiation during human spermiogenesis. *Biol. Open* 1, 446–457. doi: 10.1242/bio.2012844

Delucia, F., Faraonemennella, M. R., Derme, M., Quesada, P., Caiafa, P., and Farina, B. (1994). Histone-induced condensation of rat testis chromatin—testis-specific H1t versus somatic H1 variants. *Biochem. Biophys. Res. Commun.* 198, 32–39. doi: 10.1006/bbrc.1994.1005

Deng, W., and Lin, H. F. (2002). Miwi, a murine homolog of Piwi, encodes a cytoplasmic protein essential for spermatogenesis. *Dev. Cell* 2, 819–830. doi: 10.1016/S1534-5807(02)00165-X

Dhar, S., Thota, A., and Rao, M. R. S. (2012). Insights into role of bromodomain, testis-specific (Brdt) in acetylated histone H4-dependent chromatin remodeling in mammalian spermiogenesis. *J. Biol. Chem.* 287, 6387–6405. doi: 10.1074/jbc.M111.288167

Dong, Y., Isono, K., Ohbo, K., Endo, T. A., Ohara, O., Maekawa, M., et al. (2017). EPC1/TIP60-mediated histone acetylation facilitates spermiogenesis in mice. *Mol. Cell. Biol.* 37, e00082-17. doi: 10.1128/MCB.00082-17

Dottermusch-Heidel, C., Klaus, E. S., Gonzalez, N. H., Bhushan, S., Meinhardt, A., Bergmann, M., et al. (2014). H3K79 methylation directly precedes the histone-to-protamine transition in mammalian spermatids and is sensitive to bacterial infections. *Andrology* 2, 655–665. doi: 10.1111/j.2047-2927.2014.00248.x

Doyon, Y., Selleck, W., Lane, W. S., Tan, S., and Cote, J. (2004). Structural and functional conservation of the NuA4 histone acetyltransferase complex from yeast to humans. *Mol. Cell. Biol.* 24, 1884–1896. doi: 10.1128/MCB.24.5.1884-1896.2004

Drabent, B., Benavente, R., and Hoyer-Fender, S. (2003). Histone H1t is not replaced by H1.1 or H1.2 in pachytene spermatocytes or spermatids of H1t-deficient mice. *Cytogenet. Genome Res.* 103, 307–313. doi: 10.1159/000076818

Drabent, B., Bode, C., Bramlage, B., and Doenecke, D. (1996). Expression of the mouse testicular histone gene H1t during spermatogenesis. *Histochem. Cell Biol.* 106, 247–251. doi: 10.1007/BF02484408

Drabent, B., Saftig, P., Bode, C., and Doenecke, D. (2000). Spermatogenesis proceeds normally in mice without linker histone H1t. *Histochem. Cell Biol.* 113, 433–442.

Fantz, D. A., Hatfield, W. R., Horvath, G., Kistler, M. K., and Kistler, W. S. (2001). Mice with a targeted disruption of the H1t gene are fertile and undergo normal changes in structural chromosomal proteins during spermiogenesis. *Biol. Reprod.* 64, 425–431. doi: 10.1095/biolreprod64.2.425

Gagne, J. P., Hendzel, M. J., Droit, A., and Poirier, G. G. (2006). The expanding role of poly(ADP-ribose) metabolism: current challenges and new perspectives. *Curr. Opin. Cell Biol.* 18, 145–151. doi: 10.1016/j.ceb.2006.02.013

Gaucher, J., Boussouar, F., Montellier, E., Curtet, S., Buchou, T., Bertrand, S., et al. (2012). Bromodomain-dependent stage-specific male genome programming by Brdt. *EMBO J.* 31, 3809–3820. doi: 10.1038/emboj.2012.233

Gibson, B. A., and Kraus, W. L. (2012). New insights into the molecular and cellular functions of poly(ADP-ribose) and PARPs. *Nat. Rev. Mol. Cell Biol.* 13, 411–424. doi: 10.1038/nrm3376

Godmann, M., Auger, V., Ferraroni-Aguiar, V., Di Sauro, A., Sette, C., Behr, R., et al. (2007). Dynamic regulation of histone h3 methylation at lysine 4 in mammalian spermatogenesis. *Biol. Reprod.* 77, 754–764. doi: 10.1095/biolreprod.107.062265

Gou, L. T., Kang, J. Y., Dai, P., Wang, X., Li, F., Zhao, S., et al. (2017). Ubiquitination-deficient mutations in human Piwi cause male infertility by impairing histone-to-protamine exchange during spermiogenesis. *Obstet. Gynecol. Survey* 72, 540–541. doi: 10.1097/OGX.0000000000000482

Govin, J., Caron, C., Lestrat, C., Rousseaux, S., and Khochbin, S. (2004). The role of histones in chromatin remodelling during mammalian spermiogenesis. *Eur. J. Biochem.* 271, 3459–3469. doi: 10.1111/j.1432-1033.2004.04266.x

Govin, J., Dorsey, J., Gaucher, J., Rousseaux, S., Khochbin, S., and Berger, S. L. (2010). Systematic screen reveals new functional dynamics of histones H3 and H4 during gametogenesis. *Genes Dev.* 24, 1772–1786. doi: 10.1101/gad.1954910

Govin, J., Escoffier, E., Rousseaux, S., Kuhn, L., Ferro, M., Thevenon, J., et al. (2007). Pericentric heterochromatin reprogramming by new histone variants during mouse spermiogenesis. *J. Cell Biol.* 176, 283–294. doi: 10.1083/jcb.200604141

Govin, J., Lestrat, C., Caron, C., Pivot-Pajot, C., Rousseaux, S., and Khochbin, S. (2006). Histone acetylation-mediated chromatin compaction during mouse spermatogenesis. *Cancer Ther.* 57, 155–15+. doi: 10.1007/3-540-37633-X_9

Grimes, S. R., and Henderson, N. (1984a). Acetylation of rat testis histones H2b and Th2b. *Dev. Biol.* 101, 516–521. doi: 10.1016/0012-1606(84)90165-9

Grimes, S. R. Jr., and Henderson, N. (1984b). Hyperacetylation of histone H4 in rat testis spermatids. *Exp. Cell Res.* 152, 91–97. doi: 10.1016/0014-4827(84)90232-5

Hada, M., Masuda, K., Yamaguchi, K., Shirahige, K., and Okada, Y. (2017). Identification of a variant-specific phosphorylation of TH2A during spermiogenesis. *Sci. Rep.* 7, 1–13. doi: 10.1038/srep46228

Hao, S. L., Ni, F. D., and Yang, W. X. (2019). The dynamics and regulation of chromatin remodeling during spermiogenesis. *Gene* 706, 201–210. doi: 10.1016/j.gene.2019.05.027

Happel, N., and Doenecke, D. (2009). Histone H1 and its isoforms: contribution to chromatin structure and function. *Gene* 431, 1–12. doi: 10.1016/j.gene.2008.11.003

Hazzouri, M., Pivot-Pajot, C., Faure, A. K., Usson, Y., Pelletier, R., Sele, B., et al. (2000). Regulated hyperacetylation of core histones during mouse spermatogenesis: involvement of histone-deacetylases. *Eur. J. Cell Biol.* 79, 950–960. doi: 10.1078/0171-9335-00123

Hershko, A., and Ciechanover, A. (1998). The ubiquitin system. *Annu. Rev. Biochem.* 67, 425–479. doi: 10.1146/annurev.biochem.67.1.425

Hess, R. A., and Renato De Franca, L. (2008). Spermatogenesis and cycle of the seminiferous epithelium. *Adv. Exp. Med. Biol.* 636, 1–15. doi: 10.1007/978-0-387-09597-4_1

Hoghoughi, N., Barral, S., Vargas, A., Rousseaux, S., and Khochbin, S. (2018). Histone variants: essential actors in male genome programming. *J. Biochem.* 163, 97–103. doi: 10.1093/jb/mvx079

Hou, X., Zhang, W., Xiao, Z., Gan, H., Lin, X., Liao, S., et al. (2012). Mining and characterization of ubiquitin E3 ligases expressed in the mouse testis. *BMC Genomics* 13, 495. doi: 10.1186/1471-2164-13-495

Jha, K. N., Tripurani, S. K., and Johnson, G. R. (2017). TSSK6 is required for gamma H2AX formation and the histone-to-protamine transition during spermiogenesis. *J. Cell Sci.* 130, 1835–1844. doi: 10.1242/jcs.202721

Juliano, C., Wang, J. Q., and Lin, H. F. (2011). Uniting germline and stem cells: the function of Piwi proteins and the piRNA pathway in diverse organisms. *Ann. Rev. Genet.* 45, 447–469. doi: 10.1146/annurev-genet-110410-132541

Kan, P. Y., Caterino, T. L., and Hayes, J. J. (2009). The H4 tail domain participates in intra- and internucleosome interactions with protein and DNA during folding and oligomerization of nucleosome arrays. *Mol. Cell. Biol.* 29, 538–546. doi: 10.1128/MCB.01343-08

Ketchum, C. C., Larsen, C. D., Mcneil, A., Meyer-Ficca, M. L., and Meyer, R. G. (2018). Early histone H4 acetylation during chromatin remodeling in equine spermatogenesis. *Biol. Reprod.* 98, 115–129. doi: 10.1093/biolre/iox159

Khadake, J. R., and Rao, M. R. S. (1995). DNA-condensing and chromatin-condensing properties of rat testes Hla and hit compared to those of rat-liver Hlbdec—Hlt is a poor condenser of chromatin. *Biochemistry* 34, 15792–15801. doi: 10.1021/bi00048a025

Khor, B., Bredemeyer, A. L., Huang, C. Y., Turnbull, I. R., Evans, R., Maggi, L. B., et al. (2006). Proteasome activator PA200 is required for normal spermatogenesis. *Mol. Cell. Biol.* 26, 2999–3007. doi: 10.1128/MCB.26.8.2999-3007.2006

Kimura, S., and Loppin, B. (2016). The *Drosophila* chromosomal protein Mst77F is processed to generate an essential component of mature sperm chromatin. *Open Biol.* 6, 1–12. doi: 10.1098/rsob.160207

Kolthur-Seetharam, U., Pradeepa, M. M., Gupta, N., Narayanaswamy, R., and Rao, M.R.S. (2009). Spatiotemporal organization of AT- and GC-rich DNA and their association with transition proteins TP1 and TP2 in rat condensing spermatids. *J. Histochem. Cytochem.* 57, 951–962. doi: 10.1369/jhc.2009.953414

Komander, D., and Rape, M. (2012). The ubiquitin code. *Ann. Rev. Biochem.* 81, 203–229. doi: 10.1146/annurev-biochem-060310-170328

Kowalski, A., and Palyga, J. (2012). Linker histone subtypes and their allelic variants. *Cell Biol. Int.* 36, 981–996. doi: 10.1042/CBI20120133

Krishnamoorthy, T., Chen, X., Govin, J., Cheung, W. L., Dorsey, J., Schindler, K., et al. (2006). Phosphorylation of histone H4 Ser1 regulates sporulation in yeast and is conserved in fly and mouse spermatogenesis. *Genes Dev.* 20, 2580–2592. doi: 10.1101/gad.1457006

Kuramochi-Miyagawa, S., Kimura, T., Ijiri, T. W., Isobe, T., Asada, N., Fujita, Y., et al. (2004). Mili, a mammalian member of piwi family gene, is essential for spermatogenesis. *Development* 131, 839–849. doi: 10.1242/dev.00973

Lee, J., Park, H. S., Kim, H. H., Yun, Y. J., Lee, D. R., and Lee, S. (2009). Functional polymorphism in H2BFWT-5'UTR is associated with susceptibility to male infertility. *J. Cell. Mol. Med.* 13, 1942–1951. doi: 10.1111/j.1582-4934.2009.00830.x

Levesque, D., Veilleux, S., Caron, N., and Boissonneault, G. (1998). Architectural DNA-binding properties of the spermatidal transition proteins 1 and 2. *Biochem. Biophys. Res. Commun.* 252, 602–609. doi: 10.1006/bbrc.1998.9687

Li, A., Eirin-Lopez, J., and Ausio, J. (2005). H2AX: tailoring histone H2A for chromatin-dependent genomic integrity. *Biochem. Cell Biol.* 83, 505–515. doi: 10.1139/o05-114

Liu, C., Song, Z. H., Wang, L. N., Yu, H. Y., Liu, W. X., Shang, Y. L., et al. (2017a). Sirt1 regulates acrosome biogenesis by modulating autophagic flux during spermiogenesis in mice. *Development* 144, 441–451. doi: 10.1242/dev.147074

Liu, S. M., Yu, H. J., Liu, Y. Q., Liu, X. H., Zhang, Y., Bu, C., et al. (2017b). Chromodomain protein CDYL acts as a crotonyl-CoA hydratase to regulate histone crotonylation and spermatogenesis. *Mol. Cell* 67, 853–85+. doi: 10.1016/j.molcel.2017.07.011

Liu, Z. L., Zhou, S. L., Liao, L., Chen, X., Meistrich, M., and Xu, J. M. (2010). Jmjd1a Demethylase-regulated histone modification is essential for cAMP-response element modulator-regulated gene expression and spermatogenesis. *J. Biol. Chem.* 285, 2758–2770. doi: 10.1074/jbc.M109.066845

Lu, L. Y., Wu, J. X., Ye, L., Gavrilina, G. B., Saunders, T. L., and Yu, X. C. (2010). RNF8-dependent histone modifications regulate nucleosome removal during spermatogenesis. *Dev. Cell* 18, 371–384. doi: 10.1016/j.devcel.2010.01.010

Luense, L. J., Wang, X. S., Schon, S. B., Weller, A. H., Shiao, E. L., Bryant, J. M., et al. (2016). Comprehensive analysis of histone post-translational modifications in mouse and human male germ cells. *Epigenet. Chromatin* 9, 1–15. doi: 10.1186/s13072-016-0072-6

Ma, T., Keller, J. A., and Yu, X. C. (2011). RNF8-dependent histone ubiquitination during DNA damage response and spermatogenesis. *Acta Biochim. Biophys. Sin.* 43, 339–345. doi: 10.1093/abbs/gmr016

Manterola, M., Brown, T. M., Oh, M. Y., Garyn, C., Gonzalez, B. J., and Wolgemuth, D. J. (2018). BRDT is an essential epigenetic regulator for proper chromatin organization, silencing of sex chromosomes and crossover formation in male meiosis. *PLoS Genet.* 14, 1–30. doi: 10.1371/journal.pgen.1007209

Martianov, I., Brancorsini, S., Catena, R., Gansmuller, A., Kotaja, N., Parvinen, M., et al. (2005). Polar nuclear localization of H1T2, a histone H1 variant, required for spermatid elongation and DNA condensation during spermiogenesis. *Proc. Natl Acad. Sci. U. S. A.* 102, 2808–2813. doi: 10.1073/pnas.0406060102

Mccarrey, J. R., Geyer, C. B., and Yoshioka, H. (2005). Epigenetic regulation of testis-specific gene expression. *Testicular Cell Dyn. Endocr. Signal.* 1061, 226–242. doi: 10.1196/annals.1336.025

Meistrich, M. L., Bucci, L. R., Trostleweige, P. K., and Brock, W. A. (1985). Histone variants in rat spermatogonia and primary spermatocytes. *Dev. Biol.* 112, 230–240. doi: 10.1016/0012-1606(85)90137-X

Meistrich, M. L., Mohapatra, B., Shirley, C. R., and Zhao, M. (2003). Roles of transition nuclear proteins in spermiogenesis. *Chromosoma* 111, 483–488. doi: 10.1007/s00412-002-0227-z

Meng, C., Liao, J., Zhao, D., Huang, H., Qin, J., Lee, T. L., et al. (2019). L3MBTL2 regulates chromatin remodeling during spermatogenesis. *Cell Death Differ.* 13, 1–14. doi: 10.1038/s41418-019-0283-z

Messner, S., and Hottiger, M. O. (2011). Histone ADP-ribosylation in DNA repair, replication and transcription. *Trends Cell Biol.* 21, 534–542. doi: 10.1016/j.tcb.2011.06.001

Meyer-Ficca, M. L., Ihara, M., Bader, J. J., Leu, N. A., Beneke, S., and Meyer, R. G. (2015). Spermatid head elongation with normal nuclear shaping requires ADP-ribosyltransferase PARP11 (ARTD11) in Mice. *Biol. Reprod.* 92, 1–13. doi: 10.1095/biolreprod.114.123661

Meyer-Ficca, M. L., Ihara, M., Lonchar, J. D., Meistrich, M. L., Austin, C. A., Min, W., et al. (2011). Poly(ADP-ribose) metabolism is essential for proper nucleoprotein exchange during mouse spermiogenesis. *Biol. Reprod.* 84, 218–228. doi: 10.1095/biolreprod.110.087361

Meyer-Ficca, M. L., Lonchar, J., Credidio, C., Ihara, M., Li, Y., Wang, Z. Q., et al. (2009). Disruption of poly(ADP-ribose) homeostasis affects spermiogenesis and sperm chromatin integrity in mice. *Biol. Reprod.* 81, 46–55. doi: 10.1095/biolreprod.108.075390

Meyer-Ficca, M. L., Scherthan, H., Burkle, A., and Meyer, R. G. (2005). Poly(ADP-ribosyl)ation during chromatin remodeling steps in rat spermiogenesis. *Chromosoma* 114, 67–74. doi: 10.1007/s00412-005-0344-6

Mishra, L. N., Gupta, N., and Rao, S. M. R. (2015). Mapping of post-translational modifications of spermatid-specific linker histone H1-like protein, HILS1. *J. Proteomics* 128, 218–230. doi: 10.1016/j.jprot.2015.08.001

Mishra, L. N., Shalini, V., Gupta, N., Ghosh, K., Suthar, N., Bhaduri, U., et al. (2018). Spermatid-specific linker histone HILS1 is a poor condenser of DNA and chromatin and preferentially associates with LINE-1 elements. *Epigenet. Chromatin* 11, 1–21. doi: 10.1186/s13072-018-0214-0

Montellier, E., Boussouar, F., Rousseaux, S., Zhang, K., Buchou, T., Fenaille, F., et al. (2013). Chromatin-to-nucleoprotamine transition is controlled by the histone H2B variant TH2B. *Genes Dev.* 27, 1680–1692. doi: 10.1101/gad.220095.113

Moss, S. B., and Orth, J. M. (1993). Localization of a spermatid-specific histone-2b protein in mouse spermiogenic cells. *Biol. Reprod.* 48, 1047–1056. doi: 10.1095/biolreprod48.5.1047

Nair, M., Nagamori, I., Sun, P., Mishra, D. P., Rheaume, C., Li, B., et al. (2008). Nuclear regulator Pygo2 controls spermiogenesis and histone H3 acetylation. *Dev. Biol.* 320, 446–455. doi: 10.1016/j.ydbio.2008.05.553

Okada, Y., Scott, G., Ray, M. K., Mishina, Y., and Zhang, Y. (2007). Histone demethylase JHDM2A is critical for Tnp1 and Prm1 transcription and spermatogenesis. *Nature* 450, 119–11+. doi: 10.1038/nature06236

Oliva, R., Bazett-Jones, D., Mezquita, C., and Dixon, G. H. (1987). Factors affecting nucleosome disassembly by protamines *in vitro*. Histone hyperacetylation and chromatin structure, time dependence, and the size of the sperm nuclear proteins. *J. Biol. Chem.* 262, 17016–17025.

Oliva, R., and Mezquita, C. (1986). Marked differences in the ability of distinct protamines to disassemble nucleosomal core particles in vitro. *Biochemistry* 25, 6508–6511. doi: 10.1021/bi00369a025

Padavattan, S., Shinagawa, T., Hasegawa, K., Kumasaka, T., Ishii, S., and Kumarevel, T. (2015). Structural and functional analyses of nucleosome complexes with mouse histone variants TH2a and TH2b, involved in reprogramming. *Biochem. Biophys. Res. Commun.* 464, 929–935. doi: 10.1016/j.bbrc.2015.07.070

Padavattan, S., Thiruselvam, V., Shinagawa, T., Hasegawa, K., Kumasaka, T., Ishii, S., et al. (2017). Structural analyses of the nucleosome complexes with human testis-specific histone variants, hTh2a and hTh2b. *Biophys. Chem.* 221, 41–48. doi: 10.1016/j.bpc.2016.11.013

Pentakota, S. K., Sandhya, S., Sikarwar, A. P., Chandra, N., and Rao, M. R. S. (2014). Mapping post-translational modifications of mammalian testicular specific histone variant TH2B in tetraploid and haploid germ cells and their implications on the dynamics of nucleosome structure. *J. Proteome Res.* 13, 5603–5617. doi: 10.1021/pr500597a

Pickart, C. M. (2001). Mechanisms underlying ubiquitination. *Annu. Rev. Biochem.* 70, 503–533. doi: 10.1146/annurev.biochem.70.1.503

Pivot-Pajot, C., Caron, C., Govin, M., Vion, A., Rousseaux, S., and Khochbin, S. (2003). Acetylation-dependent chromatin reorganization by BRDT, a testis-specific bromodomain-containing protein. *Mol. Cell. Biol.* 23, 5354–5365. doi: 10.1128/MCB.23.15.5354-5365.2003

Qian, M. X., Pang, Y., Liu, C. H., Haratake, K., Du, B. Y., Ji, D. Y., et al. (2013). Acetylation-mediated proteasomal degradation of core histones during DNA repair and spermatogenesis. *Cell* 153, 1012–1024. doi: 10.1016/j.cell.2013.04.032

Rafatmanesh, A., Nikzad, H., Ebrahimi, A., Karimian, M., and Zamani, T. (2018). Association of the c.-9C > T and c.368A > G transitions in H2BFWT gene with male infertility in an Iranian population. *Andrologia* 50, 1–6. doi: 10.1111/and.12805

Raja, S. J., and Renkawitz-Pohl, R. (2005). Replacement by *Drosophila melanogaster* protamines and Mst77F of histones during chromatin condensation in late spermatids and role of sesame in the removal of these proteins from the male pronucleus. *Mol. Cell. Biol.* 25, 6165–6177. doi: 10.1128/MCB.25.14.6165-6177.2005

Rathke, C., Baarends, W. M., Awe, S., and Renkawitz-Pohl, R. (2014). Chromatin dynamics during spermiogenesis. *Biochim. Biophys. Acta* 1839, 155–168. doi: 10.1016/j.bbagrm.2013.08.004

Roosen-Runge, E. C. (1962). The process of spermatogenesis in mammals. *Biol. Rev. Camb Philos. Soc.* 37, 343–377. doi: 10.1111/j.1469-185X.1962.tb01616.x

Rossetto, D., Avvakumov, N., and Cote, J. (2012). Histone phosphorylation A chromatin modification involved in diverse nuclear events. *Epigenetics* 7, 1098–1108. doi: 10.4161/epi.21975

Sabari, B. R., Zhang, D., Allis, C. D., and Zhao, Y. M. (2017). Metabolic regulation of gene expression through histone acylations. *Nat. Rev. Mol. Cell Biol.* 18, 90–101. doi: 10.1038/nrm.2016.140

Sarg, B., Chwatal, S., Talasz, H., and Lindner, H. H. (2009). Testis-specific linker histone H1t is multiply phosphorylated during spermatogenesis identification of phosphorylation siTES. *J. Biol. Chem.* 284, 3610–3618. doi: 10.1074/jbc.M805925200

Shang, E. Y., Nickerson, H. D., Wen, D. C., Wang, X. Y., and Wolgemuth, D. J. (2007). The first bromodomain of Brdt, a testis-specific member of the BET sub-family of double-bromodomain-containing proteins, is essential for male germ cell differentiation. *Development* 134, 3507–3515. doi: 10.1242/dev.004481

Shinagawa, T., Huynh, L. M., Takagi, T., Tsukamoto, D., Tomaru, C., Kwak, H. G., et al. (2015). Disruption of Th2a and Th2b genes causes defects in spermatogenesis. *Development* 142, 1287–1292. doi: 10.1242/dev.121830

Shiraishi, K., Shindo, A., Harada, A., Ohkawa, Y., Kurumizaka, H., Kimura, H., et al. (2017). Roles of histone H3.5 in human spermatogenesis and spermatogenic disorders. *J. Urol.* 197, E85–E85. doi: 10.1016/j.juro.2017.02.277

Shires, A., Carpenter, M. P., and Chalkley, R. (1975). New histones found in mature mammalian testes. *Proc. Natl. Acad. Sci. U. S. A.* 72, 2714–2718. doi: 10.1073/pnas.72.7.2714

Shires, A., Carpenter, M. P., and Chalkley, R. (1976). Cysteine-containing H2b-like histone found in mature mammalian testis. *J. Biol. Chem.* 251, 4155–4158.

Shirley, C. R., Hayashi, S., Mounsey, S., Yanagimachi, R., and Meistrich, M. L. (2004). Abnormalities and reduced reproductive potential of sperm from Tnp1- and Tnp2-null double mutant mice. *Biol. Reprod.* 71, 1220–1229. doi: 10.1095/biolreprod.104.029363

Shogren-Knaak, M., Ishii, H., Sun, J. M., Pazin, M. J., Davie, J. R., and Peterson, C. L. (2006). Histone H4-K16 acetylation controls chromatin structure and protein interactions. *Science* 311, 844–847. doi: 10.1126/science.1124000

Singh, J., and Rao, M. R. S. (1988). Interaction of rat testis protein, Tp, with nucleosome core particle. *Biochem. Int.* 17, 701–710.

Siomi, M. C., Sato, K., Pezic, D., and Aravin, A. A. (2011). PIWI-interacting small RNAs: the vanguard of genome defence. *Nat. Rev. Mol. Cell Biol.* 12, 246–258. doi: 10.1038/nrm3089

Soboleva, T. A., Nekrasov, M., Pahwa, A., Williams, R., Huttley, G. A., and Tremethick, D. J. (2012). A unique H2A histone variant occupies the transcriptional start site of active genes. *Nat. Struct. Mol. Biol.* 19, 25–U37. doi: 10.1038/nsmb.2161

Soboleva, T. A., Parker, B. J., Nekrasov, M., Hart-Smith, G., Tay, Y. J., Tng, W. Q., et al. (2017). A new link between transcriptional initiation and pre-mRNA splicing: the RNA binding histone variant H2A.B. *PloS Genet.* 13, 1–31. doi: 10.1371/journal.pgen.1006633

Song, N., Liu, J., An, S. C., Nishino, T., Hishikawa, Y., and Koji, T. (2011). Immunohistochemical analysis of histone H3 modifications in germ cells during mouse spermatogenesis. *Acta Histochem. Cytochem.* 44, 183–190. doi: 10.1267/ahc.11027

Spiridonov, N. A., Wong, L., Zerfas, P. M., Starost, M. F., Pack, S. D., Paweletz, C. P., et al. (2005). Identification and characterization of SSTK, a serine/threonine protein kinase essential for male fertility. *Mol. Cell. Biol.* 25, 4250–4261. doi: 10.1128/MCB.25.10.4250-4261.2005

Stadtmueller, B. M., and Hill, C. P. (2011). Proteasome Activators. *Mol. Cell* 41, 8–19. doi: 10.1016/j.molcel.2010.12.020

Tachiwana, H., Kagawa, W., Osakabe, A., Kawaguchi, K., Shiga, T., Hayashi-Takanaka, Y., et al. (2010). Structural basis of instability of the nucleosome containing a testis-specific histone variant, human H3T. *Proc. Natl. Acad. Sci. U. S. A.* 107, 10454–10459. doi: 10.1073/pnas.1003064107

Talbert, P. B., and Henikoff, S. (2010). Histone variants - ancient wrap artists of the epigenome. *Nat. Rev. Mol. Cell Biol.* 11, 264–275. doi: 10.1038/nrm2861

Tan, M. J., Luo, H., Lee, S., Jin, F. L., Yang, J. S., Montellier, E., et al. (2011). Identification of 67 histone marks and histone lysine crotonylation as a new type of histone modification. *Cell* 146, 1015–1027. doi: 10.1016/j.cell.2011.08.008

Tanaka, H., Iguchi, N., Isotani, A., Kitamura, K., Toyama, Y., Matsuoka, Y., et al. (2005). HANP1/H1T2, a novel histone H1-like protein involved in nuclear formation and sperm fertility. *Mol. Cell. Biol.* 25, 7107–7119. doi: 10.1128/MCB.25.16.7107-7119.2005

Tang, M. C. W., Jacobs, S. A., Mattiske, D. M., Soh, Y. M., Graham, A. N., Tran, A., et al. (2015). Contribution of the two genes encoding histone variant H3.3 to viability and fertility in mice. *PloS Genet.* 11, 1–23. doi: 10.1371/journal.pgen.1004964

Teimouri, M., Najaran, H., Hosseinzadeh, A., and Mazoochi, T. (2018). Association between two common transitions of H2BFWT gene and male infertility: a case-control, meta, and structural analysis. *Andrology* 6, 306–316. doi: 10.1111/andr.12464

Thakar, A., Gupta, P., Ishibashi, T., Finn, R., Silva-Moreno, B., Uchiyama, S., Fukui, et al. (2009). H2A.Z and H3.3 histone variants affect nucleosome structure: biochemical and biophysical studies. *Biochemistry* 48, 10852–10857. doi: 10.1021/bi901129e

Trostleweige, P. K., Meistrich, M. L., Brock, W. A., Nishioka, K., and Bremer, J. W. (1982). Isolation and characterization of Th2a, a germ cell-specific variant of histone-2a in rat testis. *J. Biol. Chem.* 257, 5560–5567.

Tse, C., Sera, T., Wolffe, A. P., and Hansen, J. C. (1998). Disruption of higher-order folding by core histone acetylation dramatically enhances transcription of nucleosomal arrays by RNA polymerase III. *Mol. Cell. Biol.* 18, 4629–4638. doi: 10.1128/MCB.18.8.4629

Ueda, J., Harada, A., Urahama, T., Machida, S., Maehara, K., Hada, M., et al. (2017). Testis-specific histone variant H3t gene is essential for entry into spermatogenesis. *Cell Rep.* 18, 593–600. doi: 10.1016/j.celrep.2016.12.065

Unni, E., Zhang, Y., Kangasniemi, M., Saperstein, W., Moss, S. B., and Meistrich, M. L. (1995). Stage-specific distribution of the spermatid-specific histone 2b in the rat testis. *Biol. Reprod.* 53, 820–826. doi: 10.1095/biolreprod53.4.820

Urahama, T., Harada, A., Maehara, K., Horikoshi, N., Sato, K., Sato, Y., et al.(2016). Histone H3.5 forms an unstable nucleosome and accumulates around transcription start sites in human testis. *Epigenet. Chromatin* 9, 1–16. doi: 10.1186/s13072-016-0051-y

Urahama, T., Horikoshi, N., Osakabe, A., Tachiwana, H., and Kurumizaka, H. (2014). Structure of human nucleosome containing the testis-specific histone variant TSH2B. *Acta Crystallogr. Sect. F-Struct. Biol. Commun.* 70, 444–449. doi: 10.1107/S2053230X14004695

Ushijima, Y., Inoue, Y. H., Konishi, T., Kitazawa, D., Yoshida, H., Shimaji, K., et al. (2012). Roles of histone H3K9 methyltransferases during *Drosophila* spermatogenesis. *Chrom. Res.* 20, 319–331. doi: 10.1007/s10577-012-9276-1

Ustrell, V., Pratt, G., Gorbea, C., and Rechsteiner, M. (2005). Purification and assay of proteasome activator PA200. *Methods Enzymol.* 398, 321–329. doi: 10.1016/S0076-6879(05)98026-9

Van Der Heijden, G. W., Derijck, A. a. H. A., Posfai, E., Giele, M., Pelczar, P., Ramos, L., et al. (2007). Chromosome-wide nucleosome replacement and H3.3 incorporation during mammalian meiotic sex chromosome inactivation. *Nat. Genet.* 39, 251–258. doi: 10.1038/ng1949

Wang, X., Kang, J. Y., Wei, L., Yang, X., Sun, H., Yang, S., et al. (2019). PHF7 is a novel histone H2A E3 ligase prior to histone-to-protamine exchange during spermiogenesis. *Development* 146, 1–11. doi: 10.1242/dev.175547

Welchman, R. L., Gordon, C., and Mayer, R. J. (2005). Ubiquitin and ubiquitin-like proteins as multifunctional signals. *Nat. Rev. Mol. Cell. Biol.* 6, 599–609. doi: 10.1038/nrm1700

Wendt, K. D., and Shilatifard, A. (2006). Packing for the germy: the role of histone H4 Ser1 phosphorylation in chromatin compaction and germ cell development. *Genes Dev.* 20, 2487–2491. doi: 10.1101/gad.1477706

Wu, J. Y., Ribar, T. J., Cummings, D. E., Burton, K. A., Mcknight, G. S., and Means, A. R. (2000). Spermiogenesis and exchange of basic nuclear proteins are impaired in male germ cells lacking Camk4. *Nat. Genet.* 25, 448–452. doi: 10.1038/78153

Yan, W., Ma, L., Burns, K. H., and Matzuk, M. M. (2003). HILS1 is a spermatid-specific linker histone H1-like protein implicated in chromatin remodeling during mammalian spermiogenesis. *Proc. Natl. Acad. Sci. U. S. A.* 100, 10546–10551. doi: 10.1073/pnas.1837812100

Ying, H. Q., Scott, M. B., and Zhou-Cun, A. (2012). Relationship of SNP of H2BFWT gene to male infertility in a Chinese population with idiopathic spermatogenesis impairment. *Biomarkers* 17, 402–406. doi: 10.3109/1354750X.2012.677066

Yoshida, K., Muratani, M., Araki, H., Miura, F., Suzuki, T., Dohmae, N., et al. (2018). Mapping of histone-binding sites in histone replacement-completed spermatozoa. *Nat. Commun.* 9, 1–11. doi: 10.1038/s41467-018-06243-9

Yu, Y. E., Zhang, Y., Unni, E., Shirley, C. R., Deng, J. M., Russell, L. D., et al. (2000). Abnormal spermatogenesis and reduced fertility in transition nuclear protein 1-deficient mice. *Proc. Natl. Acad. Sci. U. S. A.* 97, 4683–4688. doi: 10.1073/pnas.97.9.4683

Yuen, B.T.K., Bush, K. M., Barrilleaux, B. L., Cotterman, R., and Knoepfler, P. S. (2014). Histone H3.3 regulates dynamic chromatin states during spermatogenesis. *Development* 141, 3483–3494. doi: 10.1242/dev.106450

Zhang, Z. H., Mu, S. M., Guo, M. S., Wu, J. L., Li, Y. Q., Zhang, H., et al. (2016). Dynamics of histone H2A, H4 and HS1ph during spermatogenesis with a focus on chromatin condensation and maturity of spermatozoa. *Sci. Rep.* 6, 1–11. doi: 10.1038/srep25089

Zhao, M., Shirley, C. R., Mounsey, S., and Meistrich, M. L. (2004). Nucleoprotein transitions during spermiogenesis in mice with transition nuclear protein Tnp1 and Tnp2 mutations. *Biol. Reprod.* 71, 1016–1025. doi: 10.1095/biolreprod.104.028191

Zhao, M., Shirley, C. R., Yu, Y. E., Mohapatra, B., Zhang, Y., Unni, E., et al. (2001). Targeted disruption of the transition protein 2 gene affects sperm chromatin structure and reduces fertility in mice. *Mol. Cell Biol.* 21, 7243–7255. doi: 10.1128/MCB.21.21.7243-7255.2001

Zuo, X. L., Rong, B. W., Li, L., Lv, R. T., Lan, F., and Tong, M. H. (2018). The histone methyltransferase SETD2 is required for expression of acrosin-binding protein 1 and protamines and essential for spermiogenesis in mice. *J. Biol. Chem.* 293, 9188–9197. doi: 10.1074/jbc.RA118.002851

3

New Analysis Framework Incorporating Mixed Mutual Information and Scalable Bayesian Networks for Multimodal High Dimensional Genomic and Epigenomic Cancer Data

Xichun Wang, Sergio Branciamore, Grigoriy Gogoshin, Shuyu Ding and Andrei S. Rodin*

Department of Computational and Quantitative Medicine, Beckman Research Institute and Diabetes and Metabolism Research Institute of the City of Hope, Duarte, CA, United States

Correspondence:
Andrei S. Rodin
arodin@coh.org

We propose a novel two-stage analysis strategy to discover candidate genes associated with the particular cancer outcomes in large multimodal genomic cancers databases, such as The Cancer Genome Atlas (TCGA). During the first stage, we use mixed mutual information to perform variable selection; during the second stage, we use scalable Bayesian network (BN) modeling to identify candidate genes and their interactions. Two crucial features of the proposed approach are (i) the ability to handle mixed data types (continuous and discrete, genomic, epigenomic, etc.) and (ii) a flexible boundary between the variable selection and network modeling stages — the boundary that can be adjusted in accordance with the investigators' BN software scalability and hardware implementation. These two aspects result in high generalizability of the proposed analytical framework. We apply the above strategy to three different TCGA datasets (LGG, Brain Lower Grade Glioma; HNSC, Head and Neck Squamous Cell Carcinoma; STES, Stomach and Esophageal Carcinoma), linking multimodal molecular information (SNPs, mRNA expression, DNA methylation) to two clinical outcome variables (tumor status and patient survival). We identify 11 candidate genes, of which 6 have already been directly implicated in the cancer literature. One novel LGG prognostic factor suggested by our analysis, methylation of TMPRSS11F type II transmembrane serine protease, presents intriguing direction for the follow-up studies.

Keywords: The Cancer Genome Atlas, Bayesian networks, multimodal big data, variable selection, mixed mutual information, methylation, genomic and epigenomic molecular data

INTRODUCTION

The Cancer Genome Atlas (TCGA) resource contains genomic data compiled for more than 30 different types/subtypes of cancer (Tomczak et al., 2015). For each type, clinical outcome/progression data (e.g., tumor status and patient survival) for a considerable number of patients is matched to the large-scale molecular data. The latter is multimodal, ranging from genetic (e.g., somatic mutations) to expression (e.g., RNA-seq gene expression) to epigenetic (e.g., promoter methylation) data. Not surprisingly, there is substantial enthusiasm for causally linking the latter to the former using various modeling and secondary data analysis techniques (Jeong et al., 2015; Phan et al., 2016; Hou et al., 2018; Tian et al., 2018; Xu et al., 2018). The ultimate goals of these analyses are (i) to gain better mechanistic understanding of the underlying molecular biology of cancer, primarily by identifying important genes and their interactions; (ii) to construct compact and efficient clinical predictors (e.g., prognostic scores, indices and signatures); (iii) to associate the latter with the particular patient groups and subgroups, in the context of personalized/precision medicine. One of the more attractive and popular methods for such multivariate analysis is Bayesian networks (BNs) (Heckerman, 1995), a well-established fixture in computational systems biology (Friedman et al., 2000). Among the BN advantages are their probabilistic nature, model flexibility, ability to handle non-additive, higher-order, interactions, and ease of the result interpretation. However, applications of BNs to the TCGA (and TCGA-like) data (Gevaert et al., 2006; Xu et al., 2012, 2014; Wang et al., 2013; Huang et al., 2015; Zhu et al., 2015; Kaiser et al., 2016; Wu et al., 2017) face two principal difficulties: combining mixed data types in a single analysis framework, *and* achieving sufficient (for genomic data) scalability, *simultaneously*. (These, of course, are the two fundamental, and interconnected, BN modeling challenges in general, not just in the TCGA application). The latest developments in addressing these two challenges encompass more efficient computational approaches (Gogoshin et al., 2017; Ramsey et al., 2017), and mathematically rigorous and robust methods for handling mixed data, such as mixed local probability models and/or adaptive discretization (Gogoshin et al., 2017; Andrews et al., 2018; Sedgewick et al., 2018). Nevertheless, resolving both difficulties simultaneously in a generalizable toolkit (seamlessly applicable, for example, across the individual TCGA datasets) remains elusive. A promising approach to devising such a toolkit would be to precede the comparatively exhaustive NP-hard BN modeling with a variable selection procedure [for example (Zhang et al., 2014)], where the full dataset is pared down to a subset of variables most relevant to a particular clinical outcome or phenotype. While alleviating the scalability issue, this, however, could potentially "throw away the wheat with the chaff," especially if the variable selection process (Blum and Langley, 1997; Guyon and Elisseeff, 2003) is of a simplistic and overly too restrictive kind (e.g., a statistically conservative univariate filter). There are three possible ways to address this, namely: (i) increase the scalability of the BN modeling to genomic data levels (possible, but impractical for frequent/serial analyses), (ii) incorporate higher-order interactions into the variable selection step (thus "upgrading" it from the simple filter to the wrapper [Kohavi and John, 1997; Guyon and Elisseeff, 2003; Leng et al., 2010) — this is the solution implemented in Zhang et al. (2014)], or (iii) adjust the transition boundary between the variable selection step and the BN modeling step, depending on the investigators' computational resources and the nature (dimensionality, sparseness, heterogeneity) of the actual data. It is the third analytical strategy that we propose in this study, with the goal to achieve the optimal compromise between the computational practicality and modeling exhaustiveness.

In our analysis pipeline, we start with the variable selection procedure based on the mixed-type Mixed Mutual Information (MMI) forward selection filter. We compute the MMI values for all available gene-outcome (specifically, tumor status and patient survival) pairs, and use the MMI frequency distribution to select top variables/genes (or, alternatively, to remove bottom variables/genes) before moving on to the BN modeling. This mixed-type measure-based approach to gene selection is the principal innovation of this paper. We then use the maximum entropy (ME) – based discretization to construct the mixed-type BNs using our previously reported scalable BN modeling algorithm and software (Gogoshin et al., 2017). Subsequently, we concentrate on the sub-networks centered around the clinical outcome variables of interest, and identify the molecular gene components belonging to these sub-networks.

The proposed analysis strategy has been applied by us to 12 different TCGA cancer datasets. This allowed us to check for robustness, scalability and generalizability. Here, we present the results for the Brain Lower Grade Glioma (LGG), Head and Neck Squamous Cell Carcinoma (HNSC) and Stomach and Esophageal Carcinoma (STES) datasets (all three datasets being reasonably well-populated and proportionally balanced across the different outcomes and molecular data types). For the purposes of this particular analysis, we decided to concentrate on three types of molecular data, one discrete (somatic mutations) and two – continuous (RNA-seq gene expression, and promoter methylation). This selection is reflective of the recent trends in multimodal cancer data analyses (Zhang et al., 2014; Yoo et al., 2017), makes sense in the broad cancer genetics context (Phipps et al., 2016; Fang et al., 2017; Liang et al., 2017; Rajesh et al., 2017; Zhang C. et al., 2017; Koch et al., 2018), and underscores the comparative importance of the methylation molecular data (Koch et al., 2018). While focusing solely on the gene-centric modalities is inherently limiting (many disease-linked SNPs are localized in the non-coding regions), one of the primary purposes of this study was to showcase the MMI approach (enjoining three different modalities in a single measure/score), which necessitated the gene-centric analysis. In future, we plan to generalize our analytical framework to other, non-gene-centric, data.

We conclude by identifying a compact list of genes potentially associated with cancer-related clinical phenotypes (tumor status and patient survival), scrutinizing these genes in light of the current literature, and discussing the generalizability of our approach to the different datasets, diseases and molecular data types.

MATERIALS AND METHODS

Data Preprocessing

The Cancer Genome Atlas, LGG, HNSC, and STES datasets were downloaded for the clinical data ["Clinical_Pick_Tier1

(MD5)"], SNP data ["Mutation_Packager_Calls (MD5)"], expression data ["mRNAseq_Preprocess (MD5)"] and promoter-centric methylation data ["Methylation_Preprocess (MD5)"]. Patients were further subdivided into (i) two disease progression categories (according to the "tumor status" variable), and (ii) two patient survival categories (high death risk, with survival less than 2 years, and low death risk, with survival more than 2 years, which is a common cutoff point in recent cancer literature). We further excluded patients with ambiguous or missing outcome variable values (e.g., no survival status, survival status as "living" with survival time less than 2 years, tumor status neither "tumor-free" nor "with tumor," etc.). These clinical variables ("tumor status" and "2-year survival") were subsequently used for the variable selection purposes, and, eventually, to extract "tumor status" and "survival" – centered sub-networks from the full BNs. Expression data and methylation data (designated by "E" and "M" below, for brevity) were not discretized at this stage, as both variable selection and BN construction tools in our computational pipeline can, by design, accept mixed (continuous and discreet) variable types. SNP (somatic mutation) data (designated by "S" below) were compressed into a binary variable (presence or absence of at least one non-synonymous mutation in at least one sample of the particular gene).

After filtering out patient records with incomplete, partially missing, or ambiguously labeled data, the final datasets consisted of 4782 genes (LGG), 12516 genes (HNSC) and 16164 genes (STES). 273 patient records were available for LGG/tumor status analysis (140 patients with tumor, 133 without); 213 patients – for LGG/survival (120 patients with survival less than 2 years, 93 with long-term survival). Similarly, 260 patient records were available for HNSC/tumor status analysis (94 patients with tumor, 166 without); 139 patients – for HNSC/survival (40 patients with survival less than 2 years, 99 with long-term survival). Finally, 403 patient records were available for STES/tumor status analysis (147 patients with tumor, 256 without); 258 patients – for STES/survival (191 patients with survival less than 2 years, 67 with long-term survival).

Here we would like to re-emphasize that it is possible to include other different molecular data types and outcome variables, both continuous and discrete, into the proposed framework without substantial alterations to the analysis pipeline, except for some rudimentary data preprocessing.

Variable Selection

There are very few BN algorithms/software solutions that scale up to (epi)genomic levels (tens to hundreds of thousands of variables) (Gogoshin et al., 2017; Ramsey et al., 2017). Even with these, exhaustive analyses require dedicated hardware and weeks of processing time. This might be acceptable for a one-off, "final" analysis, but is clearly impractical for the exploratory research. This is why it is a common practice to carry out variable selection (or feature selection, or feature set reduction) in order to generate a comparatively compact subset of variables to be subsequently fed into the network modeling algorithm/software (Guyon and Elisseeff, 2003). Variable selection approaches range from the very simple (univariate filters) to increasingly more sophisticated; at some point, the latter become essentially indistinguishable from the multivariate modeling methods *per se*. Depending on the dataset to be analyzed, different "couplings" of variable selection and multivariate modeling methods might prove to be more or less effective, and it is difficult to devise *a priori* the objectively optimal combination for each new dataset. For a principally network-centric data analysis approach (innate to the systems biology), it would make sense to feed as many variables into the network-building module as possible, thus "delegating" the resolution of the higher-order / non-additive interactions and conditional independence relationships to the BN algorithm itself. Therefore, for the exploratory research, we suggest that the investigators first define the upper BN scalability limit that they are comfortable with (given the available software/hardware), and then adjust the variable selection cutoff point accordingly. For more "finalized" analysis, that limit should be raised higher (and the variable selection process, consequently, be made less restrictive).

In TCGA dataset (and other similar (epi)genomic resources), there are tens of thousands of potentially predictive/relevant variables (roughly proportional to the number of genes in the human genome). The "hand off" point between the variable selection and BN analysis steps should therefore vary between 100s of variables (for the exploratory and preliminary analyses) and 1,000s of variables (for the final analyses). The actual number might also depend on the shape of the variable selection curve, or on the statistical significance criteria–we stop adding increasingly less significant variables during the forward variable selection process (or stop removing increasingly more significant variables during the backward variable elimination process) when a certain statistical significance cutoff point is reached (Rodin et al., 2009). The above considerations were taken into account in the course of this study, as detailed in the section "Results" below.

It is difficult to integrate the multimodal, mixed-type, data into the variable selection process (filter or wrapper) as, until recently, there has been a paucity of the usable mixed-type metrics. In this study, a recently developed measure, Mixed Mutual Information (MMI) (Gao et al., 2018), was used to link the gene information (a mixed-type vector consisting of the S, E, and M molecular data components for each gene) to the clinical variable (tumor status or 2-year survival) in a "forward-selection-filter" variable selection procedure. MMI is a non-parametric and distribution-free measure [which makes it more attractive than the alternatives, such as linear correlation – especially in the biological networks context (Margolin et al., 2006; Asur et al., 2007)] that is based on the entropy estimates from k-nearest neighbor (k-NN) distances (Kraskov et al., 2004). It is, therefore, sensitive to the choice of the k parameter. Lower values of k (1–4) tend to lead to higher dispersion, while much higher values (>20) are associated with unnecessarily increased computational complexity and possible overfitting [, personal communication from Gao et al. (2018)]. We have evaluated different values of k on the actual TCGA datasets by measuring the Jaccard index for the pairs of consecutive (in k) post-selection variable sets as a function of k. The index appeared to stabilize in the 8–20 range in 12 different TCGA datasets analyzed (see section "Results" below); therefore, *k* was set at 15 throughout this study.

Bayesian Networks Modeling

Bayesian networks modeling, in its basic form, reconstructs a sparse graphical representation of a joint multivariate probability distribution of random variables from a "flat" dataset. Nodes in the network represent random variables, edges – dependencies. Absence of an edge between the two nodes indicates conditional independence between them. Recent work in BN methodology refinement led to significant progress in scalability – our latest BN modeling software implementation (Gogoshin et al., 2017) easily processes datasets up to ~ 1 mln variables × 1 mln datapoints. Handling mixed variable types (both continuous and discrete, in a typical application) is still not entirely seamless; it was recently suggested (Gogoshin et al., 2017; Andrews et al., 2018) that adaptive discretization (of continuous variables) might be preferable to forcing mixed local probability models. Consequently, we were using maximum entropy – based three-bin discretization throughout this study – expression data ("E" molecular data component) and methylation data ("M" molecular data component) were discretized into three bins – which has attractive mathematical properties, and has been shown by us earlier to maintain near-optimal over/under-fitting balance (Gogoshin et al., 2017).

Detailed description of the BN methodology in general and of our implementation (including applications to other types of high-dimensional biological data) in particular can be found in Gogoshin et al. (2017), Zhang X. et al. (2017); here we will only note that (1) our BN implementation uses a hybrid "sparse candidates" + "search-and-score" graduate descent algorithm coupled with various model scoring metrics and maximum entropy-based adaptive discretization; (2) in the resulting BN visualizations, numbers next to the edges and edge "thickness" indicate relative edge strengths (the numbers are the model scores' ratios for the models with/without corresponding edges, which are proportional to the marginal likelihood ratios); (3) directionality in the network (arrow points attached to the edges, when present) does not necessarily imply the causality flow, and is used predominantly for the mathematical convenience (to avoid cyclic dependencies); (4) when deciphering conditional dependence and independence patterns, it is useful to concentrate on the immediate Markov neighborhood (MN) of a particular variable of interest (such as a clinical outcome). This neighborhood can be roughly defined as all the nodes that are in immediate contact with ("one degree of separation" from) the node representing the aforementioned variable of interest. Under certain conditions, given its MN, the variable of interest is conditionally independent of the remaining variables (rest of the network). Therefore, deriving a MN for a variable of interest is analogous to the variable selection activity, specifically of the embedded variety (Guyon and Elisseeff, 2003). The central step in our computational analysis pipeline is using full BN reconstruction to generate the MN for the clinical outcome variable, and then ascertaining the interplay of the (small number of) gene-related variables (S, E and M molecular data components) within that MN. (It should be noted that MN is a simplification of the more rigorous concept of Markov Blanket – meaning, for our purposes, that sometimes "two degrees of separation" are needed for encapsulating a variable/node of interest).

RESULTS

Figure 1 depicts the variable selection process for six possible combinations of two clinical variables ("tumor status" and "survival") and three TCGA cancer datasets (LGG, HNSC, and STES). MMI (mixed mutual information) between (S, E, M) and tumor status/survival was computed for 4782 genes (LGG), 12516 genes (HNSC), and 16164 genes (STES). (All six gene lists, with corresponding MMI values, are available in **Supplementary Tables S1–S6**). The histogram representation of the MMI distribution, as shown in **Figure 1**, is convenient, as it allows to evaluate (both visually and quantitatively) the relative predictive values of the top-ranking genes with respect to the outcome variable classification. For the purposes of this study, and to make the resulting full BNs "observable," we have chosen the "top genes" cutoff value of 99.5% MMI CDF (cumulative distribution function), which leads to the selection of 24 genes (72 future BN nodes/variables in total, comprising 24 S, 24 E, and 24 M components) out of 4728 for two LGG networks, 63 genes (189 nodes/variables) out of 12516 for two HNSC networks, and 81 genes (243 nodes/variables) out of 16164 for two STES networks. Note that the S, E, and M components of each gene vector were considered as the separate nodes/variables in the subsequent BN construction, as at this time we do not have a BN scoring function that can incorporate mixed multivariate distance measures. It should also be noted that although MMI, intuitively, should not be negative, due to the way it is computed it can get into the negative range when (i) continuous variables are involved, and (ii) the number of dimensions is more than two (four, in our case). This said, all the negative MMI values in **Figure 1** reside well within the allowed algorithmic negative deviation range, and should not influence the variable rankings [personal communication from Gao et al. (2018)].

Interestingly, every histogram in **Figure 1** has a heavy right tail, which sometimes appears to follow a clear "knee point" – for example, at MMI ~ = 0.08 in **Figures 1A–C**. This suggests that MMI > 0.08 could also be used as a "natural" cutoff value, at least in these three datasets.

The variable selection distributions shown in **Figure 1** were derived with the MMI parameter *k* set at 15. **Figure 2** illustrates the motivation behind that choice, using the LGG/survival dataset example. Shown is the plot of the Jaccard index (JI, a.k.a. set "Intersection over Union," which is a common measure of sample set similarity) comparing the gene/variable sets resulting from the above variable selection procedure, with cutoff set at 99.5% MMI CDF, where JI(*k*) compares the sets obtained with *k* and *k+1*. It is clear that as k reaches ~15, the set composition somewhat stabilizes; further increase in k does not seem to offer any advantages. (JI plots for the other datasets exhibit a similar pattern).

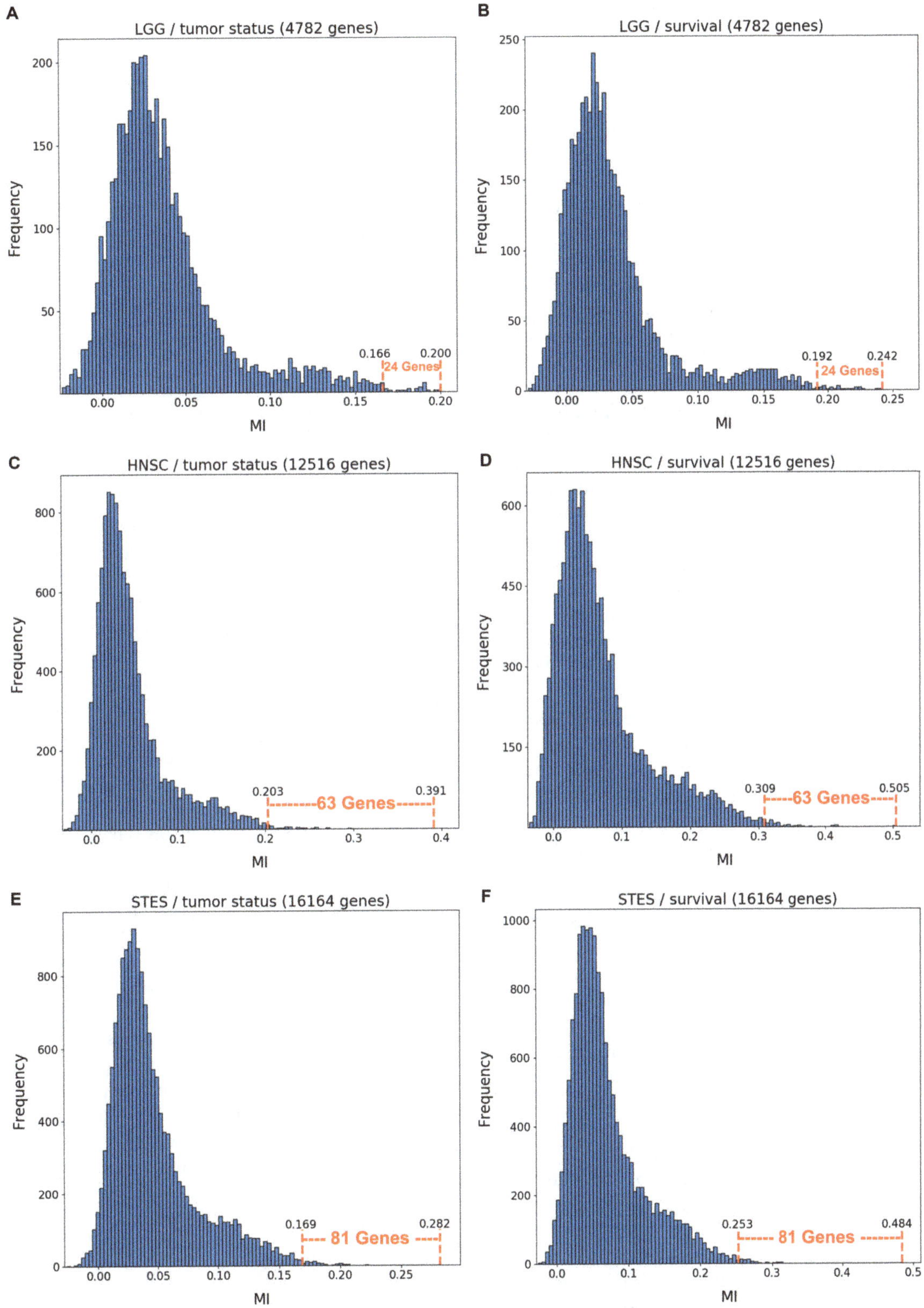

FIGURE 1 | Variable selection process for six combinations of two clinical outcome variables ("tumor status" and "survival") and three TCGA cancer datasets (LGG, HNSC, STES). MMI between the (S, E, M) molecular data vector and tumor status/survival was computed for 4782 genes (LGG), 12516 genes (HNSC) and 16164 genes (STES). The histogram representation of the MMI distribution is shown with the selection of "top" (i.e., with the MMI CDF >99.5%) genes superimposed on the right tail of the MMI frequency distribution. **(A)** LGG/tumor status; **(B)** LGG/survival; **(C)** HNSC/tumor status; **(D)** HNSC/survival; **(E)** STES/tumor status; **(F)** STES/survival.

Figures 3, 4 depict the full BNs obtained from the LGG/tumor status and LGG/survival datasets. **Supplementary Data Sheets S1–S6** depict, in PDF format, the full BNs obtained from the LGG/tumor status, LGG/survival, HNSC/tumor status, HNSC/survival, STES/tumor status, and STES/survival datasets, respectively. Six corresponding DOT (standard network / causal graphical models format) files can be found in the **Supplementary Tables S7–S12**.

While the resulting full BNs, in PDF format, are zoomable and searchable, and the DOT files can be exported into the specialized network-oriented software, the full BNs tend to be visually overwhelming for the number of variables/nodes >100. Consequently, **Figures 5–10** depict the immediate MNs of the clinical variables/nodes in the corresponding six BNs: LGG/tumor status (**Figure 5**), LGG/survival (**Figure 6**), HNSC/tumor status (**Figure 7**), HNSC/survival (**Figure 8**), STES/tumor status (**Figure 9**) and STES/survival (**Figure 10**).

It is noticeable in **Figures 5–10** that all three molecular data components (S, E, and M) are represented in the MNs. This testifies to the efficacy and proportionality of both the MMI measure (during the variable selection stage) and the maximum entropy - based discretization (during the BN construction stage). Also of note, for some genes, more than one component is present (HTR4 E and S for STES/tumor status, CHIA E and S for LGG/tumor status, AFP E and S for LGG/tumor status). Conversely, some genes are associated with both tumor status and survival (MUC4 for HNSC, TMPRSS11F, SLC6A18, and DEFB119 for LGG).

The performance of our BN reconstruction algorithm or software is discussed in general terms in Gogoshin et al. (2017); here, we will evaluate the statistical significance of the resulting MNs. While the edge strength estimates in **Figures 5–10** are useful in the relative sense, they do not immediately translate into the statistical significance measurements (such as *p*-values). Therefore, we have augmented the edge strengths with the *p*-values obtained *via* two-sample Kolmogorov–Smirnov (KS) probability distribution equality test (for continuous E and M molecular component variables) and two-sided Fisher's exact test (for discrete S molecular component variable). To illustrate the KS test application, **Figure 11** shows CDFs, separately for two "tumor status" groups, for seven continuous variables present in the MN depicted in **Figure 5** (LGG/tumor status), in order of decreasing edge strength (**Figure 11A**, MMP1_M; **Figure 11B**, DDX4_E; **Figure 11C**, AFP_E; **Figure 11D**, CHIA_E; **Figure 11E**, TMPRSS11F_M; **Figure 11F**, KERA_E; **Figure 11G**, MUC16_E). Only MMP1_M and DDX4_E appear to be statistically highly significant, with TMPRSS11F_M being arguably a borderline case.

Table 1 lists the *p*-values for all 55 potentially predictive molecular gene components present in six MNs depicted in **Figures 5–10**, in order of decreasing edge strength for each network / MN. 12 gene components were found to be statistically significant (marked with an asterisk in **Table 1**), however, we decide to exclude LCT_S (marked with ** in **Table 1**) from further scrutiny because of the very low mutation counts in both survival groups.

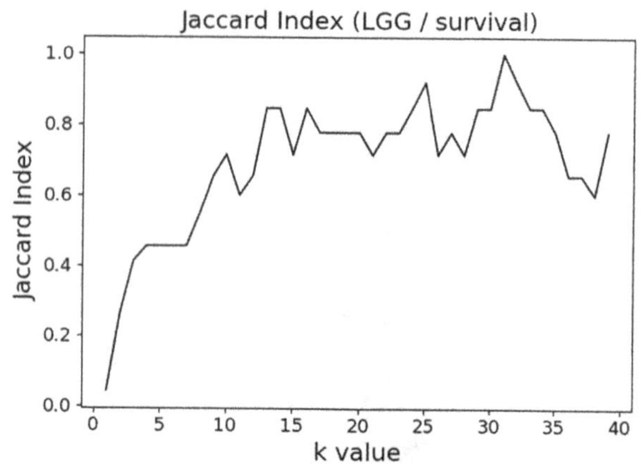

FIGURE 2 | Jaccard index (JI) ("Intersection over Union") comparing the gene/variable sets resulting from the LGG/survival dataset variable selection with the cutoff set at 99.5% MMI CDF. JI(*k*) compares the sets obtained with *k* and *k+1*.

Subsequently, we performed manual literature / database search to ascertain if any of the remaining 11 genes were previously reported in the cancer context. The following resources were used: GeneCards (Stelzer et al., 2016) and DisGeNET (Pinero et al., 2017) databases, PubMed, and Google Scholar. Six genes were found to be implicated in cancer etiology / progression / clinical outcomes with high degree of certainty: MMP1, DDX4, TRPM3, DPP6, KCNA1, and MUC17 (Senapati et al., 2010; Saied et al., 2012; Lallet-Daher et al., 2013; Kawal et al., 2016; Park et al., 2016; Schudrowitz et al., 2017). Four genes (SLC7A14, LRRIQ, SLCO1B3, and SLC9A4) were supported by weaker, circumstantial evidence (Chan-On et al., 2013; Matullo et al., 2013; Fridley et al., 2016; Tanaka et al., 2017). One gene, TMPRSS11F, has not been discussed in the cancer context before, to the best of our knowledge [see also (Kataoka et al., 2018)]. However, increased expression levels of a similar type II transmembrane serine protease, TMPRSS11D, were found to be a significant non-small cell lung cancer survival predictor (Cao et al., 2017). Therefore, we suggest that TMPRSS11F should be further investigated as a strong predictive factor playing a role in LGG patients' clinical characteristics – survival, especially. Lower TMPRSS11F methylation values correspond to a poorer long-term (2-year) survival. One possible mechanism is *via* the proteolysis of extracellular matrix which, in turn, is linked to the metastatic processes (Cao et al., 2017).

In summary, our analysis framework confirmed six well-known cancer-related genes, supplied additional evidence to support four other suspected cancer-related genes, and identified one novel potentially strongly predictive factor, methylation of TMPRSS11F.

DISCUSSION

Systems biology approach to the complex genetic and epigenetic cancer data analysis is arguably superior to the simpler single-gene (or even single-data type) alternatives. However, it is

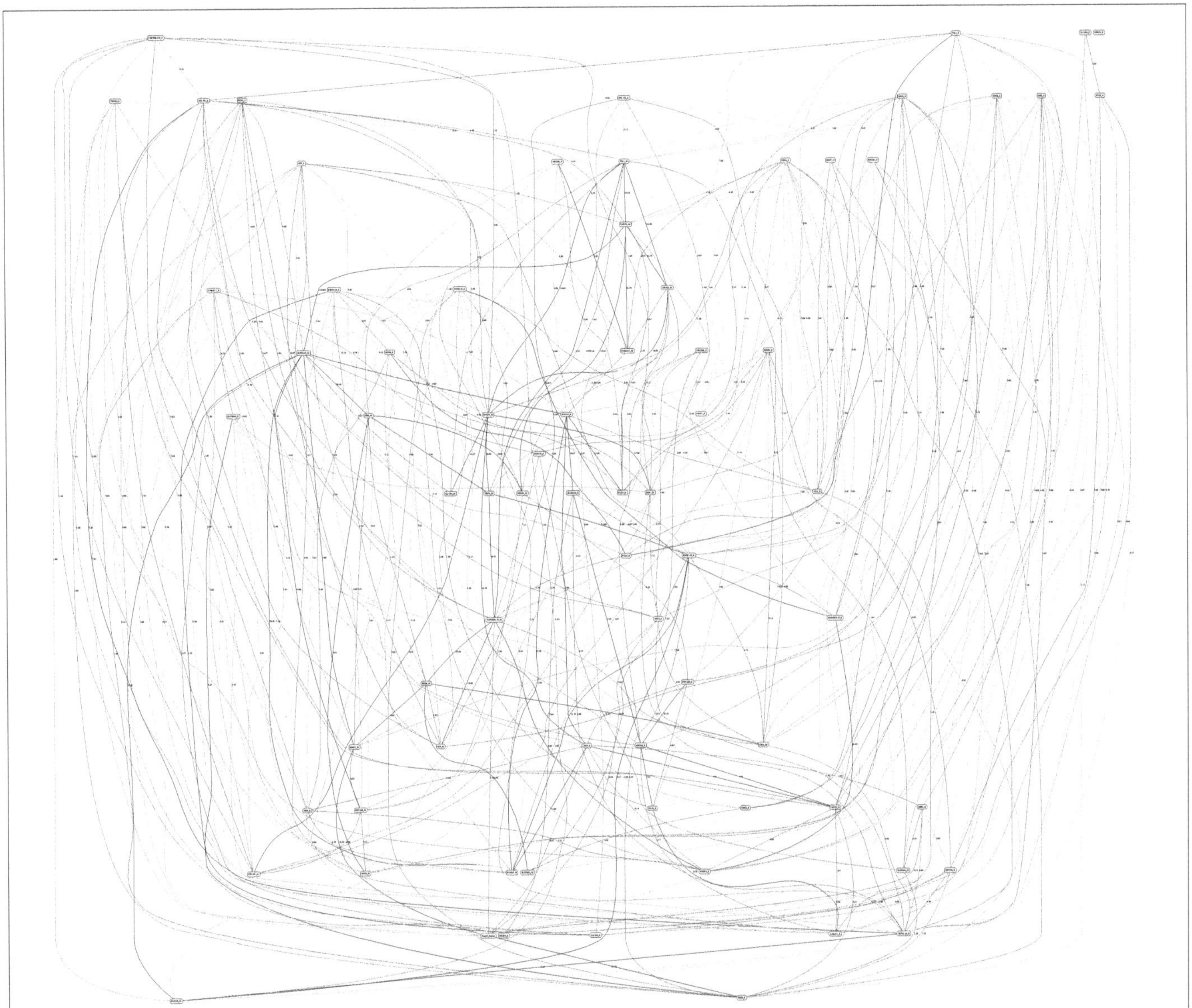

FIGURE 3 | Full BN derived from the LGG/tumor status data. "Tumor_Status" node in the BN is self-explanatory. Other nodes in the networks correspond to the genes/molecular components (gene name_S/E/M). Edges in the network correspond to the dependencies between the nodes. Directionality of the edge (arrow) is for mathematical convenience only and does not imply causation. "Boldness" of the edge is proportional to the dependency strength, also indicated by the number shown next to the edge. Note that the BN pdf image files are searchable (using gene manes), and that all the BN pdf and source files (in DOT format) are included as part of the **Supplementary Material**.

intrinsically linked to the fundamental, interrelated, challenges – scalability, "curse of dimensionality," accounting for non-additive, higher-order interactions, and visualization of the results (i.e., translation of the massive network graphs into concrete biomedical insights). In this study we propose a flexible and generalizable approach to the BN-based systems biology analysis of the multi-modal cancer data, using the TCGA database as an example. It consists of the variable selection step (which is not computationally demanding) and the BN reconstruction step (which is substantially computationally demanding). Ideally, the investigators would simply feed the complete dataset (all variables) into the BN software, obtain the full graphical model (no matter how large and complex), and then "zoom in" on the MN of the variable(s) of interest, such as a clinical outcome or a cancer phenotype. However, this is impractical for most real datasets and available hardware configurations.

Consequently, we propose starting with the variable selection step to select a (relatively) small subset of genes that are associated with the variable(s) of interest (tumor status and 2-year survival in the present study). The principal novelty of our approach lies in using the MMI measure for the variable/gene selection, in which all possible types of molecular information (discrete and continuous, genetic and epigenetic) are considered

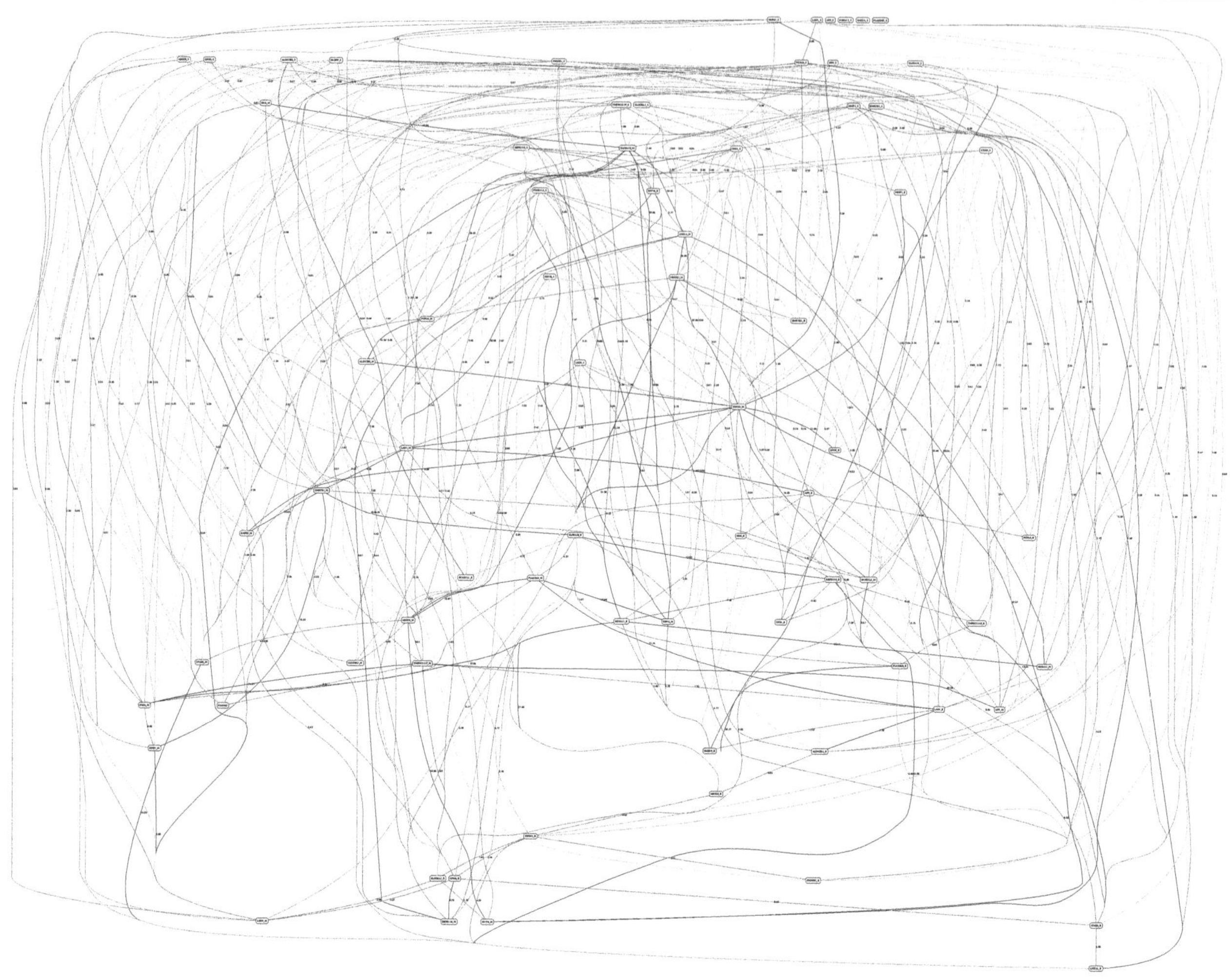

FIGURE 4 | Full BN derived from the LGG/survival data. "Survival" node in the BN is self-explanatory. Other designations are as in **Figure 3**.

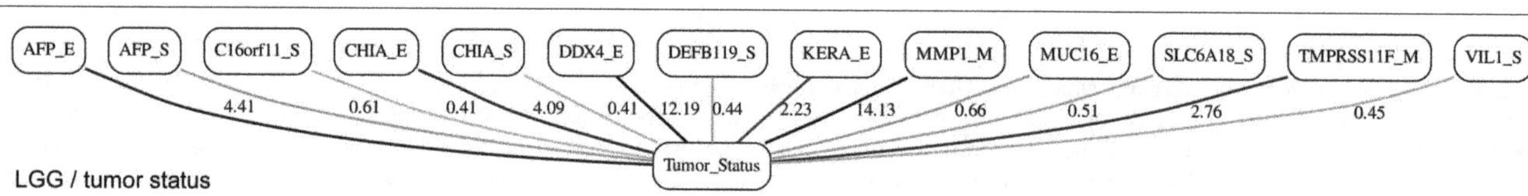

FIGURE 5 | MN of the "Tumor_Status" node in the LGG/tumor status BN.

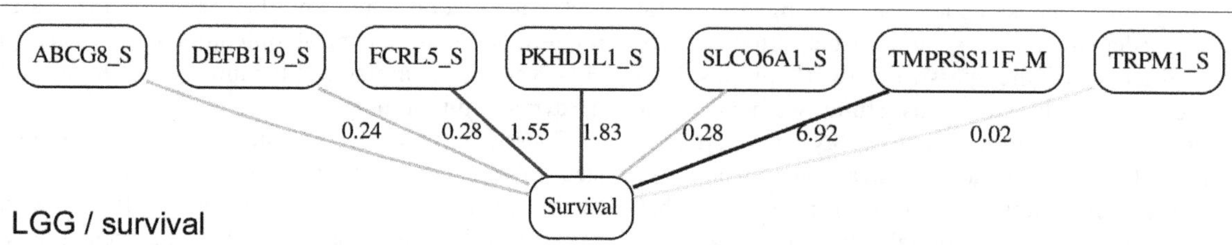

FIGURE 6 | MN of the "Survival" node in the LGG/survival BN.

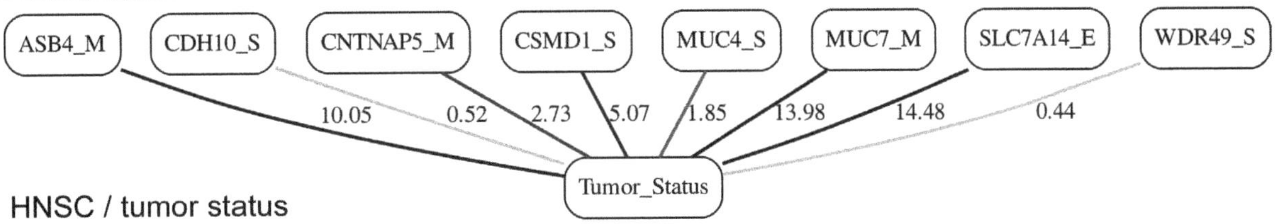

FIGURE 7 | MN of the "Tumor_Status" node in the HNSC/tumor status BN.

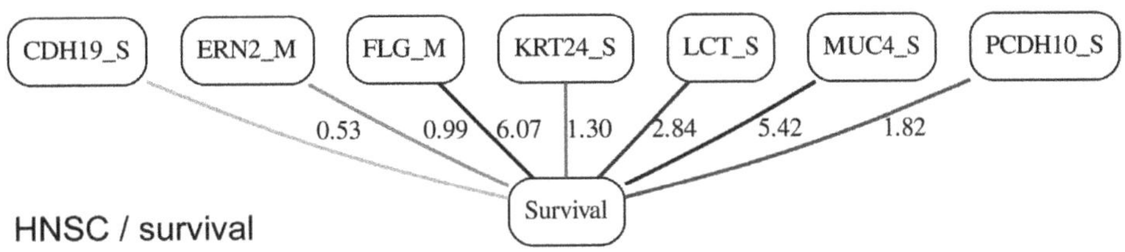

FIGURE 8 | MN of the "Survival" node in the HNSC/survival BN.

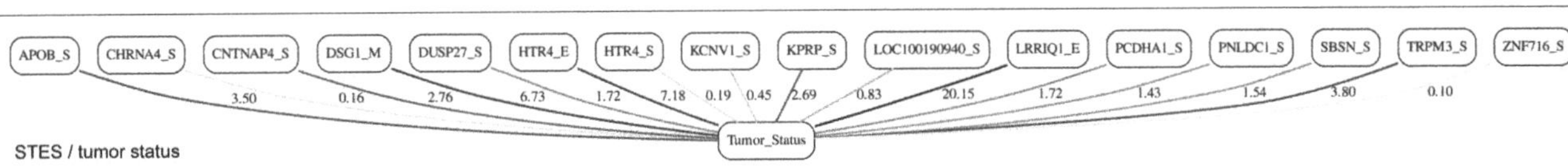

FIGURE 9 | MN of the "Tumor_Status" node in the STES/tumor status BN.

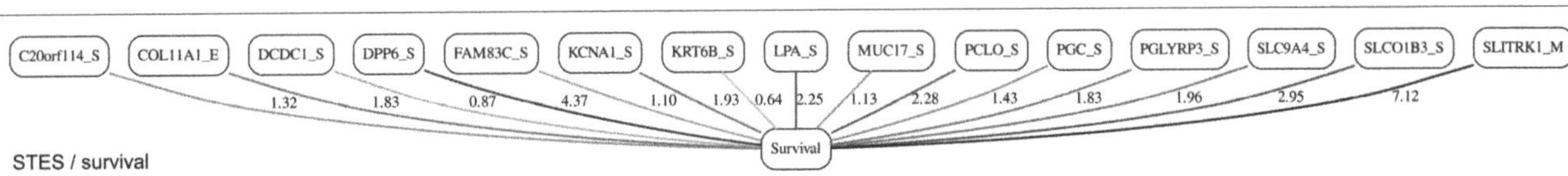

FIGURE 10 | MN of the "Survival" node in the STES/survival BN.

simultaneously. The other innovative aspect of our approach lies in the adjustability of the "hand-off" point between the variable selection and BN modeling steps. This hand-off point can depend on the investigators' computational resources, the shape of the variable selection curves, or the predefined statistical cutoff points. For example, ~20 K genes can be reduced to 100–200 genes for the subsequent BNs construction, in which case the complete analysis takes less than an hour on a mid-level PC. When feeding the complete datasets (10,000–15,000 genes, in case of TCGA and similar genomic resources) into our BN software (Gogoshin et al., 2017), without the preliminary variable selection step, it takes about 3 days to build a full BN on a dedicated multi-core workstation. Therefore, the investigators can choose the appropriate balance depending on whether they are interested in a quick, exploratory analysis or a finalized, exhaustive one.

In our analyses, the final predictive gene sets (such as shown in **Table 1**) were different from the sets (of comparable sizes) of "top" genes obtained in the variable selection step alone (otherwise there would be no need to invoke the computationally expensive BN modeling step). This was to be expected, because BN modeling is a multivariate modeling tool (which aims to reconstruct the most fitting pattern of conditional independencies in the MN of a clinical variable), while MMI ranking is a univariate variable selection "filter" that does not account for the dependencies between the (top) genes. Another reason that the two corresponding gene sets tend to be different has to do with the fact that the first analysis stage is gene-centric, whereas the second analysis stage separates the three molecular modalities. Limiting our analysis pipeline to just the first stage (MMI filter/ranking) would therefore miss the strong one-modality (but week multiple-modalities) predictors. In future, we plan to study the extent of intersection of such two sets as a function of the "hand-off" point (between MMI pre-ranking and full BN analysis) parameter.

Our computational pipeline is inherently generalizable, as it can be directly applied to any large multimodal genetic/epigenetic dataset with minimal preprocessing. The only two changeable parameters are the aforementioned variable selection / BN modeling hand-off point, and the BN discretization mechanism. The latter is currently set as the 3-bin maximum entropy-based discretization coupled with the multinomial local probability

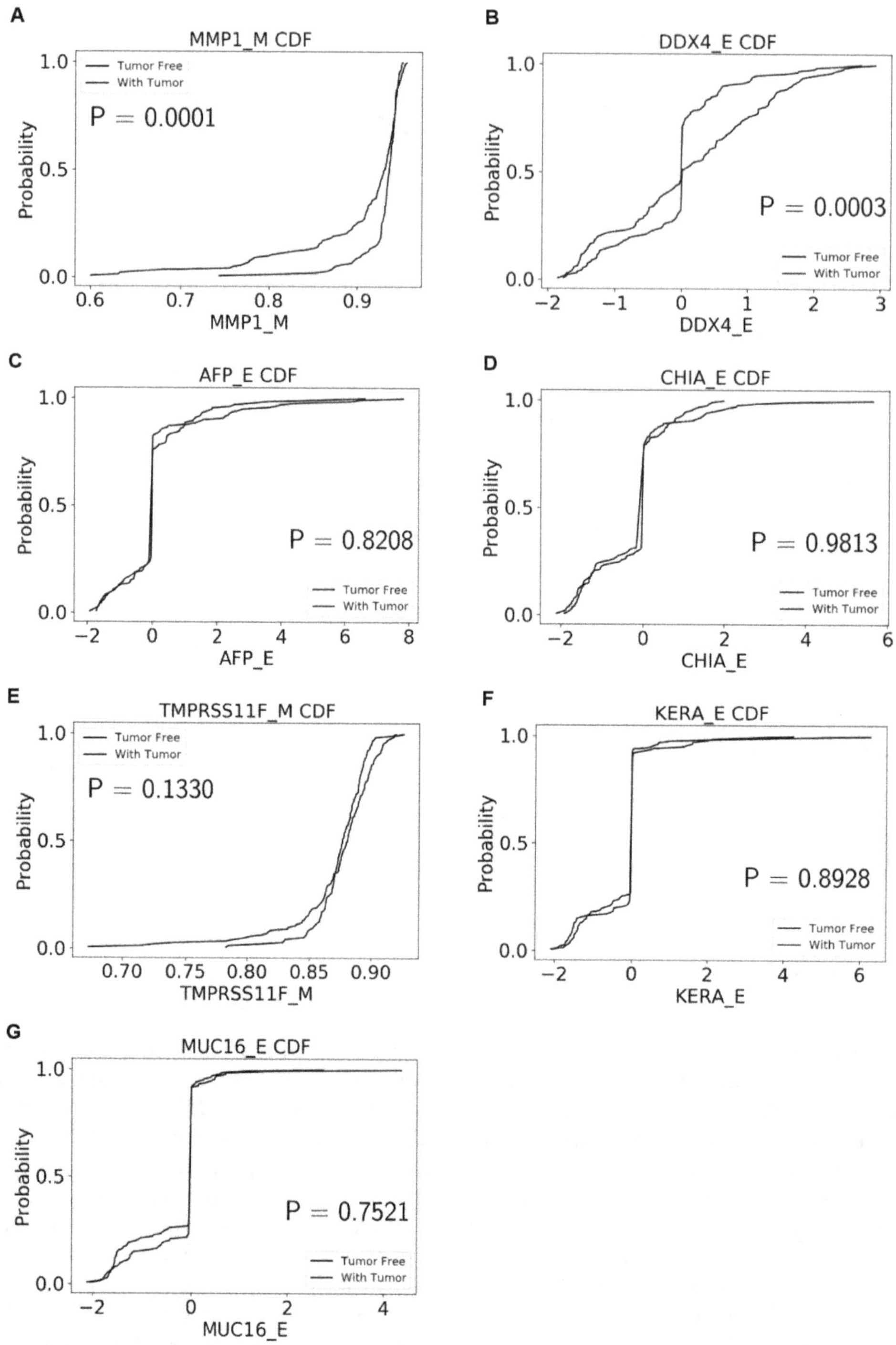

FIGURE 11 | CDFs, shown separately for two "tumor status" groups, for seven continuous variables present in the MN depicted in **Figure 5** (LGG/tumor status), in order of decreasing edge strength. **(A)** MMP1_M; **(B)** DDX4_E; **(C)** AFP_E; **(D)** CHIA_E; **(E)** TMPRSS11F_M; **(F)** KERA_E; **(G)** MUC16_E. *P*-values for the two-sample Kolmogorov-Smirnov test are shown in each chart.

model (Gogoshin et al., 2017). This is not the most elegant, or universally applicable, solution. In future, we plan to develop a novel BN model scoring function derived from a mixed distance measure (such as the MMI), or a similar metric that expresses divergence between the current network model and the data *via* mixed-type distances. The resulting two-stage analytical strategy will thus fully automatically deal with the mixed variables, in both of its stages. This has not been done before, so we plan to implement and test the MMI-based BN algorithm alongside the more established mixed-type BN solutions (hybrid local

TABLE 1 | *P*-values for 55 potentially predictive molecular gene components present in six MNs depicted in **Figures 5–10**, subdivided by six datasets, in order of decreasing edge strength for each dataset/MN.

Gene_component	BN edge strength	*p*-value
(A)		
LGG/tumor status		
MMP1_M	14.13	0.0001*
DDX4_E	12.19	0.0003*
AFP_E	4.41	0.8208
CHIA_E	4.09	0.9813
TMPRSS11F_M	2.76	0.1330
KERA_E	2.23	0.8928
MUC16_E	0.66	0.7521
AFP_S	0.61	0.4985
SLC6A18_S	0.51	~1.0
VIL1_S	0.45	0.2364
DEFB119_S	0.44	0.4872
C16orf11_S	0.41	~1.0
CHIA_S	0.41	~1.0
(B)		
LGG/survival		
TMPRSS11F_M	6.92	0.0003*
PKHD1L1_S	1.83	0.5818
FCRL5_S	1.55	0.1895
DEFB119_S	0.28	~1.0
SLCO6A1_S	0.28	~1.0
ABCG8_S	0.24	0.4366
TRPM1_S	0.02	0.1895
(C)		
HNSC/tumor status		
SLC7A14_E	14.48	2.1230e-05*
MUC7_M	13.98	0.3432
ASB4_M	10.05	0.2832
CSMD1_S	5.07	~1.0
CNTNAP5_M	2.73	0.5261
MUC4_S	1.85	0.1496
CDH10_S	0.52	~1.0
WDR49_S	0.44	~1.0
(D)		
HNSC/survival		
FLG_M	6.07	0.2427
MUC4_S	5.42	0.4103
LCT_S	2.84	0.0226**
PCDH10_S	1.82	0.3544
KRT24_S	1.3	0.4942
ERN2_M	0.99	0.4832
CDH19_S	0.53	0.5787
(E)		
STES/tumor status		
LRRIQ_E	20.15	0.0004*
HTR4_E	7.18	0.2960

(Continued)

TABLE 1 | Continued

Gene_component	BN edge strength	*p*-value
DSG1_M	6.73	0.1204
TRPM3_S	3.80	0.0245*
APOB_S	3.50	0.2723
CNTNAP4_S	2.76	0.7784
KPRP_S	2.69	~1.0
DUSP27_S	1.72	0.5480
PCDHA1_S	1.72	0.8074
SBSN_S	1.54	0.6248
PNLDC1_S	1.43	~1.0
LOC100190940_S	0.83	~1.0
KCNV1_S	0.45	~1.0
HTR4_S	0.19	0.3594
CHRNA4_S	0.16	0.3968
ZNF716_S	0.10	~1.0
(F)		
STES/survival		
SLITRK1_M	7.12	0.1082
DPP6_S	4.37	0.0280*
SLCO1B3_S	2.95	0.0059*
PCLO_S	2.28	0.7238
LPA_S	2.25	0.0549
SLC9A4_S	1.96	0.0059*
KCNA1_S	1.93	0.0108*
COL11A1_E	1.83	0.2016
PGLYRP3_S	1.83	0.1119
PGC_S	1.43	0.4527
C20orf114_S	1.32	~1.0
MUC17_S	1.13	0.0008*
FAM83C_S	1.10	0.6515
DCDC1_S	0.87	0.2051
KRT6B_S	0.64	~1.0

*Twelve gene components were found to be statistically significant (marked with *); LCT_S (marked with **) was excluded from further analysis because of the very low mutation counts (zero mutations in >2-year survival group, three mutations in <2-year survival group).*

probability models, adaptive discretization), and use both real and simulated data to investigate which method is preferable.

Another limitation of the present study has to do with its primary focus on the clinical outcomes / phenotypes; at this time, we decided to largely concentrate on the MNs of the clinical variables/nodes. In future, we intend to analyze the resulting full BNs more "holistically," paying attention to the general network topological properties, gene clusters, hub and bottleneck genes, etc. Consequently, one useful extension of our analytical framework would be to incorporate multiple clinical outcomes / phenotypes into the network analyses, to see if the inter-outcome dependencies are reflected in the resulting networks, and if they are mediated by other nodes/variables.

Application of our pipeline to TCGA data resulted in the identification of a number of candidate genes for the different clinical cancer characteristics, *via* varied molecular components. It is well known that epigenetic processes / DNA methylation play an important role in many cancers' diagnosis, progression, and outcome; our results support that notion, as many of the most statistically significant predictors generated in the present study were in fact the methylation molecular components (**Table 1**). Notably, the one novel candidate gene pinpointed in this study, TMPRSS11F, likely would not have been identified *via* any other (non-epigenetic) modality. Our results, therefore, underscore the essentiality of the simultaneous analysis of different molecular modalities, including the epigenetic ones, for the precision or personalized medicine to be effective in cancer treatment.

AUTHOR CONTRIBUTIONS

XW, SB, and AR conceptualized the study, carried out the analyses, and wrote the manuscript. GG and SD contributed to carrying out the analyses. All authors contributed to the article and approved the submitted version.

FUNDING

AR, SB, and GG are supported by NIH NCI U01 CA232216. AR is supported by the Susumu Ohno Chair in Theoretical and Computational Biology. GG is supported by Susumu Ohno Distinguished Investigator fellowship. This work was also partially supported by City of Hope funds (XW, SB, GG, and AR). The funders had no role in study design, data collection and analysis, decision to publish, or preparation of the manuscript.

ACKNOWLEDGMENTS

The authors are grateful to Arthur D. Riggs, Russell Rockne, Dustin Schones, Wendong Huang, and Weihao Gao for many stimulating discussions and useful suggestions.

SUPPLEMENTARY MATERIAL

TABLES S1–S6 | Data files, in Excel format, listing the genes analyzed in this study, together with the corresponding MMI values, in order of decreasing MMI values. **(1)** LGG/tumor status, **(2)** LGG/survival, **(3)** HNSC/tumor status, **(4)** HNSC/survival, **(5)** STES/tumor status, **(6)** STES/survival. Genes with the MMI values >99.5% MMI CDF (i.e., genes selected for further BN analyses) are shown in bold.

TABLES S7–S12 | Full Bayesian networks, in Word / DOT format, for the six datasets in this study. **(1)** LGG/tumor status, **(2)** LGG/survival, **(3)** HNSC/tumor status, **(4)** HNSC/survival, **(5)** STES/tumor status, **(6)** STES/survival.

DATA SHEETS S1–S6 | Full Bayesian networks, in PDF format, for the six datasets in this study. **(1)** LGG/tumor status, **(2)** LGG/survival, **(3)** HNSC/tumor status, **(4)** HNSC/survival, **(5)** STES/tumor status, **(6)** STES/survival. Designations are as in main text **Figure 3**.

REFERENCES

Andrews, B., Ramsey, J., and Cooper, G. F. (2018). Scoring Bayesian Networks of Mixed Variables. *Int. J. Data Sci. Anal.* 6, 3–18. doi: 10.1007/s41060-017-0085-7

Asur, S., Ucar, D., and Parthasarathy, S. (2007). An ensemble framework for clustering protein-protein interaction networks. *Bioinformatics* 23, i29–i40. doi: 10.1093/bioinformatics/btm212

Blum, A. L., and Langley, P. (1997). Selection of relevant features and examples in machine learning. *Artif. Intell.* 97, 245–271. doi: 10.1016/s0004-3702(97)00063-5

Cao, X., Tang, Z., Huang, F., Jin, Q., Zhou, X., Shi, J., et al. (2017). High TMPRSS11D protein expression predicts poor overall survival in non-small cell lung cancer. *Oncotarget* 8, 12812–12819. doi: 10.18632/oncotarget.14559

Chan-On, W., Nairismagi, M. L., Ong, C. K., Lim, W. K., Dima, S., Pairojkul, C., et al. (2013). Exome sequencing identifies distinct mutational patterns in liver fluke-related and non-infection-related bile duct cancers. *Nat. Genet.* 45, 1474–1478. doi: 10.1038/ng.2806

Fang, X., Yin, Z., Li, X., Xia, L., Quan, X., Zhao, Y., et al. (2017). Multiple functional SNPs in differentially expressed genes modify risk and survival of non-small cell lung cancer in chinese female non-smokers. *Oncotarget* 8, 18924–18934. doi: 10.18632/oncotarget.14836

Fridley, B. L., Ghosh, T. M., Wang, A., Raghavan, R., Dai, J., Goode, E. L., et al. (2016). Genome-wide study of response to platinum. taxane, and combination therapy in ovarian cancer: in vitro phenotypes, inherited variation, and disease recurrence. *Front Genet* 7:37. doi: 10.3389/fgene.2016.00037

Friedman, N., Linial, M., Nachman, I., and Pe'er, D. (2000). Using Bayesian networks to analyze expression data. *J. Comput. Biol.* 7, 601–620. doi: 10.1089/106652700750050961

Gao, W., Kannan, S., Oh, S., and Viswanath, P. (2018). Estimating mutual information for discrete-continuous mixtures. *arXiv [Preprint].* Available online at: https://arxiv.org/abs/1709.06212

Gevaert, O., De Smet, F., Timmerman, D., Moreau, Y., and De Moor, B. (2006). Predicting the prognosis of breast cancer by integrating clinical and microarray data with Bayesian networks. *Bioinformatics* 22, e184–e190. doi: 10.1093/bioinformatics/btl230

Gogoshin, G., Boerwinkle, E., and Rodin, A. S. (2017). New Algorithm and Software (BNOmics) for Inferring and Visualizing Bayesian Networks from Heterogeneous Big Biological and Genetic Data. *J. Comput. Biol.* 24, 340–356. doi: 10.1089/cmb.2016.0100

Guyon, I., and Elisseeff, A. (2003). An introduction to variable and feature selection. *J. Mach. Learn. Res.* 3, 1157–1182.

Heckerman, D. (1995). *Tutorial on Learning with Bayesian Networks.* Technical Report MSR-TR-95-96. Redmond, WA: Microsoft Research.

Hou, X., He, X., Wang, K., Hou, N., Fu, J., et al. (2018). Genome-wide network-based analysis of colorectal cancer identifies novel prognostic factors and an integrative prognostic index. *Cell Physiol. Biochem.* 49, 1703–1716. doi: 10.1159/000493614

Huang, T., Yang, J., and Cai, Y. D. (2015). Novel candidate key drivers in the integrative network of genes, microRNAs, methylations, and copy number variations in squamous cell lung carcinoma. *Biomed. Res. Int.* 2015, 358125.

Jeong, H., Leem, S., Wee, K., and Sohn, K. A. (2015). Integrative network analysis for survival-associated gene-gene interactions across multiple genomic profiles in ovarian cancer. *J. Ovarian. Res.* 8:42.

Kaiser, J. L., Bland, C. L., and Klinke, D. J. II (2016). Identifying causal networks linking cancer processes and anti-tumor immunity using Bayesian network inference and metagene constructs. *Biotechnol. Prog.* 32, 470–479. doi: 10.1002/btpr.2230

Kataoka, H., Kawaguchi, M., Fukushima, T., and Shimomura, T. (2018). Hepatocyte growth factor activator inhibitors (HAI-1 and HAI-2): emerging key players in epithelial integrity and cancer. *Pathol. Int.* 68, 145–158. doi: 10.1111/pin.12647

Kawal, P., Chandra, A., Rajkumar, Dhole, T. N., and Ojha, B. (2016). Correlations of polymorphisms in matrix metalloproteinase-1, -2, and -7 promoters to susceptibility to malignant gliomas. *Asian J. Neurosurg.* 11, 160–166.

Koch, A., Joosten, S. C., Feng, Z., de Ruijter, T. C., Draht, M. X., Melotte, V., et al. (2018). Analysis of DNA methylation in cancer: location revisited. *Nat. Rev. Clin. Oncol.* 15, 459–466. doi: 10.1038/s41571-018-0004-4

Kohavi, R., and John, G. H. (1997). Wrappers for feature subset selection. *Artif. Intell.* 97, 273–324. doi: 10.1016/s0004-3702(97)00043-x

Kraskov, A., Stögbauer, H., and Grassberger, P. (2004). Estimating mutual information. *Phys. Rev. E* 69, 066138.

Lallet-Daher, H., Wiel, C., Gitenay, D., Navaratnam, N., Augert, A., Calvé, B. L., et al. (2013). Potassium channel KCNA1 modulates oncogene-induced senescence and transformation. *Cancer Res.* 73, 5253–5265. doi: 10.1158/0008-5472.can-12-3690

Leng, J., Valli, C., and Armstrong, L. (2010). "A wrapper-based feature selection for analysis of large data sets," in *Proceedings of the Conference: 3rd International Conference on Computer and Electrical Engineering (ICCEE 2010)*, Chengdu.

Liang, A., Zhou, B., and Sun, W. (2017). Integrated genomic characterization of cancer genes in glioma. *Cancer Cell Int.* 17:90.

Margolin, A. A., Nemenman, I., Basso, K., Wiggins, C., Stolovitzky, G., Favera, R. D., et al. (2006). ARACNE: an algorithm for the reconstruction of gene regulatory networks in a mammalian cellular context. *BMC Bioinformatics* 7(Suppl. 1):S7. doi: 10.1186/1471-2105-7-S1-S7

Matullo, G., Guarrera, S., Betti, M., Fiorito, G., Ferrante, D., Voglino, F., et al. (2013). Genetic variants associated with increased risk of malignant pleural mesothelioma: a genome-wide association study. *PLoS One* 8:e61253. doi: 10.1371/journal.pone.0061253

Park, Y. R., Chun, J. N., So, I., Kim, H. J., Baek, S., Jeon, J. H, et al. (2016). Data-driven Analysis of TRP channels in cancer: linking variation in gene expression to clinical significance. *Cancer Genom. Proteom.* 13, 83–90.

Phan, J. H., Hoffman, R., Kothari, S., Wu, P. Y., and Wang, M. D. (2016). Integration of multi-modal biomedical data to predict cancer grade and patient survival. *IEEE EMBS Int. Conf. Biomed. Health Inform.* 2016, 577–580.

Phipps, A. I., Passarelli, M. N., Chan, A. T., Harrison, T. A., Jeon, J., Hutter, C. M., et al. (2016). Common genetic variation and survival after colorectal cancer diagnosis: a genome-wide analysis. *Carcinogenesis* 37, 87–95.

Pinero, J., Bravo, A., Queralt-Rosinach, N., Gutierrez-Sacristan, A., Deu-Pons, J., Centeno, E., et al. (2017). DisGeNET: a comprehensive platform integrating information on human disease-associated genes and variants. *Nucleic Acids Res.* 45, D833–D839.

Rajesh, Y., Pal, I., Banik, P., Chakraborty, S., Borkar, S. A., Dey, G., et al. (2017). Insights into molecular therapy of glioma: current challenges and next generation blueprint. *Acta Pharmacol. Sin.* 38, 591–613. doi: 10.1038/aps.2016.167

Ramsey, J., Glymour, M., Sanchez-Romero, R., and Glymour, C. (2017). A million variables and more: the Fast Greedy Equivalence Search algorithm for learning high-dimensional graphical causal models, with an application to functional magnetic resonance images. *Int. J. Data Sci. Anal.* 3, 121–129. doi: 10.1007/s41060-016-0032-z

Rodin, A. S., Litvinenko, A., Klos, K., Morrison, A. C., Woodage, T., Coresh, J., et al. (2009). Use of wrapper algorithms coupled with a random forests classifier for variable selection in large-scale genomic association studies. *J. Comput. Biol.* 16, 1705–1718. doi: 10.1089/cmb.2008.0037

Saied, M. H., Marzec, J., Khalid, S., Smith, P., Down, T. A., Rakyan, V. K., et al. (2012). Genome wide analysis of acute myeloid leukemia reveal leukemia specific methylome and subtype specific hypomethylation of repeats. *PLoS One* 7:e33213. doi: 10.1371/journal.pone.0033213

Schudrowitz, N., Takagi, S., Wessel, G. M., and Yajima, M. (2017). Germline factor DDX4 functions in blood-derived cancer cell phenotypes. *Cancer Sci.* 108, 1612–1619. doi: 10.1111/cas.13299

Sedgewick, A. J., Buschur, K., Shi, I., Ramsey, J. D., Raghu, V. K., Manatakis, D. V., et al. (2018). Mixed graphical models for integrative causal analysis with application to chronic lung disease diagnosis and prognosis. *Bioinformatics* 35, 1204–1212. doi: 10.1093/bioinformatics/bty769

Senapati, S., Ho, S. B., Sharma, P., Das, S., Chakraborty, S., Kaur, S., et al. (2010). Expression of intestinal MUC17 membrane-bound mucin in inflammatory and neoplastic diseases of the colon. *J. Clin. Pathol.* 63, 702–707. doi: 10.1136/jcp.2010.078717

Stelzer, G., Rosen, N., Plaschkes, I., Zimmerman, S., Twik, M., Fishilevich, S., et al. (2016). The genecards suite: from gene data mining to disease genome sequence analyses. *Curr. Protoc. Bioinformatics* 54:1.30.1-1.30.33.

Tanaka, H., Kanda, M., Shimizu, D., Tanaka, C., Kobayashi, D., Hayashi, M., et al. (2017). FAM46C serves as a predictor of hepatic recurrence in patients with resectable gastric cancer. *Ann. Surg. Oncol.* 24, 3438–3445. doi: 10.1245/s10434-016-5636-y

Tian, W., Li, Y., Zhang, J., Li, J., and Gao, J. (2018). Combined analysis of DNA methylation and gene expression profiles of osteosarcoma identified several prognosis signatures. *Gene* 650, 7–14. doi: 10.1016/j.gene.2018.01.093

Tomczak, K., Czerwinska, P., and Wiznerowicz, M. (2015). The Cancer Genome Atlas (TCGA): an immeasurable source of knowledge. *Contemp. Oncol.* 19, A68–A77.

Wang, W., Baladandayuthapani, V., Holmes, C. C., and Do, K. A. (2013). Integrative network-based Bayesian analysis of diverse genomics data. *BMC Bioinformatics* 14(Suppl. 13):S8. doi: 10.1186/1471-2105-14-S13-S8

Wu, S., Law, A., and Whipple, M. E. (2017). A bayesian network model of head and neck squamous cell carcinoma incorporating gene expression profiles. *Stud. Health Technol. Inform.* 245, 634–638.

Xu, P., Yang, J., Liu, J., Yang, X., Liao, J., Yuan, F., et al. (2018). Identification of glioblastoma gene prognosis modules based on weighted gene co-expression network analysis. *BMC Med. Genomics* 11:96. doi: 10.1186/s12920-018-0407-1

Xu, Y., Zhang, J., Yuan, Y., Mitra, R., Muller, P., Ji, Y., et al. (2012). A bayesian graphical model for integrative analysis of TCGA Data. *IEEE Int. Workshop Genomic Signal Process. Stat.* 2012, 135–138.

Xu, Y., Zhu, Y., Muller, P., Mitra, R., and Ji, Y. (2014). Characterizing Cancer-Specific Networks by Integrating TCGA Data. *Cancer Inform.* 13, 125–131.

Yoo, B. C., Kim, K. H., Woo, S. M., and Myung, J. K. (2017). Clinical multi-omics strategies for the effective cancer management. *J. Proteomics* 188, 97–106. doi: 10.1016/j.jprot.2017.08.010

Zhang, Q., Burdette, J. E., and Wang, J. P. (2014). Integrative network analysis of TCGA data for ovarian cancer. *BMC Syst Biol* 8:1338. doi: 10.1186/s12918-014-0136-9

Zhang, X., Branciamore, S., Gogoshin, G., Rodin, A. S., and Riggs, A. D. (2017). Analysis of high-resolution 3D intrachromosomal interactions aided by Bayesian network modeling. *Proc. Natl. Acad. Sci. U.S.A.* 114, E10359–E10368.

Zhang, C., Cheng, W., Ren, X., Wang, Z., Liu, X., Li, G., et al. (2017). Tumor purity as an underlying key factor in Glioma. *Clin. Cancer Res.* 23, 6279–6291. doi: 10.1158/1078-0432.ccr-16-2598

Zhu, Y., Xu, Y., Helseth, D. L. Jr., Gulukota, K., Yang, S., Pesce, L. L., et al. (2015). Zodiac: a comprehensive depiction of genetic interactions in cancer by integrating TCGA data. *J. Natl. Cancer Inst.* 107:djv129.

4

Detection and Comparative Analysis of Methylomic Biomarkers of Rheumatoid Arthritis

Xin Feng[1,2,3], Xubing Hao[4], Ruoyao Shi[5], Zhiqiang Xia[3], Lan Huang[6], Qiong Yu[1] and Fengfeng Zhou[3]**

[1] Department of Epidemiology and Biostatistics, School of Public Health, Jilin University, Changchun, China, [2] Jilin Institute of Chemical Technology, Jilin, China, [3] BioKnow Health Informatics Lab, College of Computer Science and Technology, and Key Laboratory of Symbolic Computation and Knowledge Engineering of Ministry of Education, Jilin University, Changchun, China, [4] BioKnow Health Informatics Lab, College of Software, and Key Laboratory of Symbolic Computation and Knowledge Engineering of Ministry of Education, Jilin University, Changchun, China, [5] BioKnow Health Informatics Lab, College of Life Sciences, Jilin University, Changchun, China, [6] College of Computer Science and Technology, and Key Laboratory of Symbolic Computation and Knowledge Engineering of Ministry of Education, Jilin University, Changchun, China

***Correspondence:**
Qiong Yu
yuqiong@jlu.edu.cn
Fengfeng Zhou
FengfengZhou@gmail.com;
ffzhou@jlu.edu.cn

Rheumatoid arthritis (RA) is a common autoimmune disorder influenced by both genetic and environmental factors. To investigate possible contributions of DNA methylation to the etiology of RA with minimum confounding genetic heterogeneity, we investigated genome-wide DNA methylation in disease-discordant monozygotic twin pairs. This study hypothesized that methylomic biomarkers might facilitate accurate RA detection. A comprehensive series of biomarker detection algorithms were utilized to find the best methylomic biomarkers for detecting RA patients using the methylomic data of the peripheral blood samples. The best model achieved 100.00% in accuracy (Acc) with 81 methylomic biomarkers and a 10-fold cross-validation (10FCV) strategy. Some of the methylomic biomarkers were experimentally confirmed to be associated with the onset or development of RA. It is also interesting to observe that many of the detected biomarkers were from chromosome Y, supporting the knowledge that RA has a significant gender discrepancy.

Keywords: feature selection, rheumatoid arthritis, methylation biomarker, methylome, chromosome Y

INTRODUCTION

The chronic autoimmune disease rheumatoid arthritis (RA) demonstrates significant changes to joints, with major symptoms like joint pain and swollenness (Triantafyllias et al., 2016). RA is strongly associated with the inflammation around major organs like lungs (Chatzidionisyou and Catrina, 2016; Farquhar et al., 2019) and heart (Crowson et al., 2013; Lazzerini et al., 2017). RA may be developed in about 1% of the population in the developed countries (Smolen et al., 2016). Moreover, females have a 2.5 times high risk than males to develop RA (Alam et al., 2011).

The cause of RA remained unclear and was hypothesized to be under the orchestrated regulation of both genetic and epigenetic factors (Villanueva-Romero et al., 2018; Khan et al., 2019). Various genetic biomarkers were detected through genome-wide association studies (Massey et al., 2018; Shadrina et al., 2018; Lopez-Mejias et al., 2019). Multiple genetic mutations were detected to be statistically associated with the susceptibility for RA, including the SNPs in the genes interferon regulatory factor 4 (IRF-4) (Lopez-Isac et al., 2016) and Solute Carrier family 8 (SLC8A3) (Julia et al., 2016). Genetic factors were also observed to be associated with the treatment responses of the tumor necrosis factor alpha inhibitors (TNFi) (Massey et al., 2018) and the methotrexate (MTX) monotherapy (Taylor et al., 2018).

Recent studies also demonstrated that the differential status of the epigenomic loci was also statistically significantly associated with RA even in a small population (Julia et al., 2017; Carnero-Montoro and Alarcon-Riquelme, 2018). The RA pathogenesis was observed to be actively regulated by the epigenetic modifications of the immune machineries in the joint tissues (Ibanez-Cabellos et al., 2019). Various environmental factors like cigarette smoking and certain oral pathogens may induce RA through epigenetic modifications (Brandt et al., 2019). Novel treatment plans were proposed to use epigenetic modulators to reverse the differentially methylated regions (Petralia et al., 2019). So the detection of RA methylation biomarkers may both facilitate the understanding of RA pathogenesis and propose more epigenetic drug targets.

There were two main types of computer algorithms to detect biomarkers, i.e., filters and wrappers (Xie et al., 2013; Singh et al., 2018; Verde and De Pietro, 2019). A filter tries to rank the features by each feature's statistical association significance with the phenotype, assuming the features are independent of each other (Lyu et al., 2017). The filter algorithm has a linear time complexity and runs fast enough for many large datasets (Xu et al., 2018). A wrapper utilizes a few heuristic rules to generate a feature subset with a performance evaluation iteratively, and the final feature subset is output if the stop criterion is met (Tekin Erguzel et al., 2015). The strategies of both filters and wrappers may be integrated to generate a hybrid feature selection algorithm (Kumar and Nirmalkumar, 2019; Wu et al., 2019).

This study hypothesized that methylomic features might reflect both the genetic and epigenetic status of RA. So a comprehensive biomarker detection procedure was carried out to find a biomarker set with the satisfying RA prediction accuracy (Acc). The best RA prediction model was also compared with the two sets of methylomic biomarkers from the previous studies. Our model demonstrated a better RA prediction Acc and interesting biological observations.

MATERIALS AND METHODS

Summary of the Dataset

This study screened 485,577 methylomic features detected from 79 RA children and their 79 healthy monozygotic twin siblings (Webster et al., 2018). The twin pairs were identified from the TwinsUK register (Moayyeri et al., 2013) and the RA status was detected in a questionnaire between 1997 and 2002. The twin volunteers were recruited after an advertisement in the National RA Society newsletter in 2013. The RA status was clinical confirmed after these twins were recruited, and only those twins with one healthy and the other RA status were kept for this study. The blood samples were stored at −80°C for DNA extraction.

The methylome was generated by the Illumina HumanMethylation450 BeadChip 15017482 v1.1. The raw data were available at the ArrayExpress database (Athar et al., 2019) with the accession number E-MTAB-6988. This methylomic dataset was formulated as a binary classification problem between the pediatric RA patients and the controls.

The data were provided in the raw format of IDAT, and the methylation level was calculated using the function getBeta() of the R package minfi version 1.28.3 (Aryee et al., 2014).

Pre-screening the Methylomic Features

Many feature selection algorithms run slow on a large dataset, and each methylome has almost half a million features. The downstream feature selection algorithms may crash if they were used directly on the methylomic datasets. So we carried out a pre-screening step to reduce the number of features to be within the capacity of the feature selection algorithms. So the classifier LinearSVC was used to select features for further feature screening. The Python package sklearn has a module SelectFromModel() for this purpose. The model can select features based on the indicators given by the LinearSVC trained on the dataset and the user may determine the number of features screened for further analysis.

Filter Algorithms

Four widely used filter algorithms were used to rank the features, assuming the features were independent of each other. *T*-test (Ttest) assumed that the data followed a normal distribution and were widely used in bioOMIC data. Ttest evaluated the statistical significance of a feature's differential values between two groups of samples (Kim, 2015; Gharbali et al., 2018; Jankowski et al., 2018). This study focused on the differential methylated residues between the RA patients and the siblings and assumed the independences between the two groups of samples (Lotsch et al., 2013; Kahl et al., 2018).

Chi-squared test (Chi2) can be used to select features with the highest values of the chi-squared statistics from a vector × relative to the classes. The chi-square test measures dependence between stochastic variables. It also checked whether a feature was statistically significantly associated with the class label under the assumption of a chi-squared distribution (Bangdiwala, 2016; Fernandez Rojas et al., 2019).

Mutual information (MI) measured the mutual dependency between a feature and the class label (Wei and Stocker, 2016; Meng et al., 2019). MI is equal to zero if and only if two random variables are independent, and a higher value means a higher dependency between the two random variables. The function relies on non-parametric methods based on entropy estimation from k-nearest-neighbor (KNN) distances.

Pearson correlation coefficient (PCC) evaluated the linear correlation between a feature and the class label with the assumption of sample independence (Liu et al., 2017). The PCC measures the linear relationship between two variables. PCC assumed that each variable be normally distributed, and do not necessarily have a zero-mean. Like the other correlation coefficients, PCC varies between −1 and +1 with 0 implying no correlation between the two variables. Correlations of −1 or +1 imply an exact negative or positive linear relationship. Positive correlations imply that as x increases, so does y. Negative correlations imply that as x increases, y decreases. The p-value roughly indicates the probability of an uncorrelated system producing variables that have a Pearson correlation at least as extreme as the one computed from these variables.

Recursive Feature Elimination Strategy

Recursive feature elimination (RFE) was a strategy to iteratively remove a feature with the least weight from the training of a classification model. The following four classification models were used to build the RFE feature selection procedure. Logistic regression (LR) (rfeLR) was a popular binary classifier and may be embedded in the RFE strategy (Pandey et al., 2018). LR is also known in the literature as logit regression, maximum-entropy classification (MaxEnt), or the log-linear classifier. In this model, the probabilities describing the possible outcomes of a single trial are modeled using a logistic function.

Lasso was a regression model and may be used to assign weights to features after a model training (rfeLasso) (Wang et al., 2019). The Lasso is a linear model that estimates sparse coefficients. It is useful in some contexts due to its tendency to prefer solutions with fewer non-zero coefficients, so Lasso can effectively reduce the number of features upon which the given solution is dependent. For this reason, Lasso and its variants are fundamental to the field of compressed sensing (Angelosante et al., 2009). Mathematically, it consists of a linear model with an added regularization term. The objective function to minimize is:

$$\min_{w} \frac{1}{2n_{\text{samples}}} ||X_{w-y}||_2^2 + \alpha||w||_1.$$

The lasso estimate thus solves the minimization of the least-squares penalty with αw_1 added, where α is a constant and w_1 is the l1-norm of the coefficient vector.

The Naïve Bayes method calculated the association probability of each feature with the class label under the assumption of inter-feature independence (rfeNBayes) (Youn and Jeong, 2009). Naive Bayes methods are a set of supervised learning algorithms based on applying Bayes' theorem with the "naive" assumption of conditional independence between every pair of features given the value of the class variable. Naive Bayes learners and classifiers can be extremely fast compared to more sophisticated methods. The decoupling of the class conditional feature distributions means that each distribution can be independently estimated as a one-dimensional distribution. This in turn helps to alleviate problems stemming from the curse of dimensionality.

The ridge regressor (rfeRidge) tried to assign minimized weights to non-associated features to a model (Barker and Brown, 2001; Rottmann and Berbeco, 2014). Ridge regression addresses some of the problems of ordinary least squares by imposing a penalty on the size of the coefficients. The ridge coefficients minimize a penalized residual sum of squares:

$$\min_{w} ||X_{w-y}||_2^2 + \alpha||w||_2^2.$$

The complexity parameter $\alpha \geq 0$ controls the amount of shrinkage: the larger the value of α, the greater the amount of shrinkage and thus the coefficients become more robust to collinearity.

Heuristic Feature Selection Strategies

Three heuristic feature selection strategies were used to generate a feature subset. The ascending feature screening (AFS) strategy started with an empty feature subset and selected the next feature with the best rank or largest weight after a model training. Then this chosen feature was removed from the remaining feature list. While the descending feature screening (DFS) strategy started with all the features and removed the next feature with the lowest rank or the least weight after a model training. Cawley and Talbot (2010) suggested that a classification model may be over-fitted if the number of training samples was smaller than that of features. We proposed a feature removal procedure BackFS to carry out an iterative removal of a feature that contributed the least prediction performance improvement. The feature subset with the best prediction performance was kept for further analysis.

All the computational experiments were conducted in the Python programming language version 3.6.5. Chi2 and MI were provided in the python sklearn version 0.19.1. PCC and Ttest were provided in the python scipy version 1.1.0. The four RFE procedures were programmed using the python sklearn version 0.19.1.

Classification Algorithms

Five widely used classifiers were utilized to measure the prediction performance of a feature subset. The discriminative power of a feature subset may be evaluated by a multivariate LR (Inzaule et al., 2018). The support vector machine (SVM) with the linear kernel function was another binary classifier that had been widely used for biomedical datasets (Citak-Er et al., 2018). SVMs are a set of supervised learning methods used for classification, regression, and outlier detection which can analyze data in classification and regression analysis. Given a set of training instances, each training instance is marked as belonging to one of the two categories, and the SVM training algorithm creates a model that assigns new instances to one of the two categories, making it a non-probability two Meta linear classifier. The SVM model represents instances as points in space, so that the mapping allows the instances of the individual categories to be separated by as wide an apparent interval as possible. Then, map new instances to the same space and predict which category they belong to based on which side of the interval they fall on. SVM may also be used to select biomarkers. After an SVM model was trained on a dataset, each input feature was assigned with a weight and the features with the default weight threshold $1e{-}5$ may be chosen for further analysis.

The simple classifier KNN had demonstrated very good prediction accuracies in some cases (Nejadgholi and Bolic, 2015; Yang et al., 2017). Neighbors-based classification is a type of instance-based learning or non-generalizing learning. It does not attempt to construct a general internal model, but simply stores instances of the training data. Classification is computed from a simple majority vote of the nearest neighbors of each point: a query point is assigned the data class which has the most representatives within the nearest neighbors of the point.

The ensembled classifier Random Forest (RF) integrated the final decision based on the prediction results of multiple random trees (Lu et al., 2017; Olsen et al., 2018; Rahman et al., 2018). The RandomForest algorithm is perturb-and-combine techniques specifically designed for trees. This means a diverse set of classifiers is created by introducing randomness in the classifier construction. The prediction of the ensemble is given as the averaged prediction of the individual classifiers. In RFs, each tree in the ensemble is built from a sample drawn with replacement (i.e., a bootstrap sample) from the training set. The Gaussian naïve Bayes classifier was used in this study as an evaluator of a feature subset (Cao et al., 2017). GaussianNB implements the Gaussian Naive Bayes algorithm for classification. The likelihood of the features is assumed to be Gaussian:

$$P(x_i|y) = \frac{1}{\sqrt{2\pi\sigma_y^2}} \exp\left(-\frac{(x_i - \mu_y)^2}{2\sigma_y^2}\right).$$

The parameters σ_y and μ_y are estimated using maximum likelihood.

The python sklearn version 0.19.1 provided the code of these five classifiers.

Performance Measurements

Three classification performance measurements, i.e., accuracy (Acc), sensitivity (Sn), and specificity (Sp), were used to evaluate how well a feature subset performed (Ye et al., 2017; Xu et al., 2018; Yokoi et al., 2018; Zhao et al., 2018). The RA children were regarded as the positive samples (P) while the matched controls were the negative samples (N). P and N were also denoted as the numbers of positive and negative samples. Sensitivity (Sn) was defined as the correctly predicted ratio of positive samples, i.e., Sn = TP/(TP + FN) = TP/P, where TP and FN were the numbers of correctly and incorrectly predicted positive samples, respectively. Specificity (Sp) was the correct prediction ratio of negative samples, i.e., Sp = TN/(TN + FP) = TN/N, where TN and FP were the numbers of negative samples with correct and incorrect predictions, respectively. The overall prediction Acc was defined as Acc = (TP + TN)/(P + N).

These measurements were used in various prediction models like the DNA and RNA functional elements (He et al., 2018; Feng et al., 2019). And they were calculated using the 10-fold cross-validation (10FCV) strategy as similar in Ye et al. (2017) and Zhao et al. (2018).

Experimental Design

The experiments were carried out in three major steps, as illustrated in **Figure 1**. The first step was to find 20,000 features with the largest variations. A methylation residue with a large variation was easier to be detected while a residue with a stable methylation level required a high-resolution technology to measure. And the downstream feature selection algorithms may crash on a dataset with a large number of features. So we have to reduce the feature dimensions to be within the capacity of the eight feature selection algorithms. So LinearSVC was used to select 147 features for further feature screening.

Then the two steps of feature selection and classification were carried out iteratively to find the best classification model using the selected features, as shown in **Figure 1**.

RESULTS AND DISCUSSION

Data Preprocessing

The raw data of this methylomic dataset was provided in the format IDAT, and was processed using the function getBeta() of the R package minfi version 1.28.3 (Aryee et al., 2014). There were 485,577 methylation features for each sample, among which 65 probes designed to interrogate SNPs within the samples and was ignored in the R package minfi. Some methylation residues had many missing values, e.g., the feature cg01550828 has no values in all the 158 samples. The feature cg01550828 was a cysteine in the N termini of the gene Ring Finger Protein 168 (RNF168), which encoded an E3 ubiquitin ligase protein. After the preprocessing, 485,511 methylomic features were detected for the following analysis.

We hypothesized that methylated residues with larger beta-value fluctuations may be easier to detect in the clinical practice. Therefore, we calculated the standard deviation of the beta-values of each methylated residue, and sorted the features in the descendental order. The top-ranked 20,000 features of the 158 samples were kept for further analysis.

Limitations the Variation Threshold 20,000

We performed the 10FCV of the classifier LinearSVC on the features with different variation thresholds, as shown in **Figure 2**. Due to that the number of features were much larger than the number of samples, only the features with the LinearSVC model weight larger than the default weight threshold 1e−5 were kept for model performance evaluation. **Figure 2** demonstrated the running time and 10FCV classification Acc of different numbers of features, i.e., 1000, 2000, 3000, . . ., 22,000. As shown in the figure, the variance threshold 20,000 achieved 0.9873 in Acc while costed a very relatively small running time 17.6620 s. But the procedure of feature selection and classification was not optimized for the final classification Acc. So the other choice of variance threshold may achieve a better final classification Acc.

The evaluation procedure was carried out in a computer with the Windows 7 operating system and Python 3.7 programming language. The computer had a 3.30GHz CPU, 32 Gb memory, and 1Tb hard disk.

Optimizing LinearSVC to Select Features

Firstly, the feature selection procedure SelectFromModel() was used to find the initial feature subset with a reasonable prediction accuracy, as shown in **Figure 3**. The screening procedure was provided by the Python package scikit-learn version 0.21.2 and Python version 3.6. The penalization was carried out by the L1 penalty. In the Python package sklearn.svm.LinearSVC, the parameter C was a float with default = 1.0. It was a regularization parameter. The strength of the regularization was inversely

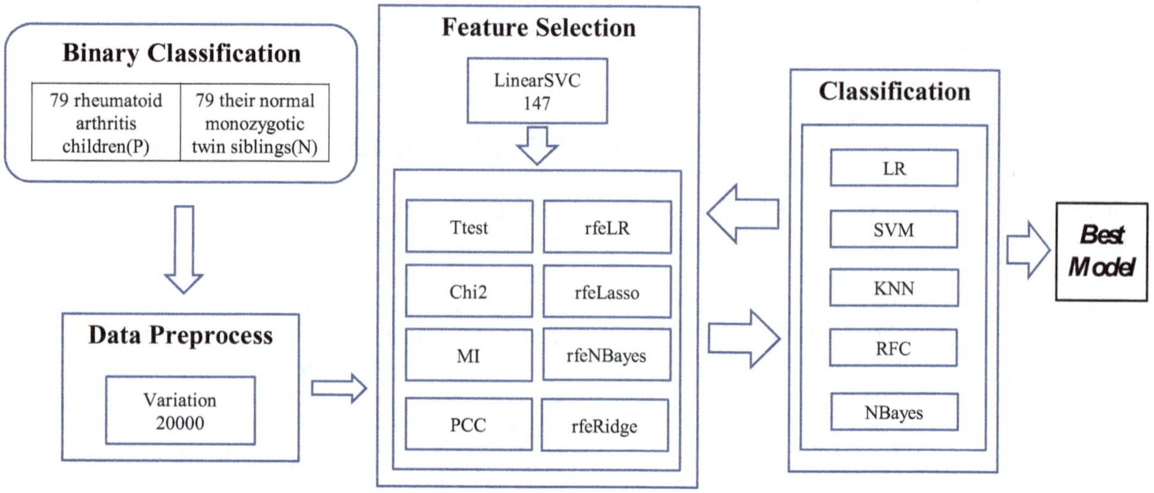

FIGURE 1 | Experiment flowchart of this study. Three major steps were carried out to find the best classification model. The first step was to find the 20,000 features with the largest variation. Then a subset of 147 features was detected using LinearSVC, and 10 feature selection algorithms were utilized to find a better feature subset. The prediction performance was evaluated using five popular binary classifiers.

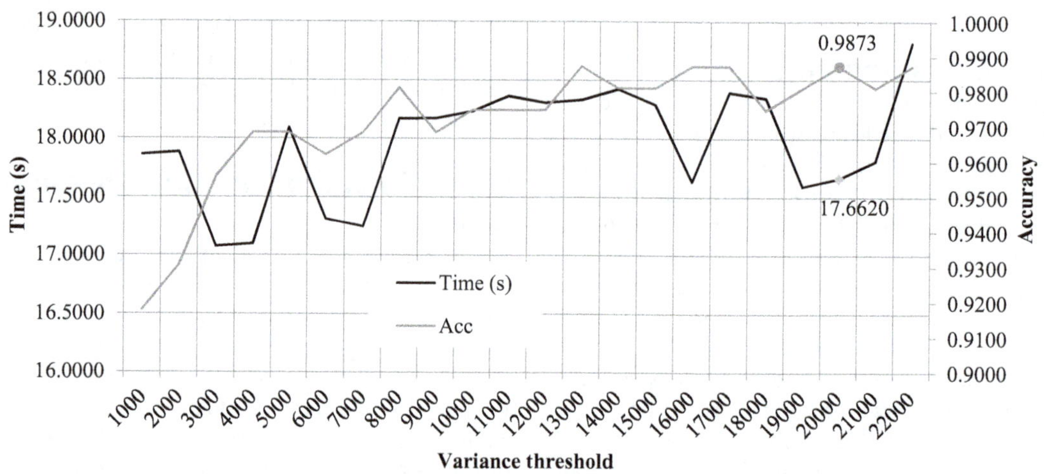

FIGURE 2 | Classification accuracy and time cost of the classifier LinearSVC with different variance thresholds. The horizontal axis was the "variance threshold." The left and right vertical axises were the computational time cost (seconds) and the classification accuracy, respectively.

proportional to C and this parameter must be strictly positive. The parameter C was screened by the values between [0.10, 5.00] with the step size 0.10, as shown in **Figure 3**.

Figure 3 demonstrated that after C reached the value 1.8, the prediction accuracy remained stable. The classifier LinearSVC achieved Acc = 0.9873 with C = 1.8 and 140 features. The best prediction accuracy 0.9937 was achieved by C = 2.4, 3.2, 3.4, 3.5, 4.3, 4.4, 4.6, and 4.7. The data demonstrated that the best Acc = 0.9937 was achieved by many choices of the parameter C, but no better performance was achieved. A smaller number of features suggested a simpler model. So C = 2.4 may be the best choice based on **Figure 3**. Its also interesting to observe that at least 155 features were chosen when C = 3.2, 3.4 and 3.5. So the following sections tried to find a smaller feature subset from this list of 147 features, which were listed in the **Supplementary Table S1**.

Selecting Features by Filters

A filter algorithm assumed the inter-feature independence and evaluated each feature separately for its association with the phenotype. So the AFS strategy selected the k-feature subset as the top-ranked k features. While the DFS strategy removed the least-ranked feature from a $(k + 1)$-feature subset based on the filter-calculated single-feature association with the class label. That is to say, the k-feature subset generated by the DFS strategy was also the top-ranked k features. The ascending and DFS strategies of a filter algorithm selected the same features for a given number of features. So this section only investigated the AFS() strategy of the four filter algorithms. The details of the

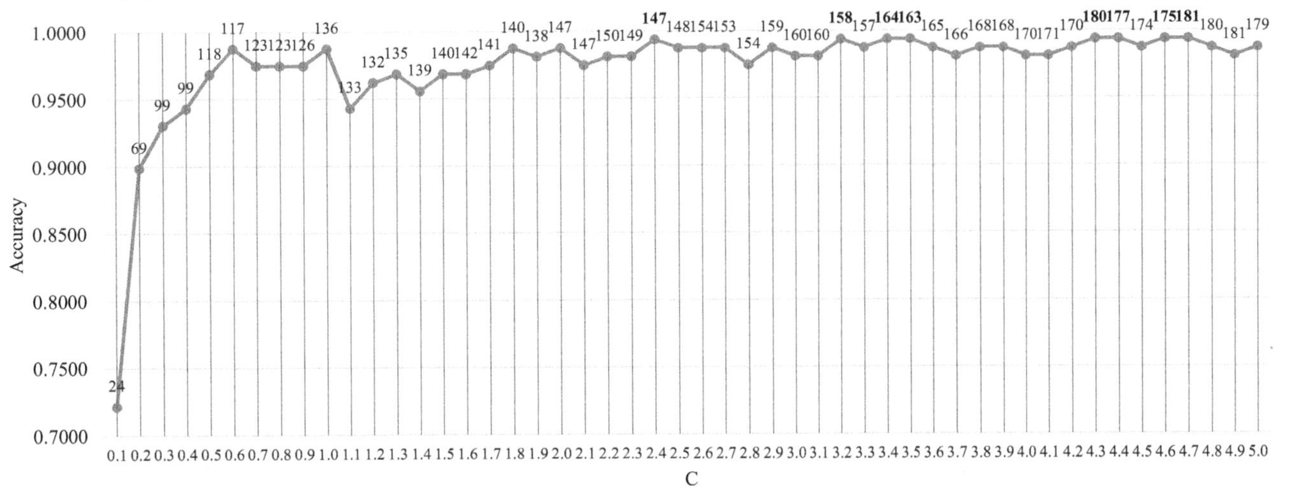

FIGURE 3 | Classification performance of the classifier LinearSVC with different values of the penalty parameter *C*. The parameter *C* was screened by the values between [0.10, 5.00] with the step size 0.10. The vertical axis was for the classification accuracy and the horizontal axis was for the values of the parameter *C*. The number of features selected was given on top of each point in the curve.

AFS strategy were described in the section "Heuristic Feature Selection Strategies."

Our data suggested that all the five classifiers performed similarly well on a feature subset with a size <50, as shown in **Figure 4**. However, the two classifiers LR and SVM kept improving the classification accuracies by adding more features. And SVM achieved the best classification accuracies on features selected by all the four filter algorithms. The best model with Acc = 1.0000 was achieved by the classifier SVM with 144 Chi2-selected methylomic features. The other three classifiers (KNN, RFC and NBayes) reached the plateau of about 0.7000 in Acc after the number of features reached 50.

Selecting Features by the RFE Strategies

We firstly evaluated the two feature selection procedures AFS(rfeLR) and DFS(rfeLR), as shown in **Supplementary Figure S1**. Filter algorithms had the assumption of the inter-feature independence. Although filters usually ran faster than the other algorithms like wrappers and RFE strategies, filters usually selected more features to achieve similar classification accuracies as the other feature selection algorithms (Srivastava et al., 2014; Suto et al., 2016).

When almost all the 147 features were kept, AFS(rfeLR) and DFS(rfeLR) performed similarly well for each of the five classifiers. The same pattern as in the previous section was observed that the two classifiers LR and SVM outperformed the other three with significantly improved accuracies, and the classifier SVM performed the best. **Supplementary Figure S1** illustrated a novel pattern that the descendent feature removal strategy (DFS) performed much better than the ascendant feature addition strategy (AFS). AFS(rfeLR) required at least 116 features to achieve Acc > 0.9000. While DFS(rfeLR) only needed 41 features to achieve Acc = 0.9114.

DFS(rfeRidge) performed even better than AFS(rfeRidge), as shown in **Figure 5** and **Supplementary Figure S4**. AFS(rfeRidge) selected 97 features to train an SVM model with Acc = 0.9051. But only 37 methylomic features were selected by DFS(rfeRidge) to train an SVM model with Acc = 0.9114. And the SVM model performed very stably with more features selected by DFS(rfeRidge), as shown in **Figure 5**. The strategy BackFS required many more features to achieve a similar prediction accuracy, as in **Figure 5C**. The classifier NBayes assumed the inter-feature independence, which may not be the case in the dataset used in this study. This might be the reason that the classifier NBayes didn't perform very well in this study, as shown in **Figure 5**.

Also, DFS(rfeLasso) performed better than AFS(rfeLasso), as shown in **Supplementary Figure S2**. AFS(rfeLasso) selected 144 features to train an SVM model with Acc = 0.9684. But 144 methylomic features were selected by DFS(rfeLasso) to train an SVM model with Acc = 0.9810. And the SVM model performed very stably with more features selected by DFS(rfeLasso).

DFS(rfeNBayes) performed similarly well for each of the five classifiers as AFS(rfeNBayes), as shown in **Supplementary Figure S3**. Both AFS(rfeNBayes) and DFS(rfeNBayes) achieved Acc = 0.9177 when selecting 101 features to train an SVM model. And the SVM model performed very stably with more features selected.

Overall, the best model achieved in this study was the SVM model (Acc = 1.0000) using the 81 features selected by the strategy DFS(rfeRidge), as shown in **Figure 5**.

Another evaluation procedure was carried out for the above-selected features. The stratified splitting strategy was used to split the samples into one-third training, one-third validation, and one-third test datasets. The SVM parameter C was evaluated for its different values from 0.1 to 3.0 with the step size 0.1, as shown in **Figure 6**. After the 81 methylomic features were selected by the strategy DFS(rfeRidge), the binary classification SVM models with different *C* values were trained on the training dataset and evaluated for the classification accuracies on the validation

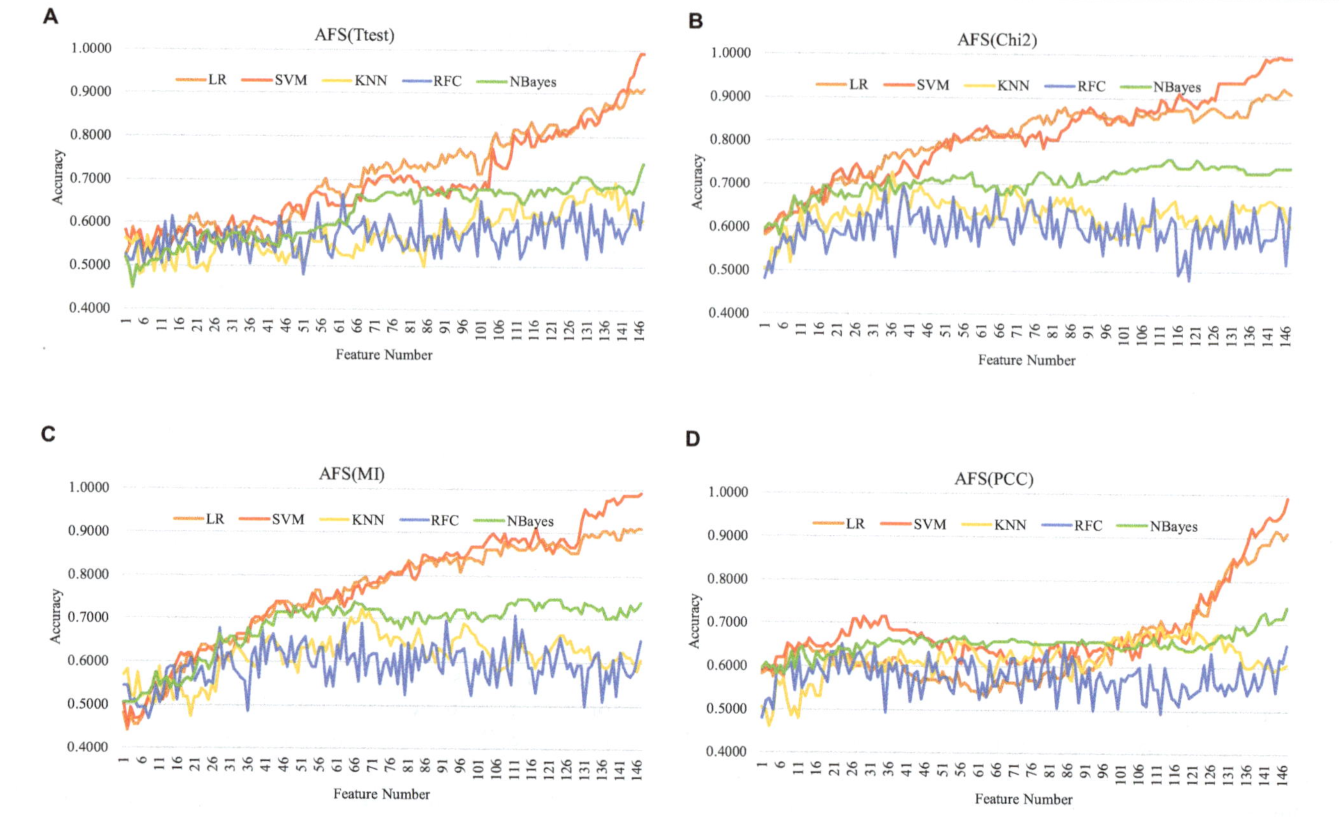

FIGURE 4 | Ascending feature screening (AFS) of four filter algorithms. The classification performance of each filter algorithm was evaluated by five classifiers. The four filter algorithms were **(A)** Ttest, **(B)** Chi2, **(C)** MI, and **(D)** PCC, and the five classifiers were LR, SVM, KNN, RFC, and NBayes.

dataset, as shown in **Figure 6**. When the parameter was 0.5, the validation accuracy reached the best value 0.8868. A similar classification accuracy 0.8679 was achieved on the test dataset. This suggested the model stability for the classification algorithm.

Refining the 147 Features With Two Other Regression Algorithms

This study evaluated how the regression-based feature selection algorithms might be improved by two other regression algorithms, i.e., sliced inverse regression (SIR) (Cook and Weisberg, 1991; Li, 1991) and group lasso (GroupLasso) (Yuan and Lin, 2006; Yuan et al., 2011). **Figure 1** demonstrated that the LinearSVC model selected 147 features and then the filters and regression-based RFE algorithms were applied. So SIR and GroupLasso were utilized to further refine the subset of 147 features.

Sliced inverse regression doesn't need to optimize the parametric or non-parametric model training process and demonstrates a significant capability to reduce the feature dimensions (Cook and Weisberg, 1991; Li, 1991). This study utilized the SIR in the Python package sliced version 0.1 (Li, 1991). Its interesting to observe that the classifier SVM from the best model achieved again Acc = 1.0000 using only the first feature engineered by SIR. Our experimental data demonstrated that SIR and the proposed feature selection procedure achieved the same classification performances on the investigated problem in this study. But the best model used only 81 original methylated residues while SIR used the one feature engineered from the 147 features.

GroupLasso is another widely used feature selection algorithm that assigns non-zero weights to groups of features instead of the individual ones like the regular lasso (Yuan and Lin, 2006; Yuan et al., 2011). This study utilized GroupLasso in the Python package group-lasso version 1.1.1 (Yuan and Lin, 2006; Yuan et al., 2011). Unfortunately no features were selected by GroupLasso.

Refining Differentially Methylated and Variable Biomarkers

Twenty differentially methylated residues were detected in the previous study, but all of them were not statistically significantly associated with RA by the adjusted *p*-values (Webster et al., 2018). This study further refined this subset of 20 methylation residues with the classification accuracy as the optimization goal.

The AFS strategy of the four filter algorithms was applied to the 20 differentially methylated residues, as shown in **Supplementary Figure S5**. The classifier NBayes achieved the best Acc = 0.7532 on the original subset of 20 features. This model may be further improved to Acc = 0.7658 using only 10 features, which was selected by the algorithm AFS(MI).

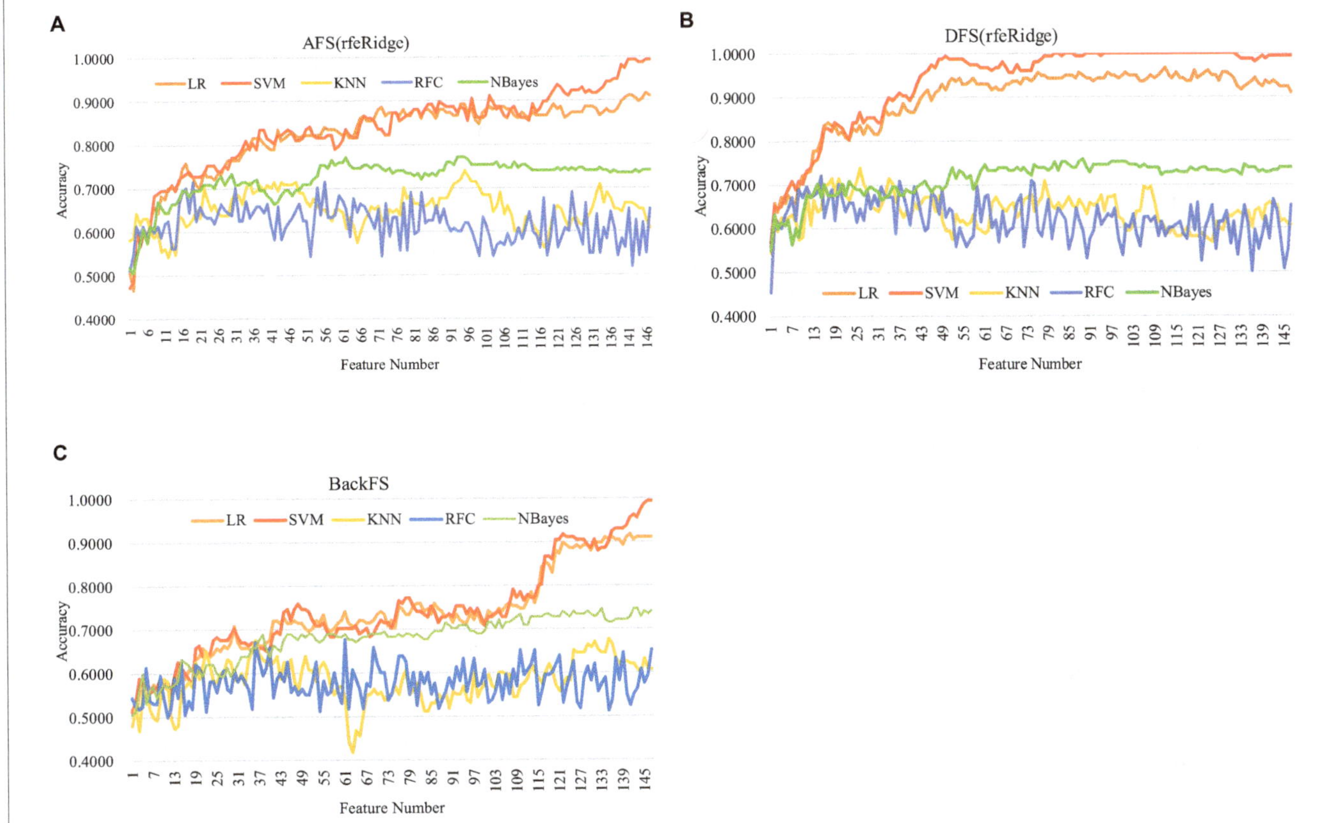

FIGURE 5 | Comparison of the three feature screening strategies of the feature selection algorithm rfeRidge. The classification performance was evaluated by five classifiers. The five classifiers were LR, SVM, KNN, RFC, and NBayes. And the three feature screening strategies were **(A)** AFS(rfeRidge), **(B)** DFS(rfeRidge), and **(C)** BackFS.

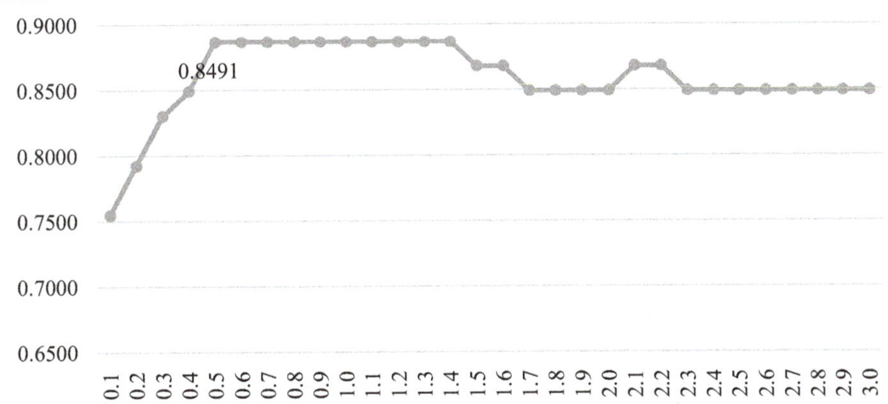

FIGURE 6 | Parameter tuning for the SVM parameter *C*. The horizontal axis was the value of the parameter *C*, and the vertical axis was the classification accuracy. Each model was trained on the training dataset and evaluated on the validation dataset.

Another algorithm AFS(Ttest) achieved the same prediction Acc = 0.7532 using only 4 and 10 features for the classifiers KNN and NBayes, respectively.

An even better improvement may be achieved by both AFS(rfeLasso) and DFS(rfeLasso), as shown in **Supplementary Figure S6.** Firstly, the original list of 20 differentially methylated residues may be reduced to 11 features to achieve Acc = 0.7658. Secondly, the best model achieved Acc = 0.8038 using only 18 features.

Webster et al. (2018) also evaluated a list of two differentially variable residues, which were refined in the same way in this study, as shown in **Supplementary Figures S7, S8.** The similar patterns were observed, and the best improved SVM model achieved Acc = 0.7722 with 12 features selected by AFS(Chi2).

Refining the Previous Biomarkers by BackFS

The two lists of RA biomarkers were further refined by a simple iterative feature elimination procedure BackFS, as shown in **Figure 7**. BackFS exhaustively removed the redundant features, so only the subset of features achieving the best prediction accuracy was kept for further analysis. The original list of 20 differentially methylated features may be further selected to achieve a better prediction Acc = 0.7658 using only 18 features for the classifier NBayes, as shown in **Figure 7A**. While the list of 20 differentially variable features may be reduced to 15 with a better prediction Acc = 0.7595 for the same classifier NBayes, as shown in **Figure 7B**.

Independent Effectiveness Evaluation of the Proposed Biomarker Detection Procedure

We further evaluated the effectiveness of the proposed biomarker detection procedure on an independent dataset. There is no simulation tool for the array-based methylomes. So another independent dataset TCGA-BRCA (Berger et al., 2018) was chosen to evaluate our biomarker detection procedure, as shown in **Figure 8**. There were 982 samples and each sample had 485,577 methylated residues. Multiple samples were extracted from some patients and only sample was randomly chosen to represent this patient. 763 samples were collected to have the clinical annotation "tumor_stage" (I/II/III/IV). The binary classification problem was formulated between the class Positive (555 samples from the stages I and II) and Negative (208 samples from the stages III and IV).

The same biomarker detection procedure was carried out on the methylomic dataset TCGA-BRCA, as shown in **Figure 6**. The initial 20,000 top-ranked features with the largest standard-deviations were screened to find the best value of the parameter C, as shown in **Figure 6**. The binary classification problem for the dataset TCGA-BRCA seemed to reach the classification accuracy 1.0000 with the parameter $C = 0.3$. There were 499 features selected in this step. Then the four filter algorithms were evaluated using the AFS strategy and the four RFE algorithms were evaluated by both AFS and DFS strategies, in the same procedure as the above. The features screened by DFS(rfeLR) achieved the best classification accuracy 1.0000 using only 240 features. Among the five classifiers, SVM achieved the best performance, as the same in the RA biomarker detection problem. The best feature selection algorithm DFS(rfeRidge) for the RA biomarker detection problem achieved a similar classification accuracy (0.9882) for the dataset TCGA-BRCA.

So overall the biomarker detection procedure in this study effectively detected methylated residues for the methylome-based classification problems.

Biological Observations of Methylomic Biomarkers

This study selected 81 methylated residues as biomarkers to separate the RA patients from their controls, as shown in **Supplementary Table S1**. Its interesting to observe that 38 of these 81 methylated residues were from the chromosome Y and many of them were within the transcriptional start sites (TSS) of non-coding RNA gene family Testis-Specific Transcript, Y-Linked (TTTY). This supported the observations in the literature about the gender discrepancy on autoimmune diseases like RA (Jansson and Holmdahl, 1994). Many of these methylated residues were in the TSS regions of these non-coding RNAs, suggesting that methylation may have played a regulatory role in the onset and development of RA (Relle et al., 2015; Houtman et al., 2018). Such reversible epigenetic modifications may serve as therapeutic candidates (Cribbs et al., 2015; Doody et al., 2017).

Another RA-associated gene HLA-DRB1 (Major Histocompatibility Complex, Class II, DR Beta 1) was also a methylation biomarker (cg27107292) detected in this study (Conigliaro et al., 2019; Okada et al., 2019). HLA-DRB1 was one of the first few RA biomarkers discovered four decades ago and harbored more than 100 RA-associated loci (Okada et al., 2019). Recently, HLA-DRB1 was also observed to be differentially methylated in RA (Liu et al., 2013) and had significant associations with the mortality and prognosis of RA (Ruyssen-Witrand et al., 2012; Viatte et al., 2015) and other autoimmune diseases (Bettencourt et al., 2012; Okayama et al., 2018). Furthermore, the pathway analysis through the KEGG Database (Kanehisa et al., 2017) demonstrated that various immune pathways were associated with HLA-DRB1 such as hsa04612 (Antigen processing and presentation pathway), hsa04659 (Th17 cell differentiation pathway), and hsa05323 (RA pathway). This suggested that the detected biomarker HLA-DRB1 was strongly connected to the autoimmune disease RA.

Furthermore, C5orf30 (a methylation biomarker cg17605604) was reported as a damaging regulator of tissue in RA, which is highly expressed in RA synovial fibroblast (RASF) involving joint destruction (Muthana et al., 2015). The clinical data analysis also demonstrated that the variant rs26232 in C5orf30 locus was testified to be associated with RA susceptibility and radiologic damage severity. These observations from the literature supported that C5orf30 may play a significant role in the progression of arthrosis damage (Teare et al., 2013).

Two gender-specific methylation biomarker genes DDX3Y and UTY which have been reported as sex-affected differentially expressed genes for inflammatory arthritis through the Wnt signaling (Kudryavtseva et al., 2012). This situation exactly matched to the gender-biased disease condition for RA. Besides DDX3Y was suggested to be differentially expressed in cartilage tissues of RA patients versus control groups with potential association with miRNA (Toraih et al., 2016). Many other genes like RPS4Y2, KDM5D, EIF1AY, and CYorf15A have also been shown as important biomarker genes in RA via the Monte Carlo cross-validation (Song et al., 2017).

Supplementary Table S1 also illustrated that the methylated biomarkers were from various genic sites, i.e., TSS, 5′-untranslated region (UTR), 3′-UTR, first exon, and genic body. This suggested that these RA methylation biomarkers contributed their regulatory roles through different biological mechanisms. Those frequently appeared genes, and non-coding RNA genes may need further wet-lab investigations of their potential biological mechanisms.

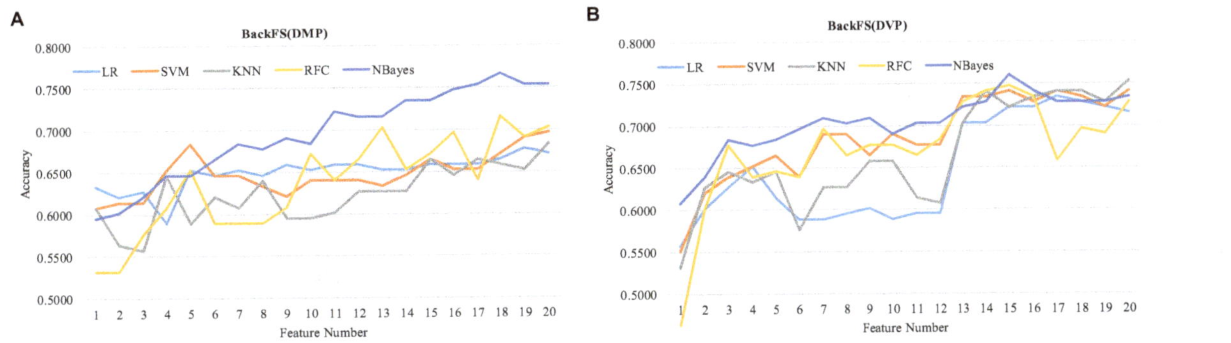

FIGURE 7 | Refine the two lists of previous methylation biomarkers of RA. The classification performance was evaluated by five classifiers. The five classifiers were LR, SVM, KNN, RFC, and NBayes. Refining procedures of **(A)** the 20 differentially methylated positions (DMP) and **(B)** the 20 differentially variable positions (DVP).

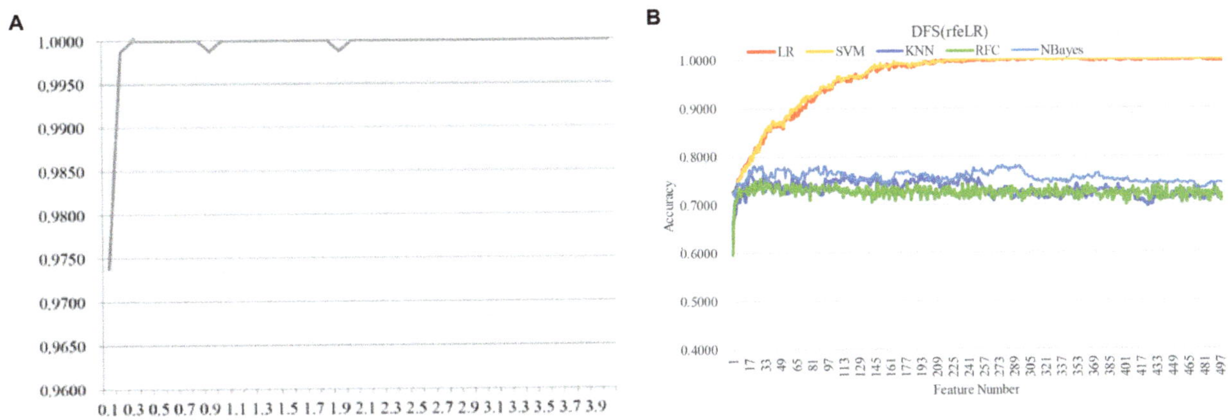

FIGURE 8 | Evaluating the proposed biomarker detection procedure with a new dataset TCGA-BRCA. The classification performance was evaluated by five classifiers. The five classifiers were LR, SVM, KNN, RFC, and NBayes. **(A)** The classification accuracies (vertical axis) of the classifier LinearSVC with different values of the parameter *C* between [0.10, 4.00] with the step size 0.10. **(B)** The classification accuracy plots of the feature selection strategy DFS(rfeLR) using the five classifiers, i.e., LR, SVM, KNN, RFC, and NBayes.

CONCLUSION

This study comprehensively utilized the widely used modeling algorithms to find the set of methylomic features with the best RA prediction accuracy. The best model used the features selected by the DFS(rfeRidge) strategy and the classifier SVM. The best accuracy 100.00% was achieved with the 81 detected methylomic biomarkers using the 10FCV strategy. The 81 methylomic biomarkers may accurately separate the RA patients from their matched controls. These biomarkers also demonstrated that chromosome Y contributed 38 methylated residues to the final model, supporting the literature about the gender-specific discrepancy. These 81 methylated biomarkers came from both regulatory regions and the gene body. So the biological mechanisms of how these 81 methylated residues were involved in RA's onset and development may vary from the transcriptional regulation to the epigenetic modifications.

The number of biomarker features was still too large for the clinical practice. Clinical data other than the methylomic features may be integrated to improve the proposed RA detection model. A weakened model may also be considered using fewer features. For example, if only 37 methylomic features selected by DFS(rfeRidge) were used to train the SVM model, the detection accuracy reached Acc = 0.9114, an acceptable accuracy in some cases. RA was a complex human disease and the subtypes may be described by fewer biomarkers. So the detection models for the RA subtypes may also use fewer biomarkers to achieve satisfying accuracies.

The samples were 70 pairs of monozygotic twins. Each twin shared the same genetic background that might reduce the noise information induced by the methylation status of genetic variations. This sample setting suggested that the detected methylomic biomarkers mainly reflected the epigenetic status of RA. Independent validation datasets might also further improve our models.

AUTHOR CONTRIBUTIONS

FZ and XF conceived the project and designed the experiments. XF, XH, RS, ZX, LH, and QY wrote the codes and conducted the experiments. XF, XH, RS, and ZX generated the experimental results and drafted the discussions. FZ and XF discussed the experimental design and polished the manuscript. FZ and XF drafted and polished the manuscript. FZ, QY, and XF designed and carried out the additional experiments according to the reviewers' comments. FZ, QY, and XF also revised and polished the revised version of the manuscript.

FUNDING

This work was supported by the Jilin Provincial Key Laboratory of Big Data Intelligent Computing (20180622002JC), Jilin Science and Technology Bureau (20190104130), the Education Department of Jilin Province (JJKH20180145KJ), and the startup grant of the Jilin University. This work was also partially supported by the Bioknow MedAI Institute (BMCPP-2018-001), the High Performance Computing Center of Jilin University, and by the Fundamental Research Funds for the Central Universities, JLU.

ACKNOWLEDGMENTS

Constructive comments from the two reviewers were much appreciated.

REFERENCES

Alam, S. M., Kidwai, A. A., Jafri, S. R., Qureshi, B. M., Sami, A., Qureshi, H. H., et al. (2011). Epidemiology of rheumatoid arthritis in a tertiary care unit, Karachi, Pakistan. *J. Pak. Med. Assoc.* 61, 123–126.

Angelosante, D., Giannakis, G. B., and Grossi, E. (2009). "Compressed sensing of time-varying signals," in *Proceedings of the 2009 16th International Conference on Digital Signal Processing* (Santorini-Hellas: IEEE), 1–8.

Aryee, M. J., Jaffe, A. E., Corrada-Bravo, H., Ladd-Acosta, C., Feinberg, A. P., Hansen, K. D., et al. (2014). Minfi: a flexible and comprehensive Bioconductor package for the analysis of Infinium DNA methylation microarrays. *Bioinformatics* 30, 1363–1369. doi: 10.1093/bioinformatics/btu049

Athar, A., Fullgrabe, A., George, N., Iqbal, H., Huerta, L., Ali, A., et al. (2019). ArrayExpress update - from bulk to single-cell expression data. *Nucleic Acids Res.* 47, D711–D715. doi: 10.1093/nar/gky964

Bangdiwala, S. I. (2016). Chi-squared statistics of association and homogeneity. *Int. J. Inj. Contr. Saf. Promot.* 23, 444–446. doi: 10.1080/17457300.2016.1228144

Barker, L., and Brown, C. (2001). Logistic regression when binary predictor variables are highly correlated. *Stat. Med.* 20, 1431–1442. doi: 10.1002/sim.680

Berger, A. C., Korkut, A., Kanchi, R. S., Hegde, A. M., Lenoir, W., Liu, W., et al. (2018). A comprehensive pan-cancer molecular study of gynecologic and breast cancers. *Cancer Cell* 33, 690–705e699. doi: 10.1016/j.ccell.2018.03.014

Bettencourt, A., da Silva, A., Pinho, E. C. P., and Martins Silva, B. (2012). Molecular genetic studies of multiple sclerosis in the portuguese population. *Acta Med. Port.* 25, 224–230.

Brandt, B., Rashidiani, S., Ban, A., and Rauch, T. A. (2019). DNA methylation-governed gene expression in autoimmune arthritis. *Int. J. Mol. Sci.* 20:5646. doi: 10.3390/ijms20225646

Cao, J., Wu, Z., Ye, W., and Wang, H. (2017). "Learning functional embedding of genes governed by pair-wised labels," in *Proceedings of the 2017 2nd IEEE International Conference on Computational Intelligence and Applications* (Beijing: IEEE), 397–401.

Carnero-Montoro, E., and Alarcon-Riquelme, M. E. (2018). Epigenome-wide association studies for systemic autoimmune diseases: the road behind and the road ahead. *Clin. Immunol.* 196, 21–33. doi: 10.1016/j.clim.2018.03.014

Cawley, G. C., and Talbot, N. L. (2010). On over-fitting in model selection and subsequent selection bias in performance evaluation. *J. Mach. Learn. Res.* 11, 2079–2107.

Chatzidionisyou, A., and Catrina, A. I. (2016). The lung in rheumatoid arthritis, cause or consequence? *Curr. Opin. Rheumatol.* 28, 76–82. doi: 10.1097/BOR.0000000000000238

Citak-Er, F., Firat, Z., Kovanlikaya, I., Ture, U., and Ozturk-Isik, E. (2018). Machine-learning in grading of gliomas based on multi-parametric magnetic resonance imaging at 3T. *Comput. Biol. Med.* 99, 154–160. doi: 10.1016/j.compbiomed.2018.06.009

Conigliaro, P., Triggianese, P., De Martino, E., Fonti, G. L., Chimenti, M. S., Sunzini, F., et al. (2019). Challenges in the treatment of rheumatoid arthritis. *Autoimmun. Rev.* 18, 706–713. doi: 10.1016/j.autrev.2019.05.007

Cook, R. D., and Weisberg, S. (1991). Sliced inverse regression for dimension reduction: comment. *J. Am. Stat. Assoc.* 86, 328–332.

Cribbs, A., Feldmann, M., and Oppermann, U. (2015). Towards an understanding of the role of DNA methylation in rheumatoid arthritis: therapeutic and diagnostic implications. *Ther. Adv. Musculoskelet. Dis.* 7, 206–219. doi: 10.1177/1759720X15598307

Crowson, C. S., Liao, K. P., Davis, J. M. III, Solomon, D. H., Matteson, E. L., Knutson, K. L., et al. (2013). Rheumatoid arthritis and cardiovascular disease. *Am. Heart J.* 166, 622.e1–628.e1. doi: 10.1016/j.ahj.2013.07.010

Doody, K. M., Bottini, N., and Firestein, G. S. (2017). Epigenetic alterations in rheumatoid arthritis fibroblast-like synoviocytes. *Epigenomics* 9, 479–492. doi: 10.2217/epi-2016-0151

Farquhar, H., Vassallo, R., Edwards, A. L., and Matteson, E. L. (2019). Pulmonary complications of rheumatoid arthritis. *Semin. Respir. Crit. Care Med.* 40, 194–207. doi: 10.1055/s-0039-1683995

Feng, X., Zhang, R., Liu, M., Liu, Q., Li, F., Yan, Z., et al. (2019). An accurate regression of developmental stages for breast cancer based on transcriptomic biomarkers. *Biomark. Med.* 13, 5–15. doi: 10.2217/bmm-2018-0305

Fernandez Rojas, R., Huang, X., and Ou, K. L. (2019). A machine learning approach for the identification of a biomarker of human pain using fNIRS. *Sci. Rep.* 9:5645. doi: 10.1038/s41598-019-42098-w

Gharbali, A. A., Najdi, S., and Fonseca, J. M. (2018). Investigating the contribution of distance-based features to automatic sleep stage classification. *Comput. Biol. Med.* 96, 8–23. doi: 10.1016/j.compbiomed.2018.03.001

He, J., Fang, T., Zhang, Z., Huang, B., Zhu, X., and Xiong, Y. (2018). PseUI: pseudouridine sites identification based on RNA sequence information. *BMC Bioinformatics* 19:306. doi: 10.1186/s12859-018-2321-0

Houtman, M., Shchetynsky, K., Chemin, K., Hensvold, A. H., Ramskold, D., Tandre, K., et al. (2018). T cells are influenced by a long non-coding RNA in the autoimmune associated PTPN2 locus. *J. Autoimmun.* 90, 28–38. doi: 10.1016/j.jaut.2018.01.003

Ibanez-Cabellos, J. S., Seco-Cervera, M., Osca-Verdegal, R., Pallardo, F. V., and Garcia-Gimenez, J. L. (2019). Epigenetic regulation in the pathogenesis of sjogren syndrome and rheumatoid arthritis. *Front. Genet.* 10:1104. doi: 10.3389/fgene.2019.01104

Inzaule, S. C., Kityo, C. M., Siwale, M., Akanmu, A. S., Wellington, M., de Jager, M., et al. (2018). Previous antiretroviral drug use compromises standard first-line HIV therapy and is mediated through drug-resistance. *Sci. Rep.* 8:15751. doi: 10.1038/s41598-018-33538-0

Jankowski, K. R. B., Flannelly, K. J., and Flannelly, L. T. (2018). The t-test: an influential inferential tool in chaplaincy and other healthcare research. *J. Health Care Chaplain.* 24, 30–39. doi: 10.1080/08854726.2017.1335050

Jansson, L., and Holmdahl, R. (1994). The Y chromosome-linked "autoimmune accelerating" yaa gene suppresses collagen-induced arthritis. *Eur. J. Immunol.* 24, 1213–1217. doi: 10.1002/eji.1830240531

Julia, A., Absher, D., Lopez-Lasanta, M., Palau, N., Pluma, A., Waite Jones, L., et al. (2017). Epigenome-wide association study of rheumatoid arthritis identifies differentially methylated loci in B cells. *Hum. Mol. Genet.* 26, 2803–2811. doi: 10.1093/hmg/ddx177

Julia, A., Gonzalez, I., Fernandez-Nebro, A., Blanco, F., Rodriguez, L., Gonzalez, A., et al. (2016). A genome-wide association study identifies SLC8A3 as a susceptibility locus for ACPA-positive rheumatoid arthritis. *Rheumatology (Oxford)* 55, 1106–1111. doi: 10.1093/rheumatology/kew035

Kahl, V. F. S., Dhillon, V. S., Simon, D., da Silva, F. R., Salvador, M., Branco, C. D. S., et al. (2018). Chronic occupational exposure endured by tobacco farmers from Brazil and association with DNA damage. *Mutagenesis* 33, 119–128. doi: 10. 1093/mutage/gex045

Kanehisa, M., Furumichi, M., Tanabe, M., Sato, Y., and Morishima, K. (2017). KEGG: new perspectives on genomes, pathways, diseases and drugs. *Nucleic Acids Res.* 45, D353–D361. doi: 10.1093/nar/gkw1092

Khan, H., Sureda, A., Belwal, T., Cetinkaya, S., Suntar, I., Tejada, S., et al. (2019). Polyphenols in the treatment of autoimmune diseases. *Autoimmun. Rev.* 18, 647–657. doi: 10.1016/j.autrev.2019.05.001

Kim, T. K. (2015). T test as a parametric statistic. *Korean J. Anesthesiol.* 68, 540–546. doi: 10.4097/kjae.2015.68.6.540

Kudryavtseva, E., Forde, T. S., Pucker, A. D., and Adarichev, V. A. (2012). Wnt signaling genes of murine chromosome 15 are involved in sex-affected pathways of inflammatory arthritis. *Arthritis Rheum.* 64, 1057–1068. doi: 10.1002/art. 33414

Kumar, N. S., and Nirmalkumar, P. (2019). A robust decision support system for wireless healthcare based on hybrid prediction algorithm. *J. Med. Syst.* 43:170. doi: 10.1007/s10916-019-1304-7

Lazzerini, P. E., Capecchi, P. L., and Laghi-Pasini, F. (2017). Systemic inflammation and arrhythmic risk: lessons from rheumatoid arthritis. *Eur. Heart J.* 38, 1717–1727. doi: 10.1093/eurheartj/ehw208

Li, K.-C. (1991). Sliced inverse regression for dimension reduction. *J. Am. Stat. Assoc.* 86, 316–327.

Liu, A. N., Wang, L. L., Li, H. P., Gong, J., and Liu, X. H. (2017). Correlation between posttraumatic growth and posttraumatic stress disorder symptoms based on pearson correlation coefficient: a meta-analysis. *J. Nerv. Ment. Dis.* 205, 380–389. doi: 10.1097/NMD.0000000000000605

Liu, Y., Aryee, M. J., Padyukov, L., Fallin, M. D., Hesselberg, E., Runarsson, A., et al. (2013). Epigenome-wide association data implicate DNA methylation as an intermediary of genetic risk in rheumatoid arthritis. *Nat. Biotechnol.* 31, 142–147. doi: 10.1038/nbt.2487

Lopez-Isac, E., Martin, J. E., Assassi, S., Simeon, C. P., Carreira, P., Ortego-Centeno, N., et al. (2016). Brief report: IRF4 newly identified as a common susceptibility locus for systemic sclerosis and rheumatoid arthritis in a cross-disease meta-analysis of genome-wide association studies. *Arthritis Rheumatol.* 68, 2338–2344. doi: 10.1002/art.39730

Lopez-Mejias, R., Carmona, F. D., Genre, F., Remuzgo-Martinez, S., Gonzalez-Juanatey, C., Corrales, A., et al. (2019). Identification of a 3'-untranslated genetic variant of RARB associated with carotid intima-media thickness in rheumatoid arthritis: a genome-wide association study. *Arthritis Rheumatol.* 71, 351–360. doi: 10.1002/art.40734

Lotsch, D., Ghanim, B., Laaber, M., Wurm, G., Weis, S., Lenz, S., et al. (2013). Prognostic significance of telomerase-associated parameters in glioblastoma: effect of patient age. *Neuro Oncol.* 15, 423–432. doi: 10.1093/neuonc/ nos329

Lu, S., Xia, Y., Cai, W., Fulham, M., Feng, D. D., and Neuroimaging Initiative, (2017). Early identification of mild cognitive impairment using incomplete random forest-robust support vector machine and FDG-PET imaging. *Comput. Med. Imaging Graph* 60, 35–41. doi: 10.1016/j.compmedimag.2017.01.001

Lyu, H., Wan, M., Han, J., Liu, R., and Wang, C. (2017). A filter feature selection method based on the maximal information coefficient and gram-schmidt orthogonalization for biomedical data mining. *Comput. Biol. Med.* 89, 264–274. doi: 10.1016/j.compbiomed.2017.08.021

Massey, J., Plant, D., Hyrich, K., Morgan, A. W., Wilson, A. G., Spiliopoulou, A., et al. (2018). Genome-wide association study of response to tumour necrosis factor inhibitor therapy in rheumatoid arthritis. *Pharmacogenomics J.* 18, 657–664. doi: 10.1038/s41397-018-0040-6

Meng, C., Wang, Q., Guan, S., Sun, K., and Liu, B. J. I. A. (2019). 2D-3D registration with weighted local mutual information in vascular interventions. *IEEE Access* 7, 162629–162638. doi: 10.1109/access.2019.2905345

Moayyeri, A., Hammond, C. J., Valdes, A. M., and Spector, T. D. (2013). Cohort profile: twinsuk and healthy ageing twin study. *Int. J. Epidemiol.* 42, 76–85. doi: 10.1093/ije/dyr207

Muthana, M., Hawtree, S., Wilshaw, A., Linehan, E., Roberts, H., Khetan, S., et al. (2015). C5orf30 is a negative regulator of tissue damage in rheumatoid arthritis. *Proc. Natl. Acad. Sci. U.S.A.* 112, 11618–11623. doi: 10.1073/pnas.1501947112

Nejadgholi, I., and Bolic, M. (2015). A comparative study of PCA, SIMCA and Cole model for classification of bioimpedance spectroscopy measurements. *Comput. Biol. Med.* 63, 42–51. doi: 10.1016/j.compbiomed.2015.05.004

Okada, Y., Eyre, S., Suzuki, A., Kochi, Y., and Yamamoto, K. (2019). Genetics of rheumatoid arthritis: 2018 status. *Ann. Rheum. Dis.* 78, 446–453. doi: 10.1136/ annrheumdis-2018-213678

Okayama, T., Hashiguchi, Y., Kikuyama, H., Yoneda, H., and Kanazawa, T. (2018). Next-generation sequencing analysis of multiplex families with atypical psychosis. *Transl. Psychiatry* 8:221. doi: 10.1038/s41398-018-0272-x

Olsen, R. M., Aasvang, E. K., Meyhoff, C. S., and Dissing Sorensen, H. B. (2018). Towards an automated multimodal clinical decision support system at the post anesthesia care unit. *Comput. Biol. Med.* 101, 15–21. doi: 10.1016/j. compbiomed.2018.07.018

Pandey, G., Pandey, O. P., Rogers, A. J., Ahsen, M. E., Hoffman, G. E., Raby, B. A., et al. (2018). A nasal brush-based classifier of asthma identified by machine learning analysis of nasal RNA sequence data. *Sci. Rep.* 8:8826.

Petralia, M. C., Mazzon, E., Basile, M. S., Cutuli, M., Di Marco, R., Scandurra, F., et al. (2019). Effects of treatment with the hypomethylating agent 5-aza-2'-deoxycytidine in murine type II collagen-induced arthritis. *Pharmaceuticals (Basel)* 12:174. doi: 10.3390/ph12040174

Rahman, M. M., Bhuiyan, M. I. H., and Hassan, A. R. (2018). Sleep stage classification using single-channel EOG. *Comput. Biol. Med.* 102, 211–220. doi: 10.1016/j.compbiomed.2018.08.022

Relle, M., Foehr, B., and Schwarting, A. (2015). Epigenetic aspects of systemic lupus erythematosus. *Rheumatol. Ther.* 2, 33–46. doi: 10.1007/s40744-015-0014-y

Rottmann, J., and Berbeco, R. (2014). Using an external surrogate for predictor model training in real-time motion management of lung tumors. *Med. Phys.* 41:121706. doi: 10.1118/1.4901252

Ruyssen-Witrand, A., Constantin, A., Cambon-Thomsen, A., and Thomsen, M. (2012). New insights into the genetics of immune responses in rheumatoid arthritis. *Tissue Antigens* 80, 105–118. doi: 10.1111/j.1399-0039.2012.01939.x

Shadrina, A., Tsepilov, Y., Sokolova, E., Smetanina, M., Voronina, E., Pakhomov, E., et al. (2018). Genome-wide association study in ethnic Russians suggests an association of the MHC class III genomic region with the risk of primary varicose veins. *Gene* 659, 93–99. doi: 10.1016/j.gene.2018. 03.039

Singh, N. P., Bapi, R. S., and Vinod, P. K. (2018). Machine learning models to predict the progression from early to late stages of papillary renal cell carcinoma. *Comput. Biol. Med.* 100, 92–99. doi: 10.1016/j.compbiomed.2018. 06.030

Smolen, J. S., Aletaha, D., and McInnes, I. B. (2016). Rheumatoid arthritis. *Lancet* 388, 2023–2038. doi: 10.1016/S0140-6736(16)30173-8

Song, W., Zhang, Y. M., Ma, T., Wang, J., and Wang, K. Z. (2017). Identification of significant pathway cross-talk in rheumatoid arthritis by the Monte Carlo cross-validation method. *Genet. Mol. Res.* 16:gmr16029142. doi: 10.4238/ gmr16029142

Srivastava, B., Srivastava, R., and Jangid, M. (2014). "Filter vs. wrapper approach for optimum gene selection of high dimensional gene expression dataset: an analysis with cancer datasets," in *Proceedings of the 2014 International Conference on High Performance Computing and Applications* (Bhubaneswar: IEEE), 1–6.

Suto, J., Oniga, S., and Sitar, P. P. (2016). "Comparison of wrapper and filter feature selection algorithms on human activity recognition," in *Proceedings of the 2016 6th International Conference on Computers Communications and Control* (Oradea: IEEE), 124–129.

Taylor, J. C., Bongartz, T., Massey, J., Mifsud, B., Spiliopoulou, A., Scott, I. C., et al. (2018). Genome-wide association study of response to methotrexate in early rheumatoid arthritis patients. *Pharmacogenomics J.* 18, 528–538. doi: 10.1038/s41397-018-0025-5

Teare, M. D., Knevel, R., Morgan, M. D., Kleszcz, A., Emery, P., Moore, D. J., et al. (2013). Allele-dose association of the C5orf30 rs26232 variant with joint damage in rheumatoid arthritis. *Arthritis Rheum.* 65, 2555–2561. doi: 10.1002/art.38064

Tekin Erguzel, T., Tas, C., and Cebi, M. (2015). A wrapper-based approach for feature selection and classification of major depressive disorder-bipolar disorders. *Comput. Biol. Med.* 64, 127–137. doi: 10.1016/j.compbiomed.2015.06.021

Toraih, E. A., Ismail, N. M., Toraih, A. A., Hussein, M. H., and Fawzy, M. S. (2016). Precursor miR-499a variant but not miR-196a2 is associated with rheumatoid arthritis susceptibility in an Egyptian population. *Mol. Diagn. Ther.* 20, 279–295. doi: 10.1007/s40291-016-0194-3

Triantafyllias, K., De Blasi, M., Hoffmann, I., Thomaidis, T., Drees, P., and Schwarting, A. (2016). The count of tender rather than swollen joints correlates with aortic stiffness in patients with rheumatoid arthritis. *Springerplus* 5:428. doi: 10.1186/s40064-016-2066-z

Verde, L., and De Pietro, G. (2019). A neural network approach to classify carotid disorders from heart rate variability analysis. *Comput. Biol. Med.* 109, 226–234. doi: 10.1016/j.compbiomed.2019.04.036

Viatte, S., Plant, D., Han, B., Fu, B., Yarwood, A., Thomson, W., et al. (2015). Association of HLA-DRB1 haplotypes with rheumatoid arthritis severity, mortality, and treatment response. *JAMA* 313, 1645–1656. doi: 10.1001/jama.2015.3435

Villanueva-Romero, R., Gutierrez-Canas, I., Carrion, M., Perez-Garcia, S., Seoane, I. V., Martinez, C., et al. (2018). The anti-inflammatory mediator, vasoactive intestinal peptide, modulates the differentiation and function of Th subsets in rheumatoid arthritis. *J. Immunol. Res.* 2018:6043710. doi: 10.1155/2018/6043710

Wang, Y., Deng, H., Xin, S., Zhang, K., Shi, R., and Bao, X. (2019). Prognostic and predictive value of three DNA methylation signatures in lung adenocarcinoma. *Front. Genet.* 10:349. doi: 10.3389/fgene.2019.00349

Webster, A. P., Plant, D., Ecker, S., Zufferey, F., Bell, J. T., Feber, A., et al. (2018). Increased DNA methylation variability in rheumatoid arthritis-discordant monozygotic twins. *Genome Med.* 10:64. doi: 10.1186/s13073-018-0575-9

Wei, X. X., and Stocker, A. A. (2016). Mutual information, fisher information, and efficient coding. *Neural Comput.* 28, 305–326. doi: 10.1162/NECO_a_00804

Wu, C., Chen, J., Liu, Y., and Hu, X. (2019). Improved prediction of regulatory element using hybrid abelian complexity features with DNA sequences. *Int. J. Mol. Sci.* 20:1704. doi: 10.3390/ijms20071704

Xie, J., Lei, J., Xie, W., Shi, Y., and Liu, X. (2013). Two-stage hybrid feature selection algorithms for diagnosing erythemato-squamous diseases. *Health Inf. Sci. Syst.* 1:10. doi: 10.1186/2047-2501-1-10

Xu, C., Liu, J., Yang, W., Shu, Y., Wei, Z., Zheng, W., et al. (2018). An OMIC biomarker detection algorithm TriVote and its application in methylomic biomarker detection. *Epigenomics* 10, 335–347. doi: 10.2217/epi-2017-0097

Yang, C. H., Weng, Z. J., Chuang, L. Y., and Yang, C. S. (2017). Identification of SNP-SNP interaction for chronic dialysis patients. *Comput. Biol. Med.* 83, 94–101. doi: 10.1016/j.compbiomed.2017.02.004

Ye, Y., Zhang, R., Zheng, W., Liu, S., and Zhou, F. (2017). RIFS: a randomly restarted incremental feature selection algorithm. *Sci. Rep.* 7:13013. doi: 10.1038/s41598-017-13259-6

Yokoi, A., Matsuzaki, J., Yamamoto, Y., Yoneoka, Y., Takahashi, K., Shimizu, H., et al. (2018). Integrated extracellular microRNA profiling for ovarian cancer screening. *Nat. Commun.* 9:4319. doi: 10.1038/s41467-018-06434-4

Youn, E., and Jeong, M. K. (2009). Class dependent feature scaling method using naive Bayes classifier for text datamining. *Pattern Recognit. Lett.* 30, 477–485. doi: 10.1016/j.patrec.2008.11.013

Yuan, L., Liu, J., and Ye, J. (2011). Efficient methods for overlapping group lasso. *Adv. Neural Inf. Process. Syst.* 35, 352–360.

Yuan, M., and Lin, Y. (2006). Model selection and estimation in regression with grouped variables. *J. R. Stat. Soc. Series B Stat. Methodol.* 68, 49–67. doi: 10.1111/j.1467-9868.2005.00532.x

Zhao, R., Zhang, R., Tang, T., Feng, X., Li, J., Liu, Y., et al. (2018). TriZ-a rotation-tolerant image feature and its application in endoscope-based disease diagnosis. *Comput. Biol. Med.* 99, 182–190. doi: 10.1016/j.compbiomed.2018.06.006

5

Association of Sperm Methylation at *LINE-1*, Four Candidate Genes and Nicotine/Alcohol Exposure with the Risk of Infertility

Wenjing Zhang[1,2†], Min Li[1†], Feng Sun[3†], Xuting Xu[4], Zhaofeng Zhang[1], Junwei Liu[1], Xiaowei Sun[1], Aiping Zhang[5], Yupei Shen[1], Jianhua Xu[1], Maohua Miao[1], Bin Wu[1], Yao Yuan[1], Xianliang Huang[6], Huijuan Shi[1]* and Jing Du[1]**

[1] NHC Key Laboratory of Reproduction Regulation (Shanghai Institute of Planned Parenthood Research), Fudan University, Shanghai, China, [2] Reproductive Medical Center, Changhai Hospital of Shanghai, Shanghai, China, [3] Department of Obstetrics and Gynecology, International Peace Maternity and Child Health Hospital, Shanghai Jiao Tong University, Shanghai, China, [4] Huzhou Key Laboratory of Molecular Medicine, Huzhou Central Hospital, Zhejiang, China, [5] Bio-X Institutes, Key Laboratory for the Genetics of Developmental and Neuropsychiatric Disorders, Ministry of Education, Shanghai Jiao Tong University, Shanghai, China, [6] Shanghai Institute of Planned Parenthood Research Hospital, Shanghai, China

***Correspondence:**
Xianliang Huang
hxl7400641@163.com
Huijuan Shi
shihuijuan2011@163.com
Jing Du
dujing42@126.com

†These authors have contributed equally to this work

In this study, we examined whether smoking and drinking affect sperm quality and the DNA methylation of the repetitive element *LINE-1*, *MEST*, *P16*, *H19*, and *GNAS* in sperm. Semen samples were obtained from 143 male residents in a minority-inhabited district of Guizhou province in southwest China. Quantitative DNA methylation analysis of the samples was performed using MassARRAY EpiTYPER assays. Sperm motility was significantly lower in both the nicotine-exposed (P = 0.0064) and the nicotine- and alcohol-exposed (P = 0.0008) groups. Follicle-stimulating hormone (FSH) levels were higher in the nicotine-exposed group (P = 0.0026). The repetitive element *LINE-1* was hypermethylated in the three exposed groups, while *P16* was hypomethylated in the alcohol and both the alcohol and nicotine exposure groups. Our results also show that alcohol and nicotine exposure altered sperm cell quality, which may be related to the methylation levels of *MEST* and *GNAS*. In addition, *MEST*, *GNAS*, and the repetitive element *LINE1* methylation was significantly associated with the concentration of sperm as well as FSH and luteinizing hormone levels.

Keywords: DNA methylation, nicotine/alcohol exposure, male infertility, imprint gene, sperm

INTRODUCTION

Infertility is a major public health concern that affects 10%–20% of married couples attempting to conceive, and male infertility is the only or a common factor (Sharlip et al., 2002; Dada et al., 2008). Recent epidemiological studies have provided plenty of pieces of evidence that environmental exposure, lifestyle, and DNA methylation are closely related to male infertility (Kobayashi et al., 2017; Laqqan et al., 2017; Nasri et al., 2017; Santi et al., 2017; Donkin and Barres, 2018; Siddeek et al., 2018). Our studies before had shown associations of aberrant DNA methylation of several genes in spermatozoa with male infertility, but the study before chose only an asthenozoospermia patient, and other environmental elements such as smoking and drinking were not examined (Xu et al., 2016). It has been shown that long-term alcohol consumption and tobacco use have adverse effects on fertility (Besingi and Johansson, 2014; Hamad et al., 2018). Tobacco exposure is associated with impaired fecundability (Chavarro et al., 2009), slightly lower sperm viability, and reduced ejaculate volume, and spermatocyte apoptosis and disruption of the seminiferous tubules were observed (Kunzle et al., 2003; Gunes et al., 2018). Although cigarette smoking and alcohol consumption have been shown to affect DNA methylation patterns of human sperm, be related to semen quality, and have effects on endocrine control of reproductive and sexual functions, their effects on semen parameters is controversial (Gaur et al., 2010; Hansen et al., 2012; Povey et al., 2012; Chang et al., 2017; Laqqan et al., 2017; Alkhaled et al., 2018; Al Khaled et al., 2018).

Several studies have shown that smoking and drinking have similar effects on oxidative stress and DNA methylation in males of reproductive age and animal models, as has been observed for other chemicals, such as cadmium and bisphenol A (BPA) (Besingi and Johansson, 2014; Miao et al., 2014; Pierron et al., 2014; Jenkins et al., 2017; McCarthy et al., 2018). In imprinted genes, the methylation level present at pro-meiosis should be maintained throughout the male gamete development (Yaman and Grandjean, 2006; Marques et al., 2011). Nicotine exposure may alter the methylation of imprinted and non-imprinted genes in sperm that are associated with oligozoospermia and asthenozoospermia (Dai et al., 2017; Dong et al., 2017; Laqqan et al., 2017). Studies have also shown that chronic paternal alcohol exposure induced behavioral abnormalities in offspring due to alterations in the methylation of imprinted genes in sperm (Kim et al., 2014; Liang et al., 2014; Chastain and Sarkar, 2017).

Mesoderm-specific transcript (*MEST*) and *GNAS* are two maternally imprinted genes that are expressed from the paternal allele. The germ-line differentially methylated regions (DMRs) in *MEST* and *GNAS* exhibit differences in methylation levels between sperm and egg. During spermatogenesis, sperm genomic imprinting (especially in germ-line DMRs) is vulnerable to environmental factors (Marques et al., 2008). In addition, alcohol exposure could cause hypomethylation of *H19* in the sperm of offspring and reduce the mean sperm concentration (Marques et al., 2011), and the methylation levels of *H19* are related to sperm parameters, sperm chromatin, and DNA integrity (Montjean et al., 2015; Darbandi et al., 2018).

The promoter of long interspersed nucleotide element (*LINE-1*), which is used as a surrogate for global methylation, is enriched with methylated CpG dinucleotides and is usually silenced in normal tissues (Rangwala et al., 2009). However, the methylation levels of the *LINE-1* DMRs were lower in BPA-exposed spermatozoa and asthenozoospermia (Miao et al., 2014; Xu et al., 2016). In addition, the P16 protein may inhibit mitosis in spermatogonia and is related to a loss of testicular function (Xin-Chang et al., 2002; Jeong et al., 2017), and we showed that increased methylation defects in the *P16* DMR may be associated with low sperm motility (Xu et al., 2016). The imprint and non-imprint methylation marks at these DMRs are established during gametogenesis and affected by environmental exposures (Li et al., 2016). *P16* methylation is strongly associated with smoking in different pathological conditions, including lung cancer and cervical cancer (Han et al., 2016; Han et al., 2017; Wang et al., 2017). However, the relationship between these genes, tobacco/alcohol exposure, and male infertility has not yet been elucidated.

To investigate the methylation modifications that occur under exposure to alcohol and nicotine, we performed a cohort study of the methylation at the repetitive element *LINE-1* and four genes (*MEST*, *P16*, *H19*, and *GNAS*) in 143 subjects. The aim of this study was to assess whether the DNA methylation of these five genes is associated with the risk of male infertility under tobacco/alcohol exposure.

METHODS

Subjects and Clinical Data

This study included 143 male residents from a minority-inhabited district in Sandu county of Guizhou province. All participants were interviewed by trained Chinese-speaking researchers and were asked about their demography, disease history, and lifestyle factors, including tobacco use and alcohol consumption. The standards for smokers and drinkers were as we described before (Liang et al., 2017; Yang et al., 2017). We defined smoking as consuming at least one cigarette per day for more than 6 months and drinking as consuming an alcohol beverage (beer, wine, and liquor) at least once a week for more than 6 months (Witkiewitz et al., 2017; Pang et al., 2018). As per the standards of the World Health Organization, semen samples were collected after 2 days of abstinence. Sperm counts and motility were assessed by a computer-aided sperm analysis system (Cyto-S; Alpha Innotech Corp., San Leandro, CA, USA) at 37°C. The remainder of the semen sample was stored at −80°C until further examination and DNA extraction. Our study was approved by the Ethics Committee of Shanghai Institute of Planned Parenthood Research, and the local approval of Guizhou province was not required. The individuals included in this study gave written informed consent before participating. All procedures were carried out in accordance with the approved guidelines and local regulations.

TABLE 1 | Primer sequence of five genes.

Target gene	F	R	CpG	Position
MEST	GGGTTTAGAGGTATAAGAAAGAGGG	TTTCTAAAAACAACCAAACCCCTAC	1–17	chr7:130130648–130131063
P16	GTGGGTTTTTAGTTTGTAGTTAAGGG	ATTATCTCCTCCTCCTCCTAACCTAA	1–35	chr9:21994026–21994435
H16	GAGATTTGAGGTGAATTTTAGGGA	CAAAACAAAATCCCCACAACC	1–20	chr11:2019635–2019930
LINE1	GGTGATTTTTGTATTTTTATTTGAGGT	CAAAAACAAACAAACCTCCTTAAACT	1–28	chr16:33760542–33761007
GNAS	GTTTTAGAGTTTTAGGGAAGGGGAG	ATCCCAAACTAACCAACTAAACCTC	1–19	chr20:57415713–57416072

DNA Methylation Assay

DNA was extracted from the semen samples by using the QIAamp DNA Mini Kit (Qiagen, Valencia, CA, USA) stored at −80°C. Bisulfite conversion of DNA was carried out using the Epitect Bisulfite Kit (Qiagen). Quantitative analysis of DNA methylation was performed using MassARRAY EpiTYPER assays (Sequenom, San Diego, CA, USA) according to a published protocol (He et al., 2013). Primers used in this study were designed using Methprimer (http://epidesigner.com; **Table 1**). CpG units that yielded data in >90% of the samples passed the initial quality control assessment. Epigenetic changes at DMRs are important in controlling the levels of gene expression. Thus methylation was measured at 76 CpG dinucleotides in the DMRs at the repetitive element *LINE-1* and four genes (*LINE-1*: 20 CpG sites; *MEST*: 7q32, 130486175–130506297, 12 CpG sites; *P16*: 9p21, 21967752–21995043, 18 CpG sites; *H19*: 11p15.5, 142575532–142578146, 14 CpG sites; and *GNAS*: 20q13.3, 58839740–58911195, 12 CpG sites; **Table 1**).

Statistical Analysis

All data were analyzed with peak picking spectra interpretation tools to generate the ratios of methyl CpG/total CpG. EpiTyper software (Sequenom, San Diego, CA, USA) was used to quantify the methylated fraction of all CpG units. Statistics 18.0 software (SPSS, Inc., Somers, NY, USA) was used to perform all the statistical analyses in this study. Pearson's correlation coefficient test and analysis of variance followed by Dunnett's *post hoc t* test were used to compare the categorical variables and the differences in the mean values of continuous variables between the two groups. All tests were two-tailed. Principal component analysis (PCA) was performed to identify underlying factors. Kaiser–Meyer–Olkin (KMO) value and Bartlett's test of sphericity were checked to confirm that the data were suitable for factor analysis. The criterion of eigenvalue >1.0 was applied to determine the number of factors retained. Items were included in the factor on which they loaded highest (minimum accepted 0.4).

RESULTS

The results of the sperm motility assessment and the levels of follicle-stimulating hormone (FSH), luteinizing hormone (LH), and testosterone (T) are shown in **Table 2**. Sperm motility was significantly lower in the nicotine-exposed ($P = 0.0064$) and the nicotine- and alcohol-exposed ($P = 0.0008$) groups than in the control group. FSH levels were higher in the nicotine-exposed group ($P = 0.0026$). Methylation of each CpG site and adjusted linear regression of alcohol and nicotine exposure are shown in **Suppl 1** and **Suppl 2**.

As shown in **Figure 1**, the average methylation levels of the repetitive element *LINE-1* and four assessed genes in sperm from 143 minority male residents were compared. In general, the methylation levels in the repetitive element *LINE-1* were higher in the three exposed groups ($P < 0.001$, $P = 0.017$, and $P < 0.001$, respectively) than in the control group, whereas methylation levels were lower in *P16* in the nicotine-exposed group and in the nicotine- and alcohol-exposed group after correction of multiple testing ($P < 0.001$, **Figure 1**). Individual CpG sites within the same gene showed similar trends in methylation level. Compared to the controls, the methylation levels of nine CpG sites in the repetitive element *LINE-1* (sites 2, 4.5.6, 7, 9, 14, 19, 20, 23, 25.26, and 27) were higher in the alcohol-exposed group, while the methylation levels of three CpG sites in the repetitive element *LINE-1* (sites 7, 8, and 9) were higher in the nicotine-exposed group, and the levels of 14 CpG sites were significantly higher in the nicotine- and alcohol-exposed group (**Figure 2**).

Among the imprinted genes, we found that the methylation levels of two CpG sites in the *GNAS* DMR (sites 1 and 3) were significantly lower in the alcohol-exposed and the nicotine- and alcohol-exposed groups, and only one site (site 11) in the *MEST* was lower in the nicotine-exposed group. However, the methylation levels of most CpGs in *H19* did not show obvious differences among the three groups (**Figure 2**).

Our results showed that the methylation levels of eight CpGs in *P16* in the nicotine-exposed and nicotine- and

TABLE 2 | Characteristics of all subjects.

Items mean (SD)	Neither nicotine nor alcohol exposed	Alcohol exposed only	Nicotine exposed only	Both nicotine and alcohol exposed	*P1*	*P2*	*P3*
N	48	16	16	63			
Age, years	30.13 (5.52)	36.56 (7.29)	39.60 (4.53)	38.68 (6.31)	**0.0004**	**<0.001**	**<0.001**
Marriage age, years,	24.35 (4.11)	21.07 (2.99)	27.92 (5.71)	24.69 (5.69)	**0.0064**	**0.0242**	0.7351
Body mass index	23.10 (4.02)	22.01 (2.05)	22.48 (2.71)	22.52 (2.42)	0.3186	0.6952	0.3651
Sexual absence, days	7.02 (5.70)	4.56 (4.29)	7.00 (7.48)	5.56 (8.47)	0.1196	0.9909	0.3039
Semen volume, ml,	2.96 (1.21)	2.50 (1.64)	2.90 (1.57)	2.52(1.39)	0.2366	0.8802	0.0869
Sperm concentration, $\times 10^6$/ml	65.47 (45.30)	65.40 (55.79)	55.31 (42.42)	58.23(47.94)	0.9958	0.4445	0.4213
Motility (moving forward), %	49.13 (12.20)	42.64 (17.97)	37.03 (20.34)	37.86(19.86)	0.1091	**0.0064**	**0.0008**
Vitality, %	68.50 (15.39)	63.00 (15.09)	62.38 (18.06)	67.30(16.20)	0.3733	0.3408	0.7583
LH, IU/L	5.32 (2.36)	4.25 (2.28)	6.02 (3.05)	4.94(3.97)	0.1181	0.3552	0.5603
T, IU/L	5.34 (1.96)	4.51 (2.47)	5.75 (1.81)	5.00(2.60)	0.1744	0.4735	0.4574
FSH, IU/L	5.05 (2.39)	4.16 (2.36)	7.87 (4.50)	5.69(5.74)	0.2003	**0.0026**	0.4734

P1: neither nicotine nor alcohol exposed vs alcohol exposed only; P2: neither nicotine- nor alcohol exposed vs nicotine exposed only; P3: neither nicotine nor alcohol exposed vs both nicotine and alcohol exposed. The bold represent p <0.05.

BMI, body mass index; FSH, Follicle-stimulating hormone, LH, luteinizing hormone; T, testosterone.

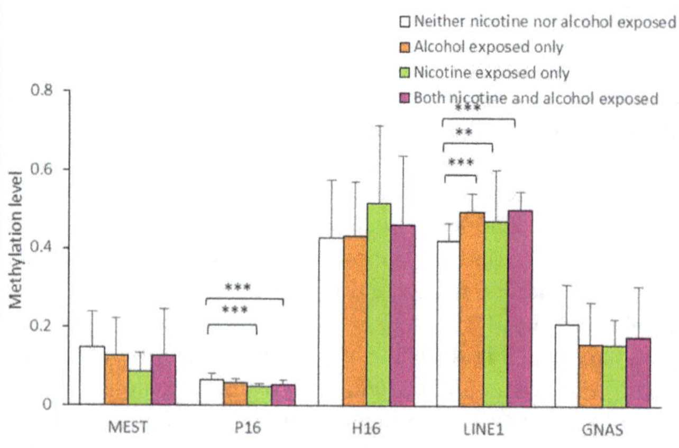

FIGURE 1 | Average methylation level of the five genes in all the subjects. The comparison of average methylation levels at *MEST, P16, H19, LINE1*, and *GNAS* in human sperms of 143 minority male residents, respectively. Data are means ± SD. Statistically significant differences are represented with asterisks: **P < 0.01, ***P < 0.001. Not significant, P > 0.05.

Correlation tests for gene modulation levels and phenotypic indices showed that the average methylation levels of *MEST* and *GNAS* were inversely correlated with sperm concentration [r = −0.522 (P = 0.038) and r = −0.557 (P = 0.025), respectively; **Figure 3A**] in the alcohol-exposed group. The average methylation levels of *MEST* and *GNAS* were positively correlated with LH levels [r = 0.344 (P = 0.012) and r = 0.365 (P = 0.006), respectively], and the methylation of the repetitive element *LINE1* was positively correlated with FSH level (r = 0.436, P = 0.001; **Figure 3B**) in the nicotine- and alcohol-exposed group. However, no association between gene methylation and the phenotypic indices was observed in the nicotine-exposed group (P > 0.05, **Table 3**).The multivariate correlation pattern between the variables was investigated using PCA. The KMO measure was 0.669, indicating that sufficient correlation existed between these variables to proceed with factor analysis. Five components were extracted by factor analysis using PCA (**Suppl 4**). Variables located near each other such as MEST, GNAS, FSH, and LH were strongly correlated (**Figure 4**).

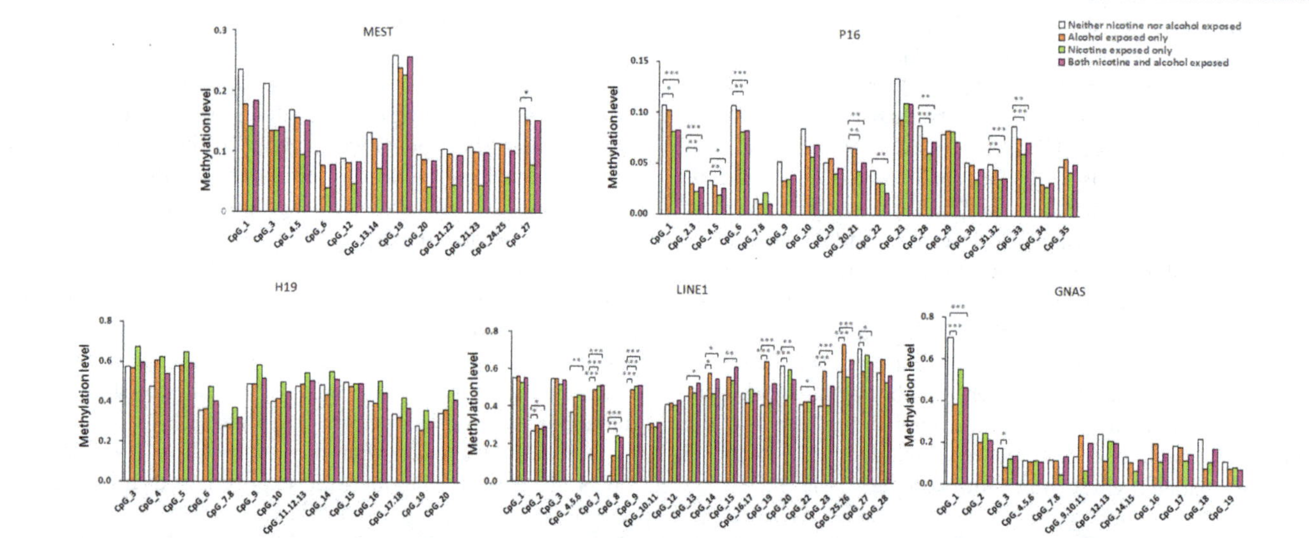

FIGURE 2 | Methylation level of the five genes in all the subjects. The comparison of site-specific methylation levels at *MEST, P16, H19, LINE1*, and *GNAS* DMR of the neither nicotine- nor alcohol-exposed controls (N = 48) with alcohol-exposed only cases (N = 16), nicotine-exposed only cases (N = 16), both nicotine- and alcohol-exposed cases (N = 63), respectively. The data are the geometric mean ratios of methylation levels at each CpG site. *P < 0.05, **P < 0.01, ***P < 0.001. Not significant, P > 0.05

alcohol-exposed groups were lower than in the controls. In contrast, there were only one CpG sites with lower methylation levels in the alcohol-exposed group when compared to the control group (**Figure 2**).

The data were checked for normal distributions using the Shapiro–Wilk test. The correlations in methylation between loci were analyzed using the Pearson's test. The methylation between *MEST* and *P16*, and *MEST* and *GNAS* were positively correlated, respectively (**Suppl 3**). The correlations between the average methylation levels and seminological parameters or hormones were analyzed using the Pearson's (normal distributions) or Spearman's correlation (abnormal distributions), respectively.

DISCUSSION

In this study, we observed that alcohol and nicotine exposure altered sperm cell quality, which may be related to the methylation levels of *MEST* and *GNAS*. The methylation levels of *MEST, GNAS*, and the repetitive element *LINE1* were significantly associated with sperm concentration and FSH and LH levels.

Recent studies have shown that tobacco use and alcohol consumption may increase the risk of global aberrant DNA methylation (Hamid et al., 2009; Semmler et al., 2015). Aberrant methylation of *LINE-1* has been reported in many recent studies on aging (Cho et al., 2015) and cancer

(Pattamadilok et al., 2008; Suzuki et al., 2013; Suter et al., 2004), and *LINE-1* methylation status could reflect the influence of environmental conditions or lifestyle habits on the genome (Schernhammer et al., 2010). High tobacco use might lead to a high risk of *LINE-1* hypermethylation-related cancers in men (Andreotti et al., 2014; Karami et al., 2015). To the best of our knowledge, our study showed, for the first time, that hypermethylation of the *LINE-1* gene in sperm was associated with alcohol and nicotine exposure. However, the association between *LINE-1* methylation level and alcohol and tobacco exposure in sperm needs to be further explored in future studies.

In our study, compared to the control group, hypomethylation of *P16* was observed in the tobacco-exposed group. In addition, we found that *GNAS* methylation was decreased in the alcohol-exposed group, and *P16* methylation was decreased in the nicotine- and alcohol-exposed group. Previous studies have suggested that chronic paternal alcohol exposure might contribute to mental deficits in offspring *via* abnormal methylation of imprinted genes (such as *H19* and *Peg3*) in sperm (Liang et al., 2014) and that methylation levels could be easily modified by air pollution, heavy metals, and other environmental factors, both *in vivo* and *in vitro* (Baccarelli and Bollati, 2009; Haggarty, 2013). An association between nicotine/alcohol exposure and methylation has been demonstrated in pregnant women (Barua and Junaid, 2015; Lee et al., 2015). In this study, we studied the influence of nicotine/alcohol exposure in male residents from Guizhou province, a population with a low fertility rate. The relationship between nicotine/alcohol exposure and the methylation of these five genes in male residents of Guizhou has not been previously reported. Abnormal DNA methylation in spermatozoa seems to be involved in environmental factor-induced transgenerational disruptive spermatogenesis (Anway et al., 2005; Anway et al., 2006). The impact of environmental factors on the epigenetic phenotype might affect offspring through abnormal spermatozoa methylation (Anway and Skinner, 2006). Some evidence has suggested that abnormal DNA methylation of imprinted genes may be associated with spermatogenesis failure (Boissonnas et al., 2010), and an observable decrease in the concentration of sperm was reported in patients with *H19* hypomethylation (Stouder et al., 2011). In addition, aberrant *MEST* DNA methylation has been shown to be significantly associated with increased FSH levels (Klaver et al., 2013). However, we found that alcohol exposure altered sperm cell quality and was related to the hypomethylation of *MEST* and *GNAS*. *MEST* and *GNAS* methylation levels were significantly associated with increased LH levels, and *LINE1* methylation was significantly associated with increased FSH levels. However, further studies are needed to explore the mechanisms underlying the association between chronic nicotine and alcohol exposure and aberration methylation of *MEST*, *GNAS*, and *LINE1* with sperm quality and abnormal FSH and LH levels.

Our study has several limitations. First, our study had a small sample size, which restricts the generalizability of our results. Therefore, our results must be verified in larger cohorts using different techniques. In addition, further studies are needed

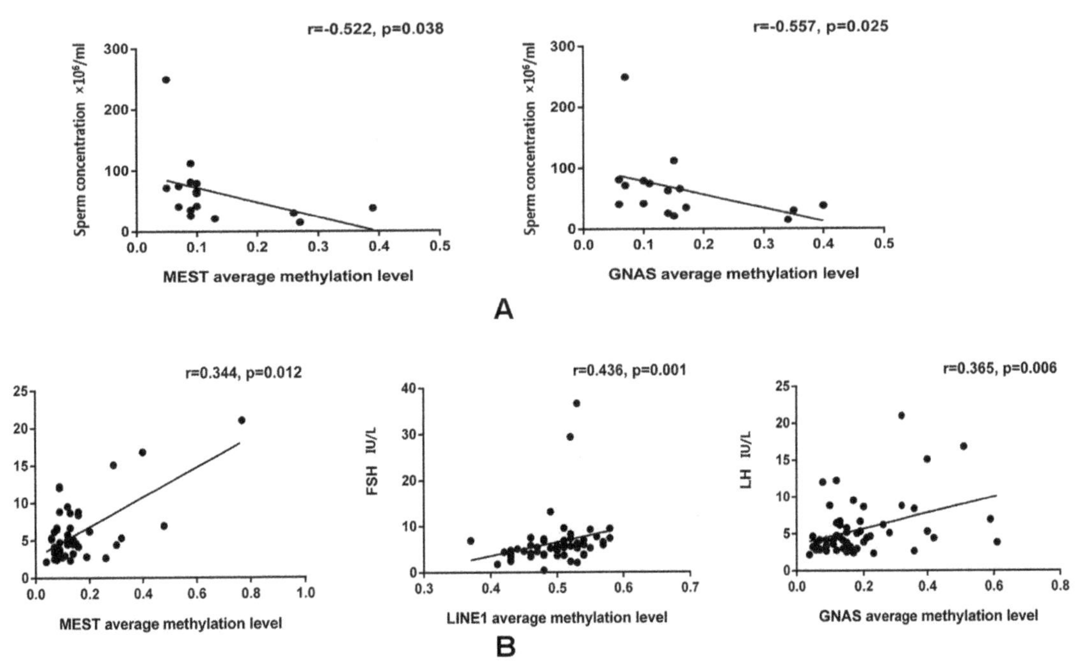

FIGURE 3 | Comparison of the gene methylation levels and semen quality/hormone level. **(A)** The significant correlations between the average methylation levels, seminological parameters and hormones in the alcohol exposed only group. **(B)** The significant correlations between the average methylation levels, seminological parameters and hormones in the both nicotine and alcohol exposed group. The dots are the intersection points between the average methylation levels, seminological parameters and hormones.

TABLE 3 | Comparison of 5 gene methylation levels and semen quality/hormone level in all subjects.

	Sperm motility (% moving forward)		Concentration (106 spermatozoa/ml)		Sperm vitality (% alive)		FSH		LH		T	
	r	P	r	P	r	P	r	P	r	P	r	P
Neither nicotine nor alcohol Exposed												
MEST	−0.033	0.828	0.317	0.030	0.121	0.525	0.022	0.886	0.051	0.735	0.025	0.867
P16	−0.024	0.872	0.020	0.894	−0.119	0.524	0.211	0.154	−0.181	0.223	−0.006	0.970
H19	−0.276	0.061	−0.147	0.323	−0.373	0.039	0.263	0.078	0.177	0.240	0.027	0.857
LINE1	−0.101	0.496	−0.224	0.125	−0.171	0.357	0.071	0.635	−0.059	0.695	−0.040	0.789
GNAS	−0.171	0.246	−0.248	0.090	−0.199	0.283	0.081	0.586	0.120	0.420	0.072	0.628
Alcohol exposed only												
MEST	0.082	0.763	−0.522	**0.038**	0.024	0.955	−0.143	0.626	0.262	0.366	−0.389	0.169
P16	−0.114	0.674	−0.291	0.274	0.582	0.130	0.026	0.930	0.333	0.245	0.019	0.949
H19	−0.284	0.286	−0.350	0.184	0.306	0.461	−0.266	0.359	0.207	0.478	−0.089	0.761
LINE1	0.169	0.531	0.016	0.953	0.518	0.188	−0.082	0.780	0.113	0.701	−0.448	0.108
GNAS	−0.054	0.843	−0.557	**0.025**	−0.005	0.986	−0.207	0.478	0.176	0.547	0.044	0.881
Nicotine exposed only												
MEST	0.041	0.884	−0.474	0.075	−0.333	0.347	0.088	0.745	−0.044	0.871	−0.362	0.169
P16	−0.354	0.196	−0.104	0.712	0.034	0.925	−0.108	0.692	−0.327	0.216	0.219	0.415
H19	−0.134	0.633	−0.427	0.113	0.604	0.064	−0.076	0.778	−0.071	0.795	−0.062	0.820
LINE1	0.056	0.849	0.041	0.890	−0.240	0.534	0.046	0.869	0.175	0.532	−0.122	0.664
GNAS	0.382	0.160	0.062	0.825	−0.544	0.104	0.209	0.438	0.482	0.058	−0.358	0.173
Both nicotine and alcohol exposed												
MEST	−0.062	0.648	−0.196	0.144	−0.023	0.889	0.241	0.082	0.344	**0.012**	0.016	0.910
P16	0.064	0.631	0.072	0.589	−0.050	0.761	0.097	0.481	0.019	0.892	−0.074	0.593
H19	−0.140	0.295	−0.103	0.441	−0.065	0.685	−0.059	0.673	0.024	0.864	0.184	0.186
LINE1	−0.037	0.780	−0.077	0.561	−0.067	0.676	0.436	**0.001**	0.173	0.206	0.168	0.221
GNAS	−0.187	0.159	−0.218	0.101	−0.087	0.593	0.194	0.156	0.365	**0.006**	0.066	0.630

The bold represent p<0.05.

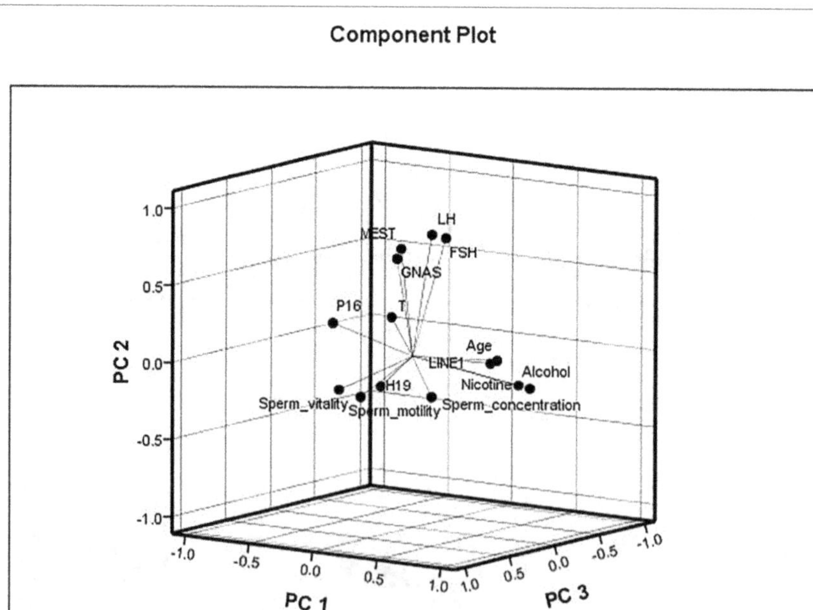

FIGURE 4 | Multivariate correlation patterns. The Kaiser–Meyer–Olkin measure was 0.669, indicating that sufficient correlation existed between these variables to proceed with factor analysis. Three components were extracted by factor analysis using principal component analysis. Factor 1 labeled as "PC1" contains nicotine exposed, alcohol exposed, age, LINE1, P16, and sperm motility and had loadings of 0.852, 0.829, 0.678, 0.578, −0.516, and −0.403, respectively. This factor explained 20.0% of the total variance. Factor 2 labeled as "PC2" contains MEST, GNAS, follicle-stimulating hormone (FSH), and luteinizing hormone (LH) and had loadings of 0.672, 0.629, 0.775, and 0.789, respectively, explaining 17.5% of the total variance. Factor 3 labeled as "PC3" contains sperm vitality, H19, and sperm concentration and had loadings of 0.746, and 0.632, and −0.516, respectively, explaining 9.3% of the total variance.

to explore how changes in methylation due to smoking and drinking affect fertility.

In conclusion, our results show that the different methylation levels of four genes, *MEST*, *P16*, *LINE-1*, and *GNAS*, alter the sperm cells of patients who consume alcohol and use nicotine. Both smoking and drinking impair sperm/semen quality and hormone levels. Thus, methylation of *MEST*, *GNAS*, and *LINE1* may be associated with sperm concentration and FSH and LH levels.

ETHICS STATEMENT

Our study was approved by the Ethics Committee of Shanghai Institute of Planned Parenthood Research (SIPPR) and the local approval of Guizhou province was not required.

AUTHOR CONTRIBUTIONS

Designed and coordinated the study: WZ, AZ, HS, JD. Performed the experiments: FS, ZZ, YS, JX, ML. Analyzed the data: XX, JL, XS, MM, JD. Contributed reagents/materials/analysis tools: YY, FS, BW. Wrote the paper: WZ, FS, JD. Helped in critical revision of the manuscript for important intellectual content: DJ, XH, ML.

ACKNOWLEDGMENTS

We thank Chunli Zhong, Yuan Yang, Kanglian Chen, and Jiang Zhu for help in collecting samples from the Population and Family Planning Institute of Guizhou Province. We would like to acknowledge research support from the National Nature Science Foundation of China (Nos. 81571503, 81270744, and 81771655) and the Major State Basic Research Development Program of China (973 Program, 2014CB943104).

REFERENCES

Al Khaled, Y., Tierling, S., Laqqan, M., Lo Porto, C., and Hammadeh, M. E. (2018). Cigarette smoking induces only marginal changes in sperm DNA methylation levels of patients undergoing intracytoplasmic sperm injection treatment. *Andrologia* 50. doi: 10.1111/and.12818

Alkhaled, Y., Laqqan, M., Tierling, S., Lo Porto, C., Amor, H., and Hammadeh, M. E. (2018). Impact of cigarette-smoking on sperm DNA methylation and its effect on sperm parameters. *Andrologia*. doi: 10.1111/and.12950

Andreotti, G., Karami, S., Pfeiffer, R. M., Hurwitz, L., Liao, L. M., Weinstein, S. J., et al. (2014). LINE1 methylation levels associated with increased bladder cancer risk in pre-diagnostic blood DNA among US (PLCO) and European (ATBC) cohort study participants. *Epigenetics* 9, 404–415. doi: 10.4161/epi.27386

Anway, M. D., and Skinner, M. K. (2006). Epigenetic transgenerational actions of endocrine disruptors. *Endocrinology* 147, S43–S49. doi: 10.1210/en.2006-0640

Anway, M. D., Cupp, A. S., Uzumcu, M., and Skinner, M. K. (2005). Epigenetic transgenerational actions of endocrine disruptors and male fertility. *Science* 308, 1466–1469. doi: 10.1126/science.1108190

Anway, M. D., Memon, M. A., Uzumcu, M., and Skinner, M. K. (2006). Transgenerational effect of the endocrine disruptor vinclozolin on male spermatogenesis. *J. Androl.* 27, 868–879. doi: 10.2164/jandrol.106.000349

Baccarelli, A., and Bollati, V. (2009). Epigenetics and environmental chemicals. *Curr. Opin. Pediatr.* 21, 243–251. doi: 10.1097/MOP.0b013e32832925cc

Barua, S., and Junaid, M. A. (2015). Lifestyle, pregnancy and epigenetic effects. *Epigenomics* 7, 85–102. doi: 10.2217/epi.14.71

Besingi, W., and Johansson, A. (2014). Smoke-related DNA methylation changes in the etiology of human disease. *Hum Mol. Genet.* 23, 2290–2297. doi: 10.1093/hmg/ddt621

Boissonnas, C. C., Abdalaoui, H. E., Haelewyn, V., Fauque, P., Dupont, J. M., Gut, I., et al. (2010). Specific epigenetic alterations of IGF2-H19 locus in spermatozoa from infertile men. *Eur. J. Hum. Genet.* 18, 73–80. doi: 10.1038/ejhg.2009.117

Chang, R. C., Skiles, W. M., Chronister, S. S., Wang, H., Sutton, G. I., Bedi, Y. S., et al. (2017). DNA methylation-independent growth restriction and altered developmental programming in a mouse model of preconception male alcohol exposure. *Epigenetics* 12, 841–853. doi: 10.1080/15592294.2017.1363952

Chastain, L. G., and Sarkar, D. K. (2017). Alcohol effects on the epigenome in the germline: role in the inheritance of alcohol-related pathology. *Alcohol* 60, 53–66. doi: 10.1016/j.alcohol.2016.12.007

Chavarro, J. E., Rich-Edwards, J. W., Rosner, B. A., and Willett, W. C. (2009). Caffeinated and alcoholic beverage intake in relation to ovulatory disorder infertility. *Epidemiology* 20, 374–381. doi: 10.1097/EDE.0b013e31819d68cc

Cho, Y. H., Woo, H. D., Jang, Y., Porter, V., Christensen, S., Hamilton, R. F., Jr., et al. (2015). The Association of LINE-1 Hypomethylation with Age and Centromere Positive Micronuclei in Human Lymphocytes. *PLoS One* 10, e0133909. doi: 10.1371/journal.pone.0133909

Dada, R., Kumar, R., Shamsi, M. B., Tanwar, M., Pathak, D., Venkatesh, S., et al. (2008). Genetic screening in couples experiencing recurrent assisted procreation failure. *Indian J. Biochem. Biophys.* 45, 116–120.

Dai, J., Wang, Z., Xu, W., Zhang, M., Zhu, Z., Zhao, X., et al. (2017). Paternal nicotine exposure defines different behavior in subsequent generation via hyper-methylation of mmu-miR-15b. *Sci. Rep.* 7, 7286. doi: 10.1038/s41598-017-07920-3

Darbandi, M., Darbandi, S., Agarwal, A., Baskaran, S., Dutta, S., Sengupta, P., et al. (2018). Reactive oxygen species-induced alterations in H19-Igf2 methylation patterns, seminal plasma metabolites, and semen quality. *J. Assist. Reprod. Genet.* doi: 10.1007/s10815-018-1350-y

Dong, H., Wang, Y., Zou, Z., Chen, L., Shen, C., Xu, S., et al. (2017). Abnormal methylation of imprinted genes and cigarette smoking: assessment of Their association with the risk of male infertility. *Reprod. Sci.* 24, 114–123. doi: 10.1177/1933719116650755

Donkin, I., and Barres, R. (2018). Sperm epigenetics and influence of environmental factors. *Mol. Metabol.* 14, 1–11. doi: 10.1016/j.molmet.2018.02.006

Gaur, D. S., Talekar, M. S., and Pathak, V. P. (2010). Alcohol intake and cigarette smoking: impact of two major lifestyle factors on male fertility. *Indian J Pathol Microbiol* 53, 35–40. doi: 10.4103/0377-4929.59180

Gunes, S., Metin Mahmutoglu, A., Arslan, M. A., and Henkel, R. (2018). Smoking-induced genetic and epigenetic alterations in infertile men. *Andrologia* 50, e13124. doi: 10.1111/and.13124

Haggarty, P. (2013). Epigenetic consequences of a changing human diet. *Proc. Nutr. Soc.* 72, 363–371. doi: 10.1017/S0029665113003376

Hamad, M. F., Dayyih, W. A. A., Laqqan, M., AlKhaled, Y., Montenarh, M., and Hammadeh, M. E. (2018). The status of global DNA methylation in the spermatozoa of smokers and non-smokers. *Reprod. Biomed. Online* 37, 581–589. doi: 10.1016/j.rbmo.2018.08.016

Hamid, A., Wani, N. A., and Kaur, J. (2009). New perspectives on folate transport in relation to alcoholism-induced folate malabsorption-association with epigenome stability and cancer development. *FEBS J.* 276, 2175–2191. doi: 10.1111/j.1742-4658.2009.06959.x

Han, J. C., Xu, F., Chen, N., Qi, G. B., Wei, Y. J., Li, H. B., et al. (2016). Promoter methylations of RASSF1A and p16 is associated with clinicopathological features in lung cancers. *J. Cancer Res. Ther.* 12, 340–349. doi: 10.4103/0973-1482.154926

Han, Y. D., Wang, X. B., Cui, N. H., Zhang, S., Wang, C., and Zheng, F. (2017). Associations of P16INK4a promoter hypermethylation with squamous intra-epithelial lesion, cervical cancer and their clinicopathological features: a meta-analysis. *Oncotarget* 8, 1871–1883. doi: 10.18632/oncotarget.12202

Hansen, M. L., Thulstrup, A. M., Bonde, J. P., Olsen, J., Hakonsen, L. B., and Ramlau-Hansen, C. H. (2012). Does last week's alcohol intake affect semen quality or reproductive hormones? A cross-sectional study among healthy young Danish men. *Reprod. Toxicol.* 34, 457–462. doi: 10.1016/j.reprotox.2012.06.004

He, J., Zhang, A., Fang, M., Fang, R., Ge, J., Jiang, Y., et al. (2013). Methylation levels at IGF2 and GNAS DMRs in infants born to preeclamptic pregnancies. *BMC Genomics* 14, 472. doi: 10.1186/1471-2164-14-472

Jenkins, T. G., James, E. R., Alonso, D. F., Hoidal, J. R., Murphy, P. J., Hotaling, J. M., et al. (2017). Cigarette smoking significantly alters sperm DNA methylation patterns. *Andrology* 5, 1089–1099. doi: 10.1111/andr.12416

Jeong, M. G., Song, H., Shin, J. H., Jeong, H., Kim, H. K., and Hwang, E. S. (2017). Transcriptional coactivator with PDZ-binding motif is required to sustain testicular function on aging. *Aging Cell* 16, 1035–1042. doi: 10.1111/acel.12631

Karami, S., Andreotti, G., Liao, L. M., Pfeiffer, R. M., Weinstein, S. J., Purdue, M. P., et al. (2015). LINE1 methylation levels in pre-diagnostic leukocyte DNA and future renal cell carcinoma risk. *Epigenetics* 10, 282–292. doi: 10.1080/15592294.2015.1006505

Kim, P., Choi, C. S., Park, J. H., Joo, S. H., Kim, S. Y., Ko, H. M., et al. (2014). Chronic exposure to ethanol of male mice before mating produces attention deficit hyperactivity disorder-like phenotype along with epigenetic dysregulation of dopamine transporter expression in mouse offspring. *J. Neurosci. Res.* 92, 658–670. doi: 10.1002/jnr.23275

Klaver, R., Tuttelmann, F., Bleiziffer, A., Haaf, T., Kliesch, S., and Gromoll, J. (2013). DNA methylation in spermatozoa as a prospective marker in andrology. *Andrology* 1, 731–740. doi: 10.1111/j.2047-2927.2013.00118.x

Kobayashi, N., Miyauchi, N., Tatsuta, N., Kitamura, A., Okae, H., Hiura, H., et al. (2017). Factors associated with aberrant imprint methylation and oligozoospermia. *Sci. Rep.* 7, 42336. doi: 10.1038/srep42336

Kunzle, R., Mueller, M. D., Hanggi, W., Birkhauser, M. H., Drescher, H., and Bersinger, N. A. (2003). Semen quality of male smokers and nonsmokers in infertile couples. *Fertil. Steril.* 79, 287–291. doi: 10.1016/S0015-0282(02)04664-2

Laqqan, M., Tierling, S., Alkhaled, Y., LoPorto, C., and Hammadeh, M. E. (2017). Alterations in sperm DNA methylation patterns of oligospermic males. *Reprod. Biol.* 17, 396–400. doi: 10.1016/j.repbio.2017.10.007

Laqqan, M., Tierling, S., Alkhaled, Y., Porto, C. L., Solomayer, E. F., and Hammadeh, M. E. (2017). Aberrant DNA methylation patterns of human spermatozoa in current smoker males. *Reprod. Toxicol.* 71, 126–133. doi: 10.1016/j.reprotox.2017.05.010

Lee, B. Y., Park, S. Y., Ryu, H. M., Shin, C. Y., Ko, K. N., Han, J. Y., et al. (2015). Changes in the methylation status of DAT, SERT, and MeCP2 gene promoters in the blood cell in families exposed to alcohol during the periconceptional period. *Alcohol. Clin. Exp. Res.* 39, 239–250. doi: 10.1111/acer.12635

Li, Y., Xie, C., Murphy, S. K., Skaar, D., Nye, M., Vidal, A. C., et al. (2016). Lead exposure during early human development and DNA methylation of imprinted gene regulatory elements in adulthood. *Environ. Health Perspect.* 124, 666–673. doi: 10.1289/ehp.1408577

Liang, F., Diao, L., Liu, J., Jiang, N., Zhang, J., Wang, H., et al. (2014). Paternal ethanol exposure and behavioral abnormities in offspring: associated alterations in imprinted gene methylation. *Neuropharmacology* 81, 126–133. doi: 10.1016/j.neuropharm.2014.01.025

Liang, H., Xu, W., Chen, J., Shi, H., Zhu, J., Liu, X., et al. (2017). The Association between exposure to environmental bisphenol A and gonadotropic hormone levels among men. *PLoS One* 12, e0169217. doi: 10.1371/journal.pone.0169217

Marques, C. J., Costa, P., Vaz, B., Carvalho, F., Fernandes, S., Barros, A., et al. (2008). Abnormal methylation of imprinted genes in human sperm is associated with oligozoospermia. *Mol. Hum. Reprod.* 14, 67–74. doi: 10.1093/molehr/gam093

Marques, C. J., Joao Pinho, M., Carvalho, F., Bieche, I., Barros, A., and Sousa, M. (2011). DNA methylation imprinting marks and DNA methyltransferase expression in human spermatogenic cell stages. *Epigenetics* 6, 1354–1361. doi: 10.4161/epi.6.11.17993

McCarthy, D. M., Morgan, T. J., Jr., Lowe, S. E., Williamson, M. J., Spencer, T. J., Biederman, J., et al. (2018). Nicotine exposure of male mice produces behavioral impairment in multiple generations of descendants. *PLoS Biol.* 16, e2006497. doi: 10.1371/journal.pbio.2006497

Miao, M., Zhou, X., Li, Y., Zhang, O., Zhou, Z., Li, T., et al. (2014). LINE-1 hypomethylation in spermatozoa is associated with Bisphenol A exposure. *Andrology* 2, 138–144. doi: 10.1111/j.2047-2927.2013.00166.x

Montjean, D., Zini, A., Ravel, C., Belloc, S., Dalleac, A., Copin, H., et al. (2015). Sperm global DNA methylation level: association with semen parameters and genome integrity. *Andrology* 3, 235–40. doi: 10.1111/andr.12001

Nasri, F., Gharesi-Fard, B., Namavar Jahromi, B., Farazi-Fard, M. A., Banaei, M., Davari, M., et al. (2017). Sperm DNA methylation of H19 imprinted gene and male infertility. *Andrologia* 49. doi: 10.1111/and.12766

Pang, Y., Holmes, M. V., Guo, Y., Yang, L., Bian, Z., Chen, Y., et al. (2018). Smoking, alcohol, and diet in relation to risk of pancreatic cancer in China: a prospective study of 0.5 million people. *Cancer Med.* 7, 229–239. doi: 10.1002/cam4.1261

Pattamadilok, J., Huapai, N., Rattanatanyong, P., Vasurattana, A., Triratanachat, S., Tresukosol, D., et al. (2008). LINE-1 hypomethylation level as a potential prognostic factor for epithelial ovarian cancer. *Int. J. Gynecol. Cancer* 18, 711–717. doi: 10.1111/j.1525-1438.2007.01117.x

Pierron, F., Baillon, L., Sow, M., Gotreau, S., and Gonzalez, P. (2014). Effect of low-dose cadmium exposure on DNA methylation in the endangered European eel. *Environ. Sci. Technol. Lett.* 48, 797–803. doi: 10.1021/es4048347

Povey, A. C., Clyma, J. A., McNamee, R., Moore, H. D., Baillie, H., Pacey, A. A., et al. (2012). Modifiable and non-modifiable risk factors for poor semen quality: a case-referent study. *Hum. Reprod.* 27, 2799–2806. doi: 10.1093/humrep/des183

Rangwala, S. H., Zhang, L., and Kazazian, Jr, H. H. (2009). Many LINE1 elements contribute to the transcriptome of human somatic cells. *Genome Biol.* 10, R100. doi: 10.1186/gb-2009-10-9-r100

Santi, D., De Vincentis, S., Magnani, E., and Spaggiari, G. (2017). Impairment of sperm DNA methylation in male infertility: a meta-analytic study. *Andrology* 5, 695–703. doi: 10.1111/andr.12379

Schernhammer, E. S., Giovannucci, E., Kawasaki, T., Rosner, B., Fuchs, C. S., and Ogino, S. (2010). Dietary folate, alcohol and B vitamins in relation to LINE-1 hypomethylation in colon cancer. *Gut* 59, 794–799. doi: 10.1136/gut.2009.183707

Semmler, A., Heese, P., Stoffel-Wagner, B., Muschler, M., Heberlein, A., Bigler, L., et al. (2015). Alcohol abuse and cigarette smoking are associated with global DNA hypermethylation: results from the German Investigation on Neurobiology in Alcoholism (GINA). *Alcohol* 49, 97–101. doi: 10.1016/j.alcohol.2015.01.004

Sharlip, I. D., Jarow, J. P., Belker, A. M., Lipshultz, L. I., Sigman, M., Thomas, A. J., et al. (2002). Best practice policies for male infertility. *Fertil Steril* 77, 873–882. doi: 10.1016/S0015-0282(02)03105-9

Siddeek, B., Mauduit, C., Simeoni, U., and Benahmed, M. (2018). Sperm epigenome as a marker of environmental exposure and lifestyle, at the origin of diseases inheritance. *Mutat Res* 778, 38–44. doi: 10.1016/j.mrrev.2018.09.001

Stouder, C., Somm, E., and Paoloni-Giacobino, A. (2011). Prenatal exposure to ethanol: a specific effect on the H19 gene in sperm. *Reprod. Toxicol.* 31, 507–512. doi: 10.1016/j.reprotox.2011.02.009

Suter, C. M., Martin, D. I., and Ward, R. L. (2004). Hypomethylation of L1 retrotransposons in colorectal cancer and adjacent normal tissue. *Int J Colorectal Dis* 19, 95–101. doi: 10.1007/s00384-003-0539-3

Suzuki, M., Shiraishi, K., Eguchi, A., Ikeda, K., Mori, T., Yoshimoto, K., et al. (2013). Aberrant methylation of LINE-1, SLIT2, MAL and IGFBP7 in non-small cell lung cancer. *Oncol. Rep.* 29, 1308–1314. doi: 10.3892/or.2013.2266

Wang, B. H., Li, Y. Y., Han, J. Z., Zhou, L. Y., Lv, Y. Q., Zhang, H. L., et al. (2017). Gene methylation as a powerful biomarker for detection and screening of non-small cell lung cancer in blood. *Oncotarget* 8, 31692–31704. doi: 10.18632/oncotarget.15919

Witkiewitz, K., Hallgren, K. A., Kranzler, H. R., Mann, K. F., Hasin, D. S., Falk, D. E., et al. (2017). Clinical validation of reduced alcohol consumption after treatment for alcohol dependence using the World Health Organization risk drinking levels. *Alcohol. Clin. Exp. Res.* 41, 179–186. doi: 10.1111/acer.13272

Xin-Chang, Z., Peng, W., Zhao-Yuan, H., Xiao-Bin, H., Ru-Jin, Z., and Yi-Xun, L. (2002). Expression of P16(INK4a) in testis of rhesus monkey during heat stress and testosterone undecanoate induced azoospermia or oligozoospermia. *Contraception* 65, 251–255. doi: 10.1016/S0010-7824(01)00305-5

Xu, J., Zhang, A., Zhang, Z., Wang, P., Qian, Y., He, L., et al. (2016). DNA methylation levels of imprinted and nonimprinted genes DMRs associated with defective human spermatozoa. *Andrologia* 48, 939–947. doi: 10.1111/and.12535

Yaman, R., and Grandjean, V. (2006). Timing of entry of meiosis depends on a mark generated by DNA methyltransferase 3a in testis. *Mol. Reprod. Dev.* 73, 390–397. doi: 10.1002/mrd.20430

Yang, F., Li, L., Chen, J. P., Liu, X. Q., Zhong, C. L., Yang, Y., et al. (2017). Couple's infertility in relation to male smoking in a Chinese rural area. *Asian J. Androl.* 19, 311–315 doi: 10.4103/1008-682X.168685.

6

Perspectives on miRNAs as Epigenetic Markers in Osteoporosis and Bone Fracture Risk: A Step Forward in Personalized Diagnosis

*Michela Bottani[1], Giuseppe Banfi[1,2] and Giovanni Lombardi[1,3]**

[1] IRCCS Istituto Ortopedico Galeazzi, Laboratory of Experimental Biochemistry & Moelcular Biology, Milano, Italy, [2] Vita-Salute San Raffaele University, Milano, Italy, [3] Department of Physiology & Pharmacology, Gdańsk University of Physical Education & Sport, Gdańsk, Poland

***Correspondence:**
Giovanni Lombardi
giovanni.lombardigrupposandonato.it;
giovanni.lombardi@awf.gda.pl

Aging is associated with an increased incidence of age-related bone diseases. Current diagnostics (e.g., conventional radiology, biochemical markers), because limited in specificity and sensitivity, can distinguish between healthy or osteoporotic subjects but they are unable to discriminate among different underlying causes that lead to the same bone pathological condition (e.g., bone fracture risk). Among recent, more sensitive biomarkers, miRNAs — the non-coding RNAs involved in the epigenetic regulation of gene expression, have emerged as fundamental post-transcriptional modulators of bone development and homeostasis. Each identified miRNA carries out a specific role in osteoblast and osteoclast differentiation and functional pathways (osteomiRs). miRNAs bound to proteins or encapsulated in exosomes and/or microvesicles are released into the bloodstream and biological fluids where they can be detected and measured by highly sensitive and specific methods (e.g., quantitative PCR, next-generation sequencing). As such, miRNAs provide a prompt and easily accessible tool to determine the subject-specific epigenetic environment of a specific condition. Their use as biomarkers opens new frontiers in personalized medicine. While miRNAs circulating levels are lower than those found in the tissue/cell source, their quantification in biological fluids may be strategic in the diagnosis of diseases that affect tissues, such as bone, in which biopsy may be especially challenging. For a biomarker to be valuable in clinical practice and support medical decisions, it must be (easily) measurable, validated by independent studies, and strongly and significantly associated with a disease outcome. Currently, miRNAs analysis does not completely satisfy these criteria, however. Starting from *in vitro* and *in vivo* observations describing their biological role in bone cell development and metabolism, this review describes the potential use of bone-associated circulating miRNAs as biomarkers for determining predisposition, onset, and development of osteoporosis and bone fracture risk. Moreover, the review focuses on their clinical relevance and discusses the pre-analytical, analytical, and post-analytical issues in their measurement, which still limits their routine application. Taken together, research and clinical findings may be helpful for creating miRNA-based diagnostic tools in the diagnosis and treatment of bone diseases.

Keywords: biomarkers, circulating miRNAs, miRNA signature, extra-analytical variability, sensitivity and specificity, osteopenia/osteoporosis, fracture risk

INTRODUCTION

Biogenesis of miRNAs and Their Biological Role

MicroRNAs (miRNAs) are short, single-stranded non-coding RNAs (18–22 nucleotides in length) that inhibit gene expression. Lee et al. (1993) discovered in *Caenorhabditis elegans* — a short, single-stranded non-coding RNA (lin-4) that downregulated lin-14 gene expression through a direct antisense RNA–RNA interaction. Since then, miRNAs have been discovered in all living kingdoms (Lagos-Quintana et al., 2001; Reinhart et al., 2002; Cerutti and Casas-Mollano, 2006; Dang et al., 2011; Bloch et al., 2017) and in viruses, as well (Grundhoff and Sullivan, 2011). Among the databases that record the ever growing number of miRNAs being discovered, miRBase (www.mirbase.org) is a comprehensive and constantly updated miRNAs database that provides universal nomenclature, information about sequence, predicted target genes, and additional annotations (Griffiths-Jones et al., 2006). Currently, it contains 38,589 entries, more than 1,900 of which are human.

Though widely discussed, miRNAs biogenesis is not yet fully understood. Briefly, miRNAs are transcribed by RNA polymerase II (Pol II) from encoding sequences (miRNA genes) located within non-coding DNA sequences, introns or untranslated regions (UTR) of protein-coding genes (Ha and Kim, 2014; Hammond, 2015). miRNA genes can be found in clusters within a chromosomal locus; they are transcribed as polycistronic primary transcripts and subsequently processed as single miRNA precursors. miRNAs within the same cluster are thought to target related mRNAs (Lee et al., 2002; Wang et al., 2016). Furthermore, the same miRNA encoding genes can be duplicated in different loci: the derived mature miRNAs (grouped within a miRNA family) have an identical seed region and share the same mRNA targets (Bartel, 2009). A long primary transcript (pri-miRNA) is processed in the nucleus by the RNase III DROSHA-DGCR8 cofactor complex that removes the stem loop-flanking structure generating the ~60 nt hairpin pre-miRNA.

After its exportation into the cytosol in a process mediated by exportin 5 (EXP5), RNase III DICER cleaves the loop to generate a double stranded (ds) miRNA. One miRNA strand, the passenger strand, is incorporated into the RNA-induced silencing complex (RISC) as a mature miRNA, while the other, the star strand, is degraded. Both strands in some miRNAs are bioactive and each strand is loaded into a RISC. The RISC protein argonaute-2 (AGO-2) is responsible for targeting a specific mRNA based on the complementarity of a 7-nt miRNA sequence ("seed region," position 2-to-7). The ds miRNA–mRNA complex induces degradation of the target mRNA, inhibition of its translation, and consequent modulation of the downstream cellular processes. Other DICER- or DROSHA-independent non-canonical miRNA biogenesis pathways exist (Ha and Kim, 2014; Hammond, 2015). Finally, miRNAs expression undergoes multilevel regulation: epigenetically in DNA methylation and histone modifications (e.g., histone acetylation) (Saito et al., 2006; Scott et al., 2006; Lujambio et al., 2008; Lujambio and Esteller, 2009) and through the regulation of proteins involved in miRNAs maturation (Davis-Dusenbery and Hata, 2010). Beside their more known inhibitory function, there are evidence suggesting that at least some miRNAs can induce gene expression under specific conditions. In this process, miRNA-associated ribonucleoproteins (miRNPs) play a key role as reviewed in (Valinezhad Orang et al., 2014).

One of the first demonstrations of the key role of miRNAs was the embryonic lethality of the DICER-1- and DGCR8-double knockout (KO) in mice (Bernstein et al., 2003; Wang et al., 2007). Conditional inactivation of DICER in mice embryonic stem (ES) impaired proliferation and differentiation and compromised miRNA biogenesis (Suh et al., 2004; Murchison et al., 2005). Several miRNAs display a cell- or tissue-specific expression profile, while others are more widely expressed (Ludwig et al., 2016). Since they are also present in human biological fluids (Weber et al., 2010), their abundance and stability in human serum and plasma prompted the idea for their potential use as biomarkers (Chen et al., 2008).

Figure 1 illustrates the canonical miRNA biogenetic pathway and notions about their nomenclature.

Aim

Based on the potentialities of miRNAs as biomarkers, research efforts have been spent in studying and defining the relationships between their altered expression and human disease, particularly bone diseases (Bellavia et al., 2019; Hadjiargyrou and Komatsu, 2019; Van Meurs et al., 2019). The search term "miRNA" on PubMed retrieves 83,067 records, 53,240 (64%) of which were published in the last 5 years.

Different from previous reviews, the aim of this paper is to comprehensively review the available data about the potential next use, or even the actual use, of circulating miRNAs as biological indexes for osteoporosis and bone fracture risk. We gleaned information from each article that claimed miRNAs diagnostic, prognostic, and/or predictive properties, including information about the pre-analytical phase, quantification platforms, and normalization methods used. Several articles also reported the sensitivity and specificity parameters in evaluating the clinical potential of a specific miRNA as a biomarker to assess the presence of disease and, at the same time, the absence of the disease in healthy individuals. Since sensitivity and specificity are inversely correlated, they can be plotted on a receiver operating characteristic (ROC) curve as 1-specificity vs. sensitivity (Hajian-Tilaki, 2013).

miRNA can be found in human biofluids and in blood as free (mainly protein-associated) and exosome-/microvesicle-/LDL-associated miRNAs. These two distinct subsets are believed to exert different functions: the free fraction is somehow passively released from cells during normal recycling of the subcellular components, whereas the encapsulated fraction is actively released and finely packaged together with other components with specific functions addressed to other target tissues. In these terms, free-miRNAs can be considered classical biomarkers, while encapsulated miRNAs more likely act as endocrine-like factors (Bayraktar et al., 2017). This review will discuss bone tissue and bone-associated free-circulating miRNAs in relation to osteoporosis and the related risk of bone fracture. In addition, the review will systematically

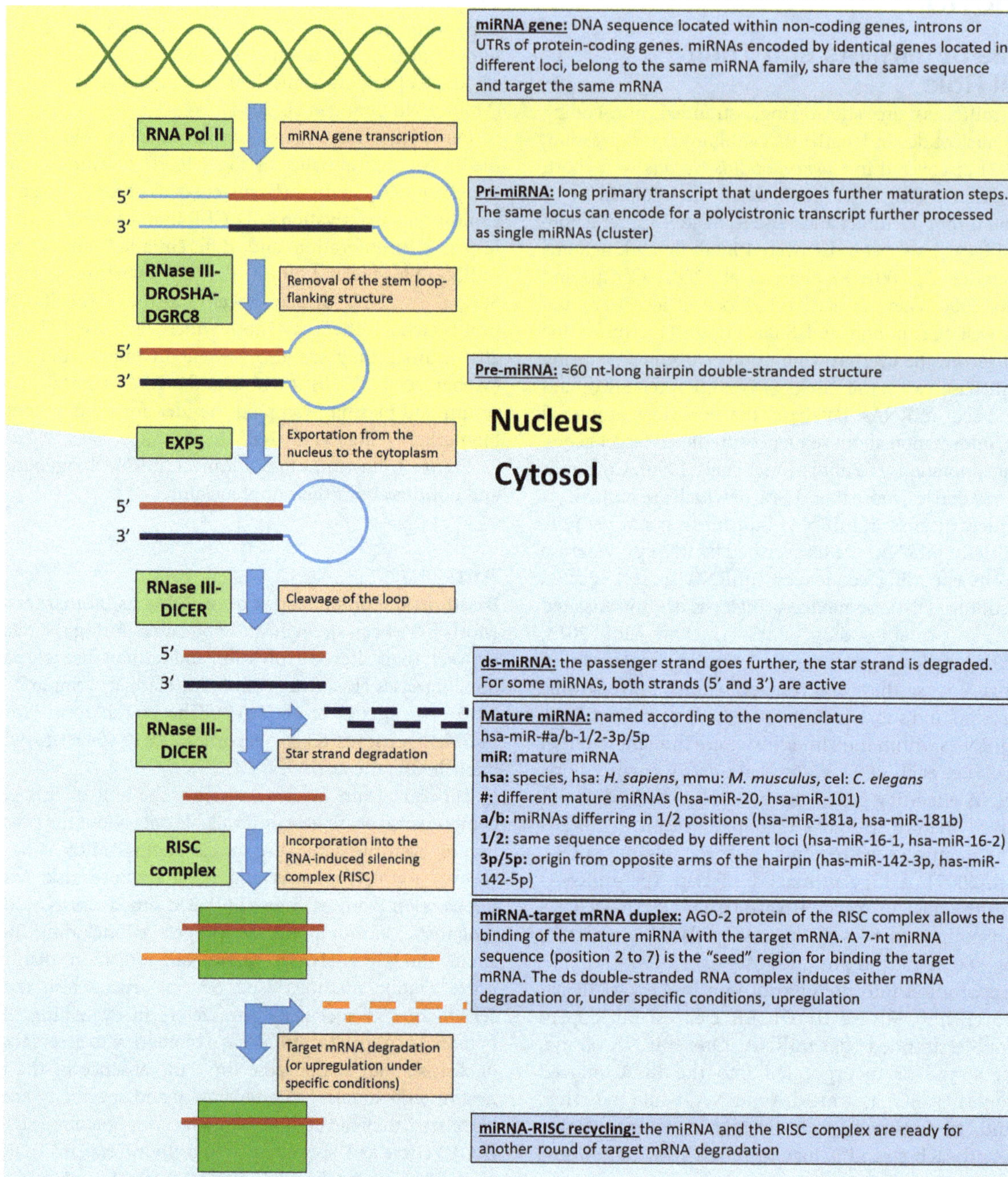

FIGURE 1 | miRNA biogenesis and nomenclature. The figure illustrates the key steps in miRNAs biogenetic canonical pathways. The light orange boxes indicate the step, the green boxes the key enzyme/enzyme complexes involved in the process, and the light blue boxes the miRNAs and miRNAs precursor nomenclature and specifications (according to Griffiths-Jones et al., 2006). RNA Pol II, RNA polymerase II; EXP5, exportin 5; RISC, RNA-induced silencing complex; AGO-2, argonaute-2 protein.

describe the *in vivo–in vitro* evidence for the role, the pathways, and the putative target genes of these miRNAs.

MIRNAS AS BIOMARKERS

Borrowing from Morrow and de Lemos (2007), the three essential features of a novel cardiovascular biomarker for clinical use are: measurability in a certain clinical setting; validation by multiple studies; and direct impact on medical decision making and patient management.

The measurability criterion requires an accurate and reproducible analytical method that can provide reliable measures rapidly and at reasonable cost. Furthermore, pre-analytical issues (conditions of measurement and sample handling, type, and stability) must be known and solved beforehand in order to control for variables in the biomarker's measurability/detectability. The validation criterion requires a strong and consistent association between the outcome/disease of interest and the biomarker level based on evidence from multiple clinical studies. Moreover, in order to directly impact medical decision making, a novel biomarker must perform better than existing tests and the associated risk might be modified by a specific therapy (Morrow and de Lemos, 2007). These criteria are still burdened by several issues regarding the pre-analytical, analytical, and post-analytical phases in miRNAs.

miRNAs as Biomarkers: Strengths

These limitations notwithstanding, the use of circulating (or also tissue) miRNAs as biomarkers is nearly ready for implementation in clinical practice. Interest in these molecules arises from the fact that, as epigenetic regulators of gene expression, they act as modulators rather than effectors of a specific biological function. As such, they provide a prompt and easily accessible tool to determine the epigenetic environment of a specific condition. And as subject-specific epigenetic determinants of a condition, they can be considered a personalized signature for tailor-made diagnosis and/or treatment. Circulating miRNAs are easily detectable in biofluids such as (but not only) plasma, serum, and urine, which are minimal/non-invasive sources of biomarkers with broad applicability in clinical research and repositories (Weber et al., 2010; Hackl et al., 2016). Although circulating miRNAs levels are lower than those found in tissues and cells (Jarry et al., 2014), this feature is advantageous, especially in diseases affecting tissues such as bone in which biopsy may be problematic (Hackl et al., 2016). Furthermore, circulating miRNAs can be detected with reliable methods based on polymerase chain reaction (PCR); reverse transcription quantitative PCR (RT-qPCR) is the most widely used owing to its high sensitivity, specificity, and reproducibility (Bustin and Nolan, 2004). Another important advantage of miRNAs as biomarkers is their stability in biofluids due to their encapsulation in extracellular vesicles (ectosomes or exosomes) and in high-density lipoproteins (HDL) and their association with proteins (Argonaute2 or nucleophosmin); miRNAs packaging is correlated with the way they are taken up by target cells (Arroyo et al., 2011; Chen et al., 2012; Li et al., 2012). miRNAs concentration in plasma, as evaluated by qPCR, is highly variable. El-Hefnawy et al. (2004) detected miRNAs concentration in the range of 1–10 μg/L, while Weber et al. (2010) reported a median concentration of 308 μg/L. Differences among healthy humans are physiological and any variation in blood processing conditions can affect circulating miRNA levels (Mitchell et al., 2008; Kroh et al., 2010; Cheng et al., 2013a).

miRNAs as Biomarkers: Weaknesses

Pre-Analytical Issues in miRNA Evaluation

In the pre-analytical phase, two sets of variables can affect miRNAs evaluation: patient-related and sampling-related factors.

Patient-related factors: lifestyle habits and diseases

Among patient-related factors, lifestyle habits and diseases affect circulating miRNA levels. Studies have shown that cigarette smoking (Takahashi et al., 2013), physical activity (Baggish et al., 2011; Faraldi et al., 2019), diet (Witwer, 2012), vitamin D levels (Bellavia et al., 2016; Bellavia et al., 2019), and head-down tilt (HDT) bed rest (Ling et al., 2017) can modify the level of a specific miRNA in circulation, whereas gender does not seem to significantly contribute to total variability (Chen et al., 2008). Also, miRNA levels are affected by circadian rhythm (Shende et al., 2011).

The total amount of circulating miRNAs is reduced in chronic kidney disease patients (Neal et al., 2011), while its correlation with liver disease is unknown (Hackl et al., 2016). As a consequence, any clinical study validating a panel of circulating miRNAs as biomarkers must follow pre-analytical protocols with strict criteria for sample collection (preferentially in the morning) and for patient inclusion and exclusion (type of diet, glomerular filtration rate, and fasting time before sample collection) to minimize the effect of variables on the validation process (Hackl et al., 2016).

Sampling-related factors: source/matrix, sample collection, and handling

A key step in the validation of a novel biomarker is selection of the correct matrix (Livesey et al., 2008; Kavsak and Hammett-Stabler, 2014). Serum and plasma miRNAs evaluated in the same blood sample are stable, and measurements in healthy individuals are reproducible, consistent, and linkable (Chen et al., 2008; Mitchell et al., 2008). In blood sample collection and handling, phlebotomy is the chief source of variability and contamination with non-circulating miRNAs (Kroh et al., 2010; Cheng et al., 2013a). In detail, miRNA quantification can be affected by the type of collection tube and anticoagulant coating, in addition to blood cell count, needle gauge (Kroh et al., 2010), and hemolysis (Kirschner et al., 2011). Since the total amount of miRNAs contained in cells is considerably higher than in circulation, quantification of circulating miRNAs can be affected by the signal coming from non-circulating miRNA contamination (e.g., the skin contaminant within the needle). In addition, miRNAs can be released by activated platelets or by hemolytic erythrocytes (Kirschner et al., 2011; Willeit et al., 2013). Another often unconsidered source of variability is tourniquet application, together with clenching the fist and maintaining it closed, that can alter blood levels of electrolytes, muscle enzymes, free hemoglobin, water, and low-molecular-weight molecules. Also at the needle insert site the concentration of some blood analytes may be increased (Lima-Oliveira et al., 2013; Lima-Oliveira et al., 2016). For the collection of plasma samples, it is important to use the right anticoagulant: heparin, potassium ethylendiaminotetraacetate (K2/K3 EDTA), sodium fluoride/potassium oxalate (NaF/KOx), or sodium citrate. Heparin (Garcia et al., 2002; Boeckel et al., 2013) and sodium citrate are not recommended for RT-qPCR-based miRNA quantification because they alter the activity of the enzymes used in PCR-based assays (Hackl et al., 2016). Conversely, EDTA is considered the right choice for PCR-based miRNA evaluation because it is easily removed from the PCR mastermix (Zampetaki and Mayr, 2012). Alternatively,

NaF/KOx may be used when EDTA is not available, although it can increase the miRNA detection rate (Kim et al., 2012). Centrifugation speed and length to separate plasma can affect miRNAs detection in EDTA-plasma possibly due to platelet-derived miRNAs (Cheng et al., 2013a), while miRNAs evaluation in serum samples is less sensitive to this process (Hackl et al., 2016). miRNAs in blood samples are stable up to 24 h at room temperature (Mitchell et al., 2008) due to their association with proteins or extracellular vesicles. This is important in clinical routine, especially when unexpected delays prolong turnaround time. Interestingly, miRNAs are reported to be stable also in extreme conditions (e.g., low and high pH) or after repeated freezing/thawing cycles (Chen et al., 2008). The ongoing discovery of novel miRNAs, together with the limited number of stability tests, calls for the need of standardized protocols in sample collection and handling in order to minimize pre-analytical sources of error (Cheng et al., 2013a). Samples can be stored for decades at low temperatures (i.e., < −70°C), which facilitates the retrieval of reliable data in retrospective studies (Zampetaki and Mayr, 2012).

Analytical and Post-Analytical Issues in miRNA Evaluation

In their study comparing 12 commercially available platforms for evaluating miRNA expression levels (7 PCR-based, 3 microarrays, and 2 next generation sequencing [NGS] technologies), Mestdagh et al. (2014) observed marked differences between the platforms. Because different technologies are often used during the validation process, platform choice will affect a method's reproducibility and specificity. For any platform combination, the average validation rate for deregulated miRNA expression is 54.6%, indicating that screening studies and validation studies on different platforms and/or technologies must be performed. Sensitivity is more technology-correlated, with qPCR platforms showing the best score and, as a consequence, higher accuracy and more reliable results. These observations suggest that analytical protocols and platforms must be the same for the discovery and the validation of a biomarker and that further efforts are required to aid in the migration to a final commercial platform (Hackl et al., 2016).

The major post-analytical issues in miRNAs evaluation are data normalization and choice of the right reference gene. Presently, there is no consensus on either issue. The amount of miRNAs in a biofluid is expressed in relative rather than absolute terms by volume unit. This makes it hard to compare results across different labs or across different studies performed in the same lab (Nelson et al., 2008; Hackl et al., 2016). The most common normalization methods for miRNAs expression of RT-qPCR data (reviewed in Faraldi et al., 2018) are based on: exogenous synthetic oligonucleotides; endogenous reference genes; and the average of all the miRNA expressed. The right choice of normalization strategy is crucial to reduce analytical variability and to obtain reliable and reproducible results. Exogenous reference genes are non-human synthetic oligonucleotides usually added to the analyzed biological sample to monitor the efficiency and quality of RNA processing.

In miRNAs quantification, the normalization strategies adopted for RT-qPCR data calculation are based on the use of a single reference gene (i.e., cel-miR-238, cel-miR-39, cel-miR-54) (Ho et al., 2010; Wang et al., 2015; Yang et al., 2017) or on the average of multiple reference exogenous oligonucleotides (Mitchell et al., 2008; Sourvinou et al., 2013). These normalization methods have an important limitation, however: unlike endogenous miRNAs, exogenous oligonucleotides are not affected by pre-analytical variables, consequently, they reduce the analytical but not the pre-analytical variability. The use of one or more endogenous reference genes satisfies this criterion because the genes are affected by the same pre-analytical variables as the same analytical procedures of the target miRNA(s); therefore, this is the most suitable normalization strategy for miRNAs data from RT-qPCR-based quantification techniques (Faraldi et al., 2018).

In human samples, the most commonly used endogenous reference gene is has-miR-16 (Faraldi et al., 2018), but several studies have shown very variable expression between cases and controls and the effect of hemolysis on its levels in blood samples (Hu et al., 2012; Liu et al., 2012; Kirschner et al., 2013). Also for endogenous sequences, the normalization method based on the use of multiple reference genes, identified with the aid of informatics tools, is thought to reduce post-analytical variability (Vandesompele et al., 2002; Andersen et al., 2004). With this procedure, however, the miRNAs set as reference cannot be used later in the analysis as targets (Faraldi et al., 2018). Finally, for large amounts of data or in the absence of an *a priori* reference gene, a commonly applied strategy is to calculate the average expression of all the evaluated endogenous miRNA (Mestdagh et al., 2009). Based on these considerations, it is of key importance to standardize the normalization method by determining the most stable reference gene(s) in each experimental setting (Faraldi et al., 2018). Recently, we demonstrated large differences in results obtained by applying different normalization strategies to RT-qPCR data from a panel of 179 circulating miRNAs. Based on analysis of the between-assay coefficients of variation (CV) and of the CV distribution frequencies, we defined the normalization of a specific miRNA (hsa-miR-320d) as the best strategy in that specific setting (Faraldi et al., 2019).

Specific guidelines to standardize pre-analytical, analytical, and post-analytical variables are desirable in order to obtain reliable and comparable miRNA expression data and to accelerate the definitive clinical implementation of miRNAs-based tests.

MIRNAS AS BIOMARKERS FOR BONE DISEASES

While the multiple roles exerted by tissue and exome/microvesicle-associated miRNAs in bone pathophysiology have been identified and validated, the clinical usefulness of circulating miRNAs in skeletal and muscle-skeletal diseases has not yet been established. This is because studies so far have been designed with a mechanistic purpose in mind and not for identifying circulating miRNAs with diagnostic/prognostic abilities for bone fracture risk or treatment response (Hackl et al., 2016). The potential role of circulating miRNAs as biomarkers for the early identification of altered bone metabolism ranks high on the clinical research agenda, given the aging population and the growing incidence of age-associated diseases (e.g., metabolic bone diseases and osteoporosis) and the related risk of bone fracture. Reliable diagnostic tools that can prognosticate a subject-specific risk of disease onset or, if already overt, a subject-specific risk of progression and response to therapy are currently lacking. Furthermore, the natural history of age-associated bone diseases is, as never before, tied to a plethora of subject-specific variables. miRNAs and their circulating fraction hold promise: as epigenetic modifiers of gene expression they act much more upstream of the expression process than classical protein markers. This means that changes in their expression, which are likely to be mirrored by changes in their circulating levels, are effective far before their translation into metabolic and structural changes (Materozzi et al., 2018).

Circulating miRNAs and Postmenopausal Osteoporosis

Osteoporosis (OP), one of the most prevalent bone diseases, is characterized by impaired bone strength and quality that increase the risk of bone fracture (NIH, 2001). Currently, dual energy X-ray absorptiometry (DXA) is the diagnostic gold standard, while bone turnover markers are useful in framing the metabolic activity of bone cells [e.g., C-terminal cross-link (CTx), N-terminal pro-peptide of type I collagen (PINP), parathyroid hormone (PTH), bone alkaline phosphatase (BAP), osteocalcin, and tartrate-resistant acid phosphatase 5b (TRAP5b), pyridonline/deoxypyridinoline] and in evaluating the effectiveness of anti-resorptive therapies (Lombardi et al., 2012; Vasikaran and Chubb, 2016). Although valuable, these diagnostic tools have several practical flaws that partially limit their utility: on the one hand, radiological methods can reveal only already established bony architectural modifications, which take several weeks or months to become detectable, and on the other, bone turnover markers are not fully specific for either bone or the metabolic process they are associated with (i.e., formation or resorption) (Lombardi et al., 2012).

Despite limitations in pre-analytical, analytical, and post-analytical standardization, miRNAs still have enormous potential in this setting. Indeed, based on their role as highly sensitive fine-tuners of biological processes, when assayed in combination with conventional diagnostics, they may give a more detailed clinical framing and a prompt measure of response to therapy (Faraldi et al., 2018; Sansoni et al., 2018). This is particularly desirable in complex syndromic conditions, such as OP, in which the prognosis (i.e., bone fracture) depends not only upon the bony metabolic status but also on the whole-body metabolism. Circulating miRNAs can much better describe such a complex network. The still limited information about the role of miRNAs in OP is derived from different types of human samples [serum, circulating monocytes or bone marrow-derived mesenchymal stem cells (BM-MSCs), and bone tissue] obtained from patients of different ethnic groups with low bone mineral density (BMD) or bone fractures and compared with healthy controls or osteoarthritis (OA) patients. Furthermore, differences in quantification platforms and normalization processes make it very hard to compare the study data.

Early evidence that OP correlates with altered expression of circulating miRNAs stems from a microarray analysis of 365 miRNAs in human circulating monocytes collected from postmenopausal Caucasian women with either low or high BMD. Of the 365 miRNAs screened by RT-qPCR analysis, only miR-133a was found significantly upregulated in the low-BMD subjects compared with their normal BMD counterparts (Wang et al., 2012). Using the same experimental protocol, the same authors found another marginally expressed miRNA associated with low BMD: miR-422a (Cao et al., 2014). Supporting the hypothesis for their tissue-specificity, subsequent analysis of miR-133a and miR-422a expression in isolated circulating B cells derived from the same subjects disclosed no difference between the two groups (Wang et al., 2012; Cao et al., 2014). Based on these results, the authors speculated that these two miRNAs might be monocyte-specific biomarkers for postmenopausal OP. Mature miR-133a is transcribed from two different loci (18q11.2 and 20q13.33). It was previously described as an inhibitor of osteoblast differentiation by directly targeting RUNX2 in murine pre-myogenic C2C12 and pre-osteoblastic MC3T3-E1 cells (Li et al., 2008; Zhang et al., 2011b). The miR-422a expression level in osteoblast-like cells was described to be decreased after treatment with peptide-15, a factor that increases bone development (Palmieri et al., 2008). Since monocytes are osteoclast precursors, a bioinformatics analysis has highlighted three osteoclast-related potential target genes for miR-133a (CXCL11, CXCR3, and SLC39A1) and five for miR-422a (CBL, CD226, IGF1, PAG1, TOB2) (Wang et al., 2012; Cao et al., 2014). The latter studies, however, suffered from several limitations: limited sample size (10 subjects per group); no evidence of a correlation between miR-133a or miR-422a and target gene expression; and no information about the stem-loop arm of origin of these miRNAs.

In another study, Chen et al. (2014a) evaluated the expression profile of 721 human miRNAs in CD14+ mononuclear cells from peripheral blood (PBMCs) collected from postmenopausal OP women. They found seven differentially expressed miRNAs compared with the non-OP group: four (miR-218, miR-503, miR-305, and miR-618) were downregulated and three (miR-107, miR-133a, and miR-411) were upregulated. Also, miR-133a was confirmed as upregulated in circulating monocytes from postmenopausal OP women (Wang et al., 2012); however, only miR-503, the most deregulated one, was validated by RT-qPCR, and its anti-osteoclastogenic effects were investigated *in vivo* and *in vitro*. Overexpression of miR-503, after pre-miR-503 transfection in OP-derived CD14+, drastically inhibited M-CSF/RANKL-induced osteoclastogenesis, while its suppression by antagomiR-503 promoted osteoclast differentiation. The authors identified and validated RANK mRNA as a target for miR-503. Furthermore, in ovariectomized (OVX) mice, antagomiR-503 increased RANK protein expression, and promoted bone loss and resorption, whereas agomiR-503 prevented bone loss and resorption (Chen et al., 2014a). Because miR-503 downregulation has a key role in postmenopausal OP onset, it may be a target for new therapeutic strategies for OP.

Using a different approach, a study evaluated the miRNA profile differences in human *bone marrow*-derived mesenchymal stromal cells (BM-MCSs) from OP patients and non-OP controls. In this case, 1,040 miRNAs were screened using a microarray in BM-MCSs collected from healthy premenopausal women (control group, n = 5) and postmenopausal OP women (n = 5) (Yang et al., 2013). Following RT-qPCR validation, miR-21 was found downregulated in the OP women, as confirmed in the MSCs from OVX mice. Further experiments revealed that Spry1 negatively regulates fibroblast growth factor (FGF) and extracellular signal-regulated kinase–mitogen-activated protein kinase (ERK-MAPK) signaling pathways and that it is directly targeted by miR-21. As a consequence, the TNFα-mediated inhibition of miR-21 may impair bone formation, as observed in OP induced by estrogen deficiency. This mRNA seems to be a main regulator of osteoblastic differentiation of MSCs and in postmenopausal OP onset (Yang et al., 2013). Moreover, osteoclast precursors express miR-21, which is upregulated during TNF-α/RANKL-induced osteoclastogenesis (Sugatani et al., 2011; Kagiya and Nakamura, 2013). miR-21 expression is upregulated by the osteoclastogenesis transcription factor c-Fos that binds the miR-21 promoter (Kagiya and Nakamura, 2013) which, in turn, downregulates c-Fos inhibitor-programmed cell death 4 (PDCD4). This positive c-Fos/miR-21/PDCD4 feedback loop regulates and promotes RANKL-induced osteoclastogenesis (Sugatani et al., 2011). In addition, miR-21 is involved in estrogen-induced osteoclasts apoptosis: estrogens inhibit miR-21 expression by inducing Fas-ligand (FasL), another miR-21 target, which in turn inhibits osteoclastogenesis and promotes osteoclast apoptosis (Garcia Palacios et al., 2005; Sugatani and Hruska, 2013).

More recent studies have been focused on whole blood, serum or plasma miRNA profiling in patients with or without OP. Circulating levels of miR-133a, miR-146a, and miR-21 have been assayed by RT-qPCR in plasma samples of Chinese postmenopausal women, grouped as normal, osteopenic or OP. miR-21 was downregulated while miR133a was upregulated in the OP and osteopenic women compared with the controls and both correlated with BMD; miR-146a was unchanged (Li et al., 2014). miR-21 was found downregulated in the BM-MCSs of postmenopausal OP women (Yang et al., 2013), while the monocyte expression of miR-133a was associated with low BMD values (Wang et al., 2012). A study investigated the discriminatory potential between OP and osteopenia of six miRNAs (miR-130b-3p, miR-151a-3p, miR-151b, miR-194-5p, and miR-590-5p) which were found upregulated in OP. Of these six, miR-194-5p was the most upregulated and its expression negatively correlated with BMD. The association between miR-194-5p circulating levels and BMD was later confirmed in a wider cohort of Chinese postmenopausal women with normal, osteopenia, and OP ranges of BMD. The study also reported that miR-194-5p may influence the TGF-β and Wnt signaling pathways, thus acting as a critical factor in the pathophysiology of postmenopausal OP (Meng et al., 2015).

The overexpression of miR-194-5p in mice BM-MSCs was correlated with osteogenesis by targeting both COUP-TFII (chicken ovalbumin upstream promoter-transcription factor II) (Jeong et al., 2014) and STAT1 (signal transducer and activator of transcription 1) (Li et al., 2015b). In parallel, among other 851 miRNAs, miR-27a was validated as the most downregulated one in the serum of postmenopausal OP women compared with their healthy counterparts (You et al., 2016). The MSCs collected from these OP patients displayed an increased adipogenic potential at the expense of osteoblast formation. During osteogenesis, miR-27a is upregulated in MSCs, whereas the opposite occurs during adipogenesis; and indeed, miR-27a silencing in mice impairs bone formation. Myocyte enhancer factor 2c (Mef2c), a transcription factor involved in developmental processes, has been identified and validated as a miR-27a target gene (You et al., 2016). Consistent with previous observations (Lin et al., 2009; Wang and Xu, 2010; Pan et al., 2014), miR-27a expression, is essential for osteoblastic differentiation of MSCs and its downregulation *in vivo* has been associated with bone loss. Bedene et al. (2016) identified, among other nine miRNAs, miR-148a-3p as a potential biomarker for postmenopausal OP based on its significantly higher levels in the plasma samples from OP subjects compared with controls. In CD14+ PBMCs, the RANKL-induced osteoclast differentiation promotes miR-148a expression dependent on the repression of V-maf musculoaponeurotic fibrosarcoma oncogene homolog B (MAFB), a transcription factor whose expression inhibits osteoclastogenesis (Cheng et al., 2013b). miR-148-3p has been found upregulated also in CD14+ PBMCs of patients with systemic lupus erythematous (SLE) in which it was correlated with reduced BMD. Furthermore, treatment of OVX mice with antagomiR-148a slowed bone resorption and increased bone mass (Cheng et al., 2013b). The expression levels of the nine miRNAs assayed by Bedene et al. (2016) revealed that plasma miR-126-3p is also positively associated with BMD at the distal forearm and that miR-423-5p plasma levels are negatively correlated with the 10-year probability of bone fracture in OP.

Using a different approach, Chen et al. (2016) screened a wide range of miRNAs in serum samples from OP mice in order to identify the most stable reference gene (miR-25-3p) for use in data normalization in humans. Fifteen of the screened miRNAs found differentially expressed in the OP mice were then investigated in serum samples from postmenopausal women (7 osteopenic, 10 OP, and 19 healthy women). miR-30b-5p was significantly lower in both the osteopenia and OP samples, while miR-103-3p, miR-142-3p, and miR-328-3p were significantly lower in the OP group only compared with the healthy subjects. The role of miR-103-3p and miR-30b-5p in bone physiology has been validated in *in vitro* studies of osteogenesis: miR-30b-5p expression, whose target is Runx2, decreases during late-stage osteoblast differentiation (Eguchi et al., 2013), while miR-103-3p inhibits osteoblasts differentiation and proliferation by directly targeting Runx2 (Zuo et al., 2015) and Cav1.2 (Sun et al., 2015), respectively. Despite the limited sample size, the serum levels of these four miRNAs in OP patients were positively correlated with BMD. The ROC analysis revealed their diagnostic potential for OP based on the following AUC–sensitivity–specificity values: 0.800–80%–72.2% (miR-103-3p), 0.789–70%–79.0% (miR-142-3p), 0.793–70.6%–79.0% (miR-30b-5p), and 0.874–80%–100% (miR-328-3p) (Chen et al., 2016).

In a study series, circulating monocytes from 12 postmenopausal Mexican-Mestizo women, divided in normal (control group) and OP groups were assayed using a microarray platform for the expression profile of 2,578 miRNAs. The results showed that the three most upregulated miRNAs in the OP group were miR-1270, miR-548x-3p, and miR-8084, while the three most downregulated were miR-6124, miR-6165, and miR-6824-5p. Among the upregulated miRNAs, only miR-1270 was further validated. Based on bioinformatics analysis, nine genes have been identified as possible targets of miR-1270, and RT-qPCR finally validated the interferon regulatory factor-8 (IRF8) gene, an inhibitor of osteoclastogenesis (Zhao et al., 2009; Jimenez-Ortega et al., 2017; Saito et al., 2017), which was significantly downregulated in the OP group. The same research team discovered another monocytic miRNA, miR-708-5p, as a potential biomarker for postmenopausal OP. Next generation sequencing (NGS) of the 46 miRNAs found differentially regulated in the two groups revealed that miR-708-5p and miR-3161 were the two most upregulated in the OP group, whereas miR-4422 and miR-939-3p were the two most downregulated. These four miRNAs were then assayed using RT-qPCR, but only miR-708-5p was validated as it was found significantly upregulated in OP patients compared with controls. Bioinformatics analysis of miR-708-5p disclosed ten potential targets involved in osteoclastogenesis, only five of which (AKT1, AKT2, PARP1, FKBP5, and MP2K3) were effectively downregulated in the OP subjects compared with controls (De-La-Cruz-Montoya et al., 2018). The major limitations besides the small sample size in these two studies were the use of different quantification platforms (microarray and NGS) in preliminary screening of differential miRNA expression and the use of two different normalization strategies for RT-qPCR data analysis. These limitations make it difficult to correlate the data. In any case, miRNA-708-5p and miR-1270 may be suitable biomarkers for postmenopausal OP but require an independent validation study with a larger sample using the same protocol for data quantification and analysis.

The last paper published by this research group is the most complete work to date. The potential of miRNAs as biomarkers for OP was evaluated in serum samples (Ramirez-Salazar et al., 2018). The study was divided in two experimental parts: in the discovery stage, 40 postmenopausal Mexican-Mestizo women (grouped into OP subjects and healthy controls) were recruited, while the validation stage comprised Mexican-Mestizo women with OP, osteopenia, and bone fractures, plus healthy postmenopausal Mexican-Mestizo women. In the discovery stage, microarray analysis of 754 serum miRNAs identified seven miRNAs (miR-1227-3p, miR-139-5p, miR-140-3p, miR-17-5p, miR-197-3p, miR-23b-3p, and miR-885-5p) in which the levels were significantly higher in the OP than in the healthy subjects. Only the three most upregulated (miR-140-3p, miR-23b-3p, and miR-885-5p) were used in the validation stage. The study confirmed by RT-qPCR the higher serum levels of miR-140-3p and miR-23b-3p in the groups with osteopenia, OP or bone fracture, and higher levels of miR-885-5p in the osteopenia group than in healthy subjects. ROC analysis for miR-140-3p and miR-23b-3p, in which their ability to discriminate between OP and healthy women was evaluated, demonstrated that the two miRNAs might be good candidates as biomarkers for BMD loss: AUC of 0.84, 0.96, and 0.92 for miR-140-3p in the osteopenia, OP, and bone fracture group, respectively, compared with the healthy controls, and AUC of 0.73, 0.69, and 0.88, respectively, for miR-23b-3p. Furthermore, miR-140-3p and miR-23b-3p were significantly correlated with BMD in each cohort. Target genes databases predicted AKT1, AKT2, AKT3, BMP2, FOXO3, GSK3B, IL6R, PRKACB, RUNX2, and WNT5B as bone-related genes potentially targeted by miR-140-3p and miR-23b-3p. Other potential osteogenic related target genes have been validated *in vitro* and *in vivo*: SMAD3 (Liu et al., 2016) and RUNX2 (Deng et al., 2017) for miR-23b-3p, and BMP2 (Hwang et al., 2014) for miR-140-5p. The study underlined the importance of miR-140-3p and miR-23b-3p as biomarkers of bone loss and risk of fracture, despite the small sample size especially of the control group.

Table 1 presents information about circulating miRNAs associated with OP.

miRNAs, Bone Fragility, and Bone Fracture Risk in Postmenopausal Women

Bone fragility and fractures are the clinically relevant consequences of OP and have a negative impact on quality of life. Considering the objective limit of bone biopsy in healthy individuals, studies have compared the miRNA expression profile of OP bone with osteoarthritis (OA) samples as control. Thirteen of 760 miRNAs assayed by microarray cards were found differentially expressed in bone specimens from the femur heads of eight women with OP hip fracture compared to the femur heads from eight women with severe hip OA but without OP hip fracture, in seven of which the miRNAs were overexpressed in OP bones. In the following replication stage, the results showed that miR-518f was overexpressed and miR-187 downregulated in OP compared with OA bone (Garmilla-Ezquerra et al., 2015). Finally, the expression profile of 1,932 miRNAs was compared between fresh femoral neck trabecular bone from postmenopausal women with OP hip fracture and from postmenopausal women with OA non-OP hip fracture (control group). Following validation, only two (miR-320a and miR-483-5p) of the 82 miRNAs differently expressed between the two groups were significantly overexpressed in the OP vs. the OA samples (De-Ugarte et al., 2015). miRNA-320a targets RUNX2 and β-catenin (Yu et al., 2011; Sun et al., 2012), while miRNA-483-5p downregulates IGF2 expression in OP-derived human osteoblast cultures (De-Ugarte et al., 2015).

To identify circulating miRNAs as biomarkers for OP fracture, Seeliger et al. (2014) assayed a panel of 83 serum miRNAs in OP and non-OP patients with either femoral neck or pertrochanteric fracture. Eleven miRNAs (miR-100-5p, miR-122a-5p, miR-124-3p, miR-125b-5p, miR-148a-3p, miR-21-5p, miR-223-3p, miR-23-3p, miR-24-3p, miR-25-3p, and miR-27a-3p) were found at significantly higher levels in the OP sera. Together with miR-93 and miR-637, these miRNAs were subsequently validated in another set of serum samples: nine miRNAs (miR-100, miR-122a, miR-124a, miR-125b, miR-148a, miR-21, miR-23a, miR-24, and miR-93) were significantly higher in the OP sera than in the controls and they were proposed as markers to differentiate OP from non-OP bone fracture. Interestingly, miR-21 was previously

TABLE 1 | miRNAs related to postmenopausal OP.

Study	Study design	Biomarker source	Sample handling	Quantification platform	Evaluated miRNA	Normalization strategy	Validated miRNA biomarker	Potential target gene	AUC-Sensitivity(%)-Specificity(%)	Limits
(Wang et al., 2012)	20 PM Caucasian women (age 57-68 years): 10 with low BMD (hip/spine Z-score < -0.84); 10 with high BMD (hip/spine Z-score > 0.84)	Circulating monocytes	Monocytes separated by density gradients in UNI-SEP tubes (sodium metrizoate 9.6% and polysucrose 5.6% with 1.077 g/ml density), and isolated using a negative isolation kit	Screening: TaqMan Human MicroRNA Array v1.0 Validation: TaqMan RT-qPCR	Screening: 365 miRNAs tested Validation: miR-133a and miR-382	RNU48	↑miR-133a in low vs. high BMD group	CXCR3, CXCL11, and SLC39A1 (identified for miR-133a using miRDB and TargetScan database but not validated)	/	Small sample size; no significant correlation between the expression level of miR-133a and the potential target genes; no information about the stem-loop arm of miRNA origin; no ROC analysis
(Cao et al., 2014)	21 PM Caucasian women (age 57-68 years): 10 with low BMD (hip/spine Z-score < -0.84); 10 with high BMD (hip/spine Z-score > 0.84)	Circulating monocytes	Monocytes separated by density gradients in UNI-SEP tubes (sodium metrizoate 9.6% and polysucrose 5.6% with 1.077 g/ml density), and isolated using a negative isolation kit	Screening: TaqMan Human MicroRNA Array v1.0 Validation: TaqMan RT-qPCR	Screening: 365 miRNAs tested Validation: miR-27b, miR-422a, miR-151, and miR-152	RNU48	↑miR-422a in low vs. high BMD group	CD226, CBL, IGF1, TOB2, and PAG1 (identified for miR-422a using TargetScan database but not validated)	/	Small sample size; no significant correlation between miR-422a and the evaluated target genes; no information about the stem-loop arm of miRNA origin; no ROC analysis
(Chen et al., 2014a)	31 Chinese PM women with OP and 30 healthy women (age 50-59 years).	PBMCs CD14+	Ficoll-Paque separation step and CD14 antibody-coated magnetic cell sorting MicroBeads used for buffy coat PBMCs isolation and CD14⁺ purification, respectively	Screening: MicroRNA microarray by LC Sciences Validation: SYBR Green RT-qPCR	Screening: 721 miRNAs tested Validation: miR-503	snRNU6	↓miR-503 in OP group vs. non-OP group	RANK (validated as miR-503 target gene)	/	Small sample size; no information about the stem-loop arm of miRNA origin; no ROC analysis
(Yang et al., 2013)	5 OP PM women (age 53-63 years) and 5 premenopausal women (age 39-45 years)	BM-MCSs	Percoll density gradient centrifugation methodology obtaining BM-MCSs from the BM	Screening: LC Sciences microarray platform Validation: RT-qPCR	Screening: 1040 miRNAs tested Validation: miR-21	snRNU6	↓miR-21 in PM OP group vs. non-OP group	SPRY1 (identified for miR-21 using Target Scan 6.0 and Pic Tar databases and validated by *in vitro* experiments)	/	Small sample size; no information about the stem-loop arm of miRNA origin; no ROC analysis
(Li et al., 2014)	40 PM Chinese women with normal, 40 with OP, and 40 with osteopenia range BMD (age 46-69 years)	Cell-free plasma	Plasma obtained from fasting blood samples and stored in liquid nitrogen	miRCURY LNA RT-qPCR	miR-21, miR-133a, and miR-146a	miR-16	↓ miR-21 and ↑ miR-133a in OP and osteopenia groups vs. control	/	/	Small sample size; no information about the used anticoagulant; small sample size; arbitrary decision of the reference gene; no evaluation of the target genes; no information about the stem-loop arm of miRNA origin; no ROC analysis

TABLE 1 | Continued

Study	Study design	Biomarker source	Sample handling	Quantification platform	Evaluated miRNA	Normalization strategy	Validated miRNA biomarker	Potential target gene	AUC-Sensitivity(%)-Specificity(%)	Limits
(Meng et al., 2015)	Discovery cohort: 25 PM women with OP and 23 PM Chinese women with osteopenia (age 59-70 years) Validation cohort: 24 PM Chinese women with normal, 32 with OP and 30 with osteopenia range BMD (age 59-70 years)	Whole blood	Blood samples lysed using RBC lysis solution and centrifuged for 10 min at 450g	Discovery: Agilent Human miRNA microarray followed by SYBR Green RT-qPCR Validation: SYBR Green RT-qPCR	Discovery cohort: comprehensive miRNA expression analysis (Microarray); miR-130b-3p, miR-151a-3p, miR-151b, miR-194-5p, miR-590-5p, and miR-660-5p (RT-qPCR) Validation cohort: miR-194-5p	snRNU6	↑ miR-130b-3p, miR-151a-3p, miR-151b, miR-194-5p, and miR-590-5p in OP vs. osteopenia (Discovery cohort)↑ miR-194-5p in OP and osteopenia vs. control (Validation cohort)	/	/	Small sample size; no evaluation of the target genes; no ROC analysis
(You et al., 2016)	155 PM Chinese women with PM OP (n = 81, age 51-62 years) or healthy (n = 74, age 40-46 years)	Cell-free serum and BM-MSCs	/	Screening: Agilent Human miRNA Microarray Validation: TaqMan RT-qPCR	Screening: 851 miRNAs Validation: miR-27a	snRNU6	↓ miR-27a in OP vs. control	Mef2c (predicted for miR-27a using TargetScan and PicTar database and validated by *in vitro* studies)	/	The mean age of OP and healthy women is significantly different; no information about the stem-loop arm of miRNA origin; no ROC analysis
(Bedene et al., 2016)	74 PM women (age 55-65 years): 57 controls and 17 OP based on femoral neck/lumbar spine/ total hip T-score ≤-2.5 SD	Cell-free plasma	Blood samples collected in EDTA tubes, centrifuged at 2800 rpm and 4°C for 10 min, then further centrifuged at 9600g and 4°C for 15 min. Plasma samples stored at -80°C	SYBR Green RT-qPCR	miR-7d-5p, miR-7e-5p, miR-30 d-5p, miR-30e-5p, miR-126-3p, miR-148a-3p, miR-199a-3p, miR-423-5p, and miR-574-5p	Combination of let-7a-5p and miR-16-5p as identified by Normfinder	↑ miR-148a-3p in OP vs. control	/	/	Small sample size of the control group; no evaluation of the target genes; no ROC analysis
(Chen et al., 2016)	36 PM women: 19 HC, 7 osteopenic, 10 OP	Cell-free serum	Serum obtained by centrifuging blood samples in two steps: for 10 min at 2000g and 4°C and for 20 min at 12000g and 4°C. Serum stored at -80°C	SYBR RT-qPCR	miR-30a-5p, miR-30e-5p, miR-425-5p, miR-142-3p, miR-191a-3p, miR-215, miR-29b-3p, miR-30b-5p, miR-26a-5p, miR-345-5p, miR-361-5p, miR-185-5p, and miR-103-3p	NormFinder and GeNorm identified miR-25-3p as the most stable reference gene in mice models of OP	↓ miR-30b-5p in both osteopenic and OP vs. HC↓ miR-103-3p, miR-328-3p, and miR-142-3p OP vs. HC	/	0.793 (miR-30b-5p) for both OP and osteopenia vs. HC0.793-70.6-79.0 (miR-30b-5p), 0.800-80-72.2 (miR-103-3p), 0.789-70-79.0 (miR-142-3p) and 0.874-80-100 (miR-328-3p) for OP vs. HC	Different number of subjects recruited in the 3 groups; the reference gene for humans was identified in mice models; no evaluation of the target genes

(Continued)

TABLE 1 | Continued

Study	Study design	Biomarker source	Sample handling	Quantification platform	Evaluated miRNA	Normalization strategy	Validated miRNA biomarker	Potential target gene	AUC-Sensitivity(%)-Specificity(%)	Limits
(Jimenez-Ortega et al., 2017)	PM Mexican-Mestizo women: 6 with normal (control group) and 6 with OP hip BMD (age 63-85 years)	PBMCs	Histopaque-1077 kit used for obtaining PCMCs by density gradients. CD14+ obtained by density gradient centrifugation for 30 min at 400g and RT and magnetic bead isolation. negative isolation kit EasySep Human Monocyte Enrichment used for naive monocyte isolation	Screening: Affymetrix GeneChip Human U133 Plus 2.0 Array Validation: TaqMan RT-qPCR	Screening: 2.578 miRNAs tested Validation: miR-1270, miR-548x-3p, and miR-8084	Screening: quantile normalization Validation: RNU44	↑miR-1270 in OP group vs. control group	IRF8 (identified for miR-1270 using PITA v5.0, microRNA.org, miRWalk v2.0, miRDB, and TargetScan Human v7.0 database and validated in study)	/	Small sample size; no ROC analysis
(De-La-Cruz-Montoya et al., 2018)	PM Mexican-Mestizo women: 7 with normal (control group) and 7 with OP hip BMD (age 63-85 years)	Human PBMCs	Blood collected in CPT tubes and PBMCs obtained. CD14+ cells enriched by negative selection (EasySep kit)	Screening: Illumia NextSeq 500 Validation: TaqMan RT-qPCR	Validation: miR-708-5p, miR-3161, miR-939-3p, and miR-4422	Validation: RNU44 and RNU48	↑miR-708-5p in osteoporosis group vs. control group	AKT1, AKT2, FKBP5, PARP1, and MP2K3 (identified for miR-708-5p using miRTarBase and MiRNet and validated in study)	/	Small sample size; no ROC analysis
(Ramirez-Salazar et al., 2018)	Discovery cohort: 40 PM Mexican-Mestizo women: 20 with normal (controls) and 20 with OP hip BMD (age 63-85 years) Validation cohort: 22 normal, 26 OP, 28 osteopenia, 21 with hip fracture BMD	Cell-free serum	Serum obtained within 1h of collection and stored at -80°C	Discovery stage: TaqMan Array Human MicroRNA A+B Cards Set v3.0 Validation stage: TaqMan RT-qPCR	Screening: 754 miRNAs tested Validation: miR-23b-3p miR-140-3p, and miR-885-5p	snRNU6	↑ miR-23b-3p and miR-140-3p in OP, osteopenia and bone fracture group vs. control↑ miR-885-5p in osteopenia vs. control	AKT1, AKT2, AKT3, IL6R, BMP2, GSK3B, FOXO3, PRKACB, WNT5B, and RUNX2 (identified for miR-23b-3p and miR-140-3p using miRWalk v3 database)	0.84 (miR-140-3p) for osteopenia, 0.96 (miR-140-3p) for OP, and 0.92 (miR-140-3p) for fracture vs. HC0.73 (miR-23b-3p) for osteopenia, 0.69 (miR-23b-3p) for OP, and 0.88 (miR-23b-3p) for fracture vs. HC0.69 (miR-885-5p) for osteopenia vs. HC	No validation of the identified target genes

AKT1, AKT serine/threonine kinase 1; AKT2, AKT serine/threonine kinase 2; AKT3, AKT serine/threonine kinase 3; BMD, bone mineral density; BM-MCSs, bone marrow mesenchymal stem cells; BMP2, bone morphogenic protein 2; CBL, casitas B-lineage lymphoma proto oncogene; CD226, cluster of differentiation 226; CXCL11, chemokine (C-X-C motif) ligand 11; CXCR3, chemokine (C-X-C motif) receptor 3; FKBP5, FK506 binding protein 5; FOXO3, forkhead box O3; FZD3, frizzled-3; GSK3B, glycogen synthase kinase 3 beta; HC, healthy controls; IGF1, insulin-like growth factor 1; IL6R, interleukin 6 receptor; IRF8, interferon regulatory factor-8; Mef2c, myocyte enhancer factor 2 c; MP2K3, mitogen-activated protein kinase kinase 3; OP, osteoporosis; OSX, osterix; PAG1, phosphoprotein associated with glycosphingolipid microdomains 1; PARP1, poly(ADP-ribose) polymerase 1; PBMCs, peripheral blood mononuclear cells; PM, postmenopausal; PRKACB, protein kinase cAMP-activated catalytic subunit beta; RANK, receptor activator of nuclear factor κ B; RANKL, receptor activator of nuclear factor k B ligand; RT, room temperature; RT-qPCR, real-time quantitative polymerase chain reaction; RUNX2, runt-related transcription factor 2; SLC39A1, solute carrier family (zinc transporter), member 1; SPRY1, protein sprouty homolog 1; TOB2, transducer of ERBB2, 2; WNT5B, Wnt family member 5B.

found downregulated in both the BM-MCSs and the plasma of OP patients (Yang et al., 2013; Li et al., 2014); these opposite results could be ascribed to the different experimental protocols used, which identified miRNAs that regulate osteoclast/osteoblast differentiation and activity, as previously demonstrated. miR-21 is highly expressed in osteoclast precursors and it is upregulated in the course of TNF-α/RANKL-induced osteoclastogenesis (Fujita et al., 2008; Kagiya and Nakamura, 2013); it stimulates osteoclastogenesis by overcoming PDCD4-mediated c-Fos inhibition (Fujita et al., 2008; Sugatani et al., 2011), while its expression is inhibited by estrogens (Garcia Palacios et al., 2005; Sugatani and Hruska, 2013). miR-23 and miR-24 belong to the miR-23a~27a~24-2 cluster and act as negative regulators of osteoblast differentiation by targeting SATB2 that cooperates with RUNX2 to induce osteogenesis, while miR-23a also inhibits RUNX2 (Hassan et al., 2010). miR-93 inhibits osteoblast mineralization by targeting OSX (Yang et al., 2012). miR-100 negatively regulates BMPR2, a key osteogenic factor for MSCs (Zeng et al., 2012). The overexpression of miR-125b is associated with impaired osteoblast differentiation and proliferation through the modulation of OSX expression (Mizuno et al., 2008; Chen et al., 2014b). miR-124 is progressively downregulated during RANKL-induced osteoclastogenesis and its overexpression affects the maturation of osteoclast precursors *via* suppression of the key osteoclastogenic factor NFATc1, and their migration *via* inhibition of RhoA/Rac1 (Lee et al., 2013).

Following the identification of nine miRNAs whose circulating levels were higher in OP patients than in controls, Seelinger et al. evaluated their expression in the bone tissues: miR-100, miR-125b, miR-21, miR-23a, miR-24, and miR-25 were upregulated also in the OP bone samples. They defined the potential diagnostic value of these miRNAs by means of ROC curve analysis. All the identified serum miRNAs showed significant AUC, sensitivity and specificity in discriminating OP from non-OP subjects: 0.69–62.9%–61.7% (miR-100), 0.77–74.1%–72.1% (miR-122a), 0.69–61.4%–61.0% (miR-124a), 0.76–76.4%–75.0% (miR-125b), 0.61–62.5%–62.3% (miR-148a), 0.63–61.3%–61.7% (miR-21), 0.63–57.4%–56.7% (miR-23a), 0.63–60.3%–60.4% (miR-24), and 0.68–69.0%–68.3% (miR-93). Consequently, the five miRNAs identified in both tissue and serum samples can be used as biomarkers for OP and related hip fractures (Seeliger et al., 2014).

Another study attempted to search for potential miRNAs marking for OP bone fractures. In the discovery stage, Caucasian women with either OP sub-capital hip fracture (n = 8) or severe hip OA (control group, n = 5), which required arthroplasty, were recruited (Panach et al., 2015). The serum levels of 179 miRNAs were analyzed by RT-qPCR. Among the 42 differently regulated miRNAs, six (miR-122-5p, miR-125b-5p, miR-143-3p, miR-21-5p, miR-210, and miR-34a-5p) were selected for the replication stage. miR-122-5p, miR-125b-5p, and miR-21-5p were significantly higher in the OP bone fracture group than the controls. miR-125b-5p and miR-21-5p have been correlated with bone metabolic indexes (Fujita et al., 2008; Mizuno et al., 2008; Sugatani and Hruska, 2013), and the upregulation of miR-21 was consistent with previous observations (Seeliger et al., 2014). ROC analysis of the diagnostic value of the serum miRNAs revealed that miR-122-5p, miR-125b-5p, and miR-21-5p consistently discriminated between the OP patients with fractures (n = 15) and the controls (n = 12) (AUC 0.87 for miR-122-5p, 0.76 for miR-125-5p, and 0.87 for miR-21-5p) (Panach et al., 2015). Using a similar protocol, Weilner et al. (2015) found three other miRNAs potentially correlated with OP fractures in postmenopausal women (n = 7 in the discovery stage, n = 12 in the validation stage) (miR-22-3p, miR-328-3p, and let-7g-5p) and that the levels were significantly lower in the serum of the cases (n = 7 in the discovery stage, n = 11 in the validation stage). Previous *in vitro* experiments demonstrated that let-7 promotes osteoblastogenesis in MSCs *in vitro*, while it induces bone formation *in vivo*. These effects are mediated by the repression of high-mobility group AT-hook 2 (HMGA2) (Wei et al., 2014). *In vitro* experiments on human unrestricted somatic stem cells (USSC) showed that miR-22-3p is upregulated during osteogenic differentiation and that its potential target is CDK6 (Trompeter et al., 2013). Finally, CD44 is a potential target of miRNA-328-3p in macrophages and it is also expressed in osteocytes (Ishimoto et al., 2014). *In vitro* experiments on MSCs collected from two OP patients with bone fracture confirmed the let-7g-5p-mediated effect and miR-22-3p downregulation, and correlated miR-328-3p repression with reduced ALP activity during osteogenic formation (Weilner et al., 2015).

Recent studies have investigated whether single or combined miRNAs discriminate bone fractures in conditions associated with bone fragility. Kocijan et al. (2016) performed a case-control study to identify serum miRNAs correlated with trauma fractures in postmenopausal OP. Three (miR-152-3p, miR-320a, and miR-335-5p) of the 187 tested miRNAs selected based on previously published studies were significantly higher, whereas sixteen (let-7b-5p, miR-140-5p, miR-16-5p, miR-186-5p, miR-19a-3p, miR-19b-3p, miR-215-5p, miR-29b-3p, miR-30e-5p, miR-324-3p, miR-365a-3p, miR-378a-5p, miR-532-5p, miR-550a-3p, miR-7-5p, and miR-93-5p) were significantly lower in postmenopausal women with bone fracture (n = 10) than in the controls without bone fracture (n = 11). ROC analysis showed that miR-140-5p, miR-152-3p, miR-19a-3p, miR-19b-3p, miR-30e-5p, miR-324-3p, miR-335-5p, and miR-550a-3p had a higher discriminating power between individuals with bone fracture and healthy individuals (AUC> 0.9) than BMD or bone turnover markers. miR-335-3p has been reported to promote osteogenic differentiation by binding and downregulating dickkopf-related protein 1 (DKK1), a soluble antagonist of the Wnt signaling pathway (Zhang et al., 2011a). miR-30e has been reported to be downregulated during osteoblastic differentiation of MSC, and its target has been identified in low-density lipoprotein receptor-related protein 6 (LRP6), a known critical factor in Wnt signaling (Wang et al., 2013b). miR-140-5p inhibits osteoblastic differentiation of hMSCs by repressing bone morphogenic protein 2 (BMP2) (Hwang et al., 2014). miR-29 family members (miR-29a-3p, miR-29b-3p, and miR-29c-3p) are upregulated during osteoclastogenesis, while their KO results in altered recruitment and migration of osteoclast precursors without any effect on osteoclast activity (Franceschetti et al., 2013). In addition, six targets (Cdc42, srGAP2, GPR85, NFIA, CD93, and CTR) of the miR-29 family are involved in cytoskeletal organization, recruitment of osteoclast precursors, and osteoclast function (Franceschetti et al., 2013). However, results for miR-29 family roles are conflicting. The administration of pre-miR-29a in rats limited the bone loss induced by glucocorticoids, while miR-29b expression was downregulated during the differentiation of CD14+ PBMCs into osteoclasts (Rossi et al., 2013; Wang et al., 2013a). These effects are probably associated with the miR-29 family action on Wnt signaling and on osteoblast activity promotion (Wang et al., 2013a). In another study, miR-29b resulted upregulated in RAW264.7 cells treated with TNF-α and RANKL to induce osteoclastogenesis (Kagiya and Nakamura, 2013). Furthermore, miR-29b has been found to promote osteogenesis and to regulate extracellular matrix proteins expression by targeting the expression of HDAC4, TGF3, ACVR2A, CTNNBIP1, DUSP2 and COL1A1, COL5A3, COL4A2, respectively (Li et al., 2009).

Recent studies have discovered other circulating miRNAs associated with OP and OP bone fracture. Chen et al. (2017) tried to find other potential serum and tissue miRNAs in Chinese OP women with hip fractures. Five of the 95 detected miRNAs were significantly upregulated in the OP patients (n = 30) compared with the healthy non-OP controls (n = 30): miR-125b, miR-30, miR-4665-3p, miR-5914, and miR-96. Only miR-125b, miR-30, and miR-5914 were subsequently validated by RT-qPCR. These three miRNAs were also found upregulated in OP bone samples compared with controls. In both cases, miR-125b was the most upregulated, and ROC analysis confirmed its diagnostic potential in postmenopausal OP (AUC 0.898) in accordance with three previous studies (Seeliger et al., 2014; Panach et al., 2015; Kelch et al., 2017).

Yavropoulou et al. (2017) investigated the expression level of fourteen serum miRNAs, previously associated with OP and OP bone fractures in the sera from postmenopausal women with low bone mass and either with (n = 35) or without (n = 35) vertebral fractures. Compared with the controls, miR-124-3p and miR-2861 were higher, whereas miR-21-5p, miR-23a-3p, and miR-29a-3p were lower in the two OP groups compared with the non-OP controls. Furthermore, in the patients with low bone mass, the levels of miR-21-5p were lowest in the patients with vertebral fractures. Together with their above- described role, miR-124-3p, miR-21-5p, miR-23a-3p, miR-2861, and miR-29a-3p are known to positively regulate osteoblast differentiation by targeting HDAC5, a transcriptional factor that affects bone formation mediated by Runx2 (Hu et al., 2011). ROC analysis showed that the associated AUC of miR-21-5p was 0.66, with 66% sensitivity and 71% specificity (Yavropoulou et al., 2017). These results contrasted with those from previous studies that found an association between miR-21-5p and miR-23-3p upregulation with bone fractures in OP (Seeliger et al., 2014; Panach et al., 2015; Kelch et al., 2017). Wang et al. (2018) identified eight out of ten miRNAs in sera and bone tissue samples from OP patients with bone fracture. miR-100, miR-122a, miR-125b, miR-24-3p, and miR-27a-3p levels were higher in serum and upregulated in the bone samples of OP patients (n = 45) than in the non-OP subjects (n = 15), while miR-128 was upregulated only in the OP bone samples. Conversely, miR-145 expression was increased only in the OP serum compared with non-OP, while miR-144-3p was downregulated in the OP serum and the bone samples. Since miR-144-3p has not been associated with OP, the authors further investigated its role in osteoclastogenesis. miR-144 was found to affect osteoclast differentiation by targeting RANK, as well as proliferation and apoptosis.

Recently, Li et al. (2018) conducted a study to validate serum miR-133a as a biomarker for postmenopausal OP with bone fracture. miR-133a upregulation in circulating monocytes and in serum has been associated with postmenopausal OP (Wang et al., 2012; Li et al., 2014). The study reported that serum miR-133a was significantly higher in the postmenopausal OP women with hip fracture than in the healthy controls, and that it negatively correlated with BMD at the lumbar spine. *In vitro*, miR-133a expression was significantly upregulated during RANKL/M-CSF-induced osteoclastogenesis in RAW264.7 and THP-1 cells and its overexpression upregulated NFATc1, c-Fos, and TRAP protein expression (Li et al., 2018). Previous studies have also demonstrated that miR-133a overexpression in the osteoblast cell line MC3T3 suppressed osteoclastogenesis by directly targeting RUNX2 (Zhang et al., 2011b). *In vivo*, miR-133a KO in OVX rats altered the circulating levels of osteoclastogenesis-related factors and prevented bone loss (Li et al., 2018). Taken together, these findings support the diagnostic potential for miR-133a in postmenopausal OP and related bone fracture and highlight the potential of miR-133a as a clinical therapeutic target for postmenopausal OP.

Table 2 summarizes information about circulating miRNAs associated with bone fracture risk in OP.

miRNAs, Fracture Risk, and Physical Activity

Physical activity (PA) is a therapeutic strategy to reduce bone fracture risk, improve bone metabolic status and, eventually, to increase bone mass during childhood, adolescence, and early adulthood or to limit the age-associated decrease in peak bone mass in older age (Xu et al., 2016). PA affects miRNAs expression in tissues and organs, the circulating miRNAs profile reflects this situation as a consequence (Lombardi et al., 2016a). The literature on PA-dependent modifications of osteoporosis- or fracture risk-associated miRNAs is scarce (Lombardi et al., 2016a). The suboptimal understanding of these mechanisms stems from failure to appreciate the complex network of interactions accompanying the metabolic response of bone to PA. This multilevel relationship contemplates: direct effects of PA on bone; whole-body metabolic effects of PA on bone; specific effects of PA on tissues (e.g., skeletal muscle, adipose tissue, immune system, nervous system) besides the release of mediators from bone (e.g., myokines, adipokines, cytokines, and neurotransmitters) that affect bone both directly and indirectly; and PA-dependent release of mediators by bone (osteokines) that affect the expression of bone-acting mediators released by other tissues (Lombardi et al., 2016b; Lombardi, 2019). Recently, we demonstrated that seven from a panel of ten fracture risk-associated miRNAs (miR-100, miR-122-5p, miR-125-5p, miR148a-3p, miR-23a-3p, miR-24-3p, and miR-93-5p) responded to a protocol of PA (8-week repeated sprint training in young healthy males) in a more sensitive way than standard bone metabolism markers, metabolic hormones, and cytokines (Sansoni et al., 2018).

TABLE 2 | miRNAs related to bone fracture risk in postmenopausal OP.

Study	Study design	Biomarker source	Sample handling	Quantification platform	Evaluated miRNA	Normalization strategy	Reported miRNA biomarker	Potential target gene	AUC-Sensitivity (%)-Specificity (%)	Limits
(Garmilla-Ezquerra et al., 2015)	Discovery cohort: 8 women with OP hip fracture, 8 women with severe hip OA without OP fractures (control group) Replication cohort: 19 women with OP hip fracture, 19 women with severe hip OA without OP fractures (control group)	Bone specimens	Trabecular bone cylinders obtained from central part of femoral head using a trephine. Fragments cut into small pieces, washed with PBS, snap-frozen in liquid nitrogen, and stored at -70°C	Discovery stage: TaqMan array human miRNA A + B cards v3 Replication stage: TaqMan RT-qPCR	Discovery stage: 760 miRNAs tested Replication stage: miR-187, miR-193a-3p, miR-214, miR-518f, miR-636, and miR-210	NormFinder and GeNorm programs identified miR-222 and let-7b as most stable normalizators.	↑ miR-518f in OP fractures group vs. control group↑ miR-187 in control group vs. OP fractures group	IGFBP1, DKK1, WISP1, CTNNBIP1 (identified for miR-518f using microRNA.org, mirbase.org, and targetscan. org prediction algorithms but not validated by *in vitro* experiments)	/	Small sample size; OA patients as control group; no validation of the identified target genes; no information about the stem-loop arm of miRNA origin; no ROC analysis.
(De-Ugarte et al., 2015)	Discovery cohort: 6 PM OP women and 6 PM OA women (control group) both with femoral neck fracture Replication cohort: 7 PM OP women and 6 PM OA women (control group) both with femoral neck fracture	Fresh bone specimens	Bone fragments from femoral neck transcervical region reduced to small pieces, washed three times with PBS, and stored at -80°C	Discovery stage: miRCURY LNA™ microRNA Array performed by Exiqon Services Replication stage: RT-qPCR performed by Exiqon Services	Discovery stage: 1932 miRNAs tested Replication stage: miR-675-5p, miR-30c-1-3p, miR-483-5p, miR-542-5p, miR-142-3p, miR-223-3p, miR-32-3p, and miR-320a	Discovery stage: Lowess (Locally Weighted Scatterplot Smoothing) global regression algorithm. Replication stage: average of miR-let-7e-5p expression in each sample	↑ miR-320a and miR-483-5p in OP fractures vs. control group	ARPP-19, BMP3 and 6, BMPR1A, CAMTA1, DNER, ESRRG, IGF1, IGF1R, IL6R, JAK2, PPARGC1A, LEPR, MAPK1, MCL, NR3C1, PDGFD, PTGER3, RARG, RXRA, SGK, SP1, SRF, TFR1 (identified for miR-320a using PicTar, TargetScan Human, miRDB, MiRanda, DIANA-TarBase, and miRTarBase database)SRF and MAPK3 (identified for miR-483-5p using mirTArBase)	/	Small sample size; OA patients as control group; no validation of the identified target genes; no ROC analysis
(Seeliger et al., 2014)	Discovery cohort: 10 OP (7 women and 3 men) and 10 non-OP (10 women) as control group, both with femoral neck or pertrochanteric fracture Replication cohort: 30 OP women and 30 non-OP women (control group), both with femoral neck or pertrochanteric fracture	Discovery stage: cell-free serum Replication stage: cell-free serum and bone tissue	/	Screening: human Serum & Plasma miRNA PCR Array MIHS-106Z Validation: SYBR RT-qPCR	Screening: 83 miRNAs tested Validation: miR-21-5p, miR-23-3p, miR-24-3p, miR-25-3p, miR-27a-3p, miR-93, miR-100-5p, miR-122a-5p, miR-124-3p, miR-125b-5p, miR-148a-3p, miR-223-3p, and miR-637	Average of SNORD96a and snRNU6	↑ miR-21, miR-23a, miR-24, miR-93, miR-100, miR-122a, miR-124a, miR-125b, and miR-148a in OP fracture serum vs. controls↑ miR-21, miR-23a, miR-24, miR-25, miR-100, and miR-125b in bone tissue from OP fracture patients vs. control	PDCD4, cFos (miR-21); RUNX2 (miR-23a/miR-24-2/ miR-27a complex); OSX (miR-93); BMPR2 (miR-100); VCAN (miR-124a); RANKL (miR-148a) (identified from previous papers but not validated in this paper)	0.63-61.3-61.7 (miR-21), 0.63-57.4-56.7 (miR-23a), 0.63-60.3-60.4 (miR-24), 0.68-69.0-68.3 (miR-93), 0.69-62.9-61.7 (miR-100), 0.77-74.1-72.1 (miR-122a), 0.69-61.4-61.0 (miR-124a), 0.76-76.4-75.0 (miR-125b), 0.61-62.5-62.3 (miR-148a) for OP fracture vs. non-OP	Small sample size; no validation of the target genes.

(*Continued*)

TABLE 2 | Continued

Study	Study design	Biomarker source	Sample handling	Quantification platform	Evaluated miRNA	Normalization strategy	Reported miRNA biomarker	Potential target gene	AUC-Sensitivity (%)-Specificity (%)	Limits
(Panach et al., 2015)	Discovery stage: 8 Caucasian women with OP subcapital hip fracture and 5 with severe OA of hip requiring surgery (control group) Replication stage: 15 Caucasian women with OP subcapital hip fracture and 12 with severe OA of hip requiring surgery (control group)	Cell-free serum	Serum samples obtained from fasting blood stored at -80°C	Discovery stage: miRCURY LNA Universal RT microRNA PCR, Serum/Plasma Focus microRNA PCR Panel Replication stage: Exiqon LNA RT-qPCR	Screening: 179 miRNAs tested Validation: miR-143-3p, miR-122-5p, miR-125b-5p, miR-210, miR-21-5p, and miR-34a-5p	GeNorm identified miR-93-5p	↑ miR-122-5p, miR-125b-5p, and miR-21-5p in OP fracture vs. control group	/	0.87 (miR-122-5p), 0.76 (miR-125-5p), and 0.87 (miR-21-5p) for OP fracture vs. control group	Small sample size, OA patients as control group; no evaluation of the target genes
(Weilner et al., 2015)	Discovery stage: 7 PM Caucasian women with femoral neck OP fracture and 7 PM women without femoral fracture (control group) Replication stage: 12 PM Caucasian women with femoral neck OP fracture and 11 PM women without femoral fracture (control group)	Cell-free serum	Serum obtained from blood samples centrifugied at RT and 2000g for 15 min, after incubation at RT for 30 min, and stored at -80°C	Screening: Exiqon serum/plasma focus panels Validation: RT-qPCR	Screening: 175 miRNAs tested Validation: miR-10a-5p, miR-10b-5p, miR-22-3p, miR 133b, miR-328-3p, and let-7g-5p	Normalization of Cp-values based on average Cp of the detected miRNAs	↓ miR-22-3p, miR-328-3p, and let-7g-5p in OP fracture serum vs. control group	/	/	Small sample size; no evaluation of the target genes; the mean age of patients recruited for the discovery and validation study was significantly different (71 years and 80 years, respectively); no ROC analysis
(Kocijan et al., 2016)	10 women with PM OP low trauma fracture and 11 healthy PM women without low-trauma fracture	Cell-free serum	Fasting blood samples immediately centrifuged and serum stored a -80°C	SYBR Green RT-qPCR	187 miRNAs tested	Global mean	↑ miR-152-3p, miR-335-5p, miR-320a and↓ let-7b-5p, miR-7-5p, miR-16-5p, miR-19a-3p, miR-19b-3p, miR-29b-3p, miR-30e-5p, miR-93-5p, miR-140-5p, miR-215-5p, miR-186-5p, miR-324-3p, miR-365a-3p, miR-378a-5p, miR-532-5p, and miR-550a-3p in fractured group vs. control group	/	0.962 (miR-152-3p), 0.959 (miR-30e-5p), 0.950 (miR-324-3p), 0.947(miR-140-5p), 0.944 (miR-19b-3p), 0.939 (miR-335-5p), 0.929 (miR-19a-3p), 0.909 (miR-550a-3p), 0.898 (miR-186-5p), 0.898 (miR-532-5p), 0.872 (miR-378a-5p), 0.870 (miR-320a), 0.879 (miR-93-5p), 0.857 (miR-16-5p), 0.853 (miR-215-5p), 0.852 (let-7b-5p), 0.824 (miR-7-5p), 0.838 (miR-29b-3p), and 0.809 (miR-365a-3p) for fracture group vs. control group	Small sample size; no evaluation of the target genes; arbitrary choice of the screened miRNAs

(Continued)

TABLE 2 | Continued

Study	Study design	Biomarker source	Sample handling	Quantification platform	Evaluated miRNA	Normalization strategy	Reported miRNA biomarker	Potential target gene	AUC-Sensitivity (%)-Specificity (%)	Limits
(Chen et al., 2017)	30 PM Chinese women with OP and 30 PM Chinese women without OP (control group) both with hip fracture	Cell-free serum and bone tissues	Blood samples allowed to clot, centrifuged at 1500g, then serum isolated and stored.	Screening: Microarray Validation: TaqMan RT-qPCR	Validation: miR-30, miR- 96, miR-125b, miR-4665-3p, and miR-5914	snRNU6	↑ miR-125b, miR-30 and miR-5914 in serum and bone tissues from OP fracture vs. control group	/	0.699 (miR-5914), 0.757 (miR-30), and 0.898 (miR-125b) for OP fracture vs. controls	Small sample size; no target genes evaluation; no information about the stem-loop arm of miRNA origin
(Yavropoulou et al., 2017)	35 PM women with low bone mass without vertebral fractures, 35 with low bone mass and vertebral fractures, 30 HC	Cell-free serum	Blood samples collected in clot activator tubes, placed at RT for 10-60 min, centrifuged for 10 min at 1900g and 4°C. Serum samples centrifuged again for 10 min at 16000g and 4°C and frozen at -80°C	SYBR Green RT-qPCR	14 miRNAs selected based on the existing literature: miR-21-5p, miR-23a-3p, miR-24-2-5p, miR-26a-5p, miR-29a, miR-33a-5p, miR-124-3p, miR-133a, miR-135b-5p, miR-214-3p, miR-218-5p, miR-335-3p, miR-422, and miR-2861	Panel of SNORD95, SNORD96A, and snRNU6-2	↑ miR-124-3p, miR-2861, and ↓ miR-21-5p, miR-23a-3p, miR-29a-3p in OP vs. controls↓miR-21-5p in OP with vertebral fracture vs. OP without vertebral fracture	SPRY1, BMP3, DKK2, and SMAD7 (miR-21-5p); SATB2 and RUNX2 (miR-23a-3p); SATB2 and CALB1 (miR-24-2-5p); EPHA5, COL10A1, and COL19A1 (miR-26a-5p); DUSP2, COL3A1, COL5A3, and PTHLH (miR-29a); DKK2, WIF1, and OSTF1 (miR-33a-5p); HDAC5, NFATC1, and NFATC2, (miR-124-3p); ACVR1B, FOXO1, SIRT1, and SMAD5 (miR-135b-5p); ATP2A3, CTNNB1, and VDR (miR-214-3p); COL1A1, SFRP2, SOST, and EPHA5 (miR-218-5p); DKK1 and SPARC (miR-335-3p); HDAC5 (miR-2861)(Identified using miRBase, DIANA TOOLS, PicTar, miRDB, TargetScanHuman, miRGator, and microRNA database)	0.66-66-71 (miR-21-5p) for OP with vertebral fracture vs. OP without vertebral fracture	Small sample size; no validation of the identified target genes
(Wang et al., 2018)	45 OP patients, 15 non-OP (control group) both with femoral fracture	Cell-free serum and bone tissues	/	RT-qPCR	miR-7-5p, miR-24-3p, miR-27a-3p, miR-100, miR-125b, miR-128, miR-145-5p, miR-211-5p, miR-144-3p, and miR-122a	snRNU6	↑ miR-24-3p, 27a-3p, miR-100, miR-125b, miR-122a, miR-145, and ↓ miR-144-3p in serum from OP fracture vs. non-OP fracture↑ miR-24-3p, 27a-3p, miR-100, miR-125b, miR-128, miR-122a, and ↓ miR-144-3p in bone tissues form OP fracture vs. non-OP fracture	RANK (identified for miR-144-3p using TargetScan online software and validated by *in vitro* study)	/	Small sample size of the non-OP group; no ROC analysis

(Continued)

TABLE 2 | Continued

Study	Study design	Biomarker source	Sample handling	Quantification platform	Evaluated miRNA	Normalization strategy	Reported miRNA biomarker	Potential target gene	AUC-Sensitivity (%)-Specificity (%)	Limits
(Li et al., 2018)	10 PM Chinese OP women with hip fracture and 10 HC	Cell-free serum	Blood samples allowed to clot then centrifuged at 1500g to obtain serum	TaqMan RT-qPCR	miR-133a	snRNU6	↑miR-133a in OP with fractures vs. HC	c-Fos, NFATc1, and TRAP for miR-133a identified by *in vitro* experiments	/	Small sample size; no ROC analysis

ACVR1B, activin A receptor type 1B; ALPL, alkaline phosphatase; ANKH, ANKH inorganic pyrophosphate transport regulator; AR, androgen receptor; ARPP-19, cAMP-regulated phosphoprotein 19; ATF4, activating transcription factor 4; ATP2A3, sarcoplasmic/endoplasmic reticulum calcium ATPase 3; BMP2K, BMP2 inducible kinase; BMP3, bone morphogenetic protein 3; BMP6, bone morphogenetic protein 6; BMPR1A, bone morphogenetic protein receptor 1A; BMPR2, bone morphogenetic protein receptor type 2; CALB1, calbindin 1; CAMTA1, calmodulin binding transcription activator 1; CNR1, cannabinoid receptor 1; CNR2, cannabinoid receptor 2; COL10A1, collagen type X alpha 1 chain; COL19A1, collagen type XIX alpha 1 chain; COL1A1, collagen type I alpha 1 chain; COL3A1, collagen type III alpha 1 chain; COL5A3, collagen type V alpha 3 chain; CTNNB1, catenin beta 1, CTNNBIP1, catenin-interacting protein 1; DKK1, Dickkopf WNT signaling pathway inhibitor 1; DKK2, Dickkopf WNT signaling pathway inhibitor 2; DNER, delta and notch-like epidermal growth factor-related receptor; DUSP2, dual specificity phosphatase 2; EPHA5, EPH receptor A5; ESR1, estrogen receptor 1; ESRRG, estrogen related receptor gamma; FOXO1, Forkhead box O1, FSHB, follicle stimulating hormone subunit beta; HC, healthy controls; HDAC5, histone deacetylase 5; IGF1, insulin-like growth factor; IGF1R, insulin-like growth factor 1 receptor; IGFBP1, insulin-like growth factor binding protein 1; IL6R, interleukin 6 receptor, JAK2,Janus kinase 2; LEPR, leptin receptor; LRP6, LDL receptor related protein 6; MAPK1, mitogen-activated protein kinase 1; MAPK3, mitogen-activated protein kinase 3; MCL, myeloid cell leukemia; MSCs, mesenchymal stem cells; NFATC1, nuclear factor of activated T cells 1; NFATC2, nuclear factor of activated T cells 2; NR3C1, nuclear receptor subfamily 3 group C member 1; OA, osteoarthritis; OP, osteoporosis; OSTF1, osteoclast stimulating factor 1; OSX, osterix; PDCD4, programmed cell death 4; PDGFD, platelet-derived growth factor D; PM, postmenopausal; PPARGC1A, peroxisome proliferator-activated receptor gamma coactivator 1-alpha; PTGER3, prostaglandin E receptor 3; PTHLH, parathyroid hormone like hormone; RANKL, receptor activator of nuclear factor k B ligand; RARG, retinoic acid receptor gamma; RT, room temperature; RT-qPCR, real-time quantitative polymerase chain reaction; RUNX2, runt-related transcription factor 2; RXRA, retinoid X receptor alpha; SATB2, SATB homeobox 2; SFRP2, secreted frizzled related protein 2; SGK, serine/threonine protein-kinase; SIRT1, sirtuin 1; SMAD5, SMAD family member 5; SMAD7, SMAD family member 7; SOST, sclerostin; SPARC, secreted protein acidic and cysteine rich; SPRY1, protein sprouty homolog 1; SRF, serum response factor; T2DM, Type 2 diabetes mellitus; TFR1, transferrin receptor protein 1; TRAP, triiodothyronine receptor auxiliary protein; TSC22D3, TSC22 domain family member 3; VCAN, versican; VDR, vitamin D receptor; WIF1, WNT inhibitory factor 1;WISP1, WNT1-inducible-signaling pathway protein 1.

miRNAs in Other Types of OP and Related Fracture Risk

Considering senile OP, a study investigated the role of a specific miRNA (miR-125b) in osteoblast differentiation (Chen et al., 2014b). miR-125b was selected due to its crucial involvement in the epigenetic regulation of proliferation/differentiation of cell lineages (Liu et al., 2011). miR-125b expression levels in BM-MSCs was found upregulated in small mixed gender populations of senile Chinese OP patients (n = 4, 3 women and 1 man) compared with subjects with normal BMD (control group, n = 5, 2 women and 3 men). miR-125b upregulation was associated with impaired BM-MSCs proliferation and osteogenic differentiation and, consistent with these observations, the antagonism of miR-125b in non-OP BM-MSCs promoted proliferation, osteoblast differentiation, and mineralization. In these cells, miR-125b also targeted Osterix (OSX), a key transcription factor for osteogenic differentiation (Chen et al., 2014b). Weilner et al. (2016) found that the presence of miR-31 in circulating microvesicles derived from senescent endothelial cells negatively impacted on the osteogenic differentiation capacity of adipose tissue-derived MSCs. Circulating miR-31 levels were higher in the plasma samples from elderly healthy donors than in young healthy controls, as well as in the plasma from OP patients compared with healthy age-matched controls. miR-31 directly inhibits osteoblast formation by targeting Frizzled-3 (FZD3). Also SATB2, Osx, and RUNX2 have been validated as targets of miR-31 (Baglio et al., 2013; Deng et al., 2014; Xie et al., 2014). This miRNA is involved in osteoclastogenesis: its expression has been found strongly upregulated during RANKL-induced osteoclast differentiation and its inhibition by specific antagomirs results in impaired osteoclast differentiation, actin ring formation, and bone resorption (Mizoguchi et al., 2013). These alterations depend upon the overexpression of the miR-31 target gene RhoA, a GTPase involved in the transduction of extracellular signals to the cytoskeleton (Mizoguchi et al., 2013). This study showed, for the first time, that the miRNA content from senescent cells-derived microvesicles might correlate with the impairment of bone formation and that miR-31 can be used as a biomarker for age-associated diseases such as OP (Weilner et al., 2016). Nonetheless, a larger cohort is needed to confirm these data.

Studies have attempted to correlate circulating and tissue-altered miRNAs expression with the risk of bone fracture in senile OP patients. In bone tissue samples from elderly Chinese patients with bone fracture, miRNA quantification by RT-PCR revealed that miR-214 expression correlated positively with age and negatively with bone formation marker levels (osteocalcin and alkaline phosphatases) (Wang et al., 2013c). The major limitations of the study were: small sample size, unclear comparison between aged and control groups, and missing information about the screened miRNAs and data normalization. In murine pre-osteoblast MC3T3-E1 cells, miR-214 negatively affected osteoblast activity and matrix mineralization by targeting activating transcription factor 4 (ATF4); these features were restored by antagomiR-214 and further accentuated by agomiR-214. Furthermore, miR-214 inhibition improved the bone phenotype in OVX and hind limb-unloaded mice, whereas osteoblast activity was limited and bone mass reduced in miR-214 transgenic mice (Wang et al., 2013c). In 2017, the nine serum miRNAs associated with OP found by Seeliger et al. (2014) were validated also in serum, bone specimens, and cultured osteoblasts and osteoclasts from another cohort of OP (n = 14, 7 women and 7 men) and OA patients (n = 14, 7 women and 7 men) with hip fractures (Kelch et al., 2017). The expression levels of miR-100-5p, miR-122-5p, miR-124-3p, miR-125b-5p, and miR-148a-3p, miR-21-5p, miR-23a-3p, miR-24-3p, and miR-93-5p were assayed by RT-qPCR. The results showed that circulating miR-100-5p, miR-122-5p, miR-124-3p, miR-148a-3p, miR-21-5p, miR-23a-3p, miR-24-3p, and miR-93-5p were significantly upregulated in the OP women and men compared with the controls, but miR-93-5p failed to discriminate between OP and non-OP male patients. Furthermore, miR-125b-5p expression was gender-related. In the OP bone samples, miR-100-5p, miR-125b-5p, miR-21-5p, miR-24-3p, and miR-93-5p were significantly upregulated in the OP patients compared with the controls and correlated with BMD. In particular, miR-21-5p expression values discriminated between osteopenia and OP. miR-100-5p, miR-125b-5p, miR-21-5p, miR-23a-3p, miR-24-3p, and miR-93-5p were upregulated in OP osteoblasts, while miR-100-5p, miR-122-5p, miR-124-3p, miR-125b-5p, miR-148a-3p, miR-21-5p, and miR-93-5p were upregulated in OP osteoclasts. Among these miRNAs, miR-122-5p was previously identified as being upregulated in serum samples from OP patients with bone fracture (Panach et al., 2015). The role of the other miRNAs and their potential target genes have been described above. These results identify miRNAs with high potential as biomarkers for OP, as well as targets for OP therapeutic treatment (Kelch et al., 2017). Recent studies have investigated whether single or combined miRNAs discriminate bone fractures in conditions associated with bone fragility. Interestingly, the nineteen serum miRNAs found altered in postmenopausal women by Kocijan et al. (2016), as previously described, were found altered also in serum samples from trauma fractures in idiopathic OP (premenopausal women, n = 10, and men, n = 16) compared to their controls (n = 28, 12 premenopausal women and 16 men) without bone fracture. Also in these cases, ROC analysis revealed that miR-140-5p, miR-152-3p, miR-19a-3p, miR-19b-3p, miR-30e-5p, miR-324-3p, miR-335-5p, and miR-550a-3p had a higher discriminating power between bone fracture and controls (AUC> 0.9) than BMD or bone turnover markers. Mandourah et al. (2018) recruited 139 subjects and divided them into 5 groups: healthy controls, osteopenic subjects with or without bone fractures, and OP patients with or without bone fractures. Fifteen of the 370 miRNAs screened in the pooled sera were differently regulated in the females with OP and the healthy females, and twenty-five were up or downregulated in the OP females compared with the osteopenic females. Following RT-qPCR validation, miR-122-5p and miR-4516 levels differed between the healthy subjects and the osteopenic/OP patients. Moreover, serum miR-122-5p and miR-4516 levels were lower in the OP patients than the healthy controls and osteopenic patients. miR-4516 was also found to be downregulated in the OP patients with bone fracture and associated with BMD. ROC analysis revealed that only miR-4516 had an acceptable diagnostic value for OP: AUC 0.727, 71% sensitivity, and 62% specificity. Furthermore, the diagnostic value of these two miRNAs increased when combined (AUC 0.752). Overall, these findings indicate that miR-122-5p and miR-4516 downregulation in patient samples may be associated with OP progression. However, miR-122-5p has been found upregulated in the sera of OP patients with hip fracture (Panach et al., 2015).

In order to discriminate between type 2 diabetes (T2DM)- and OP-associated bone fracture, serum levels of 375 miRNAs were evaluated using a low-density qPCR array. Forty-eight miRNAs were differentially expressed between T2DM patients with bone fracture and healthy controls, and 23 miRNAs differentially expressed between OP with bone fracture and healthy controls. Eighteen of these showed the same regulation pattern in the T2DM and the OP patients. Considering the top ten ranking miRNAs (i.e., four-miRNA model signatures with AUC values >0.9 for identifying the T2DM or OP fragility fracture groups), the most abundant miRNAs were miR-382-3p, miR-550a-5p, and miR-96-5p for the T2DM group and miR-188-3p, miR-382-3p, miR-942 for the OP group. miR-382-3p was downregulated in both groups with bone fracture compared with the controls; miR-550a-5p and miR-96-5p were significantly upregulated in the T2DM patients with bone fractures, while miR-188-3p and miR-942 were downregulated, although without reaching statistical significance, in OP bone fractures compared with the controls: these last two miRNAs are associated with bone metabolism (Heilmeier et al., 2016). miR-188 is recognized as a main modulator of the BM-MSCs age-associated osteogenesis-to-adipogenesis shift by targeting histone deacetylase 9 (HDAC9) and the RPTOR-independent companion of mTOR complex 2 (RICTOR). In particular, miR-188 suppression induces osteoblast differentiation and bone formation (Li et al., 2015a). By targeting the heparin-binding EGF-like growth factor (HB-EGF), miR-96 is able to promote osteoblast differentiation (Yang et al., 2014). Analyzing the *in vitro* effects of miR-188-3p, miR-382-3p, and miR-550a-5p on cell proliferation, osteogenesis, and adipogenesis, the authors demonstrated that miR-382-3p and miR-550a-5p enhance and inhibit, respectively, osteogenic differentiation and both affect adipogenesis, whereas miR-188-3p does not impair it. Thus, miR-382-3p and miR-550a-5p have been identified as potential circulating biomarkers for T2DM-associated bone disease, and miR-188-3p and miR-382-2p for bone fractures in OP (Heilmeier et al., 2016).

Table 3 presents information about circulating miRNAs associated with other types of OP and related fracture risk.

Conclusions

The growing body of evidence for the fundamental modulatory role exerted by miRNAs in biological functions, along with aberrant expression in disease onset, underline their potential as biomarkers for the onset and progression of disease. Based on current evidence, age-related bone diseases, especially in OP and OP fractures, may be correlated with altered levels of circulating and tissue miRNA. In

TABLE 3 | miRNAs associated with other types of OP and related fracture risk.

Study	Study design	Biomarker source	Sample handling	Quantification platform	Evaluated miRNA	Normalization strategy	Validated miRNA biomarker	Potential target gene	AUC-Sensitivity(%)-Specificity(%)	Limits
(Chen et al., 2014b)	4 Chinese OP patients (3 women and 1 man, age 76-88 years) and 5 Chinese subjects with normal BMD (2 women and 3 men, age 19-44 years)	BM-MCSs	Bone marrow aspirated from iliac crest and used for BM-MCSs isolation	SYBR Green RT-qPCR	miR-125b	snRNU6	↑miR-125b in OP group vs. non-OP group	OSX (Identified using TargetScan and PicTar database, and validated by *in vitro* experiments) and RUNX2 for miR-125b	/	Small sample size; no information about the stem-loop arm of miRNA origin; no ROC analysis
(Weilner et al., 2016)	14 men (mean age ~53 years) with idiopathic osteoporosis and 11 age-matched HC	Cell-free plasma and plasma microvesicles	Filtration and differential centrifugation methodologies for microvescicle purification	TaqMan RT-qPCR	miR-31	snRNU6	↑miR-31 in OP group vs. HC	FZD3 (validated by *in vitro* experiments for miR-31)	/	Small sample size; no information about the stem-loop arm of miRNA origin; study mainly focused on miRNA evaluation by *in vitro* studies; no ROC analysis
(Wang et al., 2013c)	40 Chinese patients with fracture (age 60-90 years) and 9 Chinese HC (control group)	Bone specimens	Femurs collected during surgery	RT-PCR	Not specified	Not specified in this paper	↑miR-214a in older individuals	ATF4 (identified for miR-214a using miRBase and validated by *in vitro-in vivo* experiments)	/	Small sample size of the HC group; confusing information about the comparisons done among groups; evaluated miRNAs and data normalization not explained in this paper; no information about the stem-loop arm of miRNA origin; no ROC analysis
(Kelch et al., 2017)	28 patients with hip fracture: 7 men + 7 women with OP and 7 men + 7 women with AO (control group)	Cell-free serum and bone tissue	Blood collected 2 h post-fracture (OP) or pre-operation (non-OP) into S-Monovette polypropylene tubes, placed for 30 min at RT upright, centrifuged for 10 min at 1900g, serum stored at -80°CFemoral head samples collected during surgery (within 8 h after fracture in OP group). Cylindrical bone samples obtained from middle of each femoral head, cut into small pieces with Luer forceps, rinsed with D-PBS, collected in TRI-Reagent, snap frozen in liquid nitrogen, and mechanically ground. The bone powder collected with TRI-Reagent and stored at -80°C	miScript SYBR Green RT-qPCR	miR-21-5p, miR-23a-3p, miR-24-3p, miR-93-5p, miR-100-5p, miR-122-5p, miR-124-3p, miR-125b-5p, and miR-148a-3p	SNORD96a	↑ miR-21-5p, miR-23a-3p, miR-24-3p, miR-93-5p, miR-100-5p, miR-122-5p, miR-124-3p, and miR-148a-3p in OP serum vs. control↑ miR-21-5p, miR-24-3p, miR-93-5p, miR-100-5p and miR-125b-5p in OP tissues vs. control↑ miR-21-5p, miR-23a-3p, miR-24-3p, miR-93-5p, miR-100-5p, and miR-125b-5p in OP osteoblasts vs. control↑ miR-21-5p, miR-93-5p, miR-100-5p, miR-122-5p, miR-124-3p, miR-125b-5p, and miR-148a-3p in OP osteoclasts vs. control	/	/	no evaluation of the target genes; no ROC analysis

(Continued)

TABLE 3 | Continued

Study	Study design	Biomarker source	Sample handling	Quantification platform	Evaluated miRNA	Normalization strategy	Validated miRNA biomarker	Potential target gene	AUC-Sensitivity(%)-Specificity(%)	Limits
(Kocijan et al., 2016)	Patients with idiopathic (16 men and 10 premenopausal women); HC without low-trauma fracture (16 men and 12 premenopausal women).	Cell-free serum	Fasting blood samples immediately centrifuged and serum stored a -80°C	SYBR Green RT-qPCR	187 miRNAs tested	Global mean	↑ miR-152-3p, miR-335-5p, miR-320a and↓ let-7b-5p, miR-7-5p, miR-16-5p, miR-19a-3p, miR-19b-3p, miR-29b-3p, miR-30e-5p, miR-93-5p, miR-140-5p, miR-215-5p, miR-186-5p, miR-324-3p, miR-365a-3p, miR-378a-5p, miR-532-5p, and miR-550a-3p in fractured groups vs. their control groups	/	0.962 (miR-152-3p), 0.959 (miR-30e-5p), 0.950 (miR-324-3p), 0.947(miR-140-5p), 0.944 (miR-19b-3p), 0.939 (miR-335-5p), 0.929 (miR-19a-3p), 0.909 (miR-550a-3p), 0.898 (miR-186-5p), 0.898 (miR-532-5p), 0.872 (miR-378a-5p), 0.870 (miR-320a), 0.879 (miR-93-5p), 0.857 (miR-16-5p), 0.853 (miR-215-5p), 0.852 (let-7b-5p), 0.824 (miR-7-5p), 0.838 (miR-29b-3p), and 0.809 (miR-365a-3p) for fracture groups vs. control groups	No evaluation of the target genes; arbitrary choice of the screened miRNAs
(Mandourah et al., 2018)	12 (1 male/11 females) non-OP controls, 61 (9 males/52 females) osteopenia without fracture, 15 (2 males/13 females) osteopenia with fracture, 33 (6 males/27 females) OP without fracture, and 18 (2 males/16 females) OP with fracture	Cell-free serum and plasma	Serum/plasma samples obtained by centrifuging at 2500g and RT for 30 min. Supernatants further centrifuged at 14000g and 4°C for 30 min. Samples stored at -80°C	Screening: Human Serum and Plasma miRNA PCR arrays Validation: miScript SYBR Green RT-qPCR	Screening: 370 miRNAs tested Validation: 40 miRNAs tested	SNORD96A and RNU6-6P	↓ miR-122-5p and miR-4516 in OP vs. non-OP and osteopenia patients	BMP2K, FSHB, IGF1R, VDR, SPARC, TSC22D3 and RUNX2 (miR-122-5p and miR-4516); ANKH, ALPL, CNR2, CD44, LRP6, and ESR1 (miR-122-5p); AR and CNR1 (miR-4516) (identified using miRWalk2.0 database but not validated in the study)	0.727-71-62 (miR-4516) and 0.752 (miR-122-5p+miR-4516) for OP	Small sample size; confusing information about the comparisons done among groups; no validation of the identified target genes
(Heilmeier et al., 2016)	80 PM women; two study arms with two groups each:T2DM arm composed of T2DM women with (n = 20) and without (n = 20) fragility fractures since T2DM onsetOP arm composed of healthy non-T2DM PM women with OP fragility fracture (n = 20), and control group of fracture-free PM women (n = 20).	Cell-free serum	Fasting blood placed for 40 min upright and centrifuged for 15 min at 2000g.	SYBR Green Low-density qPCR platform	375 miRNAs tested	Cq values computed using second derivative maximum method provided with LC480 II software.	Most abundant miRNAs among the top 10 four-miRNAs models:↓ miR-382-3p in T2DM and OP with fragility fracture vs. respective controls↑ miR-550a-5p and miR-96-5p in T2DM fragility fracture group vs. controls↓ miR-188-3p and miR-942 in OP fracture group vs. controls	/	10 candidate four-miRNA models displayed AUC values (0.922 -0.965) for identifying fracture status in T2DM.10 candidate four-miRNA models displayed AUC values (0.972 -0.991) for identifying fracture status in OP group.	No evaluation of the target genes; arbitrary choice of the screened miRNAs

ALPL, alkaline phosphatase; ANKH, ANKH inorganic pyrophosphate transport regulator; AR, androgen receptor; ATF4, activating transcription factor 4; BMD, bone mineral density; BM-MCSs, bone marrow mesenchymal stem cells; BMP2K, BMP2 inducible kinase; CNR2, cannabinoid receptor 2; ESR1, estrogen receptor 1; FSHB, follicle stimulating hormone subunit beta;FZD3, frizzled-3; HC, healthy controls; IGF1R, insulin-like growth factor 1 receptor;OA, osteoarthritis; OP, osteoporosis; OSX, osterix; RT-qPCR, real-time quantitative polymerase chain reaction; RUNX2, runt-related transcription factor 2; RUNX2, runt-related transcription factor 2; SPARC, secreted protein acidic and cysteine rich; T2DM, type 2 diabetes mellitus; TSC22D3, TSC22 domain family member 3; VDR, vitamin D receptor; WIF1, WNT inhibitory factor 1; WISP1, WNT1-inducible-signaling pathway protein 1.

addition, the essential regulatory role exerted by miRNAs in bone homeostasis, as revealed by *in vitro* and *in vivo* studies, underscores their huge potential as biomarkers for diagnosis, prognosis, and personalized treatment of age-associated bone-related disease. Unfortunately, clinical studies for identifying circulating miRNAs as markers for bone diseases have employed various different experimental protocols, making it difficult to compare the results obtained from different labs and even from the same lab in some cases. Furthermore, the great majority of the published studies, here reviewed, are featured by limited (and sometimes statistically unjustifiably too limited) sample sizes. For these reasons, more effort must be spent in standardizing the pre-analytical, analytical, and post-analytical stage of miRNAs discovery and validation to obtain valuable biomarkers for clinical practice and to improve the significance by validating, at least the most promising biomarkers, on wide and real life-adherent populations.

AUTHOR CONTRIBUTIONS

MB: Drafting the work, final approval. GB: Conception of the work, critical revision, final approval. GL: Conception of the work, drafting the work, critical revision, final approval.

FUNDING

This study was funded by the Italian Ministry of Health (Ricerca Corrente).

REFERENCES

Andersen, C. L., Jensen, J. L., and Orntoft, T. F. (2004). Normalization of real-time quantitative reverse transcription-PCR data: a model-based variance estimation approach to identify genes suited for normalization, applied to bladder and colon cancer data sets. *Cancer Re.s* 64 (15), 5245–5250. doi: 10.1158/0008-5472.CAN-04-0496

Arroyo, J. D., Chevillet, J. R., Kroh, E. M., Ruf, I. K., Pritchard, C. C., Gibson, D. F., et al. (2011). Argonaute2 complexes carry a population of circulating microRNAs independent of vesicles in human plasma. *Proc. Natl. Acad. Sci. U. S. A.* 108 (12), 5003–5008. doi: 10.1073/pnas.1019055108

Baggish, A. L., Hale, A., Weiner, R. B., Lewis, G. D., Systrom, D., Wang, F., et al. (2011). Dynamic regulation of circulating microRNA during acute exhaustive exercise and sustained aerobic exercise training. *J. Physiol.* 589 (Pt 16), 3983–3994. doi: 10.1113/jphysiol.2011.213363

Baglio, S. R., Devescovi, V., Granchi, D., and Baldini, N. (2013). MicroRNA expression profiling of human bone marrow mesenchymal stem cells during osteogenic differentiation reveals Osterix regulation by miR-31. *Gene* 527 (1), 321–331. doi: 10.1016/j.gene.2013.06.021

Bartel, D. P. (2009). MicroRNAs: target recognition and regulatory functions. *Cell* 136 (2), 215–233. doi: 10.1016/j.cell.2009.01.002

Bayraktar, R., Van Roosbroeck, K., and Calin, G. A. (2017). Cell-to-cell communication: microRNAs as hormones. *Mol. Oncol.* 11 (12), 1673–1686. doi: 10.1002/1878-0261.12144

Bedene, A., Mencej Bedrač, S., Ješe, L., Marc, J., Vrtačnik, P., Preželj, J., et al. (2016). MiR-148a the epigenetic regulator of bone homeostasis is increased in plasma of osteoporotic postmenopausal women. *Wien. Klin. Wochenschr.* 128 (Suppl 7), 519–526. doi: 10.1007/s00508-016-1141-3

Bellavia, D., Costa, V., De Luca, A., Maglio, M., Pagani, S., et al. (2016). Vitamin D level between calcium-phosphorus homeostasis and immune system: new perspective in osteoporosis. *Curr. Osteoporos Rep.* doi: 10.1007/s11914-016-0331-2

Bellavia, D., De Luca, A., Carina, V., Costa, V., Raimondi, L., Salamanna, F., et al. (2019). Deregulated miRNAs in bone health: Epigenetic roles in osteoporosis. *Bone* 122, 52–75. doi: 10.1016/j.bone.2019.02.013

Bernstein, E., Kim, S. Y., Carmell, M. A., Murchison, E. P., Alcorn, H., Li, M. Z., et al. (2003). Dicer is essential for mouse development. *Nat Genet.* 35 (3), 215–217. doi: 10.1038/ng1253

Bloch, S., Wegrzyn, A., Wegrzyn, G., and Nejman-Falenczyk, B. (2017). Small and Smaller-sRNAs and MicroRNAs in the Regulation of Toxin Gene Expression in Prokaryotic Cells: a mini-review. *Toxins. (Basel)* 9 (6). doi: 10.3390/toxins9060181

Boeckel, J. N., Thome, C. E., Leistner, D., Zeiher, A. M., Fichtlscherer, S., and Dimmeler, S. (2013). Heparin selectively affects the quantification of microRNAs in human blood samples. *Clin. Chem.* 59 (7), 1125–1127. doi: 10.1373/clinchem.2012.199505

Bustin, S. A., and Nolan, T. (2004). Pitfalls of quantitative real-time reverse-transcription polymerase chain reaction. *J. Biomol. Tech.* 15 (3), 155–166.

Cao, Z., Moore, B. T., Wang, Y., Peng, X. H., Lappe, J. M., Recker, R. R., et al. (2014). MiR-422a as a potential cellular microRNA biomarker for postmenopausal osteoporosis. *PLoS One* 9 (5), e97098. doi: 10.1371/journal.pone.0097098

Cerutti, H., and Casas-Mollano, J. A. (2006). On the origin and functions of RNA-mediated silencing: from protists to man. *Curr. Genet.* 50 (2), 81–99. doi: 10.1007/s00294-006-0078-x

Chen, C., Cheng, P., Xie, H., Zhou, H. D., Wu, X. P., Liao, E. Y., et al. (2014a). MiR-503 regulates osteoclastogenesis via targeting RANK. *J. Bone Miner. Res.* 29 (2), 338–347. doi: 10.1002/jbmr.2032

Chen, H., Jiang, H., Can, D., Xu, H., Zhang, K., and Guo, S. (2017). Evaluation of MicroRNA 125b as a potential biomarker for postmenopausal osteoporosis. *Trop. J. Pharm. Res.* 16 (3), 641–647. doi: 10.4314/tjpr.v16i3.20

Chen, J., Li, K., Pang, Q., Yang, C., Zhang, H., Wu, F., et al. (2016). Identification of suitable reference gene and biomarkers of serum miRNAs for osteoporosis. *Sci Rep.* 6, 36347. doi: 10.1038/srep36347

Chen, S., Yang, L., Jie, Q., Lin, Y. S., Meng, G. L., Fan, J. Z., et al. (2014b). MicroRNA125b suppresses the proliferation and osteogenic differentiation of human bone marrowderived mesenchymal stem cells. *Mol. Med. Rep.* 9 (5), 1820–1826. doi: 10.3892/mmr.2014.2024

Chen, X., Ba, Y., Ma, L., Cai, X., Yin, Y., Wang, K., et al. (2008). Characterization of microRNAs in serum: a novel class of biomarkers for diagnosis of cancer and other diseases. *Cell Res.* 18 (10), 997–1006. doi: 10.1038/cr.2008.282

Chen, X., Liang, H., Zhang, J., Zen, K., and Zhang, C. Y. (2012). Secreted microRNAs: a new form of intercellular communication. *Trends Cell Biol.* 22 (3), 125–132. doi: 10.1016/j.tcb.2011.12.001

Cheng, H. H., Yi, H. S., Kim, Y., Kroh, E. M., Chien, J. W., Eaton, K. D., et al. (2013a). Plasma processing conditions substantially influence circulating microRNA biomarker levels. *PLoS One* 8 (6), e64795. doi: 10.1371/journal.pone.0064795

Cheng, P., Chen, C., He, H. B., Hu, R., Zhou, H. D., Xie, H., et al. (2013b). miR-148a regulates osteoclastogenesis by targeting V-maf musculoaponeurotic fibrosarcoma oncogene homolog B. *J. Bone Miner. Res.* 28 (5), 1180–1190. doi: 10.1002/jbmr.1845

Dang, Y., Yang, Q., Xue, Z., and Liu, Y. (2011). RNA interference in fungi: pathways, functions, and applications. *Eukaryot Cell* 10 (9), 1148–1155. doi: 10.1128/EC.05109-11

Davis-Dusenbery, B. N., and Hata, A. (2010). Mechanisms of control of microRNA biogenesis. *J. Biochem.* 148 (4), 381–392. doi: 10.1093/jb/mvq096

De-La-Cruz-Montoya, A. H., Ramirez-Salazar, E. G., Martinez-Aguilar, M. M., Gonzalez-de-la-Rosa, P. M., Quiterio, M., Abreu-Goodger, C., et al. (2018). Identification of miR-708-5p in peripheral blood monocytes: Potential marker for postmenopausal osteoporosis in Mexican-Mestizo population. *Exp. Biol. Med. (Maywood)* 243 (13), 1027–1036. doi: 10.1177/1535370218806828

Deng, L., Hu, G., Jin, L., Wang, C., and Niu, H. (2017). Involvement of microRNA-23b in TNF-alpha-reduced BMSC osteogenic differentiation via targeting runx2. *J. Bone Miner. Metab.* 36 (6), 648–660. doi: 10.1007/s00774-017-0886-8

Deng, Y., Bi, X., Zhou, H., You, Z., Wang, Y., Gu, P., et al. (2014). Repair of critical-sized bone defects with anti-miR-31-expressing bone marrow stromal stem cells and poly(glycerol sebacate) scaffolds. *Eur. Cell Mater* 27, 13–24. doi: 10.22203/eCM.v027a02

De-Ugarte, L., Yoskovitz, G., Balcells, S., Guerri-Fernandez, R., Martinez-Diaz, S., Mellibovsky, L., et al. (2015). MiRNA profiling of whole trabecular bone: identification of osteoporosis-related changes in MiRNAs in human hip bones. *BMC Med. Genomics* 8, 75. doi: 10.1186/s12920-015-0149-2

Eguchi, T., Watanabe, K., Hara, E. S., Ono, M., Kuboki, T., and Calderwood, S. K. (2013). OstemiR: a novel panel of microRNA biomarkers in osteoblastic and osteocytic differentiation from mesencymal stem cells. *PLoS One* 8 (3), e58796. doi: 10.1371/journal.pone.0058796

El-Hefnawy, T., Raja, S., Kelly, L., Bigbee, W. L., Kirkwood, J. M., Luketich, J. D., et al. (2004). Characterization of amplifiable, circulating RNA in plasma and its potential as a tool for cancer diagnostics. *Clin. Chem.* 50 (3), 564–573. doi: 10.1373/clinchem.2003.028506

Faraldi, M., Gomarasca, M., Banfi, G., and Lombardi, G. (2018). Free Circulating miRNAs measurement in clinical settings: the still unsolved issue of the normalization. *Adv. Clin. Chem.* 87, 113–139. doi: 10.1016/bs.acc.2018.07.003

Faraldi, M., Gomarasca, M., Sansoni, V., Perego, S., Banfi, G., and Lombardi, G. (2019). Normalization strategies differently affect circulating miRNA profile associated with the training status. *Sci Rep.* 9 (1), 1584. doi: 10.1038/s41598-019-38505-x

Franceschetti, T., Kessler, C. B., Lee, S. K., and Delany, A. M. (2013). miR-29 promotes murine osteoclastogenesis by regulating osteoclast commitment and migration. *J. Biol. Chem.* 288 (46), 33347–33360. doi: 10.1074/jbc.M113.484568

Fujita, S., Ito, T., Mizutani, T., Minoguchi, S., Yamamichi, N., Sakurai, K., et al. (2008). miR-21 Gene expression triggered by AP-1 is sustained through a double-negative feedback mechanism. *J. Mol. Biol.* 378 (3), 492–504. doi: 10.1016/j.jmb.2008.03.015

Garcia Palacios, V., Robinson, L. J., Borysenko, C. W., Lehmann, T., Kalla, S. E., and Blair, H. C. (2005). Negative regulation of RANKL-induced osteoclastic differentiation in RAW264.7 Cells by estrogen and phytoestrogens. *J. Biol. Chem.* 280 (14), 13720–13727. doi: 10.1074/jbc.M410995200

Garcia, M. E., Blanco, J. L., Caballero, J., and Gargallo-Viola, D. (2002). Anticoagulants interfere with PCR used to diagnose invasive aspergillosis. *J. Clin. Microbiol.* 40 (4), 1567–1568. doi: 10.1128/JCM.40.4.1567-1568.2002

Garmilla-Ezquerra, P., Sanudo, C., Delgado-Calle, J., Perez-Nunez, M. I., Sumillera, M., and Riancho, J. A. (2015). Analysis of the bone microRNome in osteoporotic fractures. *Calcif. Tissue Int.* 96 (1), 30–37. doi: 10.1007/s00223-014-9935-7

Griffiths-Jones, S., Grocock, R. J., van Dongen, S., Bateman, A., and Enright, A. J. (2006). miRBase: microRNA sequences, targets and gene nomenclature. *Nucleic Acids Res.* 34 (Database issue), D140–144. doi: 10.1093/nar/gkj112 (Database issue).

Grundhoff, A., and Sullivan, C. S. (2011). Virus-encoded microRNAs. *Virology* 411 (2), 325–343. doi: 10.1016/j.virol.2011.01.002

Ha, M., and Kim, V. N. (2014). Regulation of microRNA biogenesis. *Nat. Rev. Mol. Cell Biol.* 15 (8), 509–524. doi: 10.1038/nrm3838

Hackl, M., Heilmeier, U., Weilner, S., and Grillari, J. (2016). Circulating microRNAs as novel biomarkers for bone diseases - complex signatures for multifactorial diseases? *Mol. Cell Endocrinol.* 432, 83–95. doi: 10.1016/j.mce.2015.10.015

Hadjiargyrou, M., and Komatsu, D. E. (2019). The therapeutic potential of MicroRNAs as orthobiologics for skeletal fractures. *J. Bone Miner. Res.* 34 (5), 797–809. doi: 10.1002/jbmr.3708

Hajian-Tilaki, K. (2013). Receiver operating characteristic (ROC) curve analysis for medical diagnostic test evaluation. *Caspian J. Int. Med.* 4 (2), 627–635.

Hammond, S. M. (2015). An overview of microRNAs. *Adv. Drug Delivery Rev.* 87, 3–14. doi: 10.1016/j.addr.2015.05.001

Hassan, M. Q., Gordon, J. A., Beloti, M. M., Croce, C. M., van Wijnen, A. J., Stein, J. L., et al. (2010). A network connecting Runx2, SATB2, and the miR-23a~27a~24-2 cluster regulates the osteoblast differentiation program. *Proc. Natl. Acad. Sci. U. S. A.* 107 (46), 19879–19884. doi: 10.1073/pnas.1007698107

Heilmeier, U., Hackl, M., Skalicky, S., Weilner, S., Schroeder, F., Vierlinger, K., et al. (2016). Serum miRNA signatures are indicative of skeletal fractures in postmenopausal women with and without type 2 diabetes and influence osteogenic and adipogenic differentiation of adipose tissue-derived mesenchymal stem cells in vitro. *J. Bone Miner. Res.* 31 (12), 2173–2192. doi: 10.1002/jbmr.2897

Ho, A. S., Huang, X., Cao, H., Christman-Skieller, C., Bennewith, K., Le, Q. T., et al. (2010). Circulating miR-210 as a novel hypoxia marker in pancreatic cancer. *Transl. Oncol.* 3 (2), 109–113. doi: 10.1593/tlo.09256

Hu, R., Liu, W., Li, H., Yang, L., Chen, C., Xia, Z. Y., et al. (2011). A Runx2/miR-3960/miR-2861 regulatory feedback loop during mouse osteoblast differentiation. *J. Biol. Chem.* 286 (14), 12328–12339. doi: 10.1074/jbc.M110.176099

Hu, Z., Dong, J., Wang, L. E., Ma, H., Liu, J., Zhao, Y., et al. (2012). Serum microRNA profiling and breast cancer risk: the use of miR-484/191 as endogenous controls. *Carcinogenesis* 33 (4), 828–834. doi: 10.1093/carcin/bgs030

Hwang, S., Park, S. K., Lee, H. Y., Kim, S. W., Lee, J. S., Choi, E. K., et al. (2014). miR-140-5p suppresses BMP2-mediated osteogenesis in undifferentiated human mesenchymal stem cells. *FEBS Lett.* 588 (17), 2957–2963. doi: 10.1016/j.febslet.2014.05.048

Ishimoto, T., Sugihara, H., Watanabe, M., Sawayama, H., Iwatsuki, M., Baba, Y., et al. (2014). Macrophage-derived reactive oxygen species suppress miR-328 targeting CD44 in cancer cells and promote redox adaptation. *Carcinogenesis* 35 (5), 1003–1011. doi: 10.1093/carcin/bgt402

Jarry, J., Schadendorf, D., Greenwood, C., Spatz, A., and van Kempen, L. C. (2014). The validity of circulating microRNAs in oncology: five years of challenges and contradictions. *Mol. Oncol.* 8 (4), 819–829. doi: 10.1016/j.molonc.2014.02.009

Jeong, B. C., Kang, I. H., Hwang, Y. C., Kim, S. H., and Koh, J. T. (2014). MicroRNA-194 reciprocally stimulates osteogenesis and inhibits adipogenesis via regulating COUP-TFII expression. *Cell Death Dis.* 5, e1532. doi: 10.1038/cddis.2014.485

Jimenez-Ortega, R. F., Ramirez-Salazar, E. G., Parra-Torres, A. Y., Munoz-Montero, S. A., Rangel-Escareno, C., Salido-Guadarrama, I., et al. (2017). Identification of microRNAs in human circulating monocytes of postmenopausal osteoporotic Mexican-Mestizo women: A pilot study. *Exp. Ther. Med.* 14 (6), 5464–5472. doi: 10.3892/etm.2017.5260

Kagiya, T., and Nakamura, S. (2013). Expression profiling of microRNAs in RAW264.7 cells treated with a combination of tumor necrosis factor alpha and RANKL during osteoclast differentiation. *J. Periodontal Res.* 48 (3), 373–385. doi: 10.1111/jre.12017

Kavsak, P. A., and Hammett-Stabler, C. A. (2014). Clinical biochemistry year in review - the clinical "good", the analytical "bad", and the "ugly" laboratory practices. *Clin. Biochem.* 47 (18), 255–256. doi: 10.1016/j.clinbiochem.2014.11.015

Kelch, S., Balmayor, E. R., Seeliger, C., Vester, H., Kirschke, J. S., and van Griensven, M. (2017). miRNAs in bone tissue correlate to bone mineral density and circulating miRNAs are gender independent in osteoporotic patients. *Sci Rep.* 7 (1), 15861. doi: 10.1038/s41598-017-16113-x

Kim, D. J., Linnstaedt, S., Palma, J., Park, J. C., Ntrivalas, E., Kwak-Kim, J. Y., et al. (2012). Plasma components affect accuracy of circulating cancer-related microRNA quantitation. *J. Mol. Diagn.* 14 (1), 71–80. doi: 10.1016/j.jmoldx.2011.09.002

Kirschner, M. B., Edelman, J. J., Kao, S. C., Vallely, M. P., van Zandwijk, N., and Reid, G. (2013). The impact of hemolysis on cell-free microRNA biomarkers. *Front. Genet.* 4, 94. doi: 10.3389/fgene.2013.00094

Kirschner, M. B., Kao, S. C., Edelman, J. J., Armstrong, N. J., Vallely, M. P., van Zandwijk, N., et al. (2011). Haemolysis during sample preparation alters microRNA content of plasma. *PLoS One* 6 (9), e24145. doi: 10.1371/journal.pone.0024145

Kocijan, R., Muschitz, C., Geiger, E., Skalicky, S., Baierl, A., Dormann, R., et al. (2016). Circulating microRNA Signatures in patients with idiopathic and postmenopausal osteoporosis and fragility fractures. *J. Clin. Endocrinol. Metab.* 101 (11), 4125–4134. doi: 10.1210/jc.2016-2365

Kroh, E. M., Parkin, R. K., Mitchell, P. S., and Tewari, M. (2010). Analysis of circulating microRNA biomarkers in plasma and serum using quantitative reverse transcription-PCR (qRT-PCR). *Methods* 50 (4), 298–301. doi: 10.1016/j.ymeth.2010.01.032

Lagos-Quintana, M., Rauhut, R., Lendeckel, W., and Tuschl, T. (2001). Identification of novel genes coding for small expressed RNAs. *Science* 294 (5543), 853–858. doi: 10.1126/science.1064921

Lee, R. C., Feinbaum, R. L., and Ambros, V. (1993). The C. elegans heterochronic gene lin-4 encodes small RNAs with antisense complementarity to lin-14. *Cell* 75 (5), 843–854. doi: 10.1016/0092-8674(93)90529-Y

Lee, Y., Jeon, K., Lee, J. T., Kim, S., and Kim, V. N. (2002). MicroRNA maturation: stepwise processing and subcellular localization. *EMBO J.* 21 (17), 4663–4670. doi: 10.1093/emboj/cdf476

Lee, Y., Kim, H. J., Park, C. K., Kim, Y. G., Lee, H. J., Kim, J. Y., et al. (2013). MicroRNA-124 regulates osteoclast differentiation. *Bone* 56 (2), 383–389. doi: 10.1016/j.bone.2013.07.007

Li, C. J., Cheng, P., Liang, M. K., Chen, Y. S., Lu, Q., Wang, J. Y., et al. (2015a). MicroRNA-188 regulates age-related switch between osteoblast and adipocyte differentiation. *J. Clin. Invest.* 125 (4), 1509–1522. doi: 10.1172/JCI77716

Li, H., Wang, Z., Fu, Q., and Zhang, J. (2014). Plasma miRNA levels correlate with sensitivity to bone mineral density in postmenopausal osteoporosis patients. *Biomarkers* 19 (7), 553–556. doi: 10.3109/1354750X.2014.935957

Li, J., He, X., Wei, W., and Zhou, X. (2015b). MicroRNA-194 promotes osteoblast differentiation via downregulating STAT1. *Biochem. Biophys. Res. Commun.* 460 (2), 482–488. doi: 10.1016/j.bbrc.2015.03.059

Li, L., Zhu, D., Huang, L., Zhang, J., Bian, Z., Chen, X., et al. (2012). Argonaute 2 complexes selectively protect the circulating microRNAs in cell-secreted microvesicles. *PLoS One* 7 (10), e46957. doi: 10.1371/journal.pone.0046957

Li, Z., Hassan, M. Q., Jafferji, M., Aqeilan, R. I., Garzon, R., Croce, C. M., et al. (2009). Biological functions of miR-29b contribute to positive regulation of osteoblast differentiation. *J. Biol. Chem.* 284 (23), 15676–15684. doi: 10.1074/jbc.M809787200

Li, Z., Hassan, M. Q., Volinia, S., van Wijnen, A. J., Stein, J. L., Croce, C. M., et al. (2008). A microRNA signature for a BMP2-induced osteoblast lineage commitment program. *Proc. Natl. Acad. Sci. U. S. A.* 105 (37), 13906–13911. doi: 10.1073/pnas.0804438105

Li, Z., Zhang, W., and Huang, Y. (2018). MiRNA-133a is involved in the regulation of postmenopausal osteoporosis through promoting osteoclast differentiation. *Acta Biochim. Biophys. Sin. (Shanghai)* 50 (3), 273–280. doi: 10.1093/abbs/gmy006

Lima-Oliveira, G., Guidi, G. C., Salvagno, G. L., Brocco, G., Danese, E., and Lippi, G. (2016). Estimation of the imprecision on clinical chemistry testing due to fist clenching and maintenance during venipuncture. *Clin. Biochem.* 49 (18), 1364–1367. doi: 10.1016/j.clinbiochem.2016.07.007

Lima-Oliveira, G., Lippi, G., Salvagno, G. L., Montagnana, M., Picheth, G., and Guidi, G. C. (2013). The effective reduction of tourniquet application time after minor modification of the CLSI H03-A6 blood collection procedure. *Biochem. Med. (Zagreb)* 23 (3), 308–315. doi: 10.11613/BM.2013.037

Lin, Q., Gao, Z., Alarcon, R. M., Ye, J., and Yun, Z. (2009). A role of miR-27 in the regulation of adipogenesis. *FEBS J.* 276 (8), 2348–2358. doi: 10.1111/j.1742-4658.2009.06967.x

Ling, S., Zhong, G., Sun, W., Liang, F., Wu, F., et al. (2017). Circulating microRNAs correlated with bone loss induced by 45 days of bed rest. *Front. Physiol.* 8, 69. doi: 10.3389/fphys.2017.00069

Liu, H., Hao, W., Wang, X., and Su, H. (2016). miR-23b targets Smad 3 and ameliorates the LPS-inhibited osteogenic differentiation in preosteoblast MC3T3-E1 cells. *J. Toxicol. Sci.* 41 (2), 185–193. doi: 10.2131/jts.41.185

Liu, J., Gao, J., Du, Y., Li, Z., Ren, Y., Gu, J., et al. (2012). Combination of plasma microRNAs with serum CA19-9 for early detection of pancreatic cancer. *Int. J. Cancer* 131 (3), 683–691. doi: 10.1002/ijc.26422

Liu, L. H., Li, H., Li, J. P., Zhong, H., Zhang, H. C., Chen, J., et al. (2011). miR-125b suppresses the proliferation and migration of osteosarcoma cells through down-regulation of STAT3. *Biochem. Biophys. Res. Commun.* 416 (1-2), 31–38. doi: 10.1016/j.bbrc.2011.10.117

Livesey, J. H., Ellis, M. J., and Evans, M. J. (2008). Pre-analytical requirements. *Clin. Biochem. Rev.* 29 Suppl 1, S11–S15.

Lombardi, G. (2019). Exercise-dependent modulation of bone metabolism and bone endocrine function: new findings and therapeutic perspectives. *J. Sci. Sport. Exercise* 1 (1), 20–28. doi: 10.1007/s42978-019-0010-y

Lombardi, G., Lanteri, P., Colombini, A., and Banfi, G. (2012). Blood biochemical markers of bone turnover: pre-analytical and technical aspects of sample collection and handling. *Clin. Chem. Lab. Med.* 50 (5), 771–789. doi: 10.1515/cclm-2011-0614

Lombardi, G., Perego, S., Sansoni, V., and Banfi, G. (2016a). Circulating miRNA as fine regulators of the physiological responses to physical activity: Pre-analytical warnings for a novel class of biomarkers. *Clin. Biochem.* 49 (18), 1331–1339. doi: 10.1016/j.clinbiochem.2016.09.017

Lombardi, G., Sanchis-Gomar, F., Perego, S., Sansoni, V., and Banfi, G. (2016b). Implications of exercise-induced adipo-myokines in bone metabolism. *Endocrine* 54 (2), 284–305. doi: 10.1007/s12020-015-0834-0

Ludwig, N., Leidinger, P., Becker, K., Backes, C., Fehlmann, T., Pallasch, C., et al. (2016). Distribution of miRNA expression across human tissues. *Nucleic Acids Res.* 44 (8), 3865–3877. doi: 10.1093/nar/gkw116

Lujambio, A., and Esteller, M. (2009). How epigenetics can explain human metastasis: a new role for microRNAs. *Cell Cycle* 8 (3), 377–382. doi: 10.4161/cc.8.3.7526

Lujambio, A., Calin, G. A., Villanueva, A., Ropero, S., Sanchez-Cespedes, M., Blanco, D., et al. (2008). A microRNA DNA methylation signature for human cancer metastasis. *Proc. Natl. Acad. Sci. U. S. A.* 105 (36), 13556–13561. doi: 10.1073/pnas.0803055105

Mandourah, A. Y., Ranganath, L., Barraclough, R., Vinjamuri, S., Hof, R. V., Hamill, S., et al. (2018). Circulating microRNAs as potential diagnostic biomarkers for osteoporosis. *Sci Rep.* 8 (1), 8421. doi: 10.1038/s41598-018-26525-y

Materozzi, M., Merlotti, D., Gennari, L., and Bianciardi, S. (2018). The potential role of mirnas as new biomarkers for osteoporosis. *Int. J. Endocrinol.* 2018, 2342860. doi: 10.1155/2018/2342860

Meng, J., Zhang, D., Pan, N., Sun, N., Wang, Q., Fan, J., et al. (2015). Identification of miR-194-5p as a potential biomarker for postmenopausal osteoporosis. *PeerJ* 3, e971. doi: 10.7717/peerj.971

Mestdagh, P., Hartmann, N., Baeriswyl, L., Andreasen, D., Bernard, N., Chen, C., et al. (2014). Evaluation of quantitative miRNA expression platforms in the microRNA quality control (miRQC) study. *Nat. Methods* 11 (8), 809–815. doi: 10.1038/nmeth.3014

Mestdagh, P., Van Vlierberghe, P., De Weer, A., Muth, D., Westermann, F., Speleman, F., et al. (2009). A novel and universal method for microRNA RT-qPCR data normalization. *Genome Biol.* 10 (6), R64. doi: 10.1186/gb-2009-10-6-r64

Mitchell, P. S., Parkin, R. K., Kroh, E. M., Fritz, B. R., Wyman, S. K., Pogosova-Agadjanyan, E. L., et al. (2008). Circulating microRNAs as stable blood-based markers for cancer detection. *Proc. Natl. Acad. Sci. U. S. A.* 105 (30), 10513–10518. doi: 10.1073/pnas.0804549105

Mizoguchi, F., Murakami, Y., Saito, T., Miyasaka, N., and Kohsaka, H. (2013). miR-31 controls osteoclast formation and bone resorption by targeting RhoA. *Arthritis Res. Ther.* 15 (5), R102. doi: 10.1186/ar4282

Mizuno, Y., Yagi, K., Tokuzawa, Y., Kanesaki-Yatsuka, Y., Suda, T., Katagiri, T., et al. (2008). miR-125b inhibits osteoblastic differentiation by down-regulation of cell proliferation. *Biochem. Biophys. Res. Commun.* 368 (2), 267–272. doi: 10.1016/j.bbrc.2008.01.073

Morrow, D. A., and de Lemos, J. A. (2007). Benchmarks for the assessment of novel cardiovascular biomarkers. *Circulation* 115 (8), 949–952. doi: 10.1161/CIRCULATIONAHA.106.683110

Murchison, E. P., Partridge, J. F., Tam, O. H., Cheloufi, S., and Hannon, G. J. (2005). Characterization of Dicer-deficient murine embryonic stem cells. *Proc. Natl. Acad. Sci. U. S. A.* 102 (34), 12135–12140. doi: 10.1073/pnas.0505479102

Neal, C. S., Michael, M. Z., Pimlott, L. K., Yong, T. Y., Li, J. Y., and Gleadle, J. M. (2011). Circulating microRNA expression is reduced in chronic kidney disease. *Nephrol. Dial. Transplant* 26 (11), 3794–3802. doi: 10.1093/ndt/gfr485

Nelson, P. T., Wang, W. X., Wilfred, B. R., and Tang, G. (2008). Technical variables in high-throughput miRNA expression profiling: much work remains to be done. *Biochim. Biophys. Acta.* 1779 (11), 758–765. doi: 10.1016/j.bbagrm.2008.03.012

NIH Consensus Development Panel on Osteoporosis Prevention, Diagnosis, and Therapy. (2001). Osteoporosis prevention, diagnosis, and therapy. *JAMA* 285 (6), 785–795. doi: 10.1001/jama.285.6785

Palmieri, A., Pezzetti, F., Brunelli, G., Martinelli, M., Lo Muzio, L., Scarano, A., et al. (2008). Peptide-15 changes miRNA expression in osteoblast-like cells. *Implant Dent.* 17 (1), 100–108. doi: 10.1097/ID.0b013e318166d182

Pan, W., Wang, H., Jianwei, R., and Ye, Z. (2014). MicroRNA-27a promotes proliferation, migration and invasion by targeting MAP2K4 in human osteosarcoma cells. *Cell Physiol. Biochem.* 33 (2), 402–412. doi: 10.1159/000356679

Panach, L., Mifsut, D., Tarin, J. J., Cano, A., and Garcia-Perez, M. A. (2015). Serum circulating MicroRNAs as biomarkers of osteoporotic fracture. *Calcif. Tissue Int.* 97 (5), 495–505. doi: 10.1007/s00223-015-0036-z

Ramirez-Salazar, E. G., Carrillo-Patino, S., Hidalgo-Bravo, A., Rivera-Paredez, B., Quiterio, M., Ramirez-Palacios, P., et al. (2018). Serum miRNAs miR-140-3p and miR-23b-3p as potential biomarkers for osteoporosis and osteoporotic fracture in postmenopausal Mexican-Mestizo women. *Gene* 679, 19–27. doi: 10.1016/j.gene.2018.08.074

Reinhart, B. J., Weinstein, E. G., Rhoades, M. W., Bartel, B., and Bartel, D. P. (2002). MicroRNAs in plants. *Genes Dev.* 16 (13), 1616–1626. doi: 10.1101/gad.1004402

Rossi, M., Pitari, M. R., Amodio, N., Di Martino, M. T., Conforti, F., Leone, E., et al. (2013). miR-29b negatively regulates human osteoclastic cell differentiation and function: implications for the treatment of multiple myeloma-related bone disease. *J. Cell Physiol.* 228 (7), 1506–1515. doi: 10.1002/jcp.24306

Saito, E., Suzuki, D., Kurotaki, D., Mochizuki, A., Manome, Y., Suzawa, T., et al. (2017). Down-regulation of Irf8 by Lyz2-cre/loxP accelerates osteoclast differentiation in vitro. *Cytotechnology* 69 (3), 443–450. doi: 10.1007/s10616-016-0013-z

Saito, Y., Liang, G., Egger, G., Friedman, J. M., Chuang, J. C., Coetzee, G. A., et al. (2006). Specific activation of microRNA-127 with downregulation of the proto-oncogene BCL6 by chromatin-modifying drugs in human cancer cells. *Cancer Cell* 9 (6), 435–443. doi: 10.1016/j.ccr.2006.04.020

Sansoni, V., Perego, S., Vernillo, G., Barbuti, A., Merati, G., La Torre, A., et al. (2018). Effects of repeated sprints training on fracture risk-associated miRNA. *Oncotarget* 9 (26), 18029–18040. doi: 10.18632/oncotarget.24707

Scott, G. K., Mattie, M. D., Berger, C. E., Benz, S. C., and Benz, C. C. (2006). Rapid alteration of microRNA levels by histone deacetylase inhibition. *Cancer Re.s* 66 (3), 1277–1281. doi: 10.1158/0008-5472.CAN-05-3632

Seeliger, C., Karpinski, K., Haug, A. T., Vester, H., Schmitt, A., Bauer, J. S., et al. (2014). Five freely circulating miRNAs and bone tissue miRNAs are associated with osteoporotic fractures. *J. Bone Miner. Res.* 29 (8), 1718–1728. doi: 10.1002/jbmr.2175

Shende, V. R., Goldrick, M. M., Ramani, S., and Earnest, D. J. (2011). Expression and rhythmic modulation of circulating microRNAs targeting the clock gene Bmal1 in mice. *PLoS One* 6 (7), e22586. doi: 10.1371/journal.pone.0022586

Sourvinou, I. S., Markou, A., and Lianidou, E. S. (2013). Quantification of circulating miRNAs in plasma: effect of preanalytical and analytical parameters on their isolation and stability. *J. Mol. Diagn.* 15 (6), 827–834. doi: 10.1016/j.jmoldx.2013.07.005

Sugatani, T., and Hruska, K. A. (2013). Down-regulation of miR-21 biogenesis by estrogen action contributes to osteoclastic apoptosis. *J. Cell Biochem.* 114 (6), 1217–1222. doi: 10.1002/jcb.24471

Sugatani, T., Vacher, J., and Hruska, K. A. (2011). A microRNA expression signature of osteoclastogenesis. *Blood* 117 (13), 3648–3657. doi: 10.1182/blood-2010-10-311415

Suh, M. R., Lee, Y., Kim, J. Y., Kim, S. K., Moon, S. H., Lee, J. Y., et al. (2004). Human embryonic stem cells express a unique set of microRNAs. *Dev. Biol.* 270 (2), 488–498. doi: 10.1016/j.ydbio.2004.02.019

Sun, J. Y., Huang, Y., Li, J. P., Zhang, X., Wang, L., Meng, Y. L., et al. (2012). MicroRNA-320a suppresses human colon cancer cell proliferation by directly targeting beta-catenin. *Biochem. Biophys. Res. Commun.* 420 (4), 787–792. doi: 10.1016/j.bbrc.2012.03.075

Sun, Z., Cao, X., Hu, Z., Zhang, L., Wang, H., Zhou, H., et al. (2015). MiR-103 inhibits osteoblast proliferation mainly through suppressing Cav1.2 expression in simulated microgravity. *Bone* 76, 121–128. doi: 10.1016/j.bone.2015.04.006

Takahashi, K., Yokota, S., Tatsumi, N., Fukami, T., Yokoi, T., and Nakajima, M. (2013). Cigarette smoking substantially alters plasma microRNA profiles in healthy subjects. *Toxicol. Appl. Pharmaco.l* 272 (1), 154–160. doi: 10.1016/j.taap.2013.05.018

Trompeter, H. I., Dreesen, J., Hermann, E., Iwaniuk, K. M., Hafner, M., Renwick, N., et al. (2013). MicroRNAs miR-26a, miR-26b, and miR-29b accelerate osteogenic differentiation of unrestricted somatic stem cells from human cord blood. *BMC Genomics* 14, 111. doi: 10.1186/1471-2164-14-111

Valinezhad Orang, A., Safaralizadeh, R., and Kazemzadeh-Bavili, M. (2014). Mechanisms of miRNA-mediated gene regulation from common downregulation to mRNA-specific upregulation. *Int. J. Genomics.* 2014, 970607. doi: 10.1155/2014/970607

Van Meurs, J. B., Boer, C. G., Lopez-Delgado, L., and Riancho, J. A. (2019). Role of epigenomics in bone and cartilage disease. *J. Bone Miner. Res.* 34 (2), 215–230. doi: 10.1002/jbmr.3662

Vandesompele, J., De Preter, K., Pattyn, F., Poppe, B., Van Roy, N., De Paepe, A., et al. (2002). Accurate normalization of real-time quantitative RT-PCR data by geometric averaging of multiple internal control genes. *Genome Biol.* 3 (7), 0034. doi: 10.1186/gb-2002-3-7-research0034

Vasikaran, S. D., and Chubb, S. A. (2016). The use of biochemical markers of bone turnover in the clinical management of primary and secondary osteoporosis. *Endocrine* 52 (2), 222–225. doi: 10.1007/s12020-016-0900-2

Wang, C., He, H., Wang, L., Jiang, Y., and Xu, Y. (2018). Reduced miR-144-3p expression in serum and bone mediates osteoporosis pathogenesis by targeting RANK. *Biochem. Cell Biol.* 96 (5), 627–635. doi: 10.1139/bcb-2017-0243

Wang, F. S., Chuang, P. C., Lin, C. L., Chen, M. W., Ke, H. J., Chang, Y. H., et al. (2013a). MicroRNA-29a protects against glucocorticoid-induced bone loss and fragility in rats by orchestrating bone acquisition and resorption. *Arthritis Rheum.* 65 (6), 1530–1540. doi: 10.1002/art.37948

Wang, J., Guan, X., Guo, F., Zhou, J., Chang, A., Sun, B., et al. (2013b). miR-30e reciprocally regulates the differentiation of adipocytes and osteoblasts by directly targeting low-density lipoprotein receptor-related protein 6. *Cell Death Dis.* 4, e845. doi: 10.1038/cddis.2013.356

Wang, P., Yang, D., Zhang, H., Wei, X., Ma, T., Cheng, Z., et al. (2015). Early detection of lung cancer in serum by a panel of MicroRNA biomarkers. *Clin. Lung Cancer* 16 (4), 313–319 e311. doi: 10.1016/j.cllc.2014.12.006

Wang, T., and Xu, Z. (2010). miR-27 promotes osteoblast differentiation by modulating Wnt signaling. *Biochem. Biophys. Res. Commun.* 402 (2), 186–189. doi: 10.1016/j.bbrc.2010.08.031

Wang, X., Guo, B., Li, Q., Peng, J., Yang, Z., Wang, A., et al. (2013c). miR-214 targets ATF4 to inhibit bone formation. *Nat. Med.* 19 (1), 93–100. doi: 10.1038/nm.3026

Wang, Y., Li, L., Moore, B. T., Peng, X. H., Fang, X., Lappe, J. M., et al. (2012). MiR-133a in human circulating monocytes: a potential biomarker associated with postmenopausal osteoporosis. *PLoS One* 7 (4), e34641. doi: 10.1371/journal.pone.0034641

Wang, Y., Luo, J., Zhang, H., and Lu, J. (2016). microRNAs in the same clusters evolve to coordinately regulate functionally related genes. *Mol. Biol. Evol.* 33 (9), 2232–2247. doi: 10.1093/molbev/msw089

Wang, Y., Medvid, R., Melton, C., Jaenisch, R., and Blelloch, R. (2007). DGCR8 is essential for microRNA biogenesis and silencing of embryonic stem cell self-renewal. *Nat Genet.* 39 (3), 380–385. doi: 10.1038/ng1969

Weber, J. A., Baxter, D. H., Zhang, S., Huang, D. Y., Huang, K. H., Lee, M. J., et al. (2010). The microRNA spectrum in 12 body fluids. *Clin. Chem.* 56 (11), 1733–1741. doi: 10.1373/clinchem.2010.147405

Wei, J., Li, H., Wang, S., Li, T., Fan, J., Liang, X., et al. (2014). let-7 enhances osteogenesis and bone formation while repressing adipogenesis of human stromal/mesenchymal stem cells by regulating HMGA2. *Stem Cells Dev.* 23 (13), 1452–1463. doi: 10.1089/scd.2013.0600

Weilner, S., Schraml, E., Wieser, M., Messner, P., Schneider, K., Wassermann, K., et al. (2016). Secreted microvesicular miR-31 inhibits osteogenic differentiation of mesenchymal stem cells. *Aging Cell* 15 (4), 744–754. doi: 10.1111/acel.12484

Weilner, S., Skalicky, S., Salzer, B., Keider, V., Wagner, M., Hildner, F., et al. (2015). Differentially circulating miRNAs after recent osteoporotic fractures can influence osteogenic differentiation. *Bone* 79, 43–51. doi: 10.1016/j.bone.2015.05.027

Willeit, P., Zampetaki, A., Dudek, K., Kaudewitz, D., King, A., Kirkby, N. S., et al. (2013). Circulating microRNAs as novel biomarkers for platelet activation. *Circuit Res.* 112 (4), 595–600. doi: 10.1161/CIRCRESAHA.111.300539

Witwer, K. W. (2012). XenomiRs and miRNA homeostasis in health and disease: evidence that diet and dietary miRNAs directly and indirectly influence circulating miRNA profiles. *RNA Biol.* 9 (9), 1147–1154. doi: 10.4161/rna.21619

Xie, Q., Wang, Z., Bi, X., Zhou, H., Wang, Y., Gu, P., et al. (2014). Effects of miR-31 on the osteogenesis of human mesenchymal stem cells. *Biochem. Biophys. Res. Commun.* 446 (1), 98–104. doi: 10.1016/j.bbrc.2014.02.058

Xu, J., Lombardi, G., Jiao, W., and Banfi, G. (2016). Effects of exercise on bone status in female subjects, from young girls to postmenopausal women: an overview of systematic reviews and meta-analyses. *Sports Med.* 46 (8), 1165–1182. doi: 10.1007/s40279-016-0494-0

Yang, L., Cheng, P., Chen, C., He, H. B., Xie, G. Q., Zhou, H. D., et al. (2012). miR-93/Sp7 function loop mediates osteoblast mineralization. *J. Bone Miner. Res.* 27 (7), 1598–1606. doi: 10.1002/jbmr.1621

Yang, M., Pan, Y., and Zhou, Y. (2014). miR-96 promotes osteogenic differentiation by suppressing HBEGF-EGFR signaling in osteoblastic cells. *FEBS Lett.* 588 (24), 4761–4768. doi: 10.1016/j.febslet.2014.11.008

Yang, N., Wang, G., Hu, C., Shi, Y., Liao, L., Shi, S., et al. (2013). Tumor necrosis factor alpha suppresses the mesenchymal stem cell osteogenesis promoter miR-21 in estrogen deficiency-induced osteoporosis. *J. Bone Miner. Res.* 28 (3), 559–573. doi: 10.1002/jbmr.1798

Yang, R., Fu, Y., Zeng, Y., Xiang, M., Yin, Y., Li, L., et al. (2017). Serum miR-20a is a promising biomarker for gastric cancer. *Biomed Rep.* 6 (4), 429–434. doi: 10.3892/br.2017.862

Yavropoulou, M. P., Anastasilakis, A. D., Makras, P., Tsalikakis, D. G., Grammatiki, M., and Yovos, J. G. (2017). Expression of microRNAs that regulate bone turnover in the serum of postmenopausal women with low bone mass and vertebral fractures. *Eur. J. Endocrinol.* 176 (2), 169–176. doi: 10.1530/EJE-16-0583

You, L., Pan, L., Chen, L., Gu, W., and Chen, J. (2016). MiR-27a is essential for the shift from osteogenic differentiation to adipogenic differentiation of mesenchymal stem cells in postmenopausal osteoporosis. *Cell Physiol. Biochem.* 39 (1), 253–265. doi: 10.1159/000445621

Yu, F., Cui, Y., Zhou, X., Zhang, X., and Han, J. (2011). Osteogenic differentiation of human ligament fibroblasts induced by conditioned medium of osteoclast-like cells. *Biosci. Trends* 5 (2), 46–51. doi: 10.5582/bst.2011.v5.2.46

Zampetaki, A., and Mayr, M. (2012). Analytical challenges and technical limitations in assessing circulating miRNAs. *Thromb. Haemos.t* 108 (4), 592–598. doi: 10.1160/TH12-02-0097

Zeng, Y., Qu, X., Li, H., Huang, S., Wang, S., Xu, Q., et al. (2012). MicroRNA-100 regulates osteogenic differentiation of human adipose-derived mesenchymal stem cells by targeting BMPR2. *FEBS Lett.* 586 (16), 2375–2381. doi: 10.1016/j.febslet.2012.05.049

Zhang, J., Tu, Q., Bonewald, L. F., He, X., Stein, G., Lian, J., et al. (2011a). Effects of miR-335-5p in modulating osteogenic differentiation by specifically downregulating Wnt antagonist DKK1. *J. Bone Miner. Res.* 26 (8), 1953–1963. doi: 10.1002/jbmr.377

Zhang, Y., Xie, R. L., Croce, C. M., Stein, J. L., Lian, J. B., van Wijnen, A. J., et al. (2011b). A program of microRNAs controls osteogenic lineage progression by targeting transcription factor Runx2. *Proc. Natl. Acad. Sci. U. S. A.* 108 (24), 9863–9868. doi: 10.1073/pnas.1018493108

Zhao, B., Takami, M., Yamada, A., Wang, X., Koga, T., Hu, X., et al. (2009). Interferon regulatory factor-8 regulates bone metabolism by suppressing osteoclastogenesis. *Nat. Med.* 15 (9), 1066–1071. doi: 10.1038/nm.2007

Zuo, B., Zhu, J., Li, J., Wang, C., Zhao, X., Cai, G., et al. (2015). microRNA-103a functions as a mechanosensitive microRNA to inhibit bone formation through targeting Runx2. *J. Bone Miner. Res.* 30 (2), 330–345. doi: 10.1002/jbmr.2352

7

Mutations in *KIAA1109*, *CACNA1C*, *BSN*, *AKAP13*, *CELSR2* and *HELZ2* are Associated with the Prognosis in Endometrial Cancer

Zhiwei Qiao, Ying Jiang, Ling Wang, Lei Wang, Jing Jiang and Jingru Zhang *

The Department of Gynaecology, Liaoning Cancer Hospital & Institute, Cancer Hospital of China Medical University, Shengyang, China

Correspondence:
Jingru Zhang
yi85317870@163.com

Endometrial cancer (EC) is one of the most common gynecologic malignancies. Emerging studies had demonstrated the mutations in genes could serve as diagnostic or prognostic markers for human cancers. In this study, we screened mutated genes in EC and found that the mutations in *KIAA1109, CACNA1C, BSN, AKAP13, CELSR2,* and *HELZ2* were correlated to the overall survival time in patients with EC. Bioinformatics analysis showed *KIAA1109* was involved in regulating NIK/NF-kappaB signaling, *CACNA1C* was found to regulate cell migration and proliferation, *BSN* was found to regulate Wnt signaling pathway, *CELSR2* was involved in regulating cell–cell adhesion, nuclear import, and protein folding, *HELZ2* was found to regulate multiple immune related biological processes, and *AKAP13* was involved in regulating translation, mRNA nonsense-mediated decay, rRNA processing, translational initiation, and mRNA splicing *via* spliceosome. The findings provided a novel therapeutic strategy in patients with EC.

Keywords: endometrial cancer, bioinformatics analyses, mutation, overall survival time, biomarkers

INTRODUCTION

Endometrial cancer (EC) is one of the most common gynecologic malignancies (Attarha et al., 2011). Despite the prognosis of the early stage EC is good with a 5-year survival rate of 69–88% (Gottwald et al., 2010). However, the prognosis of metastatic EC remained very poor, with a median survival of 7–12 months. Therefore, there is an urgent need to identify novel biomarkers for the prognosis of EC. Moreover, the mechanisms underlying the progression of EC remained largely unclear.

With the development of next-generation sequencing, multiple EC related mutations were identified. Emerging studies had demonstrated the mutations in genes could serve as diagnostic or prognostic markers for human cancers. For example, McConechy et al. identified a series of mutations in *PTEN, CTNNB1, PIK3CA, ARID1A, ARID5B*, and *KRAS* were associated with EC (Mcconechy et al., 2012). The mutations in FGFR2 were associated with poor outcomes in endometrioid endometrial cancer (Jeske et al., 2017). The genetic alterations in CTCF could promote EC cell survival and alter cell polarity (Marshall et al., 2017). Jing et al. found that MUC16 mutations could improve patients' prognosis by enhancing the infiltration of cytotoxic T lymphocytes in the EC microenvironment (Jing and Jing, 2014).

The present study identified prognosis related gene mutations in EC by analyzing TCGA databases (Collins, 2007). The mutations in 6 genes were correlated to the overall survival time in patients with EC. Bioinformatics analysis was used to predict the potential functions of these genes. The purpose of this study was to evaluate the impact of somatic tumor mutation on recurrence-free survival in this patient population.

MATERIALS AND METHODS

Data Mining With cBioPortal and TCGA Database

In this study, we identified the gene mutations in EC using TCGA database (https://portal.gdc.cancer.gov/). All searches were performed according to cBioPortal's online instructions (http://www.cbioportal.org/index.do) (Jianjiong et al., 2013). The survival analysis related to gene mutations was performed on the TCGA database (https://portal.gdc.cancer.gov/).

Co-Expression Network Analysis

In this study, the Pearson correlation coefficient was calculated according to the expression value between lncRNA–mRNA pair using cBioPortal's online instructions (http://www.cbioportal.org/index.do). The top 500 co-expressing genes were selected as potential targets of mutated genes in EC.

Bioinformatics Analysis

GO and KEGG pathway enrichment analysis were performed to determine the biological significance of DEGs, using the Database for Annotation, Visualization, and Integrated Discovery (Dennis et al., 2003) (DAVID; version 6.8; http://david.ncifcrf.gov/).

Patients' Prognostic Analyses

Survival curves were depicted using the Kaplan-Meier method and compared with log-rank test. Cox proportional hazards regression analysis was used for univariate and multivariate analyses to explore the association of clinical features, gene mutational status, and patients' prognosis. All the prognostic analyses were conducted by survival R package.

Statistical Analysis

The two groups were compared using Student's t-test. Overall survival time analyses were estimated using the Kaplan-Meier product-limit estimator, and then a log-rank test was conducted to compare wildtype and mutation status. Overall survival was measured from the date of surgery to the date of last contact or death. Patients alive were censored at the date of last contact or clinic visit. Stata v14.2 (College Station, TX) was used to conduct statistical analysis.

RESULTS

Screening of Mutated Genes in Endometrial Cancer

The present study analyzed TCGA database to identify mutated genes in EC. As shown in **Figure 1**, the top 50 mutated genes in EC included *TTN, MUC4, MUC16, PIK3CA, KMT2C, KMT2D, SYNE1, FLG, SYNE2, EP300, OBSCN, ADGRV1, RYR2, LRP1B, USH2A, MUC17, NEB, MDN1, MUC5B, CSMD1, PCLO, HUWE1, FBXW7, DMD, NSD1, NAV3, DNAH8, DST, PLEC, AHNAK2, LRP2, MKI67, DNAH2, TENM1, DNAH10, PRKDC, FAT1, TP53, HMCN1, ZFHX4, DNAH6, UBR4, NOTCH1, CREBBP, NIPBL, EYS, AHNAK, CSMD3, XIRP2*, and *MACF1*. Among these genes, *TTN, MUC4*, and *PIK3CA* are the most frequently mutated genes. The mutation rates in *TTN, MUC4*, and *PIK3CA* from the TCGA provisional data sets were 43.25% (125/289), 31.83% (92/289), and 29.41% (85/289), respectively.

The Somatic Mutations of *KIAA1109, CACNA1C, BSN, AKAP13, CELSR2*, and *HELZ2* Were Correlated to Overall Survival Time in Patients With EC

Next, we screened somatic mutations associated with overall survival time in patients with EC. As shown in **Figure 2**, Log-rank test showed that mutations in *KIAA1109, CACNA1C, BSN, AKAP13*, and *HELZ2* were significantly associated with the longer overall survival time in EC patients, however, mutations in CELSR2 were significantly associated with the shorter overall survival time in EC patients.

Mutation Profiles in *KIAA1109, CACNA1C, BSN, AKAP13, CELSR2*, and *HELZ2* in EC

The mutation rates in *KIAA1109, CACNA1C, BSN, AKAP13, CELSR2*, and *HELZ2* from the TCGA provisional data sets were 6.92% (20/289), 7.27% (21/289), 7.96% (23/289), 7.61% (22/289), 6.92% (20/289), and 7.27% (21/289), respectively in **Figure 3**. A, majority of mutations identified were missense and nonsense resulting in amino acid, changes and a truncation of these proteins. However, there was no evidence of a mutational hotspot in *KIAA1109, CACNA1C, BSN, AKAP13, CELSR2*, and *HELZ2* in EC patients (**Figure 4**).

The Effect of Mutations on mRNA Expressions of *KIAA1109, CACNA1C, BSN, AKAP13, CELSR2*, and *HELZ2* in EC Patients

Furthermore, we detected the effect of mutations in *KIAA1109, CACNA1C, BSN, AKAP13, CELSR2*, and *HELZ2* on mRNA expression based on the RNA-Seq data. As shown in **Figure 5**, we found the mutations in *CACNA1C, BSN, CELSR2*, and *HELZ2* did not result in a significant alteration of their mRNA levels. However, we found that the mRNA levels in *KIAA1109* and *AKAP13* mutated EC samples were lower than that in *KIAA1109* and *AKAP13* wild type EC samples.

Bioinformatics Analysis of *KIAA1109, CACNA1C, BSN, AKAP13, CELSR2*, and *HELZ2* in EC Patients

Furthermore, we performed bioinformatics analysis to reveal the potential functions of *KIAA1109, CACNA1C, BSN, AKAP13, CELSR2*, and *HELZ2* using their co-expressing mRNAs in EC patients. The present study selected the top 500 correlated genes as the potential targets of *KIAA1109, CACNA1C, BSN,*

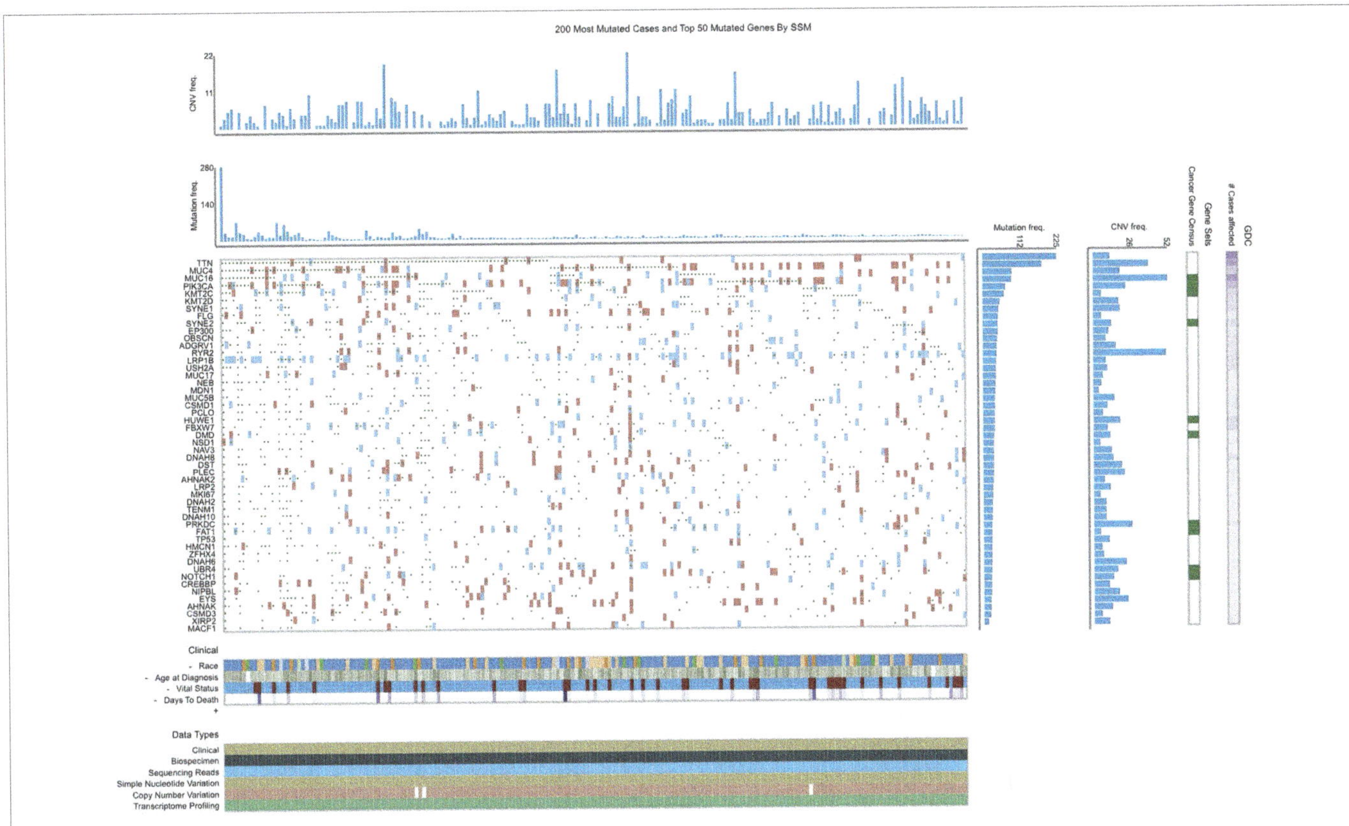

FIGURE 1 | Identification of mutated genes in EC using TCGA database.

AKAP13, CELSR2, and *HELZ2.* Bioinformatics analysis showed *KIAA1109* was involved in regulating rRNA processing, translation, transcription, NIK/NF-kappaB signaling, and histone acetylation. The results were shown in **Figure 6**. *CACNA1C* was involved in regulating collagen fibril organization, cell-matrix adhesion, cellular response to amino acid stimulus, cell adhesion, and negative regulation of cell proliferation. *BSN* was involved in regulating epidermis development, cilium movement, smoothened signaling pathway, Wnt signaling pathway, planar cell polarity pathway, and cilium morphogenesis. *AKAP13* was involved in regulating translation, mRNA nonsense-mediated decay, rRNA processing, translational initiation, and mRNA splicing *via* spliceosome. *CELSR2* was involved in regulating cell–cell adhesion, keratinocyte differentiation, spliceosomal snRNP assembly, nuclear import, and protein folding. *HELZ2* was involved in regulating type I interferon signaling pathway, innate immune response, immune response, inflammatory response, and T cell activation.

DISCUSSION

Endometrial cancer (EC) is one of the most common gynecologic malignancies. However, the mechanisms underlying EC progression remained unclear. Previous studies had showed the mutations in several genes were related to EC. For example, *MUC16* mutations improve EC prognosis through enhancing the infiltration of cytotoxic T lymphocytes. *PTEN* and *PIK3CA* mutations played crucial roles in grade 3 EC (Jing and Jing, 2014). The present study screened mutated genes in EC. Our results showed *TTN, MUC4,* and *PIK3CA* were the most frequently mutated genes in the EC, which was consistent with previous studies. Moreover, we identified the mutations in 6 genes were associated with the prognosis of EC. The results showed that mutations in *KIAA1109, CACNA1C, BSN, AKAP13,* and *HELZ2* were significantly associated with the longer overall survival time in EC patients. However, mutations in *CELSR2* were significantly associated with the shorter overall survival time in EC patients. These results suggested the important roles of these genes in the progression and prognosis of EC.

KIAA1109, located on the chromosome 4, was reported to be associated with susceptibility to celiac disease. Of note, 2 recent studies indicated *KIAA1109* was associated with the prognosis of human cancers. For example, Qing et al. reported mutations in *KIAA1109, DNAH5* and *KCNH7* were associated with poor survival of Chinese esophageal squamous cell carcinoma patients (Tao et al., 2017). Tindall et al. found genetic variation of *KIAA1109* might be associated with prostate cancer susceptibility in men with a family history of the disease (Tindall et al., 2010). *CACNA1C* gene encodes an alpha-1 subunit of a voltage-dependent calcium channel (Fayi et al., 2016). The mutations in *CACNA1C* were observed in various types of human diseases, such as ventricular fibrillation, and schizophrenia (Charles et al., 2007). Previous studies showed *CACNA1C* was

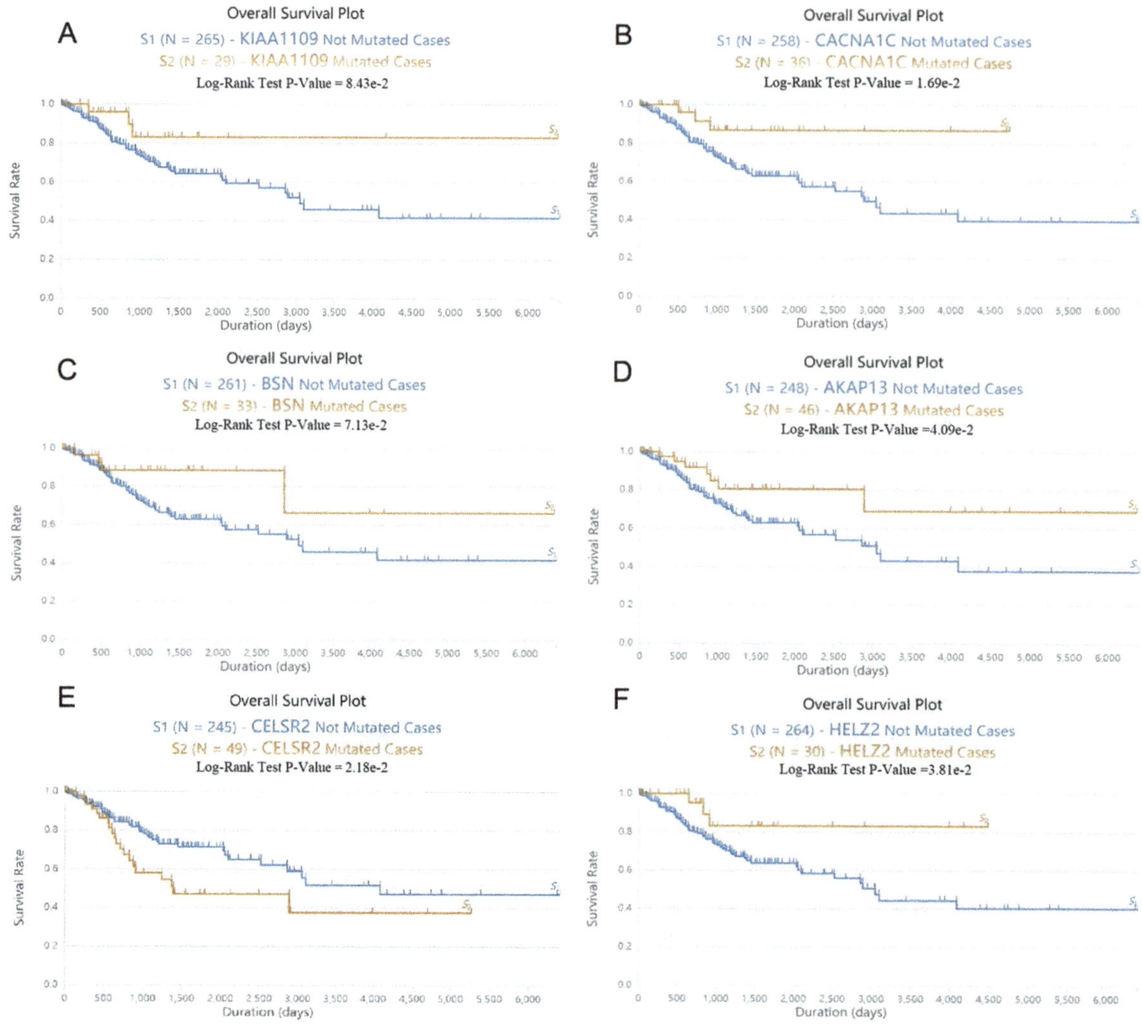

FIGURE 2 | The somatic mutations of *KIAA1109, CACNA1C, BSN, AKAP13, CELSR2*, and *HELZ2* were correlated to overall survival time in patients with EC. **(A–F)** Log-rank test showed that mutations in *KIAA1109* **(A)**, *CACNA1C* **(B)**, *BSN* **(C)**, *AKAP13* **(D)**, *CELSR2* **(E)** and *HELZ2* **(F)** were associated with the overall survival time in EC patients.

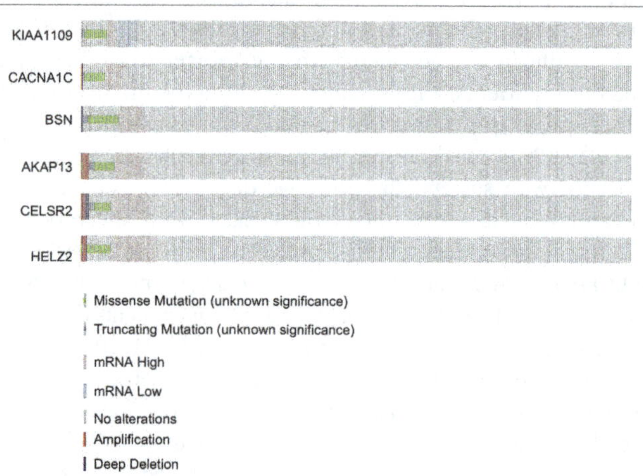

FIGURE 3 | Mutation profiles of *KIAA1109, CACNA1C, BSN, AKAP13, CELSR2* and *HELZ2* found in EC.

down-regulated in multiple human cancers (Fastje et al., 2009), including brain tumors, kidney cancers and lung cancers, suggested its regulatory roles in cancer progression. BSN encoded a scaffolding protein involved in organizing the presynaptic cytoskeleton. BSN has been demonstrated to have chemo-preventive, antiproliferative, antifungal, and anti-carcinogenic activities. In addition, *BSN* has been reported to induce G1 phase arrest through increase of p21 and p27. In PCa, *BSN* was involved in regulating cell apoptosis in cancer cells (Xu et al., 2016). The dysregulation and mutation of *AKAP13* were found to be associated with the progression of colorectal cancer and breast cancer. Bentin et al. showed *AKAP13* is essential for the phosphorylation of ERαS305 (Toaldo et al., 2015), which leads to tamoxifen resistance in breast cancer. *HELZ2* encoded b a nuclear transcriptional co-activator for peroxisome proliferator activated receptor alpha (Jakobsson et al., 2010). However, its roles in human cancers remained largely unclear. *CELSR2* was found to be dysregulated in breast cancer (Jiang et al., 2018). However, the potential functions of *CELSR2* in EC remained unknown.

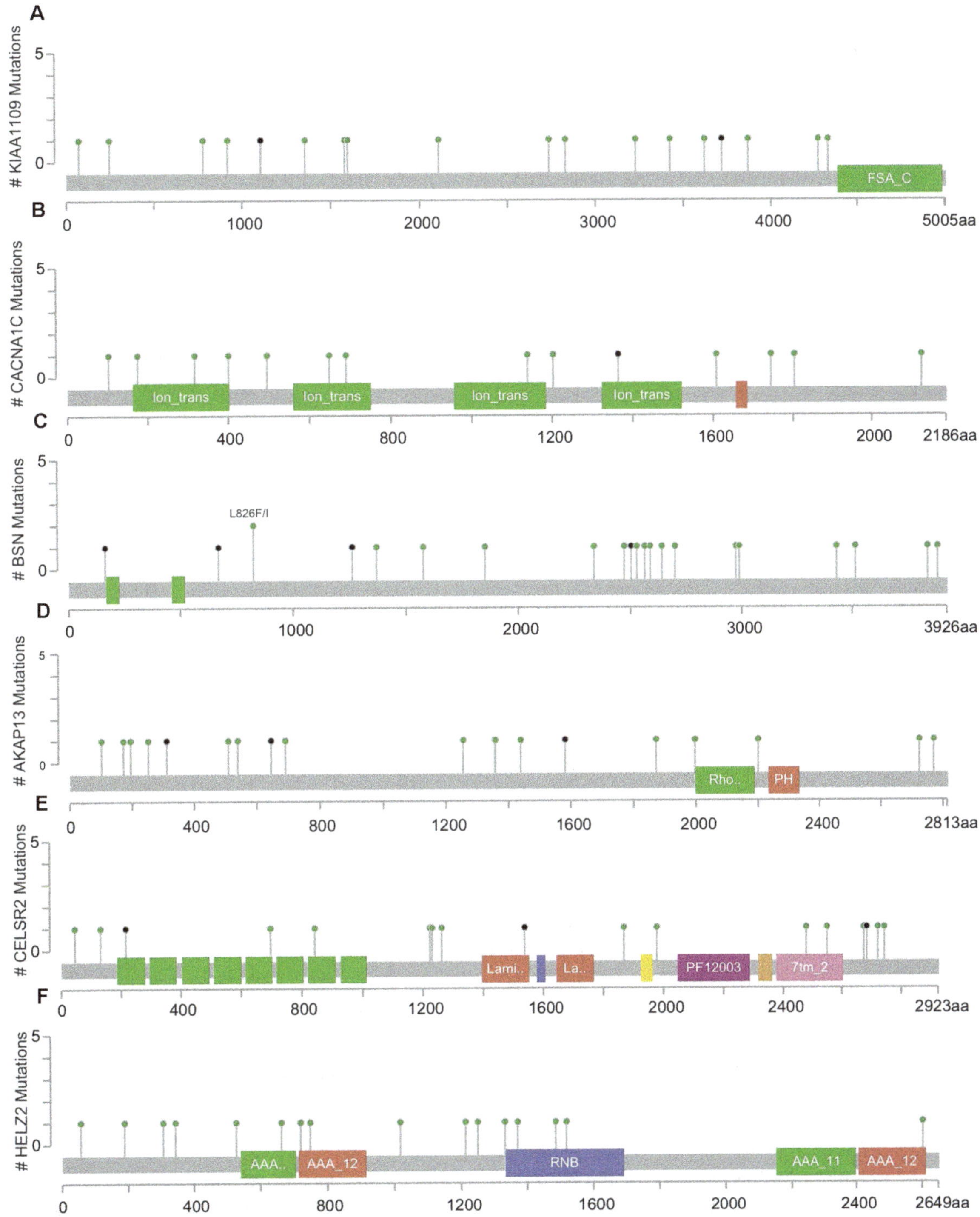

FIGURE 4 | Detailed mutation maps of *KIAA1109* **(A)**, *CACNA1C* **(B)**, *BSN* **(C)**, *AKAP13* **(D)**, *CELSR2* **(E)** and *HELZ2* **(F)** found in patients with EC. Each dot above the protein molecule represents a mutation, which spreads across the entire encoded protein of these genes.

In the present study, we performed co-expression analysis to reveal the potential roles of these mutated genes in EC. The results showed *KIAA1109* was involved in regulating NIK/NF-kappaB signaling. Of note, NF-kappaB signaling had been demonstrated to be a key regulator in cancers. Suppressing of NF-kappaB signaling could inhibit cell growth and invasion in multiple cancers. For example, NF-κB suppresses apoptosis and promotes the proliferation of bladder cancer cells. A recent study

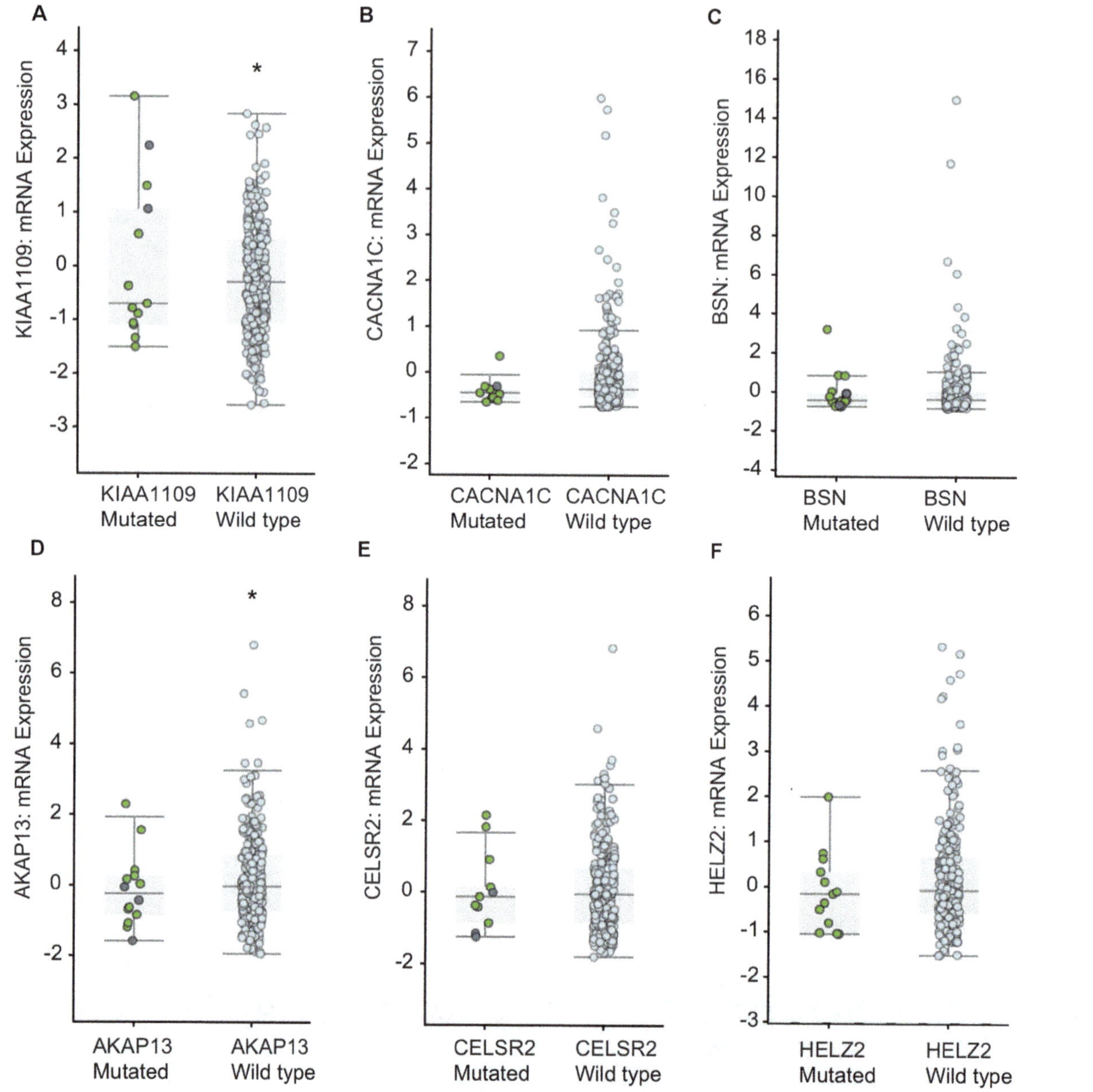

FIGURE 5 | Association between mutations in *KIAA1109* **(A)**, *CACNA1C* **(B)**, *BSN* **(C)**, *AKAP13* **(D)**, *CELSR2* **(E)** and *HELZ2* **(F)** and mRNA levels in EC samples. * *means p value < 0.05 between the two groups.*

showed liposomal curcumin targeting EC through the NF-κB Pathway. Bioinformatics analysis revealed *CACNA1C* played important roles in regulation of EC metastasis and proliferation. *BSN* was found to regulate Wnt signaling pathway. Mounting evidence has confirmed the activation of Wnt/β-catenin signaling was associated with multiple cancers, including EC. *AKAP13* was predicted as a RNA processing regulator. *CELSR2* was involved in regulating cell–cell adhesion, keratinocyte differentiation, spliceosomal snRNP assembly, nuclear import, and protein folding. *HELZ2* was involved in regulating type I interferon signaling pathway, innate immune response, immune response, inflammatory response, and T cell activation. These results suggested these mutated genes played important roles in EC tumorigenesis and progression.

Despite that bioinformatics analyses were conducted to predict the potential functions of these mutated genes in EC, several limitations still existed in this study. First, the mutated sites of these genes should be further validated in EC clinical samples using Sanger sequencing. Second, the molecular function of these key mutated genes in EC remained unclear. Therefore, gain or loss of function assays should be further conducted to investigate their important roles in EC.

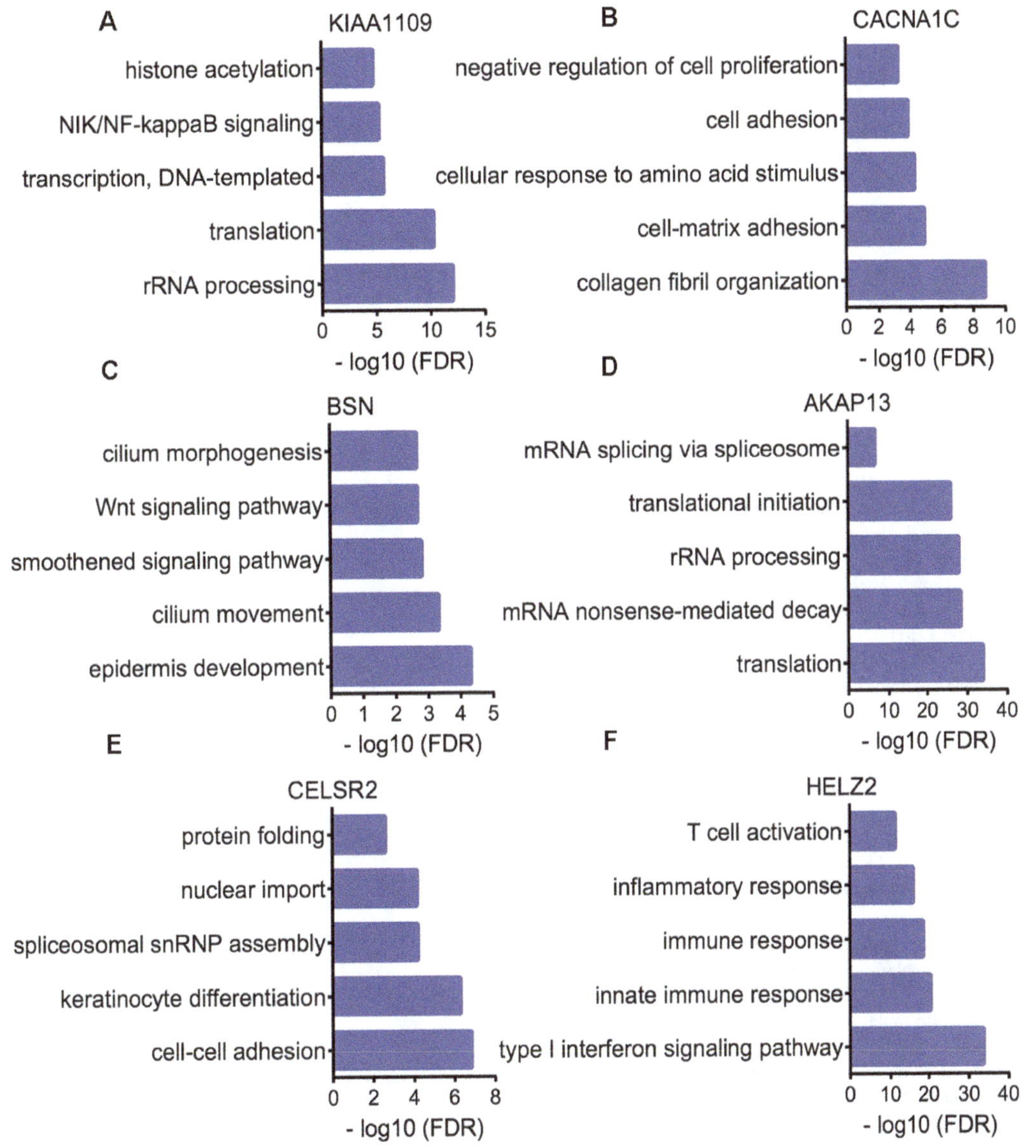

FIGURE 6 | Bioinformatics analysis of *KIAA1109* **(A)**, *CACNA1C* **(B)**, *BSN* **(C)**, *AKAP13* **(D)**, *CELSR2* **(E)** and *HELZ2* **(F)** in EC samples.

In conclusion, we screened mutated genes in EC and found that the mutations in *KIAA1109, CACNA1C, BSN, AKAP13, CELSR2*, and *HELZ2* correlated with the overall survival time in patients with EC. Bioinformatics analysis showed *KIAA1109* was involved in regulating NIK/NF-kappaB signaling, *CACNA1C* was found to regulate cell migration and proliferation, *BSN* was found to regulate Wnt signaling pathway, *CELSR2* was involved in regulating cell-cell adhesion, nuclear import, and protein folding, and *HELZ2* was found to regulate multiple immune related biological processes. The findings provided a novel therapeutic strategy in patients with EC.

AUTHOR CONTRIBUTIONS

JZ designed experiments; ZQ and YJ analyzed the data. All authors wrote and approved the manuscript.

FUNDING

This work is supported by the Natural Science Foundation of Liaoning Province, China (Grant no. 20170540570).

REFERENCES

Attarha, S., Mints, M., Andersson, S., and Souchelnytskyi, S., (2011). Endometrial cancer and application of proteomics. *Exp. Oncol.* 33, 174–177.

Charles, A., Pollevick, G. D., Cordeiro, J. M., Oscar, C., Sanguinetti, M. C., Yoshiyasu, A., et al. (2007). Loss-of-function mutations in the cardiac calcium channel underlie a new clinical entity characterized by ST-segment elevation, short QT intervals, and sudden cardiac death. *Circ.* 115, 442–449. doi: 10.1161/CIRCULATIONAHA.106.668392

Collins, A. (2007). The Cancer Genome Atlas (TCGA) pilot project. *Cancer Res.* 67.

Dennis, G., Jr., Sherman, B. T., Hosack, D. A., Yang, J., Gao, W., Lane, C. H., et al. (2003). DAVID: Database for Annotation, Visualization, and Integrated Discovery. *Genome Biol.* 4 (9) R60.

Fastje, C. D., Le, K., Sun, N. N., Wong, S. S., Sheppard, P. R., and Witte, M. L. (2009). Prenatal exposure of mice to tungstate is associated with decreased transcriptome-expression of the putative tumor suppressor gene, DMBT1: implications for childhood leukemia. *Land Contam. Reclam.* 17, 169–178. doi: 10.2462/09670513.931

Fayi, N., Xiaoli, W., Panpan, Z., Hao, Y., Wenhua, Z., Yaling, Z., et al. (2016). Genetic analysis of SNPs in *CACNA1C* and ANK3 gene with schizophrenia: a comprehensive meta-analysis. *Am. J. Med. Genet. B Neuropsychiatr. Genet.* 168, 637–648. doi: 10.1002/ajmg.b.32348

Gottwald, L., Pluta, P., Piekarski, J., Spych, M., Hendzel, K., Topczewskatylinska, K., et al. (2010). Long-term survival of endometrioid endometrial cancer patients. *Arch. Med. Sci.* 6, 937–944. doi: 10.5114/aoms.2010.19305

Jakobsson, L., Franco, C. A., Bentley, K., Collins, R. T., Ponsioen, B., Aspalter, I. M., et al. (2010). Endothelial cells dynamically compete for the tip cell position during angiogenic sprouting. *Nat. Cell Biol.* 12, 943–953. doi: 10.1038/ncb2103

Jeske, Y. W., Ali, S., Byron, S. A., Gao, F., Mannel, R. S., Ghebre, R. G., et al. (2017). FGFR2 mutations are associated with poor outcomes in endometrioid endometrial cancer: an NRG oncology/gynecologic oncology group study. *Gynecol. Oncol.* 145, 366–373. doi: 10.1016/j.ygyno.2017.02.031

Jiang, L., Zhang, X., Xiang, C., Geradts, J., Wei, Q., Liang, Y., et al. (2018). Differential cellular localization of CELSR2 and ING4 and correlations with hormone receptor status in breast cancer. *Histol. Histopathol.* 33, 11979. doi: 10.14670/HH-11-979

Jianjiong, G., Bülent Arman, A., Ugur, D., Gideon, D., Benjamin, G., Onur, S. S., et al. (2013). Integrative analysis of complex cancer genomics and clinical profiles using the cBioPortal. *Sci. Signal.* 6, pl1–pl1. doi: 10.1126/scisignal.2004088

Jing, H., and Jing, S. (2014). MUC16 mutations improve patients' prognosis by enhancing the infiltration and antitumor immunity of cytotoxic T lymphocytes in the endometrial cancer microenvironment. *Oncoimmunology*.

Marshall, A. D., Bailey, C. G., Champ, K., Vellozzi, M., O'Young, P., Metierre, C., et al. (2017). CTCF genetic alterations in endometrial carcinoma are pro-tumorigenic. *Oncogene* 36, 4100–4110. doi: 10.1038/onc.2017.25

Mcconechy, M. K., Jiarui, D., Cheang, M. C. U., Wiegand, K. C., Janine, S., Tone, A. A., et al. (2012). Use of mutation profiles to refine the classification of endometrial carcinomas. *J. Pathol.* 228, 20–30. doi: 10.1002/path.4056

Tao, Q., Zhu, S., Suo, C., Zhang, L., Zheng, Y., and Shi, L. (2017). Somatic mutations in ZFHX4 gene are associated with poor overall survival of Chinese esophageal squamous cell carcinoma patients. *Sci. Rep.* 7, 4951. doi: 10.1038/s41598-017-04221-7

Tindall, E. A., Hoang, H. N., Southey, M. C., English, D. R., Hopper, J. L., Giles, G. G., et al. (2010). The 4q27 locus and prostate cancer risk. *BMC Cancer* 10, 69. doi: 10.1186/1471-2407-10-69

Toaldo, C. B., Alexi, X., Beelen, K., Kok, M., Hauptmann, M., Jansen, M., et al. (2015). Protein Kinase A-induced tamoxifen resistance is mediated by anchoring protein AKAP13. *BMC Cancer* 15, 1–12. doi: 10.1186/s12885-015-1591-4

Xu, L., Wang, Z., He, S. Y., Zhang, S. F., Luo, H. J., Zhou, K., et al. (2016). Bax-interacting factor-1 inhibits cell proliferation and promotes apoptosis in prostate cancer cells. *Oncol. Rep.* 36, 3513. doi: 10.3892/or.2016.5172

8

Recent Advances in the Targeting of Epigenetic Regulators in B-Cell Non-Hodgkin Lymphoma

Marcelo L. Ribeiro[1,2], Diana Reyes-Garau[1], Marc Armengol[1], Miranda Fernández-Serrano[1] and Gaël Roué[1]**

[1] *Laboratory of Experimental Hematology, Department of Hematology, Vall d'Hebron Institute of Oncology (VHIO), Vall d'Hebron University Hospital, Autonomous University of Barcelona, Barcelona, Spain,* [2] *Laboratory of Immunopharmacology and Molecular Biology, Sao Francisco University Medical School, Braganca Paulista, São Paulo, Brazil*

***Correspondence:**
Marcelo L. Ribeiro
mlribeiro@vhio.net
Gaël Roué
groue@vhebron.net

In the last 10 years, major advances have been made in the diagnosis and development of selective therapies for several blood cancers, including B-cell non-Hodgkin lymphoma (B-NHL), a heterogeneous group of malignancies arising from the mature B lymphocyte compartment. However, most of these entities remain incurable and current treatments are associated with variable efficacy, several adverse events, and frequent relapses. Thus, new diagnostic paradigms and novel therapeutic options are required to improve the prognosis of patients with B-NHL. With the recent deciphering of the mutational landscapes of B-cell disorders by high-throughput sequencing, it came out that different epigenetic deregulations might drive and/or promote B lymphomagenesis. Consistently, over the last decade, numerous epigenetic drugs (or epidrugs) have emerged in the clinical management of B-NHL patients. In this review, we will present an overview of the most relevant epidrugs tested and/or used so far for the treatment of different subtypes of B-NHL, from first-generation epigenetic therapies like histone acetyl transferases (HDACs) or DNA-methyl transferases (DNMTs) inhibitors to new agents showing selectivity for proteins that are mutated, translocated, and/or overexpressed in these diseases, including EZH2, BET, and PRMT. We will dissect the mechanisms of action of these epigenetic inhibitors, as well as the molecular processes underlying their lack of efficacy in refractory patients. This review will also provide a summary of the latest strategies being employed in preclinical and clinical settings, and will point out the most promising lines of investigation in the field.

Keywords: B-cell lymphoma, DNMT, EZH2, HDAC, PRMT inhibitor, BET bromodomain inhibitor (BETi), combination therapy

INTRODUCTION

Characteristics of B-Cell Non-Hodgkin Lymphoma (B-NHL)

At the origin of 4% of all cancers and more than 90% of the cases of lymphoma, B-NHLs comprise a heterogeneous group of lymphoid neoplasms. According to the last World Health Organization hematopoietic and lymphoid tumor classification, more than 40 distinct entities are categorized, according to a combination of morphological, immunophenotypic, genetic, and clinical features, having each entity its own clinical course and requiring specific treatments (**Table 1**)

TABLE 1 | Classification of B-cell non-Hodgkin lymphoma.

Name	Cell of origin	Genetic aberration	Involved genes	Frequency (%)	References
B-ALL	Hematopoietic stem cell or B-cell progenitor	Hyperdiploidy	–	31*	(Yeoh et al., 2002)
		t(12;21)(p13.2;q22.1)	*ETV6/RUNX1*	28*	
		t(1;19)(q23;p13.3)	*TCF3/PBX1*	9*	
		t(9;22)(q34.1;q11.2)	*BCR/ABL1*	5*	
CLL/SLL	Naïve (unmutated IGHV subset) or memory (mutated IGHV subset) B cell	del(13q14.3)	–	54	(Haferlach et al., 2007)
		–	*SF3B1*	21	(Landau et al., 2015)
		Trisomy of 12	–	14	
		del(11q)	*ATM*	12	
LPL	Post-follicular B cell	–	*MYD88*	90	(Hunter et al., 2014)
		del(6q)	–	43	
		–	*CXCR4*	27	
			ARID1A	17	
NMZL	Post-germinal center marginal zone B cell	Gains of 3p	–	24	(Rinaldi et al., 2011)
		Gains of 18q	–	24	
		del(6q23)	*TNFAIP3*	16	
EMZL-MALT	Post-germinal center marginal zone B cell	Trisomy of 3	–	31	(Streubel et al., 2004)
		del(6q23)	*TNFAIP3*	30	(Rinaldi et al., 2011)
		t(11;18)(q21;q21)	*BIRC3/MALT1*	13	
		Trisomy of 18	–	11	
SMZL	Marginal zone B cell with or without antigen exposure	del(7q)	–	26	(Rinaldi et al., 2011)
		Gains of 3q	–	20	(Parry et al., 2015)
		del(17p13) or mutation	*TP53*	16	
		–	*KLF2*	12	
HCL	Late activated memory B cell	–	*BRAF*	100	(Tiacci et al., 2011)
		–	*MAP2K1*	48	(Waterfall et al., 2013)
FL	Germinal center B cell	t(14;18)(q32;q21)	*IGH/BCL2*	89	(Horsman et al., 1995)
		–	*KMT2D*	82	(Okosun et al., 2014)
		–	*CREBBP*	64	
		–	*TNFRSF14*	35	
MCL	Peripheral B cell of the inner mantle zone	t(11;14)(q13;q32)	*IGH/CCND1*	57	(Beà et al., 1999)
		Gain of 3q26	–	49	(Beà et al., 2013)
		del(11q) or mutation	*ATM*	41	
		del(17p13) or mutation	*CCND1*	34	
			TP53	27	
DLBCL-GCB	Peripheral mature B cell of germinal center origin	–	*KMT2D*	46	(Dubois et al., 2016)
		del(1p36) or mutation	*TNFRSF14*	38	(Scholtysik et al., 2015)(Roulland et al., 2018)
		Gains of 2p16	*REL*	30	
		t(18q21)	*BCL2*	28	
DLBCL-ABC	Peripheral mature B cell of germinal center exit or post-germinal center	del(9p21)	*CDKN2A*	47	(Scholtysik et al., 2015)(Dubois et al., 2016)
		del(6q21) or mutation	*PRDM1*	41	
		–	*KMT2D*	41	
		–	*MYD88*	28	
BL	Germinal center B cell	t(8;14)(q24;q32)	*MYC/IGH*	77	(Toujani et al., 2009)
		–Other t(8q24)	*ID3*	58	(Schmitz et al., 2012)
			TCF3	29	
			MYC	8–15	

**Frequency in pediatric cases. B-ALL, B-cell acute lymphocytic leukemia; CLL/SLL, chronic lymphocytic leukemia/small lymphocytic lymphoma; LPL, lymphoplasmacytic lymphoma; NMZL, nodal marginal zone lymphoma; EMZL-MALT, extranodal marginal zone lymphoma of mucosa-associated lymphoid tissue; SMZL, splenic marginal zone lymphoma; HCL, hairy cell leukemia; FL, follicular lymphoma; MCL, mantle cell lymphoma; DLBCL-GCB, diffuse large B-cell lymphoma of germinal center B-cell subtype; DLBCL-ABC, diffuse large B-cell lymphoma of activated B-cell subtype; BL, Burkitt lymphoma.*

(Campo et al., 2011; Scott and Gascoyne, 2014; Swerdlow et al., 2016). Originated from either mature or immature B cells, B-NHLs are characterized by the proliferation of lymphocytes, mainly in lymphoid organs and in extranodal tissues. Their diversity can often be traced to a particular stage of differentiation, from the bone marrow where the normal precursor B cell is originated to secondary lymphoid tissues where B cells undergo multiple rounds of selection before their differentiation into plasma cells or memory B cells. During these processes, the VDJ heavy chain is formed, followed by VJ light-chain gene rearrangement, which allows the pre-B cells to express intracytoplasmic μ-heavy chains. Subsequently, immature immunoglobulin (Ig)-positive B cells are formed. Within the lymph node, and in contact with a determined antigen, naïve B cells can mature into IgM-secreting plasma cells or may proliferate into primary follicles to form germinal center (GC) centroblasts. Upon maturation, they further differentiate into centrocytes, which give place to memory B cells or plasma cells. Within the GC, somatic hypermutation in the *Ig heavy or light chain variable region (IGHV* or *IGHL)* genes leads to increased antigen affinity.

Although tightly regulated, the B-cell differentiation process and especially the antibody diversification phase can be accompanied by inherited events that may favor lymphomagenesis, such as chromosomal translocations, oncogene activation, and/or inactivating mutations in tumor suppressor genes. Infection by determined viruses, such as the Epstein–Barr virus, has also been involved in lymphomagenesis. The malignant counterparts of the early B-cell differentiation steps account for B lymphoblastic lymphomas, which harbor high similarity with B progenitor cells. On the other hand, mantle cell lymphomas (MCLs) and a subset of chronic lymphocytic leukemia (CLL) with unmutated *IGHV* are thought to derive from naive B cells and pre-GC mature B cells expressing the CD5 surface marker. Other GC-originated lymphomas, including follicular lymphoma (FL), Burkitt's lymphoma (BL), a subset of diffuse large B-cell lymphoma (DLBCL), and Hodgkin's lymphoma (HL), present mutations in *IGHV* gene. Additional entities, including marginal zone lymphoma (MZL), lymphoplasmacytic lymphoma, CLL with somatic *IGHV* mutation, another subset of DLBCL, and multiple myeloma (MM) correspond to post-GC cells. Each lymphoma subtype retains key features of their cell of origin as judged by the similarity of immunophenotype, histological appearance, and gene expression profiles (Seifert et al., 2013) (**Table 1**). The putative normal B-cell counterpart of each B-cell lymphoma is summarized in **Figure 1**.

In the last decade, loads of evidences have suggested an association between the frequent alterations in chromatin state and epigenetic regulators observed in B-NHL patients, and disease formation and progression.

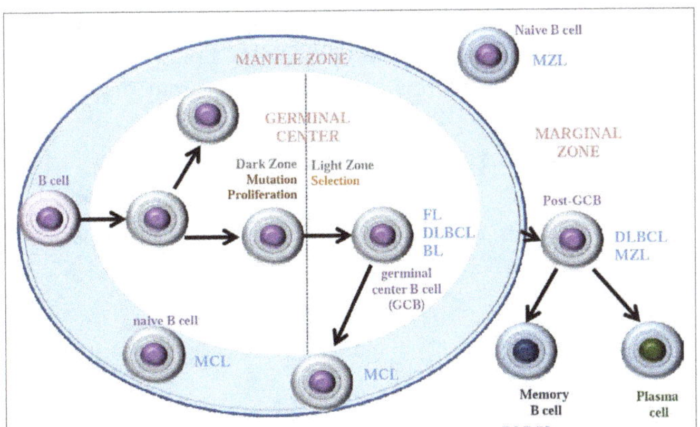

FIGURE 1 | Major B-cell non-Hodgkin lymphoma subtypes arise from different cell of origin within the lymph node. Mantle cell lymphomas (MCL) arise from naive B cells or germinal center (GC) B cells found within the mantle zone. Marginal zone lymphomas initiate from naive B cells or GCB that have entered the marginal zone. GCB are the origin of follicular lymphomas (FL), Burkitt lymphoma (BL), and diffuse large B-cell lymphomas (DLBCL) when still in the germinal center. This last DLBCL appears to also form GCB within the marginal zone or from fully developed memory B cells.

Altered Chromatin-Modifying Enzymes in B-NHL

Contrary to the general belief that only accumulations of DNA mutations might lead directly to the development of tumorigenic processes, it has been progressively reported a growing subset of epigenetic alterations lying at the basis of many malignancies, including those occurring in lymph nodes. Interestingly, in B-cell lymphomas, certain somatic mutations in chromatin-modifying enzymes account for several epigenetic alterations, suggesting that an aberrant epigenetic landscape in B-NHL may be a consequence of genetic alterations associated with a particular lymphoma subtype. For instance, deleterious and/or loss of function mutations in the histone acetyltransferase *CREB binding protein (CREBBP)* or the *E1A binding protein 300 (EP330)* have been reported in about 40% of DLBCL and FL patients as well as in other lymphoma subtypes (Morin et al., 2011; Pasqualucci et al., 2011b). Recurrent point mutations in the histone acetyl transferase (HAT) recruiting gene *myocyte enhancer binding factor 2B (MEF2B)* have been also described in 15% of FL and 13% of DLBCL patients with germinal center B cell (DLBCL-GCB) subtype (Morin et al., 2011). Although no mutations have been reported in the genes coding for histone deacetylases (HDACs), several members of this family like *HDAC1, 2,* and *6* can be overexpressed in DLBCL, in association with a decrease in the DNA accessibility to the transcription machinery (Marquard et al., 2009).

In addition to mutations in chromatin-regulatory proteins, epigenetic modifications at chromatin level are also commonly observed in B-NHL as a result of profound changes in DNA methylation patterns. Indeed, while hypo- and hyper-DNA methylation status have been linked to the pathogenesis of several cancer subtypes, somatic mutations in epigenetic genes codifying for DNA methylation regulators have been particularly well associated to a repressed chromatin state and to malignant processes in B-NHL (Esteller et al., 2001; Hassler et al., 2013). Among the main reported alterations, activating mutations in *enhancer of zeste homolog 2 (EZH2)*, a histone methyltransferase (HMT) gene, were found in 22% of DLBCL-GCB patients and 7% of FL patients (Morin et al., 2010). Further loss-of-function mutations were observed in the *histone-Lysine N-Methyltransferase 2D (MLL2/KMT2D)* gene in about 90% of FL and 30% of DLBCL patients (Morin et al., 2011; Pasqualucci et al., 2011b; Lohr et al., 2012). Concretely, *MLL2* presents a defective SET domain when mutated by either truncation or frameshift mutations, leading to a reduced H3K4 methylation activity (Shilatifard, 2008; Morin et al., 2011; Pasqualucci et al., 2011b; Lohr et al., 2012).

Hence, B-NHL occurrence as a result of disruption in epigenetic mechanisms has generated a strong rationale to target epigenetic and chromatin regulators for drug discovery attempts. To address these alterations, several Food and Drug Administration (FDA)-approved epigenetic-modulating agents, whose clinical use has been mainly restrained so far to other hematological malignancies (Popovic et al., 2013), are now being made available for their evaluation in B-NHL.

These agents include the HDAC inhibitors romidepsin (FK228, depsipeptide), vorinostat (suberanilohydroxamic acid, SAHA), panobinostat (LBH589), and belinostat (PXD101); the DNA methyltransferase (DNMT) inhibitors (hypomethylating agents, HMAs) azacitidine (5-azacytidine) and decitabine (5-aza-2′-deoxycytidine); and the isocitrate dehydrogenase (IDH) inhibitors enasidenib (AG-221) and ivosidenib (AG-120) (**Table 2**).

TARGETING WRITER EPIGENETIC ENZYMES

DNMT Inhibitors

DNA methylation is responsible for the control of gene expression and for maintaining genomic stability during embryogenesis and tissue differentiation (Meissner, 2010). This process is clonally inherited and preserved in daughter cells, and occurs through the inclusion of a methyl group at cytosine residues in CpG dinucleotides (**Figure 2**). It is carried out by the DNMTs, namely DNMT1 which primarily mediates maintenance methylation during cell division, and DNMT3A and 3B that regulate *de novo* DNA methylation (Belinsky et al., 2003; Hermann et al., 2004). DNA methylation is thought to have a significant role in the regulation of lymphoid compartment, as it has been demonstrated that differential recruitment of DNMT1, DNMT3A, and DNMT3B and consequent specific DNA methylation patterns are determined at early stages during lymphopoiesis and B-cell activation (Shaknovich et al., 2011; Lai et al., 2013).

While on the one hand, DNA methylation is essential for cell homeostasis, on the other hand, disturbance in methylation pattern have been widely described in cancer. Changes in CpG methylation are indeed commonly associated with malignant transformation and tumor progression (Berdasco and Esteller, 2010). In addition, accumulating evidences suggest that aberrant epigenetic regulation, including DNA methylation, exerts an important role in regulating each cancer's hallmarks (Flavahan et al., 2017). Illustrating this relationship in B-NHL, Shaknovich and collaborators demonstrated the relevance of DNA methylation in defining the molecular DLBCL subtypes (Shaknovich et al., 2010). It was further proposed that DNMT1 and DNMT 3B overexpression may play a role in malignant progression of these tumors (Amara et al., 2010) and also in BL neoplasm (Robaina et al., 2015). In line with this, the disruption of DNA methylation pattern is correlated with disease severity and patient survival in DLBCL and FL (De et al., 2013).

Considering that the majority of cancers, including B-NHL, harbor an altered DNA methylation pattern, and also taking into account the reversibility of this alteration, the idea to modulate the methylation machinery to restore a "normal" DNA methylation state has attracted great attention in cancer treatment (Azad et al., 2013). The first two DNA methylation epigenetic compounds (DNMTi) ratified by the FDA and the European Medicines Agency for cancer treatment, azacitidine and decitabine (Jones et al., 2016), were initially described as promising chemotherapeutic agents against myelodysplastic syndrome (MDS) and acute myeloid leukemia (AML), although with moderate efficacy and high toxicity (Li et al., 1970; Vogler et al., 1976). In further trials, low-dose decitabine and azacitidine demonstrated to be effective in these patients, improving both the response and the overall survival (OS), leading to their further approval (**Table 2** and **Figure 3**) (Silverman et al., 2002; Fenaux et al., 2009; Lübbert et al., 2016). In B-NHL patients, two phase I studies using decitabine have been completed so far, but the response to therapy and the effect on DNA methylation were moderate (Stewart et al., 2009; Blum et al., 2010). Currently, azacitidine and decitabine are being evaluated alone or in combination in approximately 10 active clinical trials involving relapsed/refractory R/R B-NHL patients (**Table 3**). Considering the preliminary data of these trials, it seems premature to conclude that DNMTis can be used as monotherapy in B-NHL.

Although the mechanism of action of DNMTi is not well understood, the activity of decitabine and azacitidine is known to involve their incorporation into the DNA of proliferating cells, followed by irreversible inhibition of DNMT1 enzymatic activity and the addressing of this latest to proteasomal degradation

TABLE 2 | FDA-approved epigenetic drugs for hematological malignancies.

Agent	Target	Indication	Year of approval	Current development
Azacitidine	DNMT	MDS CMML AML	2004	
Decitabine	DNMT	MDS AML	2006	Atherosclerosis
Vorinostat	HDAC	CTCL	2006	
Romidepsin	HDAC	CTCL PTCL	2009 2011	HIVAutism
Belinostat	HDAC	PTCL	2014	Ovarian cancer CTCL
Panobinostat	HDAC	MM	2015	CML MDS Breast cancer Prostate cancer

DNMT, DNA methyltransferase; HDAC, histone deacetylase; MDS, myelodysplastic syndrome; CMML, chronic myelomonocytic leukemia; AML, acute myeloid leukemia; CTCL, cutaneous T-cell lymphoma; PTCL, peripheral T-cell lymphoma; MM, multiple myeloma.

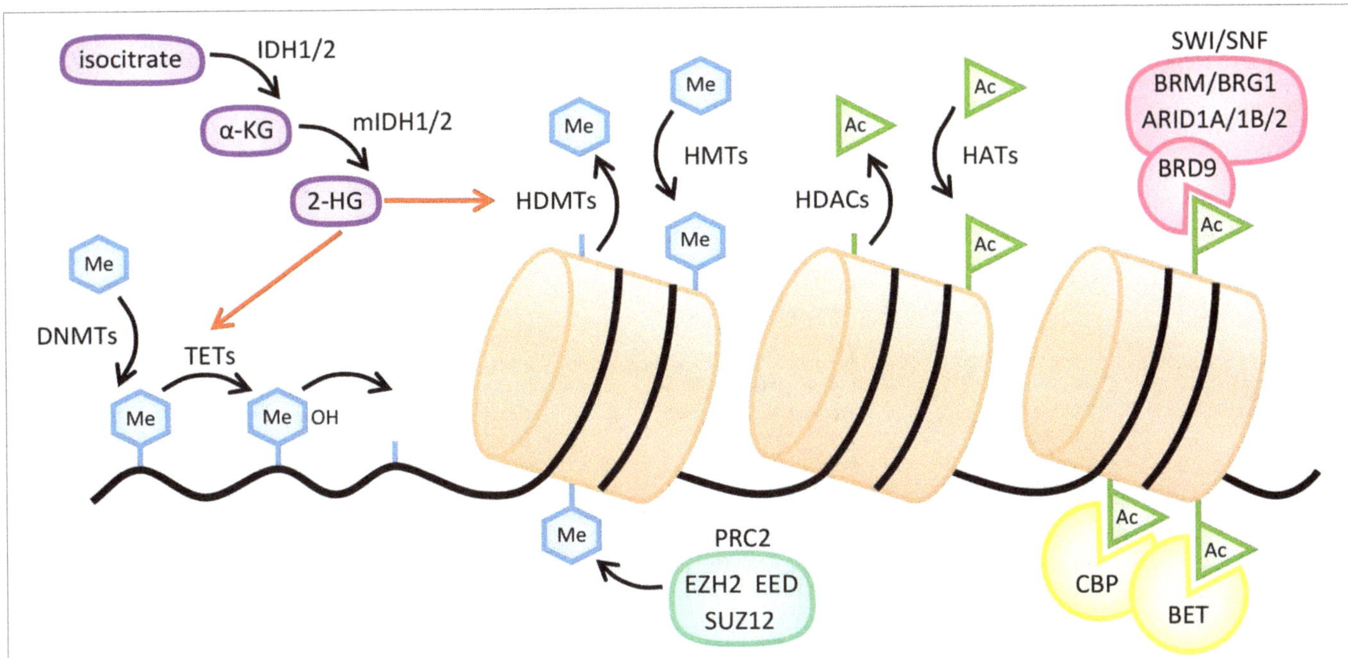

FIGURE 2 | Mechanisms of action of common epigenetic enzymes. Histone methylation is regulated by histone methyltransferases (HMTs), such as the EZH2 subunit of polycomb repressive complex 2 (PRC2), and histone demethylases (HDMTs). DNA methylation is established by DNA methyltransferases (DNMTs) and reversed by several enzymes like TET hydroxymethylases. Demethylation of both histones and DNA is inhibited by 2-hydroxyglutarate (2-HG), produced from α-ketoglutarate (α-KG) by mutant forms of IDH1/2 enzymes (mIDH). Histone acetylation is regulated by histone acetyltransferases (HATs) and histone deacetylases (HDACs). Bromodomain-containing proteins, such as CREB-binding protein (CBP), BET, or the BRD9 subunit of the SWI/SNF complex, bind to acetylated residues of histones.

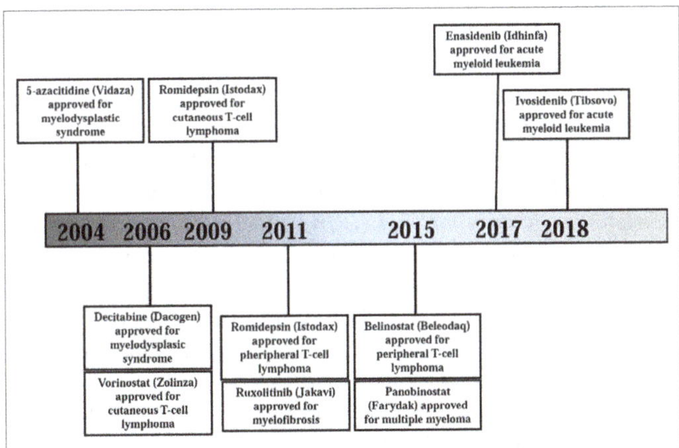

FIGURE 3 | Timeline of FDA approvals of epigenetic-modulating therapies in hematological cancers. Source: https://www.accessdata.fda.gov/scripts/cder/daf/

(Ghoshal et al., 2005; Juttermann et al., 2006). Accordingly, two main molecular effects have been described for DNMTi inhibitors: (1) a global demethylation of gene promoters (mainly tumor suppressor genes) and (2) the activation of immune system and the triggering of an anti-tumor immune response (Groudine et al., 1981; Almstedt et al., 2010; Goodyear et al., 2010; Chiappinelli et al., 2015;). As an illustration, in DLBCL it has been described that decitabine can reverse DNA methylation and restore expression of important cancer-related pathways *in vitro* and *in vivo* (Li et al., 2002; Clozel et al., 2013), although in other studies a less drastic and transient effect was observed (Karpf, 2004; McGarvey et al., 2006; Egger et al., 2007). Furthermore, DNMT inhibition is also linked to the demethylation of gene bodies, leading to oncogene downregulation (Wong et al., 2013; Yang et al., 2014).

Several new DNMTis have been developed in the last decade with potential activity in hematological malignancies. Among them, thioguanine (2-amino-1,7-dihydro-6H-purine-6-thione (6-tG)) has been approved by FDA to treat AML patients (Munshi et al., 2014). Its mechanism of action involves its incorporation into DNA, decrease in DNMT activity and DNA methylation, blockade of DNA and RNA synthesis, and ultimately cell death (Hogarth et al., 2008; Yuan et al., 2011; Flesner et al., 2014). Recently described as an experimental DNMTi, 5-fluoro-2′-deoxycytidine (FdCyd) is currently undergoing a phase I/II clinical trial in combination with other drugs (Kinders et al., 2011; Newman et al., 2015). Its mechanism of action involves the ability to block DNMT-dependent DNA methylation (Jones and Taylor, 1980; Beumer et al., 2008). 5,6-Dihydro-5-azacytidine is a reduced, hydrolytically stable form of 5-azacytidine nucleoside (Beisler et al., 1979). The mechanism of action is very similar to that described for azacytidine, with the advantage of a lower toxicity (Avramis et al., 1989). However, its evaluation in clinical settings revealed a reduced response rate and the rise of significant adverse effects (Samuels et al., 1998). Zebularine is another DNMTi, which has been previously described as tumor-selective

TABLE 3 | Selected examples of epigenetic drugs under clinical evaluation in B-NHL patients as single agents.

Epigenetic drug class	Drug	Diseases	Sponsor	Trial identifier
HDAC inhibitor	Vorinostat	FL, indolent B-NHL, MCL	Merck Sharp & Dohme Corp.	NCT00875056
	Chidamide (Epidaza)	R/R B-NHL	Sun Yat-sen University	NCT03245905
	Abexinostat	R/R FL	Xynomic Pharmaceuticals, Inc.	NCT03934567
	Mocetinostat (MGCD0103)	DLBCL, FL	Memorial Sloan Kettering Cancer Center and MethylGene Inc.	NCT02282358
	Ricolinostat(ACY-1215)	R/R NHL	Acetylon Pharmaceuticals Inc. and Columbia University	NCT02091063
	Panobinostat	CLL	Peter MacCallum Cancer Centre, Australia	NCT01658241
	CDX101	Advanced lymphomas	Cancer Research UK and Oxford University Hospitals	NCT01977638
IDH1 inhibitor	Ivosidenib(AG-120)	Advanced hematologic malignancies with an IDH1 mutation	Agios Pharmaceuticals, Inc.	NCT02074839
BET bromodomaininhibitor	CPI-0610	Progressive lymphomas	Constellation Pharmaceuticals	NCT01949883
	BMS-986158	Lymphomas	Dana-Farber Cancer Institute	NCT03936465
	Molibresib (GSK525762)	NHL	GlaxoSmithKline	NCT01943851
EZH1/2 inhibitor	DS-3201b	R/R B-NHL	Daiichi Sankyo Co., Ltd.	NCT02732275
	CPI-1205	Progressive B-cell lymphomas	Constellation Pharmaceuticals	NCT02395601
	Tazemetostat	R/R B-NHL	Eisai Co., Ltd.	NCT03009344
	Tazemetostat	R/R NHL with EZH2 gene mutations	National Cancer Institute (NCI)	NCT03213665
PRMT inhibitor	JNJ-64619178	R/R B-NHL	Janssen Research & Development, LLC	NCT03573310
	GSK3326595	MDS, AML	GlaxoSmithKline	NCT03614728
	GSK3368715	DLBCL	GlaxoSmithKline	NCT03666988
DNMT inhibitor	Decitabine	R/R DLBCL	Mingzhi Zhang, Zhengzhou University	NCT03579082
EED inhibitor	MAK683	Advanced DLBCL	Novartis Pharmaceuticals	NCT02900651

EED, embryonic ectoderm development. Source: https://clinicaltrials.gov/.

inhibitor of DNMTs (Cheng et al., 2004). Although there are a lot of evidences, both *in vitro* and *in vivo*, indicating the potential of zebularine as a demethylating agent in a wide range of tumors (Agrawal et al., 2018), its poor bioavailability has prevented its introduction into clinical trials (Ben-Kasus et al., 2005). More recently, 4′-thio-2′-deoxycytidine (TdCyd) and its 5-aza analog, 5-aza-TdCyd, have been reported to downregulate DNMT1 and to exhibit anti-tumor activity *in vitro* and in human leukemia and lung cancer xenografts (Thottassery et al., 2014). Among these last molecules, TdCyd has already entered into phase I clinical evaluation (NCT02423057 and NCT03366116). Further molecules were developed with superior anti-tumoral efficacy and included guadecitabine (SGI-110), a second-generation DNMTi that harbors an improved DNA methylation inhibition in solid tumors both *in vitro* and *in vivo* (Chuang et al., 2010; Srivastava et al., 2015). A phase I clinical trial has provided promising results in patients with MDS and AML (Issa et al., 2015). Fluorocyclopentenylcytosine (RX-3117) is a cytidine analog that presents an anti-tumor activity in a large set of tumor cells and *in vivo*. Its mechanism of action is associated with an inhibition of DNMT1 (Choi et al., 2012). This agent is being evaluated in a phase II study with R/R pancreatic or advanced bladder cancer (NCT02030067).

EZH2 Inhibitors

EZH2 constitutes the catalytic subunit of the polycomb repressive complex 2 (PRC2). Its structure is composed by a SET domain, typical in chromatin-associated regulators of gene expression (Xiao et al., 2003). It catalyzes histone H3 lysine 27 tri-methylation (H3K27me3) and the subsequent formation of heterochromatic regions and downregulation of the nearby genes (Bracken and Helin, 2009; Ferrari et al., 2014) (**Figure 2**). In B lymphocytes, EZH2 becomes expressed and inhibited in a cyclic manner. First, in pre-B lymphocytes, induction of EZH2 expression is required for an optimal V(D)J recombination. Later on, during the migration to lymphoid tissues, it is downregulated until the GC reaction occurs, after which it becomes re-expressed to allow the silencing of the anti-proliferative genes *cyclin-dependent kinase inhibitor 2A (CDKN2A)* and *cyclin-dependent kinase inhibitor 1A (CDKN1A1)* and the pro-differentiation genes *interferon regulatory factor 4 (IRF4)* and *PR domain zinc finger protein 1 (PRDM1/BLIMP1)* during the somatic hypermutation and isotype switch processes. Finally, EZH2 becomes repressed when mature B cells leave the GC (Velichutina et al., 2010; Béguelin et al., 2013). Gain-of-function mutations in *EZH2* have been reported in several solid tumors and hematological cancers. The consequence of those mutations in GC lymphocytes is the irreversible silencing of certain cell cycle checkpoint and plasma cell differentiation genes (Béguelin et al., 2013). The main gain-of-function mutation identified in DLBCL and FL patients includes a tyrosine deletion (Y641) at the EZH2 SET domain that increases the levels of H3K27me3, promoting a repressed state of cell differentiation and the repression of tumor suppressor genes (Morin et al., 2010; McCabe et al., 2012a). Similar effects have been described as a consequence of the A677G mutation in EZH2, which has been characterized in multiple human lymphoma cell lines. A change in the substrate preferences accounts for the aberrant H3K27me3 levels observed in cells bearing EZH2 mutant forms. Indeed, wt EZH2 displays preference for less methylated substrates whereas Y641 and A667G mutants prefer either substrates with higher methylation levels or show equal affinity for all three substrates (H3K73me0, me1, and me2) (McCabe et al., 2012a). Interestingly, these gain-of-function EZH2 variants expressed in GC B-cell lymphomas seem to synergize with *BCL2* deregulation, favoring the progression of these malignancies (Béguelin et al., 2013). On the other hand, overexpression of wt EZH2 has been also reported in B-NHL (Van Kemenade et al., 2001; Visser and Gunster, 2001), with a positive correlation being observed between *EZH2* transcript levels, tumor aggressiveness, and disease prognosis (Abd Al Kader et al., 2013). Taking into account these considerations, it looks reasonable that inhibiting EZH2 activity could result in a potential therapeutic strategy to treat B-NHL.

In this context, many efforts directed to develop highly selective EZH2 inhibitors have been made in the last decade. EZH2 activity was initially targeted by means of the carbocyclic adenosine analog 3-deazaneplanocin A (DZNep), an inhibitor of *S*-adenosylhomocysteine hydrolase. DZNep promotes a global increase in the levels of 5-adensylhomocystein and a further inhibition in the activity of many methyltransferases, including EZH2. Nevertheless, due to its mechanism of action, it resulted to be too unspecific as many other methyltransferases were similarly affected. In 2012, a small chemical compound named El1 with a good capacity to inhibit the Y641 mutant and wt EZH2 form was evaluated for the treatment of DLBCL. This compound was designed as a competitive inhibitor of the EZH2 methyl group donor *S*-adenosyl--methionine (SAM). Unlike DZNep, El1 showed a 10,000-fold selectivity for EZH2 over other HMTs and a 90-fold selectivity over EZH1 methyltransferase. This compound promoted a global decrease in methyl donor availability, leading to a lower global levels of H3K27me3 (Qi et al., 2012). Other subsequent compounds directed specifically against EZH2 are the dual EZH2/1 inhibitors UNC1999, with a potent capacity to suppress H3K27me3 and H3K27me2 levels and to inhibit proliferation of mixed lineage leukemia (MLL)-rearranged cells, and the OR-S1 and OR-S2 inhibitors, which were assessed for the treatment of DLBCL, AML, and MM (Konze et al., 2013; Honma et al., 2017). Later on, EPZ0005687 and GSK126, two selective and SAM-competitive EZH2 inhibitors with a higher inhibitory capacity for the mutant EZH2 form, were developed and tested in DLBCL and FL (McCabe et al., 2012b; Knutson et al., 2014). In 2014, GSK126 entered into phase I clinical trials with B-NHL and MM patients (NCT02082977) (Zeng et al., 2016; Yap et al., 2018), but unfortunately that study had to be discontinued as a consequence of insufficient therapeutic activity, evidencing the need to keep working in the improvement of those inhibitors. Also in 2014, CPI-360 and its more potent and stable analog, CPI-169, were reported to be effective EZH2 inhibitors for the treatment of several B-NHL subtypes (Vaswani et al., 2016). An improved version of these latest, CPI-1205, showed a higher oral bioavailability and was first tested in preclinical studies with xenograft mouse models generated from human B-NHL cell lines and further challenged in phase I trials for the treatment of DLBCL (NCT02395601).

Valemetostat (DS-3201) is another potent wild-type (wt) and mutant EZH1/2 inhibitor that demonstrated a strong anti-proliferative effect against NHL, DLBCL, and T-cell lymphoma (Maruyama et al., 2017). Currently, tazemetostat (EPZ-6438), another SAM competitive inhibitor with a high affinity for the wt and the mutant EZH2 forms, is being evaluated in clinical studies to treat R/R B-NHL and MM patients (NCT03456726) (Knutson et al., 2014; Gulati et al., 2018), reaching an overall response rate of 38% in a phase I clinical trial (Italiano et al., 2018).

Despite first promising results, single-agent treatment with EZH2 inhibitors is in general slightly effective in aggressive lymphomas. Among the possible mechanism(s) of resistance, overactivation of the phosphatidylinositol 3-kinase (PI3K) and mitogen-activated protein kinase (MAPK) pathways has been identified in GSK126-resistant DLBCL cells (Bisserier and Wajapeyee, 2018). Thus, it looks reasonable to prioritize the discovery of new drug combination associating EZH2 inhibitors with other compounds targeting key signaling pathways in order to prevent and/or overcome the occurrence of EZH2i resistance in lymphoid neoplasm with mutated EZH2.

PRMT Inhibitors

A conserved biological mechanism within all eukaryotic organisms, from yeast to higher mammals, is arginine methylation (Migliori et al., 2010). This post-translational modification is mediated by *N*-arginine methyltransferases (PRMTs), which catalyze the transfer of a methyl group, from SAM to the omega nitrogens found in terminus guanidine group of an arginine residue of the side chain. This transfer may occur in one or both nitrogens (Bedford and Clarke, 2009). Among the nine different members of the PRMT family (Schubert et al., 2003), PRMT1 is the major enzyme responsible for arginine methylation followed by PRMT5, according to the observation that PRMT1 and PRMT5 knockout mice die at an early stage during development whereas mice lacking any of the other seven PRMTs are fully viable (Hadjikyriacou et al., 2015). Protein modifications performed by PRMTs are traditionally related to important genetic processes such as DNA repair and gene transcription, among others. More recently, PRMT functions have been linked to carcinogenesis and metastasis, giving to these enzymes the status of potent therapeutic targets in a variety of cancers where they are overexpressed, including colon, breast, prostate, and lung cancers, neuroblastomas, leukemias, and B-cell lymphoma (Yoshimatsu et al., 2011).

Within this family, upregulation of PMRT1 and PRMT5 has been widely associated with hematological malignancies (Greenblatt et al., 2016; Smith et al., 2018). In particular, the expression and function of PMRT5 have been extensively examined during lymphomagenesis, as this enzyme is highly expressed in primary samples and cell lines from different leukemia and lymphoma subtypes, where it promotes the repression of tumor suppressors such as the retinoblastoma proteins. In these models, experimental studies have suggested that PRMT5 upregulation may be caused by overexpression of *MYC* and *NOTCH* oncogenes (Wang et al., 2008). In transformed DLBCL, the *S-methyl-5'-thioadenosine phosphorylase (MTAP)* gene encoding for a critical methionine metabolism enzyme is deleted due to its proximity to the tumor suppressor gene *CDKN2A* (Dreyling et al., 1998), and this phenomenon sensitizes cancer cells to PRMT5 inactivation

(Marjon et al., 2016). A remarkable interplay has also been described between PRMT5 and the *B cell lymphoma 6 (BCL6)* oncogene during the lymphomagenesis in the GC (Lu et al., 2018), suggesting that pharmacological inhibition of arginine methylation could be of special interest in BCL6-driven lymphoma. Regarding PRMT1, an interesting interaction exists between this enzyme and EZH2 in DLBCL-GCB tumors. Indeed, recent works have reported an increase in PRMT1-related histone arginine methylation in DLBCL-GCB cells resistant to EZH2 inhibition, in association with BCL-2 overexpression and modulation of the B-cell receptor (BCR) downstream signaling, supporting the rational association of EZH2 and PRMT1 inhibitors in DLBCL patient samples (Goverdhan et al., 2017).

Among the multiple functional inhibitors that have been developed to target the different members of the family, PRMT1 and PRMT5 small molecule inhibitors have already shown great potential against B-NHL, either alone or upon their combination with other agents. As an illustration, promising results have been obtained with the specific PRMT5 inhibitor EPZ015666 (GSK3235025) when used as single agent in *in vitro* and *in vivo* models of MCL (Chan-Penebre et al., 2015).

TARGETING ERASER EPIGENETIC ENZYMES: HDAC INHIBITORS

By favoring an open chromatin state, histone acetylation allows numerous transcription factors to bind DNA and to activate gene expression. At the same time, acetylated histones increase DNA accessibility to transcriptional activators and counteract the function of transcriptional repressors (McClure et al., 2018). Acetylation of histones and non-histone proteins is regulated through a correct balance between HAT and HDAC activities. Among these enzymes, the most advanced subfamily is human HDACs, which have been classified into four classes according to their sequence homology, activity, and subcellular localization. HDACs 1, 2, 3, and 8 constitute class I. HDAC 4, 5, 6, 7, 9, and 10 belong to class II. Class III includes sirtuin 1 (SIRT1) and sirtuin 7 (SIRT7), two NAD-dependent structurally unrelated protein deacetylases (Minucci and Pelicci, 2006). Finally, class IV is represented by HDAC11. In contrast to class II HDACs which show a heterogeneous expression pattern, class I HDACs are found at particularly high levels in lymphoid cell lines and primary tumors, suggesting a predominant role of these latest in lymphomagenesis. Accordingly, the design of HDAC inhibitors (HDACis) in lymphoid malignancies has been mainly centered on this latest group of enzymes (Gloghini et al., 2009).

Several structurally distinct classes of HDACis have been developed. These molecules can be divided into five chemical groups: hydroxamic acids, cyclic peptides, electrophilic ketones, short-chain fatty acids, and benzamides. Pan-HDACis have the capacity to inhibit almost all HDACs with the exception of class III HDACs and include the hydroxamic acid derivatives vorinostat, givinostat (ITF2357), abexinostat, panobinostat, belinostat, and trichostatin A, the carboxylate sodium butyrate, and the cyclic peptide trapoxin (Bradner et al., 2010; Di Costanzo et al., 2014). Taking into account that HDACs can also modulate the function of several non-histone proteins regulating a number of physiological processes (Lane and Chabner, 2009), and that HDACs can simultaneously exert pro- and anti-leukemic activities (Heideman et al., 2013; Santoro et al., 2013), blocking individual HDACs with isotype-selective inhibitors specific for one or two classes of HDACs might represent a strategy of choice for the treatment of lymphoid tumors. In line with this, the isotype-selective HDACis include the benzamides entinostat (MS-275, SNDX-275) and mocetinostat (MGCD0103) (Fournel et al., 2008; Vannini et al., 2004), the hydroxamic acid derivative rocilinostat (ACY-1215) (Santo et al., 2012), and the cyclic peptide romidepsin, which show preference for HDAC1-6-8, HDAC6, and HDAC1-2, respectively (Lemoine and Younes, 2010). Several HDACis like vorinostat, mocetinostat, and entinostat can be administered orally; conversely, other agents like romidepsin are given intravenously (Batlevi et al., 2016; Mann et al., 2007; Younes et al., 2011; Holkova et al., 2017). By inhibiting the catalytic activity of their target HDAC(s), these compounds impair the formation of HDAC–substrate complexes, thus altering the transcriptomic pattern of the malignant cells as well as the activity of non-histone proteins, ultimately leading to growth arrest, differentiation, and induction of apoptosis (Qiu et al., 2000). Of importance, when compared to their malignant counterparts, healthy tissues are generally unaffected by HDACis (Mai et al., 2005).

A number of preclinical studies have highlighted a role for HDACi therapy in a range of B-cell lymphoma, including DLBCL, HL, and BL, either alone or in combination with other epidrugs such as HMAs, with small molecule agents or with standard chemotherapeutics (Buglio et al., 2008; Kretzner et al., 2011; Kewitz et al., 2012; Ageberg et al., 2013; Klein et al., 2013; Rozati et al., 2016; Garrido Castro et al., 2018). Among these studies, the weak HDACi valproic acid was shown to overcome DLBCL cell resistance to the standard R-CHOP (rituximab, cyclophosphamide, doxorubicin, vincristine, prednisone) chemotherapeutic regimen (Ageberg et al., 2013). In preclinical models of DLBCL and MCL, panobinostat, belinostat, depsipeptide, and vorinostat were shown to evoke tumor growth arrest, differentiation, and/or apoptosis *in vitro* and/or *in vivo*, mediated by the accumulation of DNA damage upon PARP trapping (Valdez et al., 2018), G1 cell cycle arrest consequent to an increase in the expression of the cyclin-dependent kinase inhibitor p21, acetylation of histone H3 (Xue et al., 2016), or transcriptional activation of the BCL-2 family proapoptotic members BIM, BMF, and NOXA (Kalac et al., 2011; Xargay-Torrent et al., 2011).

Based on these preclinical studies, several HDACis have entered clinical trials under different modalities (monotherapies or in combination). Many of these trials have been conducted in DLBCLs, FLs, and HLs using HDACis, either alone or in combinatorial therapies (Watanabe et al., 2010; Stathis et al., 2011; Younes et al., 2012; Oki et al., 2013; Ogura et al., 2014; Chen et al., 2015; Morschhauser et al., 2015) (**Table 2** and **Figure 3**). As monotherapy, HDACis have shown a wide range of response in lymphoma patients, varying from complete remissions (CRs) to no response. In the absence of biomarkers for prediction of clinical outcome, the molecular mechanisms of resistance are poorly understood. Vorinostat was the first proved in relapsed B-NHL patients, including FL, MZL, and MCL. In a phase II study including relapsed FL, non-FL indolent NHL and MCL patients, oral vorinostat showed low levels as a single agent, with the exception of FL, in which an overall response rate (ORR) of 47–49% (referring to the proportion of patients with tumor size reduction of a predefined amount and for a minimum time period) and a CR rate of 23% was observed (Kirschbaum et al., 2011; Ogura et al., 2014). This agent was also tolerated, but displayed limited activity in another phase II trial against R/R DLBCL, with only 1/18 patients presenting complete response (Crump et al., 2008).

With the pan-HDACis abexinostat and quisinostat, or the class-specific mocetinostat and entinostat, the response rates were quite variable (from 12% to 56%), and mostly dependent on the drug and on the lymphoma subtype. The most robust responses were obtained with abexinostat in FL patients (56% ORR). This latest drug showed a unique pharmacokinetic profile and an optimized oral dosing schedule that allowed for a superior anti-tumoral activity. In a recent phase II study with patients with R/R B-NHL or CLL, among the evaluable patients the ORR was 28%, with highest responses observed in FL patients (ORR 56%) and DLBCL (ORR 31%) (Ribrag et al., 2017). A phase II clinical trial with mocetinostat in patients with R/R DLBCL and FL showed promising results (Batlevi et al., 2017), whereas for entinostat only one B-NHL patient has been included in phase II trial; therefore, no conclusion can be made on its efficacy in this subgroup of patients (Kummar et al., 2007).

Similar to DNMTis, the effectiveness of the first-generation HDACis carries significant toxicity and is limited to hematopoietic malignancies, which makes them challenging to combine (Suraweera et al., 2018). It is believed that part of this toxicity may be related to the capacity of HDACis to alter directly the function of many non-histone proteins. Toxicity may also be due to widespread activity across HDAC isoforms; therefore, the focus of second-generation HDACi discovery was to enhance the discrimination over HDAC family members (Galli et al., 2010; Knipstein and Gore, 2011; Younes et al., 2011; Santo et al., 2012; Evens et al., 2016). In this context, targeting HDAC6 was associated to the upregulation of CD20 and consequent enhanced efficacy of anti-CD20 monoclonal antibody therapy (Bobrowicz et al., 2017). Also, tucidinostat (CS055/chidamide), the first oral subtype-selective HDACi, was approved for the treatment of refractory/relapsed PTCL by the China Food and Drug Administration. This compound inhibits HDAC1, HDAC2, HDAC3, and HDAC10, and has entered a phase II clinical trial as single-agent treatment for patients with R/R B-NHL (NCT03245905) based on preliminary evidences of clinical activity in DLBCL (Yang et al., 2018).

Another approach to maximize efficacy with manageable toxicity consists in developing dual inhibitors. In this field, CUDC-907, a novel first-in-class oral small molecule inhibitor of both HDAC (class I and II) and PI3K (class Iα, β, and δ), has demonstrated excellent levels of activity (55% ORR) and tolerability in DLBCL patients in a phase IA clinical trial (Younes et al., 2016). In a second phase IB trial, the drug has been tested in patients with R/R DLBCL and showed a response rate of 37%, with a higher effect in MYC-altered *versus* MYC-unaltered patients (Oki et al., 2017). As a result of these encouraging initial data, this agent is currently being evaluated in a phase II study including DLBCL patients, and also in a phase I trial involving pediatric patients with lymphomas (NCT02674750 and NCT02909777).

TARGETING READER EPIGENETIC ENZYMES

BET Inhibitors

Among the post-translational modifiers with ability to orchestrate chromatin organization, bromodomain (BD)-containing proteins are readers of Ac-K residues at the N-terminal histone tails. They act as scaffolds that enable histone attachment to the chromatin and form active multi-protein transcription complexes, thereby modulating chromatin dynamics and ultimately diversifying gene expression (Filippakopoulos et al., 2012; Chaidos et al., 2015; Smith and Zhou, 2016). This family of proteins contains 46 members, comprising nuclear proteins with HAT or HMT activity, chromatin remodelers, helicases, transcription co-activators, and mediators or scaffold proteins. They are subdivided into eight subfamilies (I to VIII), based on their structure and sequence similarities. Subfamily II is the most studied one and includes the bromodomain-containing proteins mBRDT, BRD2, BRD3, and BRD4 (Padmanabhan et al., 2016). Besides the presence of two bromodomains (BD1 and BD2) that allow acetylated chromatin recognition, these proteins harbor an extra-terminal domain, which is responsible for protein–protein interactions. This bromodomain and extra-terminal (BET) subfamily has thus the capacity to act as protein adaptors facilitating the recruitment of chromatin remodelers and transcription factors for further initiation and elongation of transcription (Delmore et al., 2011; Chaidos et al., 2015; Padmanabhan et al., 2016). Several reports have highlighted the importance of the BET proteins action over DNA enhancers for the regulation of certain oncogenes expression (Lovén et al., 2013). Altogether, these studies make BET proteins attractive therapeutic targets in cancer.

As interfering with this family of proteins may serve as a strategy to address transcription irrespective of the presence of epigenetic mutations, BET proteins inhibitors have been a significant area of focus in the last decade, in cancer but also in inflammation, fibrosis, and heart diseases (Vakoc, 2015). Drug developmental studies have paid special attention to the Ac-K binding sites in the bromodomains, as these deep hydrophobic pockets with conserved asparagine and/or aspartate residues make BET proteins highly druggable (Cox et al., 2016). Indeed, the most common drug targeting approach in this family has been the development of small molecules that could block the lysine-binding pocket and disrupt the interactions between BDs and the Ac-K on chromatins (Smith and Zhou, 2016).

In 2005, a first bromodomain inhibitor developed by the Zhou laboratory, namely NP1, has the ability to target the BD of the P300/CBP-associated factor transcriptional coactivator (Zeng et al., 2005). This step was followed by the discovery in 2006 of MS7972, a weakly binding fragment specific for CREBBP-BD, hindering its binding to acetylated p53 (Sachchidanand et al., 2006). Among BET proteins, the first target considered to be druggable was BRD4, as a pioneering RNAi base unveiled its critical role in the maintenance of AML. In this study, authors found that BRD4-dependent transcriptional activity could be efficiently targeted by the pan-BET thieno-triazolo-1,4-diazepine (+)-JQ1 (Filippakopoulos et al., 2010; Zuber et al., 2011). This class of diazepine-based small molecule inhibitors, which also includes the benzodiazepine I-BET151 (GSK1210151A) (Dawson et al., 2011) and I-BET762 (GSK525762) (Mirguet et al., 2013) (NCT01943851), utilizes the methyltriazolo-diazepine ring system as the acetyl-mimetic. Further studies demonstrated that inhibition of BRD4 by (+)-JQ1 unveiled the MYC downregulation and, consequently, a genome-wide inhibition of its target genes (Filippakopoulos et al., 2010; Delmore et al., 2011). These results underlined significant preclinical activity of this inhibitor in MYC-driven B-NHL, including the aggressive, so-called "double hit" lymphoma (DHL), characterized by simultaneous oncogenic activation of *MYC* and/or *BCL2/BCL6* (Johnson-Farley et al., 2015). Accordingly, (+)-JQ1 could increase survival of mice xenografted with MYC-driven lymphoma, including those ones bearing either TP53 deletions or intrinsic resistant to the topoisomerase II inhibitor etoposide (Hogg et al., 2016).

These promising results from (+)-JQ1 encouraged the development of BET inhibitors with similar chemical structure, including the BRD4 inhibitor CPI203 characterized by a higher bioavailability profile in mice (Normant et al., 2012; King et al., 2013). This agent displayed remarkable efficacy in different preclinical models of B-NHL, either as single agent or in combination with the BCL-2 antagonist venetoclax in DHLs (Esteve-Arenys et al., 2018), in DLBCL-ABC (Ceribelli et al., 2014) and in both ABC and GCB subtypes of DLBCL in combination with blockade of the CXCR4 chemokine receptor (Recasens-zorzo et al., 2018). In these studies, BRD4i activity was mainly related to the blockade of MYC transcriptional program. This is of special interest, as despite its central role in multiple hematological malignancies, including various subtypes of B-NHL, direct targeting of MYC was considered impossible until the demonstration that BET inhibition could regulate MYC activity in varied contexts, thanks to alleviation of BRD4 occupancy on MYC super-enhancers. Importantly, beside MYC, different anti-apoptotic proteins like BCL-2 and MCL-1 are also downregulated, either by direct transcription repression or as a downstream consequence of BRD4 antagonism (Vakoc, 2015). Unlike the expected general effects of BET inhibition in the elongation of transcription of several genes, changes in the expression of only a small subset of genes was observed in cultures and/or animals receiving this therapy, suggesting that bromodomain inhibitors might be suitable modulators of certain disease-associated genes. As an illustration, high levels of BRD4 co-localize in CLL cells with super-enhancer sites of genes and microRNAs belonging to the BCR-mediated signaling pathway with possible tumor-initiating activity, including *miR-21*, *miR-15*, *TCL1*, *IL21R*, and *IL4R*. Accordingly, in a mouse model of CLL, exposure to the BET inhibitor PLX51107 promoted an expression downmodulation of several tumor-associated genes, followed by consistent reduction in tumor burden (Ozer et al., 2018).

According to these promising results, in the last years a number of clinical leads have entered into trials for the treatment of hematological patients. Nevertheless, several side effects have been reported including some bone marrow and gastrointestinal toxicity that has forced to dose discontinuation or reduction. Nowadays, 18 BET inhibitors are being assessed in clinical trials either as single agents or in combination with other compounds (**Table 4**). While the data from various solid tumor trials look mitigated, several BETis including birabresib (OTX015, MK-8628), molibresib (GSK525762), RO6870810/TEN-010, and mivebresib (ABBV-075) have demonstrated remarkable clinical efficacy in myeloproliferative disorders, while other small molecule inhibitors such as PFI-1, BI-894999, FT-1101, INCB-54329, and CPI0610, a pharmacological derivative of CPI203, are currently undergoing human clinical trials in these patients (**Table 3**). Among these different molecules, molibresib has demonstrated an 18.5% ORR in various subtypes of NHLs including a CR in a DLBCL case (Dickinson et al., 2018). CPI0610 has also been evaluated in a phase I clinical trial (NCT01949883) in 64 R/R FL, DLBCL, or HL patients, showing leading to a complete remission in one FL case and in four DLBCL patients (Blum et al., 2018). In addition, the compound INCB057643 is currently being tested in a third phase I trial involving lymphoma patients, including some FL and DLBCL cases. In this evaluation trial, a CR has been achieved in one FL case whereas in two other patients, the disease has been stabilized (Forero-Torres et al., 2017). In the dose-escalation, open-label, phase I study with OTX015,

TABLE 4 | Drug combinations with non-approved epigenetic agents in B-NHL.

Epigenetic drug class	Drug	Agent used in combination	Trial identifier
HDAC inhibitor	CUDC-907	Rituximab, venetoclax, and bendamustine	NCT01742988
	Entinostat	Isotretinoin	NCT00098891
		Molibresib	NCT03925428
	Mocetinostat	Azacitidine	NCT00543582
EZH2 inhibitor	Tazemetostat	Fluconazole, omeprazole, and repaglinide	NCT03028103
		Atezolizumab and obinutuzumab	NCT02220842
		Prednisolone	NCT01897571
	PF 06821497	SOC	NCT03460977
BET inhibitor	Molibresib	Entinostat	NCT03925428
	RO6870810	Venetoclax and rituximab	NCT03255096
INCB057643	Gemcitabine, paclitaxel, rucaparib, abiraterone, ruxolitinib, and azacitidine	NCT02711137	
	FT-1101	Azacitidine	NCT02543879

Source: https://clinicaltrials.gov/.

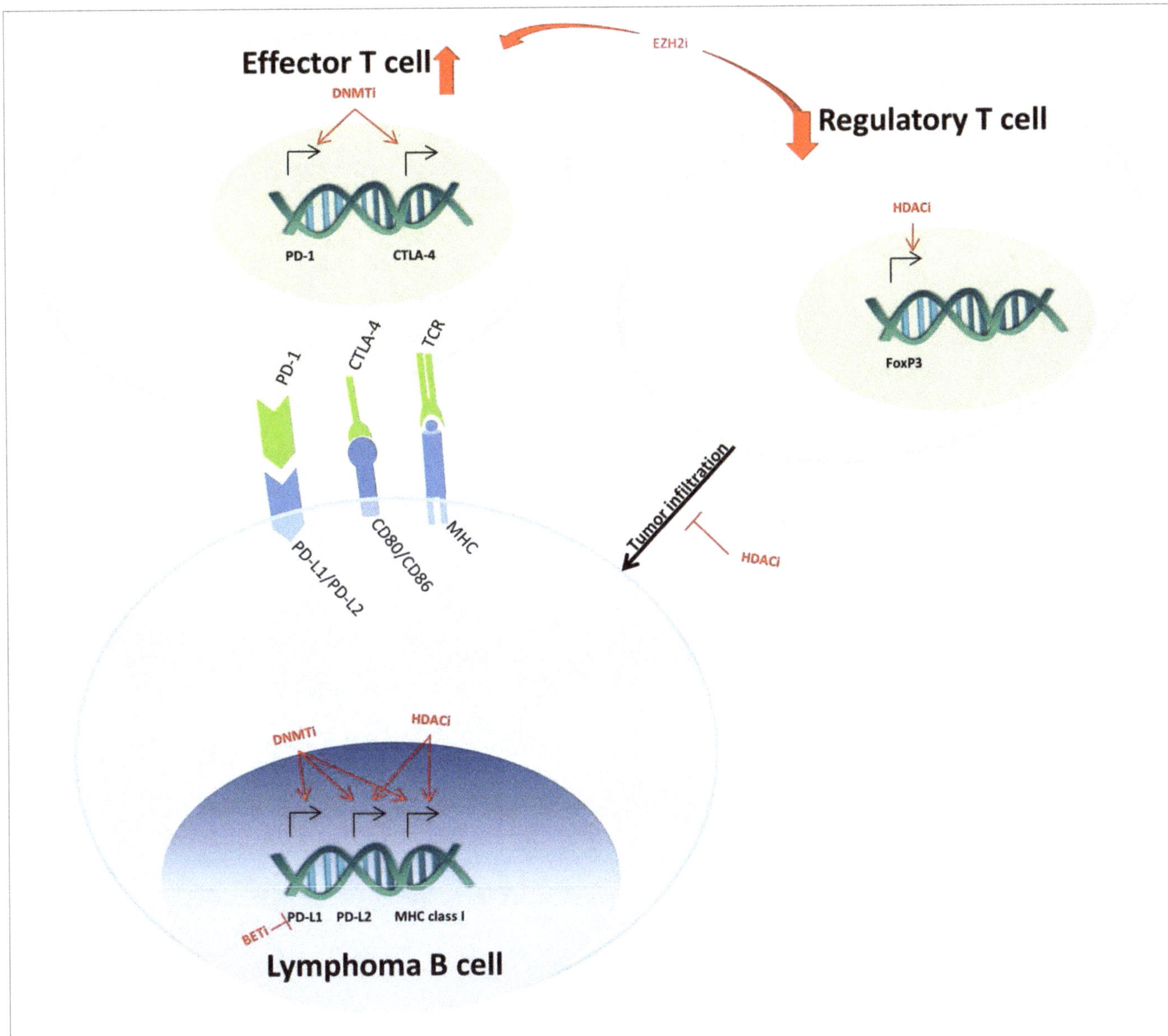

FIGURE 4 | Epigenetic-targeted effects on immuno-oncology mechanisms. In lymphoma B cells, DNMT, HDAC, and BET inhibitors (DNMTi, HDACi, BETi) regulate the expression of MHC class I and PD-1 ligands (PD-L1 and PD-L2). In effector T cells, DNMTi also upregulates the expression of PD-1 and CTLA-4, which leads to T-cell exhaustion. The effects of HDACi on FoxP3 decrease the infiltration of regulatory T cells into the tumor. Lastly, EZH2i decreases the regulatory and increases effector T-cell population in the microenvironment.

a 47% complete remission was reported in 17 DLBCL cases; however, objective responses were seen in only three DLBCL patients and clinical activity in other six B-NHL patients (NCT01713582) (Amorim et al., 2016). More recently, the BETis molibresib, CC-90010, and INCB054329 are being challenged in clinical trials including various hematological malignancies (NCT02431260, NCT01943851, and NCT03220347), but no data have been released so far.

Although at the moment most of the tested compounds aimed at inhibiting BET bromodomains are pan-BET inhibitors, many efforts are being focused in targeting BET proteins in a more specific and novel way. These new approaches include ABBV-744 (which targets bromodomain-containing protein II) (Sheppard et al., 2018), the bivalent BET inhibitors AZD5153 and MT1 (a JQ1-derived BETi) (Rhyasen et al., 2016; Tanaka et al., 2016), and the so-called BET-PROTACs (QCA570, dBET6, BETd-260, and ARV-771) that drive BET proteins to their degradation by proteolysis-targeted chimera (Raina et al., 2016; Winter et al., 2017; Qin et al., 2018). These molecules have shown both to promote apoptosis in MCL-derived cells resistant to the first-in-class Bruton's kinase (BTK) inhibitor ibrutinib as well as to increase survival compared to OTX015-treated MCL xenografts (Sun et al., 2018). Although promising results have been reported for this new generation of BET-targeting agents in preclinical

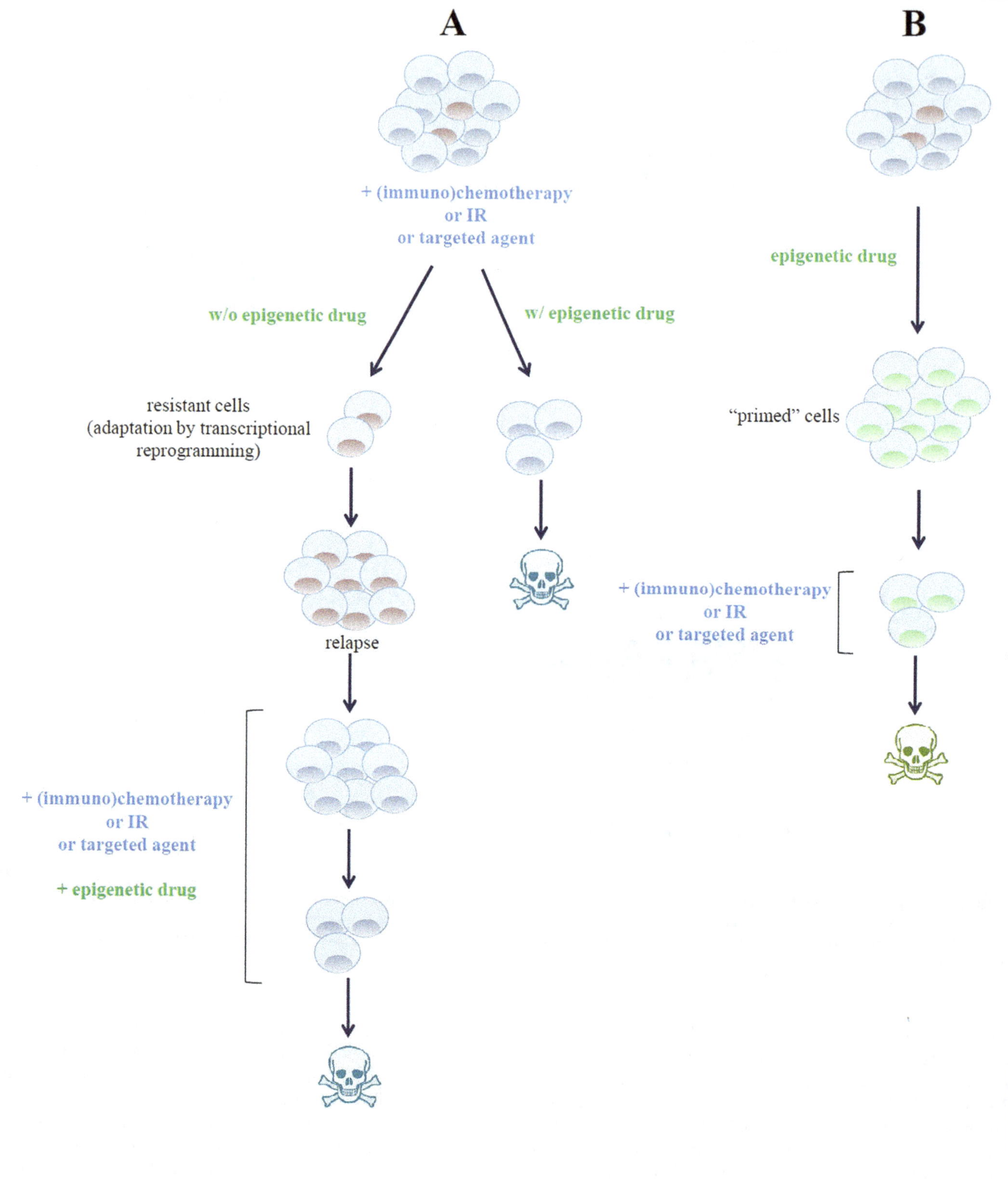

FIGURE 5 | Different strategies for combining drugs targeting epigenetic regulators in B-cell lymphoma. **(A)** Epigenetic drugs can be used to overcome (left axis) or to circumvent (right axis) malignant B-cell resistance to targeted agents or to standard chemotherapeutic regimens. **(B)** Pre-exposure of tumor cells to epigenetic drugs induces profound modifications of cell transcriptional profile, thus priming them to the cytotoxic effect of chemotherapeutic and targeted agents.

studies, their therapeutic window when moving to clinical trials has still to be evaluated.

Non-BET Bromodomain-Containing Proteins: the Histone Acetyltransferase CREB-Binding Protein (CBP)

As previously mentioned, chromatin modifications can regulate several important features of cell function. Among these modifications, histone lysine acetylation is generally associated with activation of gene expression (Shahbazian and Grunstein, 2007). HAT enzymes can deposit acetyl marks on histones and modify chromatin structure. Such marks are also recognized by bromodomains, thus adding a second level of regulation of the transcription process (Kouzarides, 2007). The transcriptional co-activators CBP/p300 are highly homologous, multifunctional proteins that encode a single bromodomain each and possess HAT activity (Chen and Li, 2011; Delvecchio et al., 2013). CBP/p300 act as transcriptional co-factors, involved in the regulation of several biological processes (Dancy and Cole, 2015). Animal studies have shown that CBP and p300 are required for the generation and activity of normal hematopoietic stem cells as well as for adult hematopoietic stem cell maintenance and function (Chan et al., 2011; Rebel et al., 2002). Consequently, CBP ablation has a direct impact on the quiescence, apoptosis, and self-renewal of adult hematopoietic stem cells (Chan et al., 2011) and CBP/p300 have a tumor suppressor role in mice models (Kung et al., 2000; Kang-Decker et al., 2004; Chan et al., 2011). This role of CBP and p300 as tumor suppressors has been also observed in B-NHL, where its inactivating mutation is a common event in FL and DLBCL, providing a rationale for employing drugs with the capacity to modulate acetylation and deacetylation processes in these tumors (Cerchietti et al., 2010; Mullighan et al., 2011; Pasqualucci et al., 2011a).

CHROMATIN REMODELERS: SWI/SNF AND BRG1 AND ARID1

The SWItch/Sucrose Non-Fermentable (SWI/SNF) complex was initially discovered in yeast. It is composed by polypeptides associated with a subset of proteins codified by the SWI1, SWI2, SNF2, SWI3, SWI5, and SWI6 genes (Pazin and Kadonaga, 1997). This complex regulates gene transcription by altering DNA–nucleosome interactions at expenses of ATP consumption, thus facilitating or impeding the accession of the transcription machinery at concrete genomic regions (Workman and Kingston, 2002). Several studies have reported its capacity to repair nucleotide excisions and DNA double-strand breaks by homologous recombination (Chai et al., 2005). The mammalian analog of the SWI/SNF complex (mSWI/SNF) is the BRG1-Associated Factors (BAF) complex. It comprised approximately 11 subunits encoded by 19 distinct genes assembled in different combinations according to its specific molecular mechanism of action, and in a concrete genomic region. Two of the BAF components are the human Brahma (hBRM, also SMARCA2) and the Brahma-related gene 1 (BRG1, also SMARCA4). These proteins are ATPase subunits (Khavari et al., 1993) and either one or the other constitute the core component of the BAF complex. They contain BDs within their structure that recognize and contact acetyl groups present in histone proteins (Wang et al., 1996). Although they share similarities in their domain composition, they interact with different families of transcription factors what confers to them specific functions in the BAF complex (Kadam and Emerson, 2003).

BRG1 has been reported to be the most frequently mutated protein of the BAF complex in cancer. Classically, it has been described as a tumor suppressor gene as inactivating mutations of its protein have been found in numerous solid tumors like breast, lung, gastric, bladder, colon, ovarian cancers, and melanomas (Atlas et al., 2012; Hodis et al., 2012; Jelinic et al., 2014), but also in determined B-NHL subtype like DLBCL and MCL (Cuadros et al., 2017). Concretely, these loss-of-function mutations lead to the upregulation of the pro-survival gene *BCL2L1* in MCL, conferring to this malignancy primary resistance to treatment or eventually relapse after dual exposure to ibutrinib and venetoclax (Agarwal et al., 2019). Other studies described BRG1 as a potent oncogene, since its function was required for AML progression in mice, through its binding to *MYC* enhancer region and consequent aberrant expression of this second oncogene (Shi et al., 2013; Buscarlet et al., 2014).

Beside BRG1, several BRG-/BRM-associated factors (BAF subunits) participate in tumoral progression. Two of these subunits, namely the AT-Rich Interaction Domain 1A (ARID1A/BAF250A) and its homologous ARID1B/BAF250B, contain domains capable of recognizing and binding to AT-enriched genomic regions and C terminus region, stimulating the activation of transcription in a glucocorticoid receptor-dependent manner. The presence of each of them in the complex is mutually exclusive, suggesting specific roles at concrete genomic regions (Wang et al., 2004).

Mutations that truncate the ARID1A sequence and promote its degradation have been widely characterized in endometrial carcinoma (Kandoth et al., 2013), colon cancer (Atlas et al., 2012), stomach cancer (Wang et al., 2011), bladder cancer (Gui et al., 2011), neuroblastoma (Sausen et al., 2013), and pancreatic or hepatocellular carcinoma (Biankin et al., 2012; Fujimoto et al., 2012), evidencing the role of this protein in preventing tumoral progression. Similar to the mutations reported for ARID1A, *truncating mutations have also been identified for ARID1B* although in a lesser frequency and *most of them associated with neurodevelopmental disorders (*Santen et al., 2012*) or neuroblastomas (*Lee et al., 2017*).* ARID1B knockdown has been reported to destabilize the SWI/SNF complex and inhibit cell proliferation in both ARID1A-mutant cancer cell lines and primary tumor cells, suggesting that this protein could constitute an interesting therapeutic target for the treatment of ARID1A-mutant tumors (Helming et al., 2014).

INDIRECT INHIBITION OF EPIGENETIC DYSREGULATION BY IDH INHIBITORS

The enzyme isocitrate dehydrogenase (IDH) catalyzes the conversion of isocitrate into α-ketoglutarate (α-KG) by oxidative decarboxylation using $NADP^+$ as a cofactor. The IDH1 isomer is located in the cytosol and the peroxisomes, whereas IDH2 is found in the mitochondria. IDH enzymes play an important role in the tricarboxylic (TCA) or Krebs' cycle, but are also related with other cellular functions such as the regulation of redox balance (Dang et al., 2016; Dang and Su, 2017). Mutations in *IDH* genes are most commonly found in the R132 codon of *IDH1* and the R172 and R140 codons of *IDH2*, which correspond to evolutionarily conserved residues in the enzyme active site which is critical for substrate binding. Mutant forms of IDH have much lower catalytic activity and are associated with metabolic alterations. More importantly, mutant IDH enzymes gain neomorphic activity as they convert α-KG into 2-hydroxyglutarate (2-HG). Under homeostatic conditions, 2-HG is only produced by errors in catalysis and it is maintained at low levels due to the action of 2-HG-hydroxigenases (2-HGHD). Unlike in bacteria and plants, 2-HG has no known physiological function in mammals (Dang and Su, 2017). 2-HG is structurally similar to α-KG and acts as a competitive inhibitor, blocking the activity of α-KG-dependent dioxygenases. This group of enzymes includes the TET family of hydroxylases, which participate in DNA demethylation, and the JMJ domain-containing histone demethylases (Dang and Su, 2017). The consequent aberrant hypermethylation of both DNA and histones has been associated to a blockade in differentiation in hematopoietic cells (Figueroa et al., 2010; Losman et al., 2013), hepatocytes (Saha et al., 2014), and mesenchymal stem cells (Jin et al., 2015), among other cell types.

Homozygous missense mutations in both *IDH1* or *IDH2* have been described in several cancer types, including glioma, cholangiocarcinoma, and hematological tumors, such as AML and MDS (Dang et al., 2016). Although infrequent, mutations have also been found in lymphoid malignancies like angioimmunoblastic T-cell lymphomas (Cairns et al., 2012) and acute lymphocytic leukemia, both in pediatric (Andersson et al., 2011; Tang et al., 2012) and adult cases (Kang et al., 2009; Abbas et al., 2010; Zhang et al., 2012). Dysregulation of the IDH pathway has also been reported in CLL, as leukemic B cells from these patients show overexpression of IDH1 and lower levels of IDH2 when compared to healthy B cells (Van Damme et al., 2016).

Two IDH inhibitors have been recently approved by the FDA for the treatment of R/R AML in adults. Enasidenib (AG-221) targets IDH2 with R172S, R172K, and R140Q mutations, whereas ivosidenib (AG-120) targets IDH1 with susceptible mutations, such as R132H and R132C (Han et al., 2019). Other non-approved IDH inhibitors are currently in clinical trials involving patients with advanced hematological cancers. Among these molecules, AG-881 is a pan-inhibitor of both IDH1 and IDH2 that can penetrate the blood–brain barrier, while IDH305, FT-2102, and BAY-1436032 are IDH1-specific inhibitors (Dang et al., 2016; Montalban-Bravo and DiNardo, 2018). At the preclinical level, the pharmacological IDH2 inhibitor AGI-6780 displayed synergistic cytotoxicity in MCL and BL cell lines in combination with the proteasome inhibitor carfilzomib, mediated by the blockade of tricarboxylic acid cycle and the decrease in ATP levels, as a consequence of enhanced IDH2 enzymatic inhibition (Bergaggio et al., 2019). Thus, although activating mutations of IDH genes are rare in B-NHL, there may be some room to evaluate, alone or in combination with standard chemotherapy, some of the molecules exhibiting clinical activity in non-lymphoid patients.

COMBINATION INVOLVING EPIGENETIC-TARGETING APPROACHES

Concomitant Targeting of Different Epigenetic Modulators

In recent years, thanks to the many works directed to characterize and get a better understanding of the human epigenome, it came out that more than 50% of the human cancers account for aberrant changes in chromatin organization at certain genomic regions, as a consequence of mutations in enzymes involved in the regulation of chromatin structure (You and Jones, 2012; The Cancer Genome Atlas Research Network, 2013). Changes in the activity of these chromatin modifiers can lead not only to the initiation of a tumor formation process but also to its progression, metastasis, development of drug resistances, and further relapse and/or escape from immune surveillance (Jones et al., 2016). Therapeutic modulation of such alterations can be achieved with chemical compounds that broadly affect the structure of the DNA such as DNMTis, histone HDACis, or BETis (**Figure 4**). While single-agent clinical trials with these compounds have been conducted with some success in MDS or R/R AML patients receiving azacitidine (Scott, 2016; Schuh et al., 2017) or in R/R FL, MZL, and MCL patients treated with vorinostat (Kirschbaum et al., 2011; Ogura et al., 2014), the association of these agents with other compounds has also been tested. As an example, the combinatorial treatment with vorinostat and the sirtuin inhibitor niacinamide was evaluated in R/R NHL and HL cases (NCT00691210) (Amengual et al., 2013), but it achieved a modest efficiency with an ORR below 50% (Olsen et al., 2007). Other examples include the combination of panobinostat with decitabine which displayed synergistic caspase-dependent cell death in DLBCL cells (Kalac et al., 2011) or the combination of romidepsin with the antimetabolite pralatrexate for the treatment of relapsed PTCL (Amengual et al., 2018).

A different therapeutic approach consists in targeting specifically certain chromatin regulatory proteins to achieve a more restricted effect in the transcription of a concrete subset of genes. Promising examples are the inhibition of the DOT1-like (DOT1L) histone H3K79 methyltransferase with pinometostat (EPZ-5676) in adults with MLL/KMT2A-driven leukemia (NCT02141828) (Stein et al., 2018) or inhibition of histone H3K4 and K9 demethylation by the lysine-specific demethylase 1 (LSD1) inhibitor seclidemstat, currently being assessed in clinical trials to treat refractory Ewing sarcomas (NCT03600649).

Combinations with chemical compounds that broadly affect an epigenetic mark and a specific inhibitor of a chromatin-modifying enzyme, such as the EZH2 inhibitor GSK126 and romidepsin, have also been assessed in preclinical studies with DLBCL-GCB cell lines, leading to synergistic tumor growth inhibition effects in mice (Lue et al., 2019). Another example of the strategies currently evaluated in clinical studies is the concomitant treatment of drug-resistant MM with panobinostat and bortezomib (NCT01083602) (Richardson et al., 2016).

Finally, and in concordance with the concept that acquired resistance to chemotherapy is tightly linked to changes in chromatin structure, many efforts have been made in identifying combinational strategies associating different types of cytotoxic drugs to small molecule regulators of chromatin modifiers. As an example, the dinitroazetidine derivative RRx-001 administered in combination with radiation, chemotherapy, or immunotherapies promotes the generation of reactive oxygen and nitrogen species, leading to the oxidation of the cysteines present at the catalytic sites of DNMTs and HDACs. This phenomenon entrains the inhibition in DNMT and HDAC enzymatic activities, with subsequent alterations in the chromatin structure. The therapeutic benefits of this compound have been assessed in phase II clinical trials both as a radio- and chemo-sensitizer, as well as a way to prone tumor response to conventional therapies (NCT02215512, NCT02452970, NCT02096341, NCT02871843) (Oronsky et al., 2017; Zhao et al., 2017).

Combination of Epigenetic Drugs With Other Classes of Anti-Tumoral Drugs

The use of epigenetic agents combined with other anti-tumoral drugs may represent the future of epigenetic-targeted therapies (**Figure 5**). The rationale of such combinations would be, on the one hand, to benefit from the transcriptional effects of targeting epigenome. Indeed, growing evidences are showing that epigenetic therapy, using DNMTi or HDACi, in combination with conventional therapy or immunotherapy, might be an up-and-coming step toward the development of new and efficient cancer treatment strategies (Brahmer et al., 2012; Sharma and Allison 2015; Topalian et al., 2015; Issa et al., 2017). Accordingly, the acquired capacity of tumors to resist chemotherapy is related with changes in the cancer cell's epigenome, which might affect directly the cell cycle and/or some key apoptosis regulators (Fodale et al., 2011).

In a phase I study, Clozel and collaborators proposed a new approach to beaten chemotherapy resistance in DLBCL patients. The authors demonstrated a high rate of complete remission when a 5-day exposure to azacitidine followed by treatment with R-CHOP was employed. Mechanistically, the treatment leads to the demethylation of the chemoresistance-associated gene SMAD1 and subsequent chemosensitization (Clozel et al., 2013). Based on these results, an ongoing phase I study using azacitidine combined with R-CHOP in therapy-naive DLBCL, grade 3B FL, or transformed FL patients is showing promising preliminary results (NCT02343536). Finally, the safety and tolerability of adding oral azacitidine to R-ICE therapy is being evaluated in R/R DLBCL patients (NCT03450343).

Regarding HDACi, *in vitro* studies have demonstrated that this class of agents can synergize with chemotherapy. Globally, these trials have had mixed heterogeneous results. Among the potently successful studies, in indolent B-NHL the vorinostat/rituximab combination exhibited a nice activity with an acceptable safety profile and durable responses (Chen et al., 2015). Ageberg and collaborators also showed that valproic acid sensitizes to CHOP and enhances the CHOP ability to induce apoptosis in DLBCL cell lines (Ageberg et al., 2013). Subsequently, it has been shown in a small set of DLBCL patients that the administration of valproate before R-CHOP treatment upregulated the CD20 levels and increased the efficacy of anti-CD20-based therapy (Damm et al., 2015). Recently, the VALFRID phase I trial (NCT01622439) showed that valproate when added to standard R-CHOP therapy is secure, tolerable, and increases OS in DLBCL patients (Drott et al., 2018). The efficacy of vorinostat combined with cyclophosphamide, etoposide, and prednisone (R-CVEP) was evaluated in aged patients with R/R DLBCL (NCT00667615); however, the R-CVEP association did not reach the criteria for cohort expansion (Straus et al., 2015). Similarly, the combination of vorinostat with R-CHOP was evaluated in the SWOG S0806 phase I/II trial (NCT00972478) without success in DLBCL patients (Persky et al., 2018). Panobinostat was tested in combination with conventional therapy and although the data from the clinical trial NCT01238692 suggested that as a single agent this drug induces a durable response in a subset of R/R DLBCL patients, its combination with rituximab did not improve the response rate (Assouline et al., 2016). Similarly, Barnes and collaborators observed that this combination was effective in a minority of DLBCL patients heavily pretreated (NTC01282476) (Barnes et al., 2018). The combination with immunomodulatory drug (IMiD) lenalidomide was assessed in a phase I/II clinical trial in patients with R/R HL (NCT01460940); however, the combination was not advantageous over single-agent treatment and raised relevant concerns regarding the toxicity (Maly et al., 2017). Finally, preclinical data have shown that belinostat exhibits synergistic cytotoxic activity in DLBCL cell lines when associated to the microtubule-interfering drug vincristine, mediated by the prevention of cell polyploidy (Havas et al., 2016).

Regarding EZH2 inhibitors, combinatorial treatments with tazemetostat and the anti-programmed death-ligand 1 (PDL1) antibody atezolizumab (NCT02220842), prednisone alone, or combined with other components of CHOP regimen are currently being evaluated in patients with refractory DLBCL (NCT02889523) (Gulati et al., 2018). Moreover, combinations with EZH2 inhibitors and inhibitors of the BCR signaling cascade such as ibrutinib, the spleen tyrosine kinase (SYK) inhibitor tamatinib, the mammalian target of rapamycin (mTOR) inhibitor everolimus, or MAPK inhibitor have also been challenged in pre-clinical models of DLBCL (Brach et al., 2017; Lue et al., 2017). Other therapeutic strategies currently assessed in pre-clinical studies for the treatment of MM consist in combining the inhibitor tazemetostat with IMiDs such as lenalidomide or pomalidomide (Dang et al., 2016), glucocorticoid receptor agonists (dexamethasone or prednisolone), proteasome inhibitors (bortezomib or ixazomib) (Drew et al., 2017), or HDACis (Issa et al., 2017).

Finally, in combination with the CDK4/6 inhibitor palbocilib, the BETi JQ1 has shown synergistic activity in MCL *in vitro* and *in vivo* (Sun et al., 2015). Another member of the CDK family, CDK9, is a core component of the assembly of the positive transcription elongation factor complex (P-TEFb), which is recruiting by BRD4.

In relation with this, the BETi BI-894999 shows profound synergy with CDK9 inhibitors alvocidib and LDC000067 in both *in vitro* and *in vivo* models of hematological malignancies (Doroshow et al., 2017). Among other promising combinations, CPI203 combined with the proteasome inhibitor bortezomib or with lenalidomide was particularly efficient in aggressive bortezomib-resistant MCL tumors (Moros et al., 2014), and GS-5829 synergistically interacted with venetoclax or with BCR-interfering agents in preclinical models of DLBCL, MCL, and/or CLL (Bates et al., 2016; Kim et al., 2017).

CONCLUSIONS

Besides the well-known genomic changes, several epigenetic modifications that result in an altered chromatin state and alterations in the DNA methylation status have been described in lymphoma cells. In general, these alterations favor the malignant transformation and/or tumor progression. Among the mechanisms that may apply to several lymphoma entities, epigenetic activation of suppressors of lineage fidelity leads to downregulation of lineage-specific genes, while additional silencing of essential transcription factors through H3K27 trimethylation avoids the restoration of the cell type characteristic expression program. Therefore, there is undoubtedly an important clinical role for epigenetic drugs across the spectrum of lymphoid malignancies, including B-NHL.

In the last decade, the progresses in the awareness of epigenetic changes in lymphoma cells have paved the way for targeted therapy alternatives employing epigenetic drugs. Treatment approaches such as HDAC inhibition or DNMT blockade have shown remarkable activity in specific subsets of lymphoma patients who remained unresponsive to or relapsed after standard therapy. These drugs have already been added into routine use for patients with a particular lymphoma/leukemia subtype and are the most broadly studied now. However, the identification of biomarkers of clinical sensitivity/resistance to these agents is still needed in order to better identify those lymphoma patients suitable for treatment with these drugs, and for the design of rationally based targeted combination therapies. Although several epigenetic drugs can be successfully combined with standard chemotherapy, allowing to decrease the chemotherapy doses and to limit toxicities and adverse effects, co-administration of two epigenetic modulators like DNA hypomethylating agents and HDAC inhibitors, for example, can also show synergistic molecular effects, resulting in increased antitumor activity.

In the light of the large number of drugs currently in clinical development in B-NHL patients, selection of the most relevant targeted therapies will be extremely important to move the field ahead. Epigenetic drugs with more specific targets, such as EZH2 inhibitors or BRD4 inhibitors, but also the newer epigenetic agents like PRMT5 and IDH inhibitors, are also of great interest, as demonstrated by a particularly rapid translation from bench to bedside within the past 5 years.

Despite these considerable advances in epigenetic drug therapy in B-cell lymphoma, there is still some way to go before reaching a complete overview of the complex landscape of the epigenetic modifications occurring during the lymphomagenesis, and much work is still to be done to improve the rationale use of epigenetic drugs in lymphoma patients. According to the promising reports from several trials involving the newest agents and the most innovative drug combinations in B-NHL patients with relapse disease, it seems that we are entering a very exciting era for the field of epigenetics in lymphoma.

AUTHOR CONTRIBUTIONS

MR, DR, MA, MF and GR made a substantial contribution to all aspects of the preparation of this manuscript.

FUNDING

The authors received financial support from Fondo de Investigación Sanitaria PI15/00102 and PI18/01383, European Regional Development Fund (ERDF) "Una manera de hacer Europa" (to GR). The authors received fundings from TG Therapeutics and Celgene Corp to support researches unrelated to the present work. Funders were involved neither in the design, nor in the writing of this review.

REFERENCES

Abbas, S., Lugthart, S., Kavelaars, F. G., Schelen, A., Koenders, J. E., Zeilemaker, A., et al. (2010). Acquired mutations in the genes encoding IDH1 and IDH2 both are recurrent aberrations in acute myeloid leukemia: prevalence and prognostic value. *Blood* 116, 2122–2126. doi: 10.1182/blood-2009-11-250878

Abd Al Kader, L., Oka, T., Takata, K., Sun, X., Sato, H., Murakami, I., et al. (2013). In aggressive variants of non-Hodgkin lymphomas, Ezh2 is strongly expressed and polycomb repressive complex PRC1.4 dominates over PRC1.2. *Virchows Arch.* 463, 697–711. doi: 10.1007/s00428-013-1428-y

Agarwal, R., Chan, Y. C., Tam, C. S., Hunter, T., Vassiliadis, D., Teh, C. E., et al. (2019). Dynamic molecular monitoring reveals that SWI-SNF mutations mediate resistance to ibrutinib plus venetoclax in mantle cell lymphoma. *Nat. Med.* 25, 119–129. doi: 10.1038/s41591-018-0243-z

Ageberg, M., Rydström, K., Relander, T., and Drott, K. (2013). The histone deacetylase inhibitor valproic acid sensitizes diffuse large B-cell lymphoma cell lines to CHOP-induced cell death. *Am. J. Transl. Res.* 5, 170–183.

Agrawal, K., Das, V., Vyas, P., and Hajdúch, M. (2018). Nucleosidic DNA demethylating epigenetic drugs —A comprehensive review from discovery to clinic. *Pharmacol. Ther.* 188, 45–89. doi: 10.1016/j.pharmthera.2018.02.006

Almstedt, M., Blagitko-Dorfs, N., Duque-Afonso, J., Karbach, J., Pfeifer, D., Jäger, E., et al. (2010). The DNA demethylating agent 5-aza-2'2'-deoxycytidine induces expression of NY-ESO-1 and other cancer/testis antigens in myeloid leukemia cells. *Leuk. Res.* 34, 899–905. doi: 10.1016/j.leukres.2010.02.004

Amara, K., Ziadi, S., Hachana, M., Soltani, N., Korbi, S., and Trimeche, M. (2010). DNA methyltransferase DNMT3b protein overexpression as a prognostic factor in patients with diffuse large B-cell lymphomas. *Cancer Sci.* 101, 1722–1730. doi: 10.1111/j.1349-7006.2010.01569.x

Amengual, J. E., Clark-Garvey, S., Kalac, M., Scotto, L., Marchi, E., Neylon, E., et al. (2013). Sirtuin and pan-class I/II deacetylase (DAC) inhibition is synergistic in preclinical models and clinical studies of lymphoma. *Blood.* 122, 2104–2113. doi: 10.1182/blood-2013-02-485441

Amengual, J. E., Lichtenstein, R., Lue, J., Sawas, A., Deng, C., Lichtenstein, E., et al. (2018). A phase 1 study of romidepsin and pralatrexate reveals marked activity in relapsed and refractory T-cell lymphoma. *Blood.* 131, 397–407. doi: 10.1182/blood-2017-09-806737

Amorim, S., Stathis, A., Gleeson, M., Iyengar, S., Magarotto, V., Leleu, X., et al. (2016). Bromodomain inhibitor OTX015 in patients with lymphoma or multiple myeloma: a dose-escalation, open-label, pharmacokinetic, phase 1 study. *Lancet Haematol.* 3, e196–e204. doi: 10.1016/S2352-3026(16)00021-1

Andersson, A. K., Miller, D. W., Lynch, J. A., Lemoff, A. S., Cai, Z., Pounds, S. B., et al. (2011). IDH1 and IDH2 mutations in pediatric acute leukemia. *Leukemia* 25, 1570–1577. doi: 10.1038/leu.2011.133

Assouline, S. E., Nielsen, T. H., Yu, S., Alcaide, M., Chong, L., MacDonald, D., et al. (2016). Phase 2 study of panobinostat with or without rituximab in relapsed diffuse large B-cell lymphoma. *Blood.* 128, 185–194. doi: 10.1182/blood-2016-02-699520

Atlas, T. C. G. N., Muzny, D., Bainbridge, M., Chang, K., Dinh, H., Drummond, J., et al. (2012). Comprehensive molecular characterization of human colon and rectal cancer. *Nature* 487, 330–337. doi: 10.1038/nature11252

Avramis, V. I., Powell, W. C., and Mecum, R. A. (1989). Cellular metabolism of 5,6-dihydro-5-azacytidine and its incorporation into DNA and RNA of human lymphoid cells CEM/O and CEM/dCk(-). (-). *Cancer Chemother. Pharmacol.* 24, 155–160. doi: 10.1007/BF00300235

Azad, N., Zahnow, C. A., Rudin, C. M., and Baylin, S. B. (2013). The future of epigenetic therapy in solid tumours - —Lessons from the past. *Nat. Rev. Clin. Oncol.* 10, 256–266. doi: 10.1038/nrclinonc.2013.42

Barnes, J. A., Redd, R., Fisher, D. C., Hochberg, E. P., Takvorian, T., Neuberg, D., et al. (2018). Panobinostat in combination with rituximab in heavily pretreated diffuse large B-cell lymphoma: Results of a phase II study. *Hematol. Oncol.* 36, 633–637. doi: 10.1002/hon.2515

Bates, J., Kusam, S., Tannheimer, S., Clarke, A., Kenney, T., Breckenridge, D., et al. (2016). Combination of the BET inhibitor GS-5829 and a BCL2 inhibitor resulted in broader activity in DLBCL and MCL cell lines. *Blood* 128, 5104.

Batlevi, C. L., Crump, M., Andreadis, C., Rizzieri, D., Assouline, S. E., Fox, S., et al. (2017). A phase 2 study of mocetinostat, a histone deacetylase inhibitor, in relapsed or refractory lymphoma. *Br. J. Haematol.* 178, 434–441. doi: 10.1111/bjh.14698

Batlevi, C. L., Kasamon, Y., Bociek, R. G., Lee, P., Gore, L., Copeland, A., et al. (2016). ENGAGE- 501: Phase II study of entinostat (SNDX-275) in relapsed and refractory Hodgkin lymphoma. *Haematologica* 101, 968–975. doi: 10.3324/haematol.2016.142406

Beà, S., Ribas, M., Hernandez, J. M., Bosch, F., Pinyol, M., Hernández, L., et al. (1999). Increased number of chromosomal imbalances and high-level DNA amplifications in mantle cell lymphoma are associated with blastoid variants. *Blood* 93, 4365–4374.

Beà, S., Valdés-Mas, R., Navarro, A., Salaverria, I., Martín-Garcia, D., Jares, P., et al. (2013). Landscape of somatic mutations and clonal evolution in mantle cell lymphoma. *Proc. Natl. Acad. Sci. U. S. A.* 110,18250–18255. doi: 10.1073/pnas.1314608110

Bedford, M. T., and Clarke, S. G. (2009). Protein arginine methylation in mammals: Who, what, and why. *Mol. Cell* 33, 1–13. doi: 10.1016/j.molcel.2008.12.013

Béguelin, W., Popovic, R., Teater, M., Jiang, Y., Bunting, K. L., Rosen, M., et al. (2013). EZH2 is required for germinal center formation and somatic EZH2 mutations promote lymphoid transformation. *Cancer Cell* 23, 677–692. doi: 10.1016/j.ccr.2013.04.011

Beisler, J. A., Abbasi, M. M., and Driscoll, J. S. (1979). Synthesis and antitumor activity of 5-azacytosine arabinoside. *J. Med. Chem.* 22, 1230–1234. doi: 10.1021/jm00196a015

Belinsky, S. A., Klinge, D. M., Stidley, C. A., Issa, J. P., Herman, J. G., March, T. H., et al. (2003). Inhibition of DNA methylation and histone deacetylation prevents murine lung cancer. *Cancer Res.* 63, 7089–7093.

Ben-Kasus, T., Ben-Zvi, Z., Marquez, V. E., Kelley, J. A., and Agbaria, R. (2005). Metabolic activation of zebularine, a novel DNA methylation inhibitor, in human bladder carcinoma cells. *Biochem. Pharmacol.* 70, 121–133. doi: 10.1016/j.bcp.2005.04.010

Berdasco, M., and Esteller, M. (2010). Aberrant epigenetic landscape in cancer: How cellular identity goes awry. *Dev. Cell.* 19, 698–711. doi: 10.1016/j.devcel.2010.10.005

Bergaggio, E., Riganti, C., Garaffo, G., Vitale, N., Mereu, E., Bandini, C., et al. (2019). IDH2 inhibition enhances proteasome inhibitor responsiveness in hematological malignancies. *Blood* 133, 156 LP–15 167. doi: 10.1182/blood-2018-05-850826

Beumer, J. H., Parise, R. A., Newman, E. M., Doroshow, J. H., Synold, T. W., Lenz, H. J., et al. (2008). Concentrations of the DNA methyltransferase inhibitor 5-fluoro-2′- deoxycytidine (FdCyd) and its cytotoxic metabolites in plasma of patients treated with FdCyd and tetrahydrouridine (THU). *Cancer Chemother. Pharmacol.* 62, 363–368. doi: 10.1007/s00280-007-0603-8

Biankin, A. V., Waddell, N., Kassahn, K. S., Gingras, M. C., Muthuswamy, L. B., Johns, A. L., et al. (2012). Pancreatic cancer genomes reveal aberrations in axon guidance pathway genes. *Nature.* 491, 399–405. doi: 10.1038/nature11547

Bisserier, M., and Wajapeyee, N. (2018). Mechanisms of resistance to ezh2 inhibitors in diffuse large B-cell lymphomas. *Blood.* 131, 2125–2137. doi: 10.1182/blood-2017-08-804344

Blum, K. A., Abramson, J., Maris, M., Flinn, I., Goy, A., Mertz, J., et al. (2018). 41OA phase I study of CPI-0610, a bromodomain and extra terminal protein (BET) inhibitor in patients with relapsed or refractory lymphoma. *Ann. Oncol.* 29, A410. doi: 10.1093/annonc/mdy048

Blum, K. A., Liu, Z., Lucas, D. M., Chen, P., Xie, Z., Baiocchi, R., et al. (2010). Phase I trial of low dose decitabine targeting DNA hypermethylation in patients with chronic lymphocytic leukaemia and non-Hodgkin lymphoma: dose-limiting myelosuppression without evidence of DNA hypomethylation. *Br. J. Haematol.* 29, 410. doi: 10.1111/j.1365-2141.2010.08213.x

Bobrowicz, M., Dwojak, M., Pyrzynska, B., Stachura, J., Muchowicz, A., Berthel, E., et al. (2017). HDAC6 inhibition upregulates CD20 levels and increases the efficacy of anti-CD20 monoclonal antibodies. *Blood* 130, 1628–1638. doi: 10.1182/blood-2016-08-736066

Brach, D., Johnston-blackwellBlackwell, D., Drew, A., Lingaraj, T., Motwani, V., Warholic, N. M., et al. (2017). EZH2 inhibition by tazemetostat results in altered dependency on B-cell activation signaling in DLBCL 16. *Mol. Cancer Ther.* 2586-2597. doi: 10.1158/1535-7163.MCT-16-0840

Bracken, A. P., and Helin, K. (2009). Polycomb group proteins: Navigators of lineage pathways led astray in cancer. *Nat. Rev. Cancer* 9, 773–784. doi: 10.1038/nrc2736

Bradner, J. E., West, N., Grachan, M. L., Greenberg, E. F., Haggarty, S. J., Warnow, T., et al. (2010). Chemical phylogenetics of histone deacetylases. *Nat. Chem. Biol.* 6, 238–243. doi: 10.1038/nchembio.313

Brahmer, J. R., Tykodi, S. S., Chow, L. Q. M., Hwu, W.-J., Topalian, S. L., Hwu, P., et al. (2012). Safety and activity of anti-PD-L1 antibody in patients with advanced cancer. *N. Engl. J. Med.* 366, 2455–2465. doi: 10.1056/NEJMoa1200694

Buglio, D., Georgakis, G. V., Hanabuchi, S., Arima, K., Khaskhely, N. M., Liu, Y.-J., et al. (2008). Vorinostat inhibits STAT6-mediated TH2 cytokine and TARC production and induces cell death in Hodgkin lymphoma cell lines. *Blood* 112, 1424–1433. doi: 10.1182/blood-2008-01-133769

Buscarlet, M., Krasteva, V., Ho, L., Simon, C., Hébert, J., Wilhelm, B., et al. (2014). Essential role of BRG, the ATPase subunit of BAF chromatin remodeling complexes, in leukemia maintenance. *Blood.* 123, 1720–1728. doi: 10.1182/blood-2013-02-483495

Cairns, R. A., Iqbal, J., Lemonnier, F., Kucuk, C., De Leval, L., Jais, J.-P., et al. (2012). IDH2 mutations are frequent in angioimmunoblastic T-cell lymphoma. *Blood* 119, 1901–1903. doi: 10.1182/blood-2011-11-391748

Campo, E., Swerdlow, S. H., Harris, N. L., Pileri, S., Stein, H., and Jaffe, E. S. (2011). The 2008 WHO classification of lymphoid neoplasms and beyond: evolving concepts and practical applications. *Blood* 117, 5019–5032. doi: 10.1182/blood-2011-01-293050

Cerchietti, L. C., Hatzi, K., Caldas-Lopes, E., Yang, S. N., Figueroa, M. E., Morin, R. D., et al. (2010). BCL6 repression of EP300 in human diffuse large B cell lymphoma cells provides a basis for rational combinatorial therapy. *J. Clin. Invest.* 120, 4569–4582. doi: 10.1172/JCI42869

Ceribelli, M., Kelly, P. N., Shaffer, A. L., Wright, G. W., Xiao, W., Yang, Y., et al. (2014). Blockade of oncogenic IκB kinase activity in diffuse large B-cell lymphoma by bromodomain and extraterminal domain protein inhibitors. *Proc. Natl. Acad. Sci. U. S. A.* 111, 11365–11370. doi: 10.1073/pnas.1411701111

Chai, B., Huang, J., Cairns, B. R., and Laurent, B. C. (2005). Distinct roles for the RSC and Swi/Snf ATP-dependent chromatin remodelers in DNA double-strand break repair. *Genes Dev.* 19, 1656–1661. doi: 10.1101/gad.1273105

Chaidos, A., Caputo, V., and Karadimitris, A. (2015). Inhibition of bromodomain and extra-terminal proteins (BET) as a potential therapeutic approach in haematological malignancies: Emerging preclinical and clinical evidence. *Ther. Adv. Hematol.* 6, 128–141. doi: 10.1177/2040620715576662

Chan-Penebre, E., Kuplast, K. G., Majer, C. R., Boriack-Sjodin, P. A., Wigle, T. J., Johnston, L. D., et al. (2015). A selective inhibitor of PRMT5 with in vivo and in vitro potency in MCL models. *Nat. Chem. Biol.* 11, 432–437. doi: 10.1038/nchembio.1810

Chan, W.-I., Hannah, R. L., Dawson, M. A., Pridans, C., Foster, D., Joshi, A., et al. (2011). The transcriptional coactivator Cbp regulates self-renewal and differentiation in adult hematopoietic stem cells. *Mol. Cell. Biol.* 31, 5046–5060. doi: 10.1128/MCB.05830-11

Chen, J., and Li, Q. (2011). Life and death of transcriptional co-activator p300. *Epigenetics*. 6, 957–961. doi: 10.4161/epi.6.8.16065

Chen, R., Frankel, P., Popplewell, L., Siddiqi, T., Ruel, N., Rotter, A., et al. (2015). A phase II study of vorinostat and rituximab for treatment of newly diagnosed and relapsed/refractory indolent non-Hodgkin lymphoma. *Haematologica* 100, 357–362. doi: 10.3324/haematol.2014.117473

Cheng, J. C., Yoo, C. B., Weisenberger, D. J., Chuang, J., Wozniak, C., Liang, G., et al. (2004). Preferential response of cancer cells to zebularine. *Cancer Cell.* 6, 151–158. doi: 10.1016/j.ccr.2004.06.023

Chiappinelli, K. B., Strissel, P. L., Desrichard, A., Li, H., Henke, C., Akman, B., et al. (2015). Inhibiting DNA methylation causes an interferon response in cancer via dsRNA including endogenous retroviruses. *Cell.* 162, 974–986. doi: 10.1016/j.cell.2015.07.011

Choi, W. J., Chung, H. J., Chandra, G., Alexander, V., Zhao, L. X., Lee, H. W., et al. (2012). Fluorocyclopentenyl-cytosine with broad spectrum and potent antitumor activity. *J. Med. Chem.* 55, 4521–4525. doi: 10.1021/jm3004009

Chuang, J. C., Warner, S. L., Vollmer, D., Vankayalapati, H., Redkar, S., Bearss, D. J., et al. (2010). S110, a 5-aza-2'2'-deoxycytidine-containing dinucleotide, is an effective DNA methylation inhibitor in vivo and can reduce tumor growth. *Mol. Cancer Ther.* 9, 1443–1450. doi: 10.1158/1535-7163.MCT-09-1048

Clozel, T., Yang, S. N., Elstrom, R. L., Tam, W., Martin, P., Kormaksson, M., et al. (2013). Mechanism-based epigenetic chemosensitization therapy of diffuse large B-cell lymphoma. *Cancer Discov.* 3, 1002–1019. doi: 10.1158/2159-8290.CD-13-0117

Cox, O. B., Krojer, T., Collins, P., Monteiro, O., Talon, R., Bradley, A., et al. (2016). A poised fragment library enables rapid synthetic expansion yielding the first reported inhibitors of PHIP(2), an atypical bromodomain. *Chem. Sci.* 7, 2322–2330. doi: 10.1039/C5SC03115J

Crump, M., Coiffier, B., Jacobsen, E. D., Sun, L., Ricker, J. L., Xie, H., et al. (2008). Phase II trial of oral vorinostat (suberoylanilide hydroxamic acid) in relapsed diffuse large-B-cell lymphoma. *Ann. Oncol. Off. J. Eur. Soc. Med. Oncol.* 19, 964–969. doi: 10.1093/annonc/mdn031

Cuadros, M., Sánchez-Martín, V., Herrera, A., Baliñas, C., Martín-Padrón, J., Boyero, L., et al. (2017). BRG1 regulation by miR-155 in human leukemia and lymphoma cell lines. *Clin. Transl. Oncol.* 19, 1010–1017. doi: 10.1007/s12094-017-1633-2

Damm, J. K., Gordon, S., Ehinger, M., Jerkeman, M., Gullberg, U., Hultquist, A., et al. (2015). Pharmacologically relevant doses of valproate upregulate CD20 expression in three diffuse large B-cell lymphoma patients in vivo. *Exp. Hematol. Oncol.* 4, eColection. doi: 10.1186/2162-3619-4-4

Dancy, B. M., and Cole, P. A. (2015). Protein lysine acetylation by p300/CBP. *Chem. Rev.* 115, 2419–2452. doi: 10.1021/cr500452k

Dang, L., and Su, S.-S. M. (2017). Isocitrate dehydrogenase mutation and (R)-2-hydroxyglutarate: from basic discovery to therapeutics development. *Annu. Rev. Biochem.* 86, 305–331. doi: 10.1146/annurev-biochem-061516-044732

Dang, L., Yen, K. E., and Attar, E. C. (2016). IDH mutations in cancer and progress toward development of targeted therapeutics. *Ann. Oncol.* 27, 599–608. doi: 10.1093/annonc/mdw013

Dawson, M. A., Prinjha, R. K., Dittmann, A., Giotopoulos, G., Bantscheff, M., Chan, W. I., et al. (2011). Inhibition of BET recruitment to chromatin as an effective treatment for MLL-fusion leukaemia. *Nature.* 478, 529–533. doi: 10.1038/nature10509

De, S., Shaknovich, R., Riester, M., Elemento, O., Geng, H., Kormaksson, M., et al. (2013). Aberration in DNA methylation in B-cell lymphomas has a complex origin and increases with disease severity. *PLoS Genet.* 9, e1003137. doi: 10.1371/journal.pgen.1003137

Delmore, J. E., Issa, G. C., Lemieux, M. E., Rahl, P. B., Shi, J., Jacobs, H. M., et al. (2011). BET bromodomain inhibition as as a therapeutic strategy to target c-Myc. *Cell* 146, 904–917. doi: 10.1016/j.cell.2011.08.017

Delvecchio, M., Gaucher, J., Aguilar-Gurrieri, C., Ortega, E., and Panne, D. (2013). Structure of the p300 catalytic core and implications for chromatin targeting and HAT regulation. *Nat. Struct. Mol. Biol.* 20, 1040–1046. doi: 10.1038/nsmb.2642

Di Costanzo, A., Del Gaudio, N., Migliaccio, A., and Altucci, L. (2014). Epigenetic drugs against cancer: an evolving landscape. *Arch. Toxicol.* 88, 1651–1668. doi: 10.1007/s00204-014-1315-6

Dickinson, M., Kamdar, M., Huntly, B. J., Larrea, C. F., De, Cordoba, R., Mateos, M.-V., et al. (2018). A phase I study of molibresib (GSK525762), a selective bromodomain (BRD) and extra terminal protein (BET) inhibitor: results from part 1 of a phase I/II open label single agent study in subjects with non-Hodgkin's lymphoma (NHL). *Blood* 132, 1682–1682. doi: 10.1182/BLOOD-2018-99-117089

Doroshow, D. B., Eder, J. P., and LoRusso, P. M. (2017). BET inhibitors: a novel epigenetic approach. *Ann. Oncol.* 28, 1776–1787. doi: 10.1093/annonc/mdx157

Drew, A. E., Motwani, V., Campbell, J. E., Tang, C., Smith, J. J., Chesworth, R., et al. (2017). Abstract 5060: activity of the EZH2 inhibitor tazemetostat as a monotherapy and in combination with multiple myeloma therapies in preclinical models. *Cancer Res.* 77, n5060. doi: 10.1158/1538-7445.AM2017-5060

Dreyling, M. H., Roulston, D., Bohlander, S. K., Vardiman, J., and Olopade, O. I. (1998). Codeletion of CDKN2 and MTAP genes in a subset of non-Hodgkin's lymphoma may be associated with histologic transformation from low-grade to diffuse large-cell lymphoma. *Genes Chromosomes Cancer* 22, 72–78. doi: 10.1002/(SICI)1098-2264(199805)22:1<72::AID-GCC10>3.3.CO;2-G

Drott, K., Hagberg, H., Papworth, K., Relander, T., and Jerkeman, M. (2018). Valproate in combination with rituximab and CHOP as first-line therapy in diffuse large B-cell lymphoma (VALFRID). *Blood Adv.* 26, 1386–1392. doi: 10.1182/bloodadvances.2018019240

Dubois, S., Viailly, P., Mareschal, S., Bohers, E., Bertrand, P., Ruminy, P., et al. (2016). Next-generation sequencing in diffuse large B-cell lymphoma highlights molecular divergence and therapeutic opportunities : a LYSA study *Clin. Cancer Res.* 22, 2919–2929. doi: 10.1158/1078-0432.CCR-15-2305

Egger, G., Aparicio, A. M., Escobar, S. G., and Jones, P. A. (2007). Inhibition of histone deacetylation does not block resilencing of p16 after 5-aza-2'-deoxycytidine treatment. *Cancer Res.* 67, 346–356. doi: 10.1158/0008-5472.CAN-06-2845

Esteller, M., Corn, P. G., Baylin, S. B., and Herman, J. G. (2001). A gene hypermethylation profile of human cancer. *Cancer Res.* 61, 3225–3229.

Esteve-Arenys, A., Valero, J. G., Chamorro-Jorganes, A., Gonzalez, D., Rodriguez, V., Dlouhy, I., et al. (2018). The BET bromodomain inhibitor CPI203 overcomes resistance to ABT-199 (venetoclax) by downregulation of BFL-1/A1 in in vitro and in vivo models of MYC+/BCL2+ double hit lymphoma. *Oncogene.* 37, 1830–1844. doi: 10.1038/s41388-017-0111-1

Evens, A. M., Balasubramanian, S., Vose, J. M., Harb, W., Gordon, L. I., Langdon, R., et al. (2016). A phase I/II multicenter, open-label study of the oral histone deacetylase inhibitor abexinostat in relapsed/refractory lymphoma. *Clin. Cancer Res.* 22, 1059–1066. doi: 10.1158/1078-0432.CCR-15-0624

Fenaux, P., Mufti, G. J., Hellstrom-Lindberg, E., Santini, V., Finelli, C., Giagounidis, A., et al. (2009). Efficacy of azacitidine compared with that of conventional care regimens in the treatment of higher-risk myelodysplastic syndromes: A randomised, open-label, phase III study. *Lancet Oncol.* 10, 223–232. doi: 10.1016/S1470-2045(09)70003-8

Ferrari, K. J., Scelfo, A., Jammula, S., Cuomo, A., Barozzi, I., Stützer, A., et al. (2014). Polycomb-dependent H3K27me1 and H3K27me2 regulate active transcription and enhancer fidelity. *Mol. Cell.* 53, 49–62. doi: 10.1016/j.molcel.2013.10.030

Figueroa, M. E., Abdel-Wahab, O., Lu, C., Ward, P. S., Patel, J., Shih, A., et al. (2010). Leukemic IDH1 and IDH2 mutations result in a hypermethylation phenotype, disrupt TET2 function, and impair hematopoietic differentiation. *Cancer Cell* 18, 553–567. doi: 10.1016/j.ccr.2010.11.015

Filippakopoulos, P., Picaud, S., Mangos, M., Keates, T., Lambert, J. P., Barsyte-Lovejoy, D., et al. (2012). Histone recognition and large-scale structural analysis of the human bromodomain family. *Cell.* 149, 214–231. doi: 10.1016/j.cell.2012.02.013

Filippakopoulos, P., Qi, J., Picaud, S., Shen, Y., Smith, W. B., Fedorov, O., et al. (2010). Selective inhibition of BET bromodomains. *Nature.* 468, 1067–1073. doi: 10.1038/nature09504

Flavahan, W. A., Gaskell, E., and Bernstein, B. E. (2017). Epigenetic plasticity and the hallmarks of cancer. *Science.* 357, p.eaal2380. doi: 10.1126/science.aal2380

Flesner, B. K., Kumar, S. R., and Bryan, J. N. (2014). 6-Thioguanine and zebularine down-regulate DNMT1 and globally demethylate canine malignant lymphoid cells. *BMC Vet. Res.* 10, 290. doi: 10.1186/s12917-014-0290-8

Fodale, V., Pierobon, M., Liotta, L., and Petricoin, E. (2011). Mechanism of cell adaptation: When and how do cancer cells develop chemoresistance? *Cancer J.* 17, 89–95. doi: 10.1097/PPO.0b013e318212dd3d

Forero-Torres, A., Rosen, S., Smith, D. C., Lesser, G., Peguero, J., Gupta, S., et al. (2017). Preliminary results from an ongoing phase 1/2 Study of INCB057643, a bromodomain and extraterminal (BET) protein inhibitor, in patients (pts) with advanced malignancies. *Blood* 130, 4048.

Fournel, M., Bonfils, C., Hou, Y., Yan, P. T., Trachy-Bourget, M.-C., Kalita, A., et al. (2008). MGCD0103, a novel isotype-selective histone deacetylase inhibitor, has broad spectrum antitumor activity in vitro and in vivo. *Mol. Cancer Ther.* 7, 759–768. doi: 10.1158/1535-7163.MCT-07-2026

Fujimoto, A., Totoki, Y., Abe, T., Boroevich, K. A., Hosoda, F., Nguyen, H. H., et al. (2012). Whole-genome sequencing of liver cancers identifies etiological influences on mutation patterns and recurrent mutations in chromatin regulators. *Nat. Genet.* 44, 760–764. doi: 10.1038/ng.2291

Galli, M., Salmoiraghi, S., Golay, J., Gozzini, A., Crippa, C., Pescosta, N., et al. (2010). A phase II multiple dose clinical trial of histone deacetylase inhibitor ITF2357 in patients with relapsed or progressive multiple myeloma. *Ann. Hematol.* 89, 185–190. doi: 10.1007/s00277-009-0793-8

Garrido Castro, P., van Roon, E. H. J., Pinhanços, S. S., Trentin, L., Schneider, P., Kerstjens, M., et al. (2018). The HDAC inhibitor panobinostat (LBH589) exerts in vivo anti-leukaemic activity against MLL-rearranged acute lymphoblastic leukaemia and involves the RNF20/RNF40/WAC-H2B ubiquitination axis. *Leukemia* 32, 323–331. doi: 10.1038/leu.2017.216

Ghoshal, K., Datta, J., Majumder, S., Bai, S., Kutay, H., Motiwala, T., et al. (2005). 5-Aza-deoxycytidine induces selective degradation of DNA methyltransferase 1 by a proteasomal pathway that requires the KEN box, bromo-adjacent homology domain, and nuclear localization signal. *Mol. Cell. Biol.* 25, 4727–4741. doi: 10.1128/MCB.25.11.4727-4741.2005

Gloghini, A., Buglio, D., Khaskhely, N. M., Georgakis, G., Orlowski, R. Z., Neelapu, S. S., et al. (2009). Expression of histone deacetylases in lymphoma: implication for the development of selective inhibitors. *Br. J. Haematol.* 147, 515–525. doi: 10.1111/j.1365-2141.2009.07887.x

Goodyear, O., Agathanggelou, A., Novitzky-Basso, I., Siddique, S., McSkeane, T., Ryan, G., et al. (2010). Induction of a CD8+ T-cell response to the MAGE cancer testis antigen by combined treatment with azacitidine and sodium valproate in patients with acute myeloid leukemia and myelodysplasia. *Blood.* 116, 1908–1918. doi: 10.1182/blood-2009-11-249474

Goverdhan, A., Lee, H.-H., Havranek, O., Davis, R. E., and Hung, M.-C., (2017). "Abstract 13: PRMT1 as a therapeutic target in diffuse large B-cell lymphoma," in *Epigenetics* (American Association for Cancer Research), 13–13. doi: 10.1158/1557-3265.HEMMAL17-13

Greenblatt, S. M., Liu, F., and Nimer, S. D. (2016). Arginine methyltransferases in normal and malignant hematopoiesis. *Exp. Hematol.* 44, 435–441. doi: 10.1016/j.exphem.2016.03.009

Groudine, M., Eisenman, R., and Weintraub, H. (1981). Chromatin structure of endogenous retroviral genes and activation by an inhibitor of DNA methylation. *Nature.* 292, 311–317. doi: 10.1038/292311a0

Gui, Y., Guo, G., Huang, Y., Hu, X., Tang, A., Gao, S., et al. (2011). Frequent mutations of chromatin remodeling genes in transitional cell carcinoma of the bladder. *Nat. Genet.* 44, 17–19. doi: 10.1038/ng.907

Gulati, N., Béguelin, W., and Giulino-Roth, L. (2018). Enhancer of zeste homolog 2 (EZH2) inhibitors. *Leuk. Lymphoma* 59, 1574–1585. doi: 10.1080/10428194.2018.1430795

Hadjikyriacou, A., Yang, Y., Espejo, A., Bedford, M. T., and Clarke, S. G. (2015). Unique features of human protein arginine methyltransferase 9 (PRMT9) and its substrate RNA splicing factor SF3B2. *J. Biol. Chem.* 290, 16723–16743. doi: 10.1074/jbc.M115.659433

Haferlach, C., Dicker, F., Schnittger, S., Kern, W., and Haferlach, T. (2007). Comprehensive genetic characterization of CLL: a study on 506 cases analysed with chromosome banding analysis, interphase FISH, IgV(H) status and immunophenotyping. *Leukemia* 21, 2442–2451. doi: 10.1038/sj.leu.2404935

Han, M., Jia, L., Lv, W., Wang, L., and Cui, W. (2019). Epigenetic enzyme mutations: role in tumorigenesis and molecular inhibitors. *Front. Oncol.* 9, 1–9. doi: 10.3389/fonc.2019.00194

Hassler, M. R., Schiefer, A.-I., and Egger, G. (2013). Combating the epigenome: epigenetic drugs against non-Hodgkin's lymphoma. *Epigenomics* 5, 397–415. doi: 10.2217/epi.13.39

Havas, A. P., Rodrigues, K. B., Bhakta, A., Demirjian, J. A., Hahn, S., Tran, J., et al. (2016). Belinostat and vincristine demonstrate mutually synergistic cytotoxicity associated with mitotic arrest and inhibition of polyploidy in a preclinical model of aggressive diffuse large B cell lymphoma. *Cancer Biol. Ther.* 17, 1240–1252. doi: 10.1080/15384047.2016.1250046

Heideman, M. R., Wilting, R. H., Yanover, E., Velds, A., de Jong, J., Kerkhoven, R. M., et al. (2013). Dosage-dependent tumor suppression by histone deacetylases 1 and 2 through regulation of c-Myc collaborating genes and p53 function. *Blood* 121, 2038–2050. doi: 10.1182/blood-2012-08-450916

Helming, K. C., Wang, X., Wilson, B. G., Vazquez, F., Haswell, J. R., Manchester, H. E., et al. (2014). ARID1B is a specific vulnerability in ARID1A-mutant cancers. *Nat. Med.* 20, 251–254. doi: 10.1038/nm.3480

Hermann, A., Goyal, R., and Jeltsch, A. (2004). The Dnmt1 DNA-(cytosine-C5)-methyltransferase methylates DNA processively with high preference for hemimethylated target sites. *J. Biol. Chem.* 279, 48350–48359. doi: 10.1074/jbc.M403427200

Herviou, L., Kassambara, A., Boireau, S., Robert, N., Requirand, G., Vincent, L., et al. (2016). Targeting EZH2 in multiple myeloma could be promising for a subgroup of MM patients in combination with IMiDs. *Blood.* 128, 311.

Hodis, E., Watson, I. R., Kryukov, G. V., Arold, S. T., Imielinski, M., Theurillat, J. P., et al. (2012). A landscape of driver mutations in melanoma. *Cell.* 150, 251–266. doi: 10.1016/j.cell.2012.06.024

Hogarth, L. A., Redfern, C. P. F., Teodoridis, J. M., Hall, A. G., Anderson, H., Case, M. C., et al. (2008). The effect of thiopurine drugs on DNA methylation in relation to TPMT expression. *Biochem. Pharmacol.* 76, 1024–1035. doi: 10.1016/j.bcp.2008.07.026

Hogg, S. J., Newbold, A., Vervoort, S. J., Cluse, L. A., Martin, B. P., Gregory, G. P., et al. (2016). BET inhibition induces apoptosis in aggressive B-cell lymphoma via epigenetic regulation of BCL-2 family members. *Mol. Cancer Ther.* 15, 2030–2041. doi: 10.1158/1535-7163.MCT-15-0924

Holkova, B., Yazbeck, V., Kmieciak, M., Bose, P., Ma, S., Kimball, A., et al. (2017). A phase 1 study of bortezomib and romidepsin in patients with chronic lymphocytic leukemia/small lymphocytic lymphoma, indolent B-cell lymphoma, peripheral T-cell lymphoma, or cutaneous T-cell lymphoma. *Leuk. Lymphoma* 58, 1349–1357. doi: 10.1080/10428194.2016.1276287

Honma, D., Kanno, O., Watanabe, J., Kinoshita, J., Hirasawa, M., Nosaka, E., et al. (2017). Novel orally bioavailable EZH1/2 dual inhibitors with greater antitumor efficacy than an EZH2 selective inhibitor. *Cancer Sci.* 108, 2069–2078. doi: 10.1111/cas.13326

Horsman, D. E., Gascoyne, R. D., Coupland, R. W., Coldman, A. J., and Adomat, S. A. (1995). Comparison of cytogenetic analysis, Southern analysis, and polymerase chain reaction for the detection of t(14; 18) in follicular lymphoma. *Am. J. Clin. Pathol.* 103, 472–478. doi: 10.1093/ajcp/103.4.472

Hunter, Z. R., Xu, L., Yang, G., Zhou, Y., Liu, X., Cao, Y., et al. (2014). The genomic landscape of Waldenström macroglobulinemia is characterized by highly recurring MYD88 and WHIM-like CXCR4 mutations, and small somatic deletions associated with B-cell lymphomagenesis. *Blood* 123, 1637–1646. doi: 10.1182/blood-2013-09-525808

Issa, J. P. J., Roboz, G., Rizzieri, D., Jabbour, E., Stock, W., O'Connell, C., et al. (2015). Safety and tolerability of guadecitabine (SGI-110) in patients with myelodysplastic syndrome and acute myeloid leukaemia: A multicentre, randomised, dose-escalation phase 1 study. *Lancet Oncol.* 16, 1099–1110. doi: 10.1016/S1470-2045(15)00038-8

Issa, M. E., Takhsha, F. S., Chirumamilla, C. S., Perez-Novo, C., Vanden Berghe, W., and Cuendet, M. (2017). Epigenetic strategies to reverse drug resistance in heterogeneous multiple myeloma. *Clin. Epigenetics.* 9, 17. doi: 10.1186/s13148-017-0319-5

Italiano, A., Soria, J., Toulmonde, M., Michot, J., Lucchesi, C., Varga, A., et al. (2018). Articles Tazemetostat , an EZH2 inhibitor , in relapsed or refractory B-cell non-Hodgkin lymphoma and advanced solid tumours : a first-in-human, open-label , phase 1 study 2045, *Lancet Oncol.* 1–11. doi: 10.1016/S1470-2045(18)30145-1

Jelinic, P., Mueller, J. J., Olvera, N., Dao, F., Scott, S. N., Shah, R., et al. (2014). Recurrent SMARCA4 mutations in small cell carcinoma of the ovary. *Nat. Genet.* 46, 424–426. doi: 10.1038/ng.2922

Jin, Y., Elalaf, H., Watanabe, M., Tamaki, S., Hineno, S., Matsunaga, K., et al. (2015). Mutant IDH1 dysregulates the differentiation of mesenchymal stem cells in association with gene-specific histone modifications to cartilage- and bone-related genes. *PLoS One* 10, 1–15. doi: 10.1371/journal.pone.0131998

Johnson-Farley, N., Veliz, J., Bhagavathi, S., and Bertino, J. R. (2015). ABT-199, a BH3 mimetic that specifically targets Bcl-2, enhances the antitumor activity of chemotherapy, bortezomib and JQ1 in ""double hit"" lymphoma cells. *Leuk. Lymphoma* 56, 2146–2152. doi: 10.3109/10428194.2014.981172

Jones, P. A., Issa, J. P. J., and Baylin, S. (2016). Targeting the cancer epigenome for therapy. *Nat. Rev. Genet.* 17, 630–641. doi: 10.1038/nrg.2016.93

Jones, P. A., and Taylor, S. M. (1980). Cellular differentiation, cytidine analogs and DNA methylation. *Cell.* 20, 85–93. doi: 10.1016/0092-8674(80)90237-8

Juttermann, R., Li, E., and Jaenisch, R. (2006). Toxicity of 5-aza-2'2'-deoxycytidine to mammalian cells is mediated primarily by covalent trapping of DNA methyltransferase rather than DNA demethylation. *Proc. Natl. Acad. Sci.* 91, 11797–11801. doi: 10.1073/pnas.91.25.11797

Kadam, S., and Emerson, B. M. (2003). Transcriptional specificity of human SWI/SNF BRG1 and BRM chromatin remodeling complexes. *Mol. Cell.* 1, 177–189. doi: 10.1016/S1097-2765(03)00034-0

Kalac, M., Scotto, L., Marchi, E., Amengual, J., Seshan, V. E., Bhagat, G., et al. (2011). HDAC inhibitors and decitabine are highly synergistic and associated with unique gene-expression and epigenetic profiles in models of DLBCL. *Blood* 118, 5506–5516. doi: 10.1182/blood-2011-02-336891

Kandoth, C., Schultz, N., Cherniack, A. D., Akbani, R., Liu, Y., Shen, H., et al. (2013). Integrated genomic characterization of endometrial carcinoma. *Nature.* 497, 67–73. doi: 10.1038/nature12113

Kang-Decker, N., Tong, C., Boussouar, F., Baker, D. J., Xu, W., Leontovich, A. A., et al. (2004). Loss of CBP causes T cell lymphomagenesis in synergy with p27 Kip1 insufficiency. *Cancer Cell.* 5, 177–189. doi: 10.1016/S1535-6108(04)00022-4

Kang, M. R., Kim, M. S., Oh, J. E., Kim, Y. R., Song, S. Y., Seo, S., et al. (2009). Mutational analysis of IDH1 codon 132 in glioblastomas and other common cancers. *Int. J. Cancer* 125, 353–355. doi: 10.1002/ijc.24379

Karpf, A. R. (2004). Limited gene activation in tumor and normal epithelial cells treated with the DNA methyltransferase Inhibitor 5-aza-2'2'-deoxycytidine. *Mol. Pharmacol.* 65, 18–27. doi: 10.1124/mol.65.1.18

Kewitz, S., Bernig, T., and Staege, M. S. (2012). Histone deacetylase inhibition restores cisplatin sensitivity of Hodgkin's lymphoma cells. *Leuk. Res.* 36, 773–778. doi: 10.1016/j.leukres.2012.02.021

Khavari, P. A., Peterson, C. L., Tamkun, J. W., Mendel, D. B., and Crabtree, G. R. (1993). BRG1 contains a conserved domain of the SWI2/SNF2 family necessary for normal mitotic growth and transcription. *Nature.* 366, 170–174. doi: 10.1038/366170a0

Kim, E., Ten Hacken, E., Clarke, A., Keating, M. J., Wierda, W. G., Ferrajoli, A., et al. (2017). The clinical BET inhibitor, GS-5829, is active against chronic lymphocytic leukemia as single agent and in combination with B-cell receptor signaling inhibitors. *Blood* 130, 3844.

Kinders R. J., Wang, L., Kummar, K. S., Balasubramanian, P., Zhu, W., Parchment, R. E., et al. (2011). Investigation of 5-fluorodeoxycytidine with tetrahydrouracil as a demethylation regimen in solid tumors. *Mol. Cancer Ther.* 10, A106. doi: 10.1158/1535-7163.TARG-11-A106

King, B., Trimarchi, T., Reavie, L., Xu, L., Mullenders, J., Ntziachristos, P., et al. (2013). The ubiquitin ligase FBXW7 modulates leukemia-initiating cell activity by regulating MYC stability. *Cell* 153, 1552–1566. doi: 10.1016/j.cell.2013.05.041

Kirschbaum, M., Frankel, P., Popplewell, L., Zain, J., Delioukina, M., Pullarkat, V., et al. (2011). Phase II study of vorinostat for treatment of relapsed or refractory indolent non-Hodgkin's lymphoma and mantle cell lymphoma. *J. Clin. Oncol.* 29, 1198–1203. doi: 10.1200/JCO.2010.32.1398

Klein, J. M., Henke, A., Sauer, M., Bessler, M., Reiners, K. S., Engert, A., et al. (2013). The histone deacetylase inhibitor LBH589 (panobinostat) modulates the crosstalk of lymphocytes with Hodgkin lymphoma cell lines. *PLoS One* 8, e79502. doi: 10.1371/journal.pone.0079502

Knipstein, J., and Gore, L. (2011). Entinostat for treatment of solid tumors and hematologic malignancies. *Expert Opin. Investig. Drugs* 20, 1455–1467. doi: 10.1517/13543784.2011.613822

Knutson, S. K., Kawano, S., Minoshima, Y., Warholic, N. M., Huang, K.-C., Xiao, Y., et al. (2014). Selective inhibition of EZH2 by EPZ-6438 leads to potent antitumor activity in EZH2-mutant non-Hodgkin lymphoma. *Mol. Cancer Ther.* 13, 842–854. doi: 10.1158/1535-7163.MCT-13-0773

Konze, K. D., Ma, A., Li, F., Barsyte-Lovejoy, D., Parton, T., MacNevin, C. J., et al. (2013). An orally bioavailable chemical probe of the lysine methyltransferases EZH2 and EZH1. *ACS Chem. Biol.* 8, 1324–1334. doi: 10.1021/cb400133j

Kouzarides, T. (2007). Chromatin modifications and their function. *Cell.* 128, 693–705. doi: 10.1016/j.cell.2007.02.005

Kretzner, L., Scuto, A., Dino, P. M., Kowolik, C. M., Wu, J., Ventura, P., et al. (2011). Combining histone deacetylase inhibitor vorinostat with aurora kinase inhibitors enhances lymphoma cell killing with repression of c-Myc, hTERT, and microRNA levels. *Cancer Res.* 71, 3912–3920. doi: 10.1158/0008-5472.CAN-10-2259

Kummar, S., Gutierrez, M., Gardner, E. R., Donovan, E., Hwang, K., Chung, E. J., et al. (2007). Phase I trial of MS-275, a histone deacetylase inhibitor, administered weekly in refractory solid tumors and lymphoid malignancies. *Clin. Cancer Res.* 13, 5411–5417. doi: 10.1158/1078-0432.CCR-07-0791

Kung, A. L., Rebel, V. I., Bronson, R. T., Ch'ng, L. E., Sieff, C. A., Livingston, D. M., et al. (2000). Gene dose-dependent control of hematopoiesis and hematologic tumor suppression by CBP. *Genes Dev.* 14, 172–177.

Lai, A. Y., Mav, D., Shah, R., Grimm, S. A., Phadke, D., Hatzi, K., et al. (2013). DNA methylation profiling in human B cells reveals immune regulatory elements and epigenetic plasticity at Alu elements during B-cell activation. *Genome Res.* 12, 2030–2041. doi: 10.1101/gr.155473.113

Landau, D. A., Tausch, E., Taylor-Weiner, A. N., Stewart, C., Reiter, J. G., Bahlo, J., et al. (2015). Mutations driving CLL and their evolution in progression and relapse. *Nature* 526, 525–530. doi: 10.1038/nature15395

Lane, A. A., and Chabner, B. A. (2009). Histone deacetylase inhibitors in cancer therapy. *J. Clin. Oncol.* 27, 5459–5468. doi: 10.1200/JCO.2009.22.1291

Lee, S. H., Kim, J.-S., Zheng, S., Huse, J. T., Bae, J. S., Lee, J. W., et al. (2017). ARID1B alterations identify aggressive tumors in neuroblastoma. *Oncotarget.* 8, 45943–45950. doi: 10.18632/oncotarget.17500

Lemoine, M., and Younes, A. (2010). Histone deacetylase inhibitors in the treatment of lymphoma. *Discov. Med.* 10, 462–470.

Li, L. H., Olin, E. J., Buskirk, H. H., and Reineke, L. M. (1970). Cytotoxicity and mode of action of 5-azacytidine on L1210 leukemia. *Cancer Res.* 30, 2760–2769.

Li, Y., Nagai, H., Ohno, T., Yuge, M., Hatano, S., Ito, E., et al. (2002). Aberrant DNA methylation of p57 KIP2 gene in the promoter region in lymphoid malignancies of B-cell phenotype. *Blood.* 100, 2572–2577. doi: 10.1182/blood-2001-11-0026

Lohr, J. G., Stojanov, P., Lawrence, M. S., Auclair, D., Chapuy, B., Sougnez, C., et al. (2012). Discovery and prioritization of somatic mutations in diffuse large B-cell lymphoma (DLBCL) by whole-exome sequencing. *Proc. Natl. Acad. Sci. U. S. A.* 109, 3879–3884. doi: 10.1073/pnas.1121343109

Losman, J.-A., Looper, R., Koivunen, P., Lee, S., Schneider, R. K., McMahon, C., et al. (2013). (R)-2-hydroxyglutarate is sufficient to promote leukemogenesis and its effects are reversible. *Science (80-.).* 339, 1621–1625. doi: 10.1126/science.1231677

Lovén, J., Hoke, H. A., Lin, C. Y., Lau, A., Orlando, D. A., Vakoc, C. R., et al. (2013). Selective inhibition of tumor oncogenes by disruption of super-enhancers. *Cell.* 153, 320–334. doi: 10.1016/j.cell.2013.03.036

Lu, X., Fernando, T. M., Lossos, C., Yusufova, N., Liu, F., Fontán, L., et al. (2018). PRMT5 interacts with the BCL6 oncoprotein and is required for germinal center formation and lymphoma cell survival. *Blood* 132, 2026–2039. doi: 10.1182/blood-2018-02-831438

Lübbert, M., Suciu, S., Hagemeijer, A., Rüter, B., Platzbecker, U., Giagounidis, A., et al. (2016). Decitabine improves progression-free survival in older high-risk MDS patients with multiple autosomal monosomies: results of a subgroup analysis of the randomized phase III study 06011 of the EORTC Leukemia cooperative group and german MDS study group. *Ann. Hematol.* 95, 191–199. doi: 10.1007/s00277-015-2547-0

Lue, J. K., Prabhu, S. A., Liu, Y., Gonzalez, Y., Verma, A., Mundi, P. S., et al. (2019). Precision targeting with EZH2 and HDAC inhibitors in epigenetically dysregulated lymphomas. *Clin. Cancer Res.* 25, 5271–5283. doi: 10.1158/1078-0432.CCR-18-3989

Lue, J. K., Prabhu, S. A., Liu, Y., Verma, A., Elemento, O., and Amengual, J. E. (2017). Dual inhibition of EZH2 and HDAC is synergistic in EZH2 Dysregulated Lymphomas. *Hematol. Oncol.* 35, 254–255. doi: 10.1002/hon.2438_120

Mai, A., Massa, S., Rotili, D., Cerbara, I., Valente, S., Pezzi, R., et al. (2005). Histone deacetylation in epigenetics: an attractive target for anticancer therapy. *Med. Res. Rev.* 25, 261–309. doi: 10.1002/med.20024

Maly, J. J., Christian, B. A., Zhu, X., Wei, L., Sexton, J. L., Jaglowski, S. M., et al. (2017). A phase I/II trial of panobinostat in combination with lenalidomide in patients with relapsed or refractory Hodgkin lymphoma. *Clin. Lymphoma Myeloma Leuk.* 17, 347–353. doi: 10.1016/j.clml.2017.05.008

Mann, B. S., Johnson, J. R., Cohen, M. H., Justice, R., and Pazdur, R. (2007). FDA approval summary: Vorinostat for treatment of advanced primary cutaneous T-cell lymphoma. *Oncologist* 12, 1247–1252. doi: 10.1634/theoncologist.12-10-1247

Marjon, K., Cameron, M. J., Quang, P., Clasquin, M. F., Mandley, E., Kunii, K., et al. (2016). MTAP deletions in cancer create vulnerability to targeting of the MAT2A/PRMT5/RIOK1 axis. *Cell Rep.* 15, 574–587. doi: 10.1016/j.celrep.2016.03.043

Marquard, L., Poulsen, C. B., Gjerdrum, L. M., de Nully Brown, P., Christensen, I. J., Jensen, P. B., et al. (2009). Histone deacetylase 1, 2, 6 and acetylated histone H4 in B- and T-cell lymphomas. *Histopathology* 54, 688–698. doi: 10.1111/j.1365-2559.2009.03290.x

Maruyama, D., Tobinai, K., Makita, S., Ishida, T., Kusumoto, S., Ishitsuka, K., et al. (2017). First-in-human study of the EZH1/2 dual inhibitor DS-3201b in patients with relapsed or refractory non-Hodgkin lymphomas — Preliminary results. *Blood.* 130, 4070.

McCabe, M. T., Graves, A. P., Ganji, G., Diaz, E., Halsey, W. S., Jiang, Y., et al. (2012a). Mutation of A677 in histone methyltransferase EZH2 in human B-cell lymphoma promotes hypertrimethylation of histone H3 on lysine 27 (H3K27). *Proc. Natl. Acad. Sci. U. S. A.* 109, 2989–2994. doi: 10.1073/pnas.1116418109

McCabe, M. T., Ott, H. M., Ganji, G., Korenchuk, S., Thompson, C., Van Aller, G. S., et al. (2012b). EZH2 inhibition as a therapeutic strategy for lymphoma with EZH2-activating mutations. *Nature.* 492, 108–112. doi: 10.1038/nature11606

McClure, J. J., Li, X., and Chou, C. J. (2018). Advances and challenges of HDAC inhibitors in cancer therapeutics. *Adv. Cancer Res.* 183–211. doi: 10.1016/bs.acr.2018.02.006

McGarvey, K. M., Fahrner, J. A., Greene, E., Martens, J., Jenuwein, T., and Baylin, S. B. (2006). Silenced tumor suppressor genes reactivated by DNA demethylation do not return to a fully euchromatic chromatin state. *Cancer Res.* 66, 3541–3549. doi: 10.1158/0008-5472.CAN-05-2481

Meissner, A. (2010). Epigenetic modifications in pluripotent and differentiated cells. *Nat. Biotechnol.* 28, 1079–1088. doi: 10.1038/nbt.1684

Migliori, V., Phalke, S., Bezzi, M., and Guccione, E. (2010). Arginine/lysine-methyl/methyl switches: biochemical role of histone arginine methylation in transcriptional regulation. *Epigenomics* 2, 119–137. doi: 10.2217/epi.09.39

Minucci, S., and Pelicci, P. G. (2006). Histone deacetylase inhibitors and the promise of epigenetic (and more) treatments for cancer. *Nat. Rev. Cancer* 6, 38–51. doi: 10.1038/nrc1779

Mirguet, O., Gosmini, R., Toum, J., Clément, C. A., Barnathan, M., Brusq, J.-M., et al. (2013). Discovery of epigenetic regulator I-BET762: lead optimization to afford a clinical candidate inhibitor of the BET bromodomains. *J. Med. Chem.* 56, 7501–7515. doi: 10.1021/jm401088k

Montalban-Bravo, G., and DiNardo, C. D. (2018). The role of IDH mutations in acute myeloid leukemia. *Futur. Oncol.* 14, 979–993. doi: 10.2217/fon-2017-0523

Morin, R. D., Johnson, N. A., Severson, T. M., Mungall, A. J., An, J., Goya, R., et al. (2010). Somatic mutations altering EZH2 (Tyr641) in follicular and diffuse large B-cell lymphomas of germinal-center origin. *Nat. Genet.* 42, 181–185. doi: 10.1038/ng.518

Morin, R. D., Mendez-Lago, M., Mungall, A. J., Goya, R., Mungall, K. L., Corbett, R. D., et al. (2011). Frequent mutation of histone-modifying genes in non-Hodgkin lymphoma. *Nature* 476, 298–303. doi: 10.1038/nature10351

Moros, A., Rodríguez, V., Saborit-Villarroya, I., Montraveta, A., Balsas, P., Sandy, P., et al. (2014). Synergistic antitumor activity of lenalidomide with the BET bromodomain inhibitor CPI203 in bortezomib-resistant mantle cell lymphoma. *Leukemia* 28, 2049–2059. doi: 10.1038/leu.2014.106

Morschhauser, F., Terriou, L., Coiffier, B., Bachy, E., Varga, A., Kloos, I., et al. (2015). Phase 1 study of the oral histone deacetylase inhibitor abexinostat in patients with Hodgkin lymphoma, non-Hodgkin lymphoma, or chronic lymphocytic leukaemia. *Invest. New Drugs* 33, 423–431. doi: 10.1007/s10637-015-0206-x

Mullighan, C. G., Zhang, J., Kasper, L. H., Lerach, S., Payne-Turner, D., Phillips, L. A., et al. (2011). CREBBP mutations in relapsed acute lymphoblastic leukaemia. *Nature.* 471, 235–239. doi: 10.1038/nature09727

Munshi, P. N., Lubin, M., and Bertino, J. R. (2014). 6-Thioguanine: a drug with unrealized potential for cancer therapy. *Oncologist.* 19, 760–765. doi: 10.1634/theoncologist.2014-0178

Newman, E. M, Morgan, R. J., Kummar, S., Beumer, J. H., Blanchard, M. S., Ruel, C., et al. (2015). A phase I, pharmacokinetic, and pharmacodynamic evaluation of the DNA methyltransferase inhibitor 5-fluoro-2'2'-deoxycytidine, administered with tetrahydrouridine. *Cancer Chemother. Pharmacol.* 75, 537–547.

Normant, E., Cummings, R., Bellon, S., Bailey, C., Albrecht, B., Hewitt, M., et al. (2012). "Abstract LB-237: in vitro and in vivo characterization of CPI-267203, a potent inhibitor of bromodomain-containing proteins," in *Experimental and molecular therapeutics* (American Association for Cancer Research), LB-237-LB-237. doi: 10.1158/1538-7445.AM2012-LB-237

Ogura, M., Ando, K., Suzuki, T., Ishizawa, K., Oh, S. Y., Itoh, K., et al. (2014). A multicentre phase II study of vorinostat in patients with relapsed or refractory indolent B-cell non-Hodgkin lymphoma and mantle cell lymphoma. *Br. J. Haematol.* 165, 768–776. doi: 10.1111/bjh.12819

Oki, Y., Buglio, D., Fanale, M., Fayad, L., Copeland, A., Romaguera, J., et al. (2013). Phase I study of panobinostat plus everolimus in patients with relapsed or refractory lymphoma. *Clin. Cancer Res.* 19, 6882–6890. doi: 10.1158/1078-0432.CCR-13-1906

Oki, Y., Kelly, K. R., Flinn, I., Patel, M. R., Gharavi, R., Ma, A., et al. (2017). CUDC-907 in relapsed/refractory diffuse large B-cell lymphoma, including patients with MYC-alterations: Results from an expanded phase I trial. *Haematologica* 102, 1923–1930. doi: 10.3324/haematol.2017.172882

Okosun, J., Bödör, C., Wang, J., Araf, S., Yang, C.-Y., Pan, C., et al. (2014). Integrated genomic analysis identifies recurrent mutations and evolution patterns driving the initiation and progression of follicular lymphoma. *Nat Genet.* 46, 176–181. doi: 10.1038/ng.2856

Olsen, E. A., Kim, Y. H., Kuzel, T. M., Pacheco, T. R., Foss, F. M., Parker, S., et al. (2007). Phase IIB multicenter trial of vorinostat in patients with persistent, progressive, or treatment refractory cutaneous T-cell lymphoma. *J. Clin. Oncol.* 25, 3109–3115. doi: 10.1200/JCO.2006.10.2434

Oronsky, B., Paulmurugan, R., Foygel, K., Scicinski, J., Knox, S. J., Peehl, D., et al. (2017). RRx-001: a systemically non-toxic M2-to-M1 macrophage stimulating and prosensitizing agent in phase II clinical trials. *Expert Opin. Investig. Drugs.* 26, 109–119. doi: 10.1080/13543784.2017.1268600

Ozer, H. G., El-Gamal, D., Powell, B., Hing, Z. A., Blachly, J. S., Harrington, B., et al. (2018). BRD4 profiling identifies critical chronic lymphocytic leukemia oncogenic circuits and reveals sensitivity to PLX51107, a novel structurally distinct BET inhibitor. *Cancer Discov.* 8, 458–477. doi: 10.1158/2159-8290.CD-17-0902

Padmanabhan, B., Mathur, S., Manjula, R., and Tripathi, S. (2016). Bromodomain and extra-terminal (BET) family proteins: new therapeutic targets in major diseases. *J. Biosci.* 41, 295–311. doi: 10.1007/s12038-016-9600-6

Parry, M., Rose-Zerilli, M. J. J., Ljungström, V., Gibson, J., Wang, J., Walewska, R., et al. (2015). Genetics and prognostication in splenic marginal zone lymphoma: revelations from deep sequencing. *Clin. Cancer Res.* 21, 4174–4183. doi: 10.1158/1078-0432.CCR-14-2759

Pasqualucci, L., Dominguez-Sola, D., Chiarenza, A., Fabbri, G., Grunn, A., Trifonov, V., et al. (2011a). Inactivating mutations of acetyltransferase genes in B-cell lymphoma. *Nature.* 471, 189–195. doi: 10.1038/nature09730

Pasqualucci, L., Trifonov, V., Fabbri, G., Ma, J., Rossi, D., Chiarenza, A., et al. (2011b). Analysis of the coding genome of diffuse large B-cell lymphoma. *Nat. Genet.* 43, 830–837. doi: 10.1038/ng.892

Pazin, M. J., and Kadonaga, J. T. (1997). SWI2/SNF2 and related proteins: ATP-driven motors that disrupt protein- -DNA interactions? *Cell.* 88, 737–740. doi: 10.1016/S0092-8674(00)81918-2

Persky, D. O., Li, H., Rimsza, L. M., Barr, P. M., Popplewell, L. L., Bane, C. L., et al. (2018). A phase I/II trial of vorinostat (SAHA) in combination with rituximab-CHOP in patients with newly diagnosed advanced stage diffuse large B-cell lymphoma (DLBCL): SWOG S0806. *Am. J. Hematol.* 93, 486–493. doi: 10.1002/ajh.25010

Popovic, R., Shah, M. Y., and Licht, J. D. (2013). Epigenetic therapy of hematological malignancies: Where are we now? *Ther. Adv. Hematol.* 4, 81–91. doi: 10.1177/2040620712466864

Qi, W., Chan, H., Teng, L., Li, L., Chuai, S., Zhang, R., et al. (2012). Selective inhibition of Ezh2 by a small molecule inhibitor blocks tumor cells proliferation. *Proc. Natl. Acad. Sci.* 109, 21360–21365. doi: 10.1073/pnas.1210371110

Qin, C., Hu, Y., Zhou, B., Fernandez-Salas, E., Yang, C.-Y., Liu, L., et al. (2018). Discovery of QCA570 as an exceptionally potent and efficacious proteolysis targeting chimera (PROTAC) degrader of the bromodomain and extra-terminal (BET) proteins capable of inducing complete and durable tumor regression. *J. Med. Chem.* 61, 6685–6704. doi: 10.1021/acs.jmedchem.8b00506

Qiu, L., Burgess, A., Fairlie, D. P., Leonard, H., Parsons, P. G., and Gabrielli, B. G. (2000). Histone deacetylase inhibitors trigger a G2 checkpoint in normal cells that is defective in tumor cells. *Mol. Biol. Cell* 11, 2069–2083. doi: 10.1091/mbc.11.6.2069

Raina, K., Lu, J., Qian, Y., Altieri, M., Gordon, D., Rossi, A. M. K., et al.. (2016). PROTAC-induced BET protein degradation as a therapy for castration-resistant prostate cancer. *Proc. Natl. Acad. Sci. U. S. A.* 113, 7124–7129. doi: 10.1073/pnas.1521738113

Rebel, V. I., Kung, A. L., Tanner, E. A., Yang, H., Bronson, R. T., and Livingston, D. M. (2002). Distinct roles for CREB-binding protein and p300 in hematopoietic stem cell self-renewal. *Proc. Natl. Acad. Sci.* 99, 14789–14794. doi: 10.1073/pnas.232568499

Recasens-zorzo, C., Cardesa-salzmann, T., Petazzi, P., Ros-blanco, L., Esteve-arenys, A., Clot, G., et al. (2018). Pharmacological modulation of CXCR4 cooperates with BET bromodomain inhibition in diffuse large B-cell lymphoma. *Haematologica* 104, 778–788. doi: 10.3324/haematol.2017.180505

Rhyasen, G. W., Hattersley, M. M., Yao, Y., Dulak, A., Wang, W., Petteruti, P., et al. (2016). AZD5153: a novel bivalent BET bromodomain inhibitor highly active against hematologic malignancies. *Mol. Cancer Ther.* 15, 2563–2574. doi: 10.1158/1535-7163.MCT-16-0141

Ribrag, V., Kim, W. S., Bouabdallah, R., Lim, S. T., Coiffier, B., Illes, A., et al. (2017). Safety and efficacy of abexinostat, a pan-histone deacetylase inhibitor, in non-Hodgkin lymphoma and chronic lymphocytic leukemia: Results of a phase II study. *Haematologica* 102, 903–909. doi: 10.3324/haematol.2016.154377

Richardson, P. G., Hungria, V. T. M., Yoon, S. S., Beksac, M., Dimopoulos, M. A., Elghandour, A., et al. (2016). Panobinostat plus bortezomib and dexamethasone in previously treated multiple myeloma: Outcomes by prior treatment. *Blood.* 15, 2563–2574. doi: 10.1182/blood-2015-09-665018

Rinaldi, A., Mian, M., Chigrinova, E., Arcaini, L., Bhagat, G., Novak, U., et al. (2011). Genome-wide DNA profiling of marginal zone lymphomas identifies subtype-specific lesions with an impact on the clinical outcome. *Blood* 117, 1595–1604. doi: 10.1182/blood-2010-01-264275

Robaina, M. C., Mazzoccoli, L., Arruda, V. O., Reis, F. R., de, S., Apa, A. G., et al. (2015). Deregulation of DNMT1, DNMT3B and miR-29s in Burkitt lymphoma suggests novel contribution for disease pathogenesis. *Exp. Mol. Pathol.* 98, 200–207. doi: 10.1016/j.yexmp.2015.03.006

Roulland, S., Kasbekar, M., Young, R. M., Shaffer, A. L., Hodson, D. J., Xiao, W., et al. (2018). Genetics and pathogenesis of diffuse large B-cell lymphoma. *N. Engl. Med.* 378, 1396–1407. doi: 10.1056/NEJMoa1801445

Rozati, S., Cheng, P. F., Widmer, D. S., Fujii, K., Levesque, M. P., and Dummer, R. (2016). Romidepsin and azacitidine synergize in their epigenetic modulatory effects to induce apoptosis in CTCL. *Clin. Cancer Res.* 22, 2020–2031. doi: 10.1158/1078-0432.CCR-15-1435

Sachchidanand, R-S, L., Yan, S., Mutjaba, S., Liu, W. J., Zeng, L., et al. (2006). Target structure-based discovery of small molecules that block human p53 and CREB binding protein association. *Chem. Biol.* 13, 81–90. doi: 10.1016/j.chembiol.2005.10.014

Saha, S. K., Parachoniak, C. A., Ghanta, K. S., Fitamant, J., Ross, K. N., Najem, M. S., et al. (2014). Mutant IDH inhibits HNF-4α to block hepatocyte differentiation and promote biliary cancer. *Nature* 513, 110–152. doi: 10.1038/nature13441

Samuels,B.L.,Herndon,J.E.,Harmon,D.C.,Carey,R.,Aisner,J.,Corson,J.M.,etal.(1998). Dihydro-5-azacytidine and cisplatin in the treatment of malignant mesothelioma: a phase II study by the Cancer and Leukemia Group B. *Cancer.* 82, 1578–1584. doi: 10.1002/(SICI)1097-0142(19980415)82:8<1578::AID-CNCR21>3.0.CO;2-0

Santen, G. W. E., Aten, E., Sun, Y., Almomani, R., Gilissen, C., Nielsen, M., et al. (2012). Mutations in SWI/SNF chromatin remodeling complex gene ARID1B cause Coffin-Siris syndrome. *Nat. Genet.* 44, 379–380. doi: 10.1038/ng.2217

Santo, L., Hideshima, T., Kung, A. L., Tseng, J.-C., Tamang, D., Yang, M., et al. (2012). Preclinical activity, pharmacodynamic, and pharmacokinetic properties of a selective HDAC6 inhibitor, ACY-1215, in combination with bortezomib in multiple myeloma. *Blood* 119, 2579–2589. doi: 10.1182/blood-2011-10-387365

Santoro, F., Botrugno, O. A., Dal Zuffo, R., Pallavicini, I., Matthews, G. M., Cluse, L., et al. (2013). A dual role for Hdac1: oncosuppressor in tumorigenesis, oncogene in tumor maintenance. *Blood* 121, 3459–3468. doi: 10.1182/blood-2012-10-461988

Sausen, M., Leary, R. J., Jones, S., Wu, J., Reynolds, C. P., Liu, X., et al. (2013). Integrated genomic analyses identify ARID1A and ARID1B alterations in the childhood cancer neuroblastoma. *Nat. Genet.* 45, 12–17. doi: 10.1038/ng.2493

Schmitz, R., Young, R. M., Ceribelli, M., Jhavar, S., Xiao, W., Zhang, M., et al. (2012). Burkitt lymphoma pathogenesis and therapeutic targets from structural and functional genomics. *Nature* 490, 116–120. doi: 10.1038/nature11378

Scholtysik, R., Kreuz, M., Hummel, M., Rosolowski, M., Szczepanowski, M., Klapper, W., et al. (2015). Characterization of genomic imbalances in diffuse large B-cell lymphoma by detailed SNP-chip analysis. *Int. J. Cancer* 136, 1033–1042. doi: 10.1002/ijc.29072

Schubert, H. L., Blumenthal, R. M., and Cheng, X. (2003). Many paths to methyltransfer: a chronicle of convergence. *Trends Biochem. Sci.* 28, 329–335. doi: 10.1016/S0968-0004(03)00090-2

Schuh, A. C., Döhner, H., Pleyer, L., Seymour, J. F., Fenaux, P., and Dombret, H. (2017). Azacitidine in adult patients with acute myeloid leukemia. *Crit. Rev. Oncol. Hematol.* 116, 159–177. doi: 10.1016/j.critrevonc.2017.05.010

Scott, D. W., and Gascoyne, R. D. (2014). The tumour microenvironment in B cell lymphomas. *Nat. Rev. Cancer* 14, 517–534. doi: 10.1038/nrc3774

Scott, L. J. (2016). Azacitidine: A review in myelodysplastic syndromes and acute myeloid leukaemia. *Drugs.* 14, 517–534. doi: 10.1007/s40265-016-0585-0

Seifert, M., Scholtysik, R., and Küppers, R., (2013). "Origin and pathogenesis of B cell lymphomas," in *Methods Mol. Biol. (Clifton, N.J.)*, 1–25. doi: 10.1007/978-1-62703-269-8_1

Shahbazian, M. D., and Grunstein, M. (2007). Functions of site-specific histone acetylation and deacetylation. *Annu. Rev. Biochem.* 76, 75–100. doi: 10.1146/annurev.biochem.76.052705.162114

Shaknovich, R., Cerchietti, L., Tsikitas, L., Kormaksson, M., De, S., Figueroa, M. E., et al. (2011). DNA methyltransferase 1 and DNA methylation patterning contribute to germinal center B-cell differentiation. *Blood.* 118, 3559–3569. doi: 10.1182/blood-2011-06-357996

Shaknovich, R., Geng, H., Johnson, N. A., Tsikitas, L., Cerchietti, L., Greally, J. M., et al. (2010). DNA methylation signatures define molecular subtypes of diffuse large B-cell lymphoma. *Blood.* 116, e81–89. doi: 10.1182/blood-2010-05-285320

Sharma, P., and Allison, J. P. (2015). Immune checkpoint targeting in cancer therapy: Toward combination strategies with curative potential. *Cell.* 161, 205–214. doi: 10.1016/j.cell.2015.03.030

Sheppard, G. S., Wang, L., Fidanze, S. D., Hasvold, L. A., Liu, D., Pratt, J. K., et al. (2018). "Abstract 931: Discovery of ABBV-744, a first-in-class highly BDII-selective BET bromodomain inhibitor," in *Cancer chemistry* (American Association for Cancer Research), 931–931. doi: 10.1158/1538-7445.AM2018-931

Shi, J., Whyte, W. A., Zepeda-Mendoza, C. J., Milazzo, J. P., Shen, C., Roe, J. S., et al. (2013). Role of SWI/SNF in acute leukemia maintenance and enhancer-mediated Myc regulation. *Genes Dev.* 27, 2648–2662. doi: 10.1101/gad.232710.113

Shilatifard, A. (2008). Molecular implementation and physiological roles for histone H3 lysine 4 (H3K4) methylation. *Curr. Opin. Cell Biol.* 20, 341–348. doi: 10.1016/j.ceb.2008.03.019

Silverman, L. R., Demakos, E. P., Peterson, B. L., Kornblith, A. B., Holland, J. C., Odchimar-Reissig, R., et al. (2002). Randomized controlled trial of azacitidine in patients with the myelodysplastic syndrome: A study of the cancer and leukemia group B. *J. Clin. Oncol.* 20, 2429–2440. doi: 10.1200/JCO.2002.04.117

Smith, E., Zhou, W., Shindiapina, P., Sif, S., Li, C., and Baiocchi, R. A. (2018). Recent advances in targeting protein arginine methyltransferase enzymes in cancer therapy. *Expert Opin. Ther. Targets* 22, 527–545. doi: 10.1080/14728222.2018.1474203

Smith, S. G., and Zhou, M.-M. (2016). The bromodomain: A new target in emerging epigenetic medicine. *ACS Chem. Biol.* 11, 598–608. doi: 10.1021/acschembio.5b00831

Srivastava, P., Paluch, B. E., Matsuzaki, J., James, S. R., Collamat-Lai, G., Taverna, P., et al. (2015). Immunomodulatory action of the DNA methyltransferase inhibitor SGI-110 in epithelial ovarian cancer cells and xenografts. *Epigenetics.* 10, 237–246. doi: 10.1080/15592294.2015.1017198

Stathis, A., Hotte, S. J., Chen, E. X., Hirte, H. W., Oza, A. M., Moretto, P., et al. (2011). Phase I study of decitabine in combination with vorinostat in patients with advanced solid tumors and non-Hodgkin's lymphomas. *Clin. Cancer Res.* 17, 1582–1590. doi: 10.1158/1078-0432.CCR-10-1893

Stein, E. M., Garcia-Manero, G., Rizzieri, D. A., Tibes, R., Berdeja, J. G., Savona, M. R., et al. (2018). The DOT1L inhibitor pinometostat reduces H3K79 methylation and has modest clinical activity in adult acute leukemia. *Blood.* 131, 2661–2669. doi: 10.1182/blood-2017-12-818948

Stewart, D. J., Issa, J. P., Kurzrock, R., Nunez, M. I., Jelinek, J., Hong, D., et al. (2009). Decitabine effect on tumor global DNA methylation and other parameters in a phase I trial in refractory solid tumors and lymphomas. *Clin. Cancer Res.* 15, 3881–3888. doi: 10.1158/1078-0432.CCR-08-2196

Straus, D. J., Hamlin, P. A., Matasar, M. J., Lia Palomba, M., Drullinsky, P. R., Zelenetz, A. D., et al.. (2015). Phase I/II trial of vorinostat with rituximab, cyclophosphamide, etoposide and prednisone as palliative treatment for elderly patients with relapsed or refractory diffuse large B-cell lymphoma not eligible for autologous stem cell transplantation. *Br. J. Haematol.* 168, 663–670. doi: 10.1111/bjh.13195

Streubel, B., Simonitsch-Klupp, I., Müllauer, L., Lamprecht, A., Huber, D., Siebert, R., et al. (2004). Variable frequencies of MALT lymphoma-associated genetic aberrations in MALT lymphomas of different sites. *Leukemia* 18, 1722–1726. doi: 10.1038/sj.leu.2403501

Sun, B., Fiskus, W., Qian, Y., Rajapakshe, K., Raina, K., Coleman, K. G., et al. (2018). BET protein proteolysis targeting chimera (PROTAC) exerts potent lethal activity against mantle cell lymphoma cells. *Leukemia* 32, 343–352. doi: 10.1038/leu.2017.207

Sun, B., Shah, B., Fiskus, W., Qi, J., Rajapakshe, K., Coarfa, C., et al. (2015). Synergistic activity of BET protein antagonist-based combinations in mantle cell lymphoma cells sensitive or resistant to ibrutinib. *Blood* 126, 1565–1574. doi: 10.1182/blood-2015-04-639542

Suraweera, A., O'Byrne, K. J., and Richard, D. J. (2018). Combination therapy with histone deacetylase inhibitors (HDACi) for the Treatment of cancer: achieving the full therapeutic potential of HDACi. *Front. Oncol.* 8, 92. doi: 10.3389/fonc.2018.00092

Swerdlow, S. H., Campo, E., Pileri, S. A., Harris, N. L., Stein, H., Siebert, R., et al. (2016). The 2016 revision of the World Health Organization classification of lymphoid neoplasms. *Blood* 127, 2375–2390. doi: 10.1182/blood-2016-01-643569

Tanaka, M., Roberts, J. M., Seo, H.-S., Souza, A., Paulk, J., Scott, T. G., et al. (2016). Design and characterization of bivalent BET inhibitors. *Nat. Chem. Biol.* 12, 1089–1096. doi: 10.1038/nchembio.2209

Tang, J.-Y., Chang, C.-C., Lin, P.-C., and Chang, J.-G. (2012). Isocitrate dehydrogenase mutation hot spots in acute lymphoblastic leukemia and oral cancer. *Kaohsiung J. Med. Sci.* 28, 138–144. doi: 10.1016/j.kjms.2011.10.023

The Cancer Genome Atlas Research Network (2013). The Cancer Genome Atlas Pan-Cancer analysis project. *Nat. Genet.* 45, 1113–1120. doi: 10.1038/ng.2764

Thottassery, J. V., Sambandam, V., Allan, P. W., Maddry, J. A., Maxuitenko, Y. Y., Tiwari, K., et al. (2014). Novel DNA methyltransferase-1 (DNMT1) depleting anticancer nucleosides, 4′-thio-2′-deoxycytidine and 5-aza-4′-thio-2′-deoxycytidine. *Cancer Chemother. Pharmacol.* 74, 291–302. doi: 10.1007/s00280-014-2503-z

Tiacci, E., Trifonov, V., Schiavoni, G., Holmes, A., Kern, W., Martelli, M. P., et al. (2011). BRAF mutations in hairy-cell leukemia. *N. Engl. J. Med.* 364, 2305–2315. doi: 10.1056/NEJMoa1014209

Topalian, S. L., Drake, C. G., and Pardoll, D. M. (2015). Immune checkpoint blockade: a common denominator approach to cancer therapy. *Cancer Cell.* 27, 450–461. doi: 10.1016/j.ccell.2015.03.001

Toujani, S., Dessen, P., Ithzar, N., Danglot, G., Richon, C., Vassetzky, Y., et al. (2009). High resolution genome-wide analysis of chromosomal alterations in Burkitt's lymphoma. *PLoS One* 4, e7089. doi: 10.1371/journal.pone.0007089

Vakoc, C. R. (2015). "BET bromodomain inhibition as a therapeutic approach in hematological malignancies," in *Histone recognition*. Ed. Zhou, M. M. (Heidelberg, Germany: Springer), 185–198. doi: 10.1007/978-3-319-18102-8_9

Valdez, B. C., Li, Y., Murray, D., Liu, Y., Nieto, Y., Champlin, R. E., et al. (2018). Combination of a hypomethylating agent and inhibitors of PARP and HDAC traps PARP1 and DNMT1 to chromatin, acetylates DNA repair proteins, down-regulates NuRD and induces apoptosis in human leukemia and lymphoma cells. *Oncotarget* 9, 3908–3921. doi: 10.18632/oncotarget.23386

Van Damme, M., Crompot, E., Meuleman, N., Maerevoet, M., Mineur, P., Bron, D., et al. (2016). Characterization of TET and IDH gene expression in chronic lymphocytic leukemia: comparison with normal B cells and prognostic significance. *Clin. Epigenetics* 8, 1–11. doi: 10.1186/s13148-016-0298-y

Van Kemenade, F. J., Raaphorst, F. M., Blokzijl, T., Fieret, E., Hamer, K. M., Satijn, D. P. E., et al. (2001). Coexpression of BMI-1 and EZH2 polycomb-group proteins is associated with cycling cells and degree of malignancy in B-cell non-Hodgkin lymphoma. *Blood.* 97, 3896–3901. doi: 10.1182/blood.V97.12.3896

Vannini, A., Volpari, C., Filocamo, G., Casavola, E. C., Brunetti, M., Renzoni, D., et al. (2004). Crystal structure of a eukaryotic zinc-dependent histone deacetylase, human HDAC8, complexed with a hydroxamic acid inhibitor. *Proc. Natl. Acad. Sci. U. S. A.* 101, 15064–15069. doi: 10.1073/pnas.0404603101

Vaswani, R. G., Gehling, V. S., Dakin, L. A., Cook, A. S., Nasveschuk, C. G., Duplessis, M., et al. (2016). Identification of (R)-N-((4-Methoxy-6-methyl-2-oxo-1,2-dihydropyridin-3-yl)methyl)-2-methyl-1-(1-(1-(2,2,2-trifluoroethyl) piperidin-4-yl)ethyl)-1H-indole-3-carboxamide (CPI-1205), a potent and selective inhibitor of histone methyltransferase EZH2, Suitabl. *J. Med. Chem.* 59, 9928–9941. doi: 10.1021/acs.jmedchem.6b01315

Velichutina, I., Shaknovich, R., Geng, H., Johnson, N. A., Gascoyne, R. D., Melnick, A. M., et al. (2010). EZH2-mediated epigenetic silencing in germinal center B cells contributes to proliferation and lymphomagenesis. *Blood.* 116, 5247–5255. doi: 10.1182/blood-2010-04-280149

Visser, H. P. J., and Gunster, M. J. (2001). "The Polycomb group protein EZH2 is upregulated in proliferating, cultured human mantle cell lymphoma - Visser - 2001," in *Br. J. of Haematol.* Mar; 112 (4), 950–958. (Wiley Online Library. Br. J). doi: 10.1046/j.1365-2141.2001.02641.x

Vogler, W. R., Miller, D. S., and Keller, J. W. (1976). 5 Azacytidine (NSC 102816): A new drug for the treatment of myeloblastic leukemia. *Blood.* 48, 331–337.

Wang, K., Kan, J., Yuen, S. T., Shi, S. T., Chu, K. M., Law, S., et al. (2011). Exome sequencing identifies frequent mutation of ARID1A in molecular subtypes of gastric cancer. *Nat. Genet.* 43, 1219–1223. doi: 10.1038/ng.982

Wang, L., Pal, S., and Sif, S. (2008). Protein arginine methyltransferase 5 suppresses the transcription of the RB family of tumor suppressors in leukemia and lymphoma cells. *Mol. Cell. Biol.* 28, 6262–6277. doi: 10.1128/MCB.00923-08

Wang, W., Côté, J., Xue, Y., Zhou, S., Khavari, P. A., Biggar, S. R., et al. (1996). Purification and biochemical heterogeneity of the mammalian SWI—SNF complex. *EMBO J.* 15, 5370–5382. doi: 10.1002/j.1460-2075.1996.tb00921.x

Wang, X., Nagl, N. G., Wilsker, D., Van Scoy, M., Pacchione, S., Yaciuk, P., et al. (2004). Two related ARID family proteins are alternative subunits of human SWI/SNF complexes. *Biochem. J.* 383, 319–325. doi: 10.1042/BJ20040524

Watanabe, T., Kato, H., Kobayashi, Y., Yamasaki, S., Morita-Hoshi, Y., Yokoyama, H., et al. (2010). Potential efficacy of the oral histone deacetylase inhibitor vorinostat in a phase I trial in follicular and mantle cell lymphoma. *Cancer Sci.* 101, 196–200. doi: 10.1111/j.1349-7006.2009.01360.x

Waterfall, J. J., Arons, E., Walker, R. L., Pineda, M., Roth, L., Killian, J. K., et al. (2013). High prevalence of MAP2K1 mutations in variant and IGHV4-34-expressing hairy-cell leukemias. *Nat. Genet.* 46, 8–10. doi: 10.1038/ng.2828

Winter, G. E., Mayer, A., Buckley, D. L., Erb, M. A., Roderick, J. E., Vittori, S., et al. (2017). BET bromodomain proteins function as master transcription elongation factors independent of CDK9 recruitment. *Mol. Cell* 67, 5–18.e19. doi: 10.1016/j.molcel.2017.06.004

Wong, Y. F., Jakt, L. M., and Nishikawa, S. I. (2013). Prolonged treatment with DNMT inhibitors Induces distinct effects in promoters and gene-bodies. *PLoS One.* 8, e71099. doi: 10.1371/journal.pone.0071099

Workman, J. L., and Kingston, R. E. (2002). Alteration of nucleosome structure as a mechanism of transcriptional regulation. *Annu. Rev. Biochem.* 67, 545–579. doi: 10.1146/annurev.biochem.67.1.545

Xargay-Torrent, S., López-Guerra, M., Saborit-Villarroya, I., Rosich, L., Campo, E., Roué, G., et al. (2011). Vorinostat-induced apoptosis in mantle cell lymphoma is mediated by acetylation of proapoptotic BH3-only gene promoters. *Clin. Cancer Res.* 17, 3956–3968. doi: 10.1158/1078-0432.CCR-10-3412

Xiao, B., Wilson, J. R., and Gamblin, S. J. (2003). SET domains and histone methylation. *Curr. Opin. Struct. Biol.* 13, 699–705. doi: 10.1016/j.sbi.2003.10.003

Xue, K., Gu, J. J., Zhang, Q., Mavis, C., Hernandez-Ilizaliturri, F. J., Czuczman, M. S., et al. (2016). Vorinostat, a histone deacetylase (HDAC) inhibitor, promotes cell cycle arrest and re-sensitizes rituximab- and chemo-resistant lymphoma cells to chemotherapy agents. *J. Cancer Res. Clin. Oncol.* 142, 379–387. doi: 10.1007/s00432-015-2026-y

Yang, D., Zhang, W.-P., Yang, J.-M., He, M.-X., Cheng, C., and Chen, J. (2018). Secondary skin involvement in gastric diffuse large B-cell lymphoma treated with chidamide: A case report. *Medicine (Baltimore)* 97, e13093. doi: 10.1097/MD.0000000000013093

Yang, X., Han, H., DeCarvalho, D. D., Lay, F. D., Jones, P. A., and Liang, G. (2014). Gene body methylation can alter gene expression and is a therapeutic target in cancer. *Cancer Cell.* 26, 577–590. doi: 10.1016/j.ccr.2014.07.028

Yap, T. A., Johnson, P. W. M., Winter, J., Leonard, J., Giulino-Roth, L., Horner, T., et al.. (2018). A phase I, open-label study of GSK2816126, an enhancer of zeste homolog 2 (EZH2) inhibitor, in patients with relapsed/refractory diffuse large B-cell lymphoma (DLBCL), transformed follicular lymphoma (tFL), other non-Hodgkin's lymphomas (NHL), multiple my. *J. Clin. Oncol.* 34, TPS2595. doi: 10.1200/jco.2016.34.15_suppl.tps2595

Yeoh, E.-J., Ross, M. E., Shurtleff, S. A., Williams, W. K., Patel, D., Mahfouz, R., et al.. (2002). Classification, subtype discovery, and prediction of outcome in pediatric acute lymphoblastic leukemia by gene expression profiling. *Cancer Cell* 1, 133–143. doi: 10.1016/S1535-6108(02)00032-6

Yoshimatsu, M., Toyokawa, G., Hayami, S., Unoki, M., Tsunoda, T., Field, H. I., et al. (2011). Dysregulation of PRMT1 and PRMT6, type I arginine methyltransferases, is involved in various types of human cancers. *Int. J. Cancer* 128, 562–573. doi: 10.1002/ijc.25366

You, J. S., and Jones, P. A. (2012). Cancer genetics and epigenetics: Two sides of the same coin? *Cancer Cell.* 22, 9–20. doi: 10.1016/j.ccr.2012.06.008

Younes, A., Berdeja, J. G., Patel, M. R., Flinn, I., Gerecitano, J. F., Neelapu, S. S., et al. (2016). Safety, tolerability, and preliminary activity of CUDC-907, a first-in-class, oral, dual inhibitor of HDAC and PI3K, in patients with relapsed or refractory lymphoma or multiple myeloma: An open-label, dose-escalation, phase 1 trial. *Lancet Oncol.* 17, 622–631. doi: 10.1016/S1470-2045(15)00584-7

Younes, A., Oki, Y., Bociek, R. G., Kuruvilla, J., Fanale, M., Neelapu, S., et al. (2011). Mocetinostat for relapsed classical Hodgkin's lymphoma: An open-label, single-arm, phase 2 trial. *Lancet Oncol.* 12, 1222–1228. doi: 10.1016/S1470-2045(11)70265-0

Younes, A., Sureda, A., Ben-Yehuda, D., Zinzani, P. L., Ong, T.-C., Prince, H. M., et al. (2012). Panobinostat in patients with relapsed/refractory Hodgkin's lymphoma after autologous stem-cell transplantation: Results of a phase II study. *J. Clin. Oncol.* 30, 2197–2203. doi: 10.1200/JCO.2011.38.1350

Yuan, B., Zhang, J., Wang, H., Xiong, L., Cai, Q., Wang, T., et al. (2011). 6-Thioguanine reactivates epigenetically silenced genes in acute lymphoblastic leukemia cells by facilitating proteasome-mediated degradation of DNMT. *Cancer Res.* 71, 1904–1911. doi: 10.1158/0008-5472.CAN-10-3430

Zeng, D., Liu, M., and Pan, J. (2016). Blocking EZH2 methylation transferase activity by GSK126 decreases stem cell-like myeloma cells. *Oncotarget.* 8, 3396–3411. doi: 10.18632/oncotarget.13773

Zeng, L., Li, J., Muller, M., Yan, S., Mujtaba, S., Pan, C., et al. (2005). Selective small molecules blocking HIV-1 Tat and coactivator PCAF association. *J. Am. Chem. Soc.* 127, 2376–2377. doi: 10.1021/ja044885g

Zhang, Y., Wei, H., Tang, K., Lin, D., Zhang, C., Mi, Y., et al. (2012). Mutation analysis of isocitrate dehydrogenase in acute lymphoblastic leukemia. *Genet. Test. Mol. Biomarkers* 16, 991–995. doi: 10.1089/gtmb.2011.0323

Zhao, H., Ning, S., Nolley, R., Scicinski, J., Oronsky, B., Knox, S. J., et al. (2017). The immunomodulatory anticancer agent, RRx-001, induces an interferon response through epigenetic induction of viral mimicry. *Clin. Epigenetics.* 9, 4. doi: 10.1186/s13148-017-0312-z

Zuber, J., Shi, J., Wang, E., Rappaport, A. R., Herrmann, H., Sison, E. A., et al. (2011). RNAi screen identifies Brd4 as a therapeutic target in acute myeloid leukaemia. *Nature.* 478, 524–528. doi: 10.1038/nature10334

9

E-Cadherin Downregulation is Mediated by Promoter Methylation in Canine Prostate Cancer

Carlos Eduardo Fonseca-Alves[1,2], Priscila Emiko Kobayashi[3], Antonio Fernando Leis-Filho[3], Patricia de Faria Lainetti[2], Valeria Grieco[4], Hellen Kuasne[5], Silvia Regina Rogatto[6†] and Renee Laufer-Amorim[2†]*

[1] Institute of Health Sciences, Paulista University—UNIP, Bauru, Brazil, [2] Department of Veterinary Surgery and Anesthesiology, School of Veterinary Medicine and Animal Science, Sao Paulo State University—UNESP, Botucatu, Brazil, [3] Department of Veterinary Clinic, School of Veterinary Medicine and Animal Science, Sao Paulo State University—UNESP, Botucatu, Brazil, [4] Department of Veterinary Medicine, Università degli studi di Milano, Milan, Italy, [5] International Center for Research (CIPE), AC Camargo Cancer Center, Sao Paulo, Brazil, [6] Department of Clinical Genetics, University Hospital of Southern Denmark, Institute of Regional Health Research, University of Southern Denmark, Vejle, Denmark

***Correspondence:**
Carlos Eduardo Fonseca-Alves
carlos.e.alves@unsp.br

†These authors have contributed equally to this work

E-cadherin is a transmembrane glycoprotein responsible for cell-to-cell adhesion, and its loss has been associated with metastasis development. Although E-cadherin downregulation was previously reported in canine prostate cancer (PC), the mechanism involved in this process is unclear. It is well established that dogs, besides humans, spontaneously develop PC with high frequency; therefore, canine PC is an interesting model to study human PC. In human PC, *CDH1* methylation has been associated with E-cadherin downregulation. However, no previous studies have described the methylation pattern of *CDH1* promoter in canine PC. Herein, we evaluated the E-cadherin protein and gene expression in canine PC compared to normal tissues. DNA methylation pattern was investigated as a regulatory mechanism of *CDH1* silencing. Our cohort is composed of 20 normal prostates, 20 proliferative inflammatory atrophy (PIA) lesions, 20 PC, and 11 metastases from 60 dogs. The E-cadherin protein expression was assessed by immunohistochemistry and western blotting and gene expression by qPCR. Bisulfite-pyrosequencing assay was performed to investigate the *CDH1* promoter methylation pattern. Membranous E-cadherin expression was observed in all prostatic tissues. A higher number of E-cadherin negative cells was detected more frequently in PC compared to normal and PIA samples. High-grade PC showed a diffuse membranous positive immunostaining. Furthermore, PC patients with a higher number of E-cadherin negative cells presented shorter survival time and higher Gleason scores. Western blotting and qPCR assays confirmed the immunohistochemical results, showing lower E-cadherin protein and gene expression levels in PC compared to normal samples. We identified *CDH1* promoter hypermethylation in PIA and PC samples. An in vitro assay with two canine prostate cancer cells (PC1 and PC2 cell lines) was performed to confirm the methylation as a regulatory mechanism of E-cadherin expression. PC1 cell line presented *CDH1* hypermethylation and after 5-Aza-dC treatment, a decreased *CDH1* methylation and increased gene expression levels were observed. Positive E-cadherin cells were massively found in metastases (mean of 90.6%). In conclusion, low levels of E-cadherin protein, gene downregulation and *CDH1* hypermethylation was detected in canine PC. However, in metastatic foci occur E-cadherin re-expression confirming its relevance in these processes.

Keywords: dog, *CDH1*, prostate, hypermethylation, surface protein

INTRODUCTION

Human prostate cancer (PC), the second cause of male cancer-related death in North America, has a variable behavior (Siegel et al., 2019). The mortality rate is associated with metastasis (Huynh et al., 2016), which more commonly affects bone, lymph node, and lung (Siegel et al., 2019). Canine PC is a very aggressive disease associated with high metastatic rate at the diagnosis (more than 85%) being bones, lungs, and iliac lymph nodes, the most common metastatic sites disease-associated (Cornell et al., 2000; Fonseca-Alves et al., 2015a).

Dogs have been reported as a model for human PC and the knowledge regarding molecular aspects of canine PC has increased in recent years (Fonseca-Alves et al., 2018a; Costa et al., 2019; Laufer-Amorim et al., 2019; Rivera-Calderón et al., 2019). These recent studies bring new evidence that canine PC can represent a model to human castration-resistant prostate cancer (CRPC) (Laufer-Amorim et al., 2019). Usually, canine PC lacks NKX3.1, PTEN (Fonseca-Alves et al., 2013; Fonseca-Alves et al., 2018a; Fonseca-Alves et al., 2018b), and androgen receptor expression (Laufer-Amorim et al., 2019) resembling human CRPC. Besides that, canine PC shows alterations in TP53, C-MYC, and MDM2 protein expression (Fonseca-Alves et al., 2013; Fonseca-Alves et al., 2018b). These findings pointed out that the clinical behavior and molecular alterations are similar in both species, making dogs an exciting model in comparative initiatives.

The carcinogenic process, from normal to pre-neoplastic and invasive carcinoma, involves the ability of epithelial cells to detach one another, survive and invade the surrounding tissues (Friedl and Wolf, 2003). Metastasis of PC is a complex process associated with loss of epithelial markers, acquirement of a mesenchymal phenotype, and ability of cells to spread through the lymphatic system or bloodstream (Staník et al., 2014). E-cadherin is a transmembrane protein that has a crucial role in cell adhesion and migration (Debelec-Butuner et al., 2014). E-cadherin also is involved in the β catenin/APC pathway, which is related to cell proliferation and epithelial-mesenchymal transition (EMT) (Tsui et al., 2016). Loss of E-cadherin is associated with poor prognosis in patients with high-grade prostate tumors in both humans (Umbas et al., 1992; Umbas et al., 1994; Abdelrahman et al., 2017; Dhar et al., 2017; Wang et al., 2017; Li et al., 2019) and canine (Fonseca-Alves et al., 2013; Fonseca-Alves et al., 2015a; Kobayashi et al., 2018).

Different mechanisms have been implicated with E-cadherin downregulation in human medicine, including copy number loss (Saramaki and Visakorpi, 2007), somatic mutations (Busch et al., 2017), methylation (Graff et al., 1995; Yoshiura et al., 1995; Li et al., 2001; Mostafavi-Pour et al., 2015), and suppression mediated by ZEB1 and SRC family kinases (Mostafavi-Pour et al., 2015). *CDH1* gene repression promoted by its promoter hypermethylation, plays a crucial role in tumor invasion and spread (Graff et al., 1995; Yoshiura et al., 1995; Li et al., 2001; Mostafavi-Pour et al., 2015). *CDH1* hypermethylation and E-cadherin downregulation have been reported in more than 75% of patients with metastatic PC (Maruyama et al., 2002; Singal et al., 2004; Hoque et al., 2005). Also, *CDH1* promoter methylation is widely studied as a cause of E-cadherin down-regulation in human PC (Graff et al., 1995; Yoshiura et al., 1995; Li et al., 2001; Mostafavi-Pour et al., 2015). However, conflicting results have been reported due to the difficulties in studying methylation (Zhang et al., 2016b). Disparities among methodologies, sample quality, regions of prostatic biopsy, and promoter region evaluated make difficult comparisons among the published studies (Zhang et al., 2016b). Besides that, neoplastic cells can induce hypomethylation and re-express the transcript and its respective protein (Chao et al., 2010), which is compatible with the reversibility phenomenon described in the methylation process.

Transcriptional E-cadherin downregulation mediated by its promoter methylation is widely investigated in human PC (Graff et al., 1995; Yoshiura et al., 1995; Li et al., 2001; Mostafavi-Pour et al., 2015), and E-cadherin plasticity has been proposed during the metastatic progression in human PC (Bae et al., 2011). In high-grade human PC, E-cadherin loss leads to the invasion of metastatic cells to lymph nodes and bones (Putzke et al., 2011). Interestingly, bone metastasis seems to express more E-cadherin than soft tissue metastasis (Putzke et al., 2011). However, few studies evaluating the molecular mechanisms related to *CDH1* silencing have been reported in dogs. Loss of E-cadherin during the lymphatic invasion by neoplastic epithelial cells and E-cadherin re-expression in metastatic foci were previously reported in canine PC (Fonseca-Alves et al., 2015a).

Herein, we investigated E-cadherin gene and protein expression in canine proliferative inflammatory atrophy (PIA), PC and its metastasis as well the methylation status of *CDH1* as a silencing mechanism responsible for the dynamic E-cadherin expression.

MATERIALS AND METHODS

Tissue Selection and Histopathological Evaluation

This cohort is composed of 60 dogs of different breeds, varying from 8 to 14 years old. We selected 20 normal canine prostates, 20 PIA lesions, and 9 PC formalin-fixed embedded-paraffin (FFPE) from the archives from the Department Veterinary Pathology, Sao Paulo State University- UNESP, Brazil. In addition, 11FFPE prostate cancer matched with 11 metastases from the same subjects were selected. All metastases were morphologically analyzed and presented PSA protein expression, as previously described (Fonseca-Alves et al., 2018b). The correspondent fresh frozen tissues from 20 normal canine prostates, 20 PIA lesions, 20 PC samples were used for pyrosequencing and Western blot. All FFPE samples were evaluated by protein and gene expression using immunohistochemistry and qPCR, respectively.

PC samples were collected during surgical or biopsy procedures from animals showing clinical signs. The metastases were identified by imaging tests (X-ray or computed tomography) followed by a biopsy. Normal and PIA samples were collected during necropsies from animals without clinical signs of prostatic disease, with an interval between death and necropsy less than 6 h. All prostate samples were from intact dogs.

The histopathological classification was performed according to the human WHO classification of Tumors of the Urinary System and Male Genital Organs (Humphrey et al., 2016). The Gleason-like system was applied according to Palmieri and Grieco (Palmieri and Grieco, 2015). Briefly, the architectural patterns are evaluated, and the sum of the primary and secondary grades is determined to result in a final Gleason score.

The study was approved by the Animal Ethics Committee according to the national and international guidelines for using animals in research. All animal owners gave written informed consent for the dog's material, clinical information and examination results to be used for research and academic matters under protocol #107/2015.

E-cadherin Expression Analysis by Immunohistochemistry

Five-micron thick sections were obtained from FFPE blocks, dewaxed in xylol and rehydrated in graded ethanol. For antigen retrieval, the slides containing the samples were incubated with citrate buffer (pH 6.0) in a pressure cooker (Pascal®; Dako, Carpinteria, CA, USA). The samples were then treated with freshly prepared 3% hydrogen peroxide in methanol for 20 min and further washed in Tris-buffered saline. The slides were incubated overnight at 4°C with 0.01µg/µL monoclonal mouse Anti-Human E-cadherin antibody (catalog number GA059, Dako, Carpinteria, CA, USA). A polymer system (catalog number K406511-2, Envision, Dako, Carpinteria, CA, USA) was applied as a secondary antibody conjugated to peroxidase. DAB (3′-diaminobenzidine tetrahydrochloride, Dako, Carpinteria, CA, USA) was used as the chromogen, for 5 min, followed by Harris hematoxylin counterstain. Negative control using mouse universal negative control (Dako, Carpinteria, CA, USA) was included according to the manufacturer's recommendation. Positive E-cadherin cells in adjacent epithelial cells were considered positive internal controls.

E-cadherin immunoexpression was evaluated according to the number of negative cells. Slides were analyzed under a light microscope (Leica Microsystems, Germany) and 10 images were taken for each slide (Leica QWin V3 software; Leica Microsystems, Germany) at high-power (40X objective) field. Representative areas were qualitatively selected for immunostaining analysis. We choose areas with minimal inflammatory cells, necrosis or connective tissue and with lower E-cadherin staining. Samples were scored based on an assessment of the number of negative cells per the total of cells in 10 high power fields (HPF), according to Hong et al. (2011). These results were expressed in a percentage of negative cells.

E-cadherin/Ki67 Double Immunostaining

E-cadherin and Ki67 double immunoexpression were performed to exclude cell proliferation as a mechanism associated with E-cadherin focal loss. The procedures were performed as previously reported (Fonseca-Alves et al., 2015b). Briefly, the paraffin sections were deparaffinated in xylol for 15 min and antigen retravel was performed using citrate buffer pH 6.0 solution in a pressure cooker (Pascal, Dako, Carpinteria, CA, USA). Then, endogenous peroxidase was blocked using 8% of hydrogen peroxidase (Dinamica, São Paulo, SP, Brazil), diluted in methanol (Dinamica, São Paulo, SP, Brazil). We used 0.02µg/µL of mouse monoclonal anti-Ki67 antibody (catalog number GA62661-2, Dako, Carpinteria, CA, USA) overnight at 4°C. The polymer system was applied as a secondary antibody for 1 h (catalog number K406511-2, Envision, Dako, Carpinteria, CA, USA) and 3′-diaminobenzidine tetrahydrochloride (DAB, Dako, Carpinteria, CA, USA) was used as the chromogen, for 5 min. The tissue sections were washed with immunohistochemistry buffer (Dako, Carpinteria, CA, USA) and 0.01µg/µL of mouse monoclonal anti-E-cadherin antibody (catalog number GA059, Dako, Carpinteria, CA, USA) was applied overnight at 4°C. After, the HRP magenta chromogen (catalog number GV925, Dako, Carpinteria, CA, USA) was used for 5 min and counterstained with Harris hematoxylin. The positive and negative controls were performed, as described above.

Immunoblotting

Western blotting was performed to quantify E-cadherin protein expression in seven normal prostates, seven PIA lesions, and seven PC. The frozen prostate samples were sectioned in a cryostat and re-analyzed to confirm the previous diagnosis. The samples were mechanically homogenized, prepared and transferred to nitrocellulose membranes, as previously described (Rivera-Calderón et al., 2016). The blots were blocked with 6% skimmed milk in TBS-T (BioRad, Hercules, CA, USA) for 2 h. Next, the Mouse monoclonal anti-human E-cadherin (0.002µg/µL; catalog number GA059, Dako, Carpinteria, CA, USA) antibody was applied and the slides were incubated at 4°C for 18 h. Goat polyclonal anti-β-actin antibody (0.001µg/µL, catalog number sc-1615, Santa Cruz Biotechnology, Santa Cruz, CA, USA) was used as a loading control. After incubation with the corresponding horseradish peroxidase-conjugated sheep anti-mouse (catalog number NA931, GE Healthcare, Chicago, IL, USA) and donkey anti-goat (catalog number NA9340, GE Healthcare, Chicago, IL, USA) secondary antibodies (0.001µg/µL), the blots were detected by means of chemiluminescence (Amersham ECL Select Western Blotting Detection Reagent, GE Healthcare). Protein bands were quantified by densitometry analysis (Imagequant LAS 500,

GE Healthcare, Chicago, IL, USA) and expressed as integrated optical density (IOD). E-cadherin protein expression was normalized using the β-actin values. Normalized data were expressed in means and standard deviations (SD).

Tumor-Derived Cell Cultures

Two cell lines (PC1 and PC2) were established in our previous study (Zhang et al., 2016). The PC1 cell line was from a 10-years-old, intact, mixed breed dog with non-metastatic PC (cribriform pattern and Gleason score 10). PC2 cell line was from an 11-year-old, intact, poodle dog with metastatic PC (tumor showed cribriform pattern and Gleason score 10). Both cell lines were cultured (the passage 30) in DMEM medium (Lonza, Basel, Switzerland) containing 10% fetal bovine serum (FBS) (LGC Bio, Cotia, SP, Brazil), 1% of penicillin-streptomycin (Thermo Fischer Scientific, Waltham, MA, USA) and amphotericin B (Thermo Fischer Scientific, Waltham, MA, USA) at 37°C in a humidified atmosphere containing 5% CO2. After reaching a minimum of 80% of confluence, both cell lines were processed to obtain DNA. DNA extraction were also performed in their respective primary tumors (fresh frozen samples) followed by pyrosequencing to evaluate the *CDH1* methylation status.

Methyl Thiazolyl Tetrazolium (MTT) Assay

The 5-Aza 2′deoxycytidine (5-Aza-dC) toxicity was investigated in canine prostatic cells based on the MTT assay. The IC_{50} values were calculated from the dose-response curves to establish the in vitro dosage that will induce demethylation instead of cell death. We used 96-well plates to grow the cancer cells at a density of 2,500 cells per well. The medium was changed every 48 h, and 5-Aza-dC (Sigma-Aldrich, Saint Louis, MO, USA) was added every 24 h. MTT analysis was performed on day 7. The medium was removed, the cells were washed with 3X PBS, and fresh medium was added in each well followed by incubation at 37°C for 4 h. The medium was removed and 200μL of dimethyl sulfoxide (DMSO) (Sigma-Aldrich, Saint Louis, MO, USA) was added in each well and formazan (Sigma-Aldrich, Saint Louis, MO, USA) was solubilized. The optical density (OD) level was measured at 570 wavelengths. Each treatment was performed in triplicate and the experiment in duplicate. Cell viability was calculated into a percentage.

CDH1 Gene Expression

Gene expression analysis was performed in our set of samples and both cell lines prior and after 5-Aza-dC treatment. Macrodissection was performed in normal, PIA, PC, and metastatic samples (FFEP) using 16-gauge needles, as previously described (Hoque et al., 2005). mRNA was extracted using RecoverAll™ Total Nucleic Acid Kit (Ambion, Life Technologies, MA, USA) according to the manufacturer's instructions. cDNA synthesis was performed using total RNA (Applied Biosystems, Foster City, CA, USA), according to the manufacturer's recommendations. The primers set for *CDH1* (Gene ID: 442858) (Forward: 5′-CAGCATGGACTCAGAAGACAGAAG-3′ and Reverse: 5′-TTCCGGGCAGCTGATAGG-3′) and *ACTB* (Gene ID: 403580) used as endogenous (ACTB, Forward: 5′-GGCATCCTGACCCTCAAGTA-3′ and Reverse: 5′-CTTCT CCATGTCGTCCCAGT-3′) genes were used for RT-qPCR assays. The reaction was conducted in a total volume of 10 μL containing Power SYBR Green PCR Master Mix (Applied Biosystems; Foster City, CA, USA), 1 μL of cDNA (1:10) and 0.3 μM of each primer pair in triplicate using QuantStudio 12K Flex Thermal Cycler equipment (Applied Biosystems; Foster City, CA, USA). A dissociation curve was included in all experiments to determine the PCR product specificity. Relative gene expression was quantified using the $2^{-\Delta\Delta CT}$ method (Livak and Schmittgen, 2001).

5-Aza-2′-Deoxycytidine Treatment

To investigate if hypermethylation is associated with *CDH1* silencing, we treated the PC cell lines with 5-Aza-dC and compared with untreated cells. As previously established by MTT assay, we added 1μg of 5-Aza-dC to the culture medium every 24 h (due to 5-Aza-dC stability) and for seven days. Treated cells were washed with PBS three times. All procedures were performed in duplicate, according to da Costa Prando et al. 2011). Subsequently, mRNA and DNA were extracted to perform RT-qPCR and pyrosequencing analysis, respectively.

Quantitative Bisulfite Pyrosequencing

The pyrosequencing analysis was performed to evaluate the frequency of *CDH1* gene promoter methylation in all frozen tissue samples (20 normal prostates, 20 PIA samples, and 20 PC) and cell lines (prior and after 5-Aza-dC treatment). Prostate samples were sectioned in a cryostat to confirm the diagnosis. The bisulfite conversion of the genomic DNA was performed using EZ DNA Methylation-Gold Kit (Zymo Research Corporation, Irvine, CA, USA). The forward (5′ TTTGGGAAGAGGAGGGGG 3′) and reverse primer (5′ CCCTTCCCCTCTCTCTCTC - BIOTIN 3′) of *CDH1* CpG island (Gene ID: 442858) were amplified by PCR (HotStarTaq Master Mix kit - Qiagen). The pyrosequencing was performed using a sequencing primer (5′ TTTGGGAAGAGGAGGGGG 3′) following the manufacturer's instructions (PyroMark ID Q96, Qiagen and Biotage, Uppsala, Sweden).

Statistical Analysis

Statistical analysis was performed using GraphPad Prism v.8.1.0 (GraphPad Software Inc., La Jolla, CA, USA). The column test was performed to evaluate data normality. For statistical purposes, the mean of E-cadherin negative cells was used as a threshold to compare the overall survival between patients with over and lower protein expression. Variance analysis (ANOVA) was applied to compare CDH1 transcript levels among normal, PIA and PC samples. Mann-Whitney test was used to evaluate the association of E-cadherin protein and gene expression between two categorical variables. Correlation among the IHC score and clinical parameters, protein expression and transcript levels were also investigated. Mann-Whitney test was applied to evaluate the differences in the methylation levels among the groups. The samples were grouped according to the Gleason score in "low Gleason score" (Gleason score 6 and 8) and "high Gleason score" (Gleason score 10).

RESULTS

Clinical Features

The clinical features of the 20 PC-affected dogs are described in **Table 1**. Survival information was not available in two of 20 PC patients. The 20 canine PC preseted Gleason scores 6 (30% of cases), 8 (15%) and 10 (55%). Eleven of 20 dogs with PC had metastasis (55%); eight of them (8/11) presented bone and lung metastasis while pelvic bones, intestine and liver were observed in one patient each. From the patients with multiple metastatic sites (bone and lung), only the bone biopsy was evaluated. Seventy-three percent (8/11) of PC patients showing Gleason score 10 had metastasis. Dogs with PC Gleason 8 had no metastasis (n = 3), while 50% (3/6) of cases with Gleason 6 showed metastasis at diagnosis. Patients with lower Gleason score (6 and 8) experienced a higher survival time (P = 0.003) than those with Gleason score 10 (**Figure 1A**).

E-cadherin Immunoexpression

We found positive epithelial cells with membranous staining in normal, PIA, PC (**Figure 2**), and metastasis. Cases with less than 10% of negative cells showed a higher survival time (P = 0.004) (**Figure 1B**). A higher number of negative cells was observed in PC (**Figure 1C**) compared to normal and PIA samples. Normal samples showed 100% E-cadherin positive cells; while a mean of 2.1% and 10.5% of negative cells was detected in PIA and PC samples, respectively. Metastases had a mean of 9.5% of negative cells. Tumors showing Gleason score 10 had a higher percentage of negative E-cadherin neoplastic cells compared to PC Gleason scores 6 and 8 and normal samples (P = 0.0003). Metastases had a higher number of negative cells in comparison with normal samples (P = 0.0003) and no statistical difference was observed between all PC samples and metastases (P > 0.05). E-cadherin pattern in each histological subtype is detailed in **Table 1**. The

TABLE 1 | Clinical information of 20 canine prostate cancer-affected patients evaluated in this study.

Case	Breed	Age (years)	Histological Pattern	Gleason-like score*	Treatment	Metastasis**	E-cadherin Negative Cells (%)	E-cadherin Positive Cells (%)	Methylation (%)	Follow-up (days)
1	Boxer	14	Cribriform	10	Piroxicam	Lung, Bone and Liver	30	70	94	90
2	Boxer	12	Cribriform	10	LDMT	Bone, Lung	15	85	94	278
3	German Shepherd	8	Small acinar	6	RP	No	2	98	95	453
4	American Cocker Spaniel	9	Small acinar	6	LDMT	No	1	99	95	523
5	Poodle	13	Small acinar	6	N/T	Bone, Lung	10	90	95	321
6	Poodle	14	Small acinar	6	LDMT	No	20	80	94	674
7	Boxer	11	Small acinar	6	Piroxicam	Bone	1	99	92	52
8	MBD	14	Small acinar	6	LDMT	Lung, Intestine	0	100	93	132
9	Poodle	13	Papillary	8	Piroxicam	No	10	90	95	463
10	MBD	12	Papillary	8	Carboplatin + Piroxicam	No	0	100	92	567
11	MBD	11	Papillary	8	LDMT	No	8	92	93	368
12	American Cocker Spaniel	10	Small acinar	10	RP	No	2	98	98	32
13	Poodle	10	Solid	10	RP	No	17	83	100	213
14	MBD	10	Solid	10	Piroxicam	Lung, Liver	0	100	95	55
15	MBD	15	Cribriform with comedonecrosis	10	Doxorrubicin + Piroxicam	Bone, Lung	10	90	94	75
16	American Cocker Spaniel	10	Solid	10	Doxorrubicin	Bone, Lung	22	78	100	78
17	MBD	9	Cribriform	10	LDMT	Bone, Lung	15	85	98	375
18	MBD	7	Cribriform with comedonecrosis	10	N/A	Bone, Lung	25	75	96	N/A
19	MBD	13	Cribriform with comedonecrosis	10	RP	Bone, Lung	5	95	97	45
20	Teckel	11	Cribriform	10	N/A	No	9	91	95	N/A

*PC, prostate cancer; MBD, Mixed Breed dog; N/A, Not Available; N/T, No Treatment; RP, Radical Prostatectomy; LDMT, Low-dose metronomic therapy. * Gleason like score was evaluated according to Palmieri and Grieco (2015). ** Metastasis identified at the diagnosis or during the follow-up.*

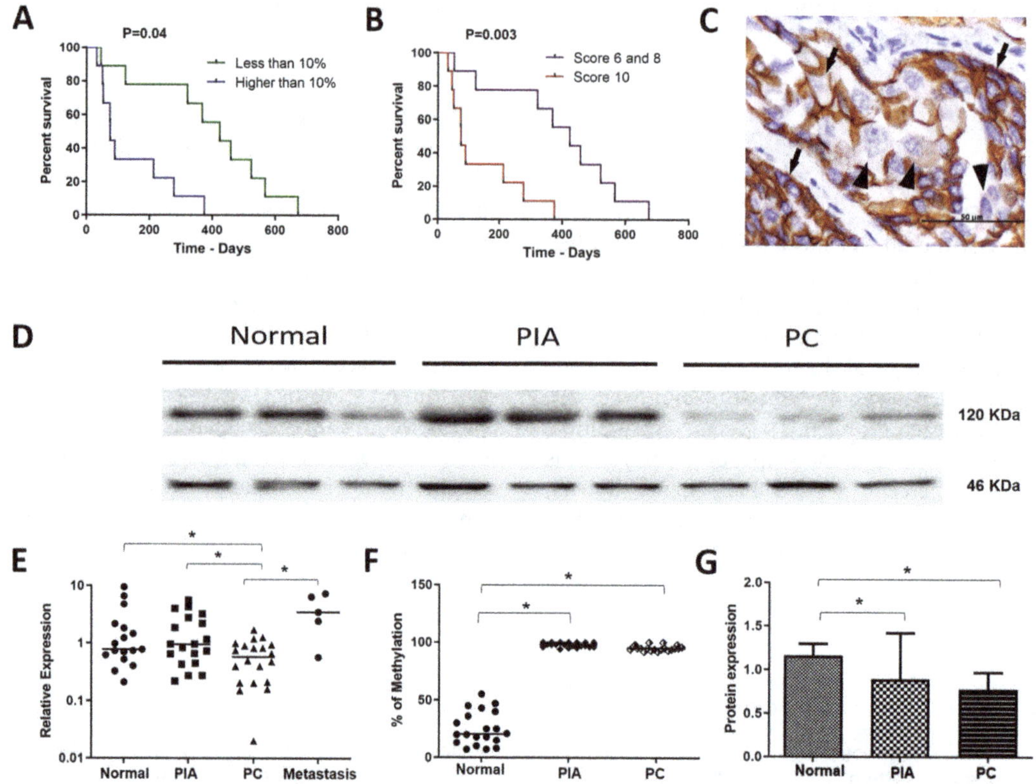

FIGURE 1 | (A) survival analysis according to the percentage of E-cadherin negative cells. Patients with over than 10% o E-cadherin negative cells experienced a shorter survival time. **(B)** survival analysis of the canine prostate cancer affected patients according to the Gleason score. Patients with Gleason score 10 experienced a shorter survival time. **(C)** E-cadherin immunohistochemistry showing positive membranous staining (arrows) in neoplastic epithelial cells. Cells were considered E-cadherin negative when partial or total (arrowhead) lack of expression. **(D)** Western blotting showing E-cadherin expression in normal, proliferative inflammatory atrophy and prostate cancer (PC) samples. It is possible to observe E-cadherin down expression in PC samples. **(E)** ANOVA analysis of *CDH1* transcripts in the different canine samples. The prostate cancer (PC) samples showed a lower *CDH1* transcript levels among normal, proliferative inflammatory atrophy (PIA) and metastasis. **(F)** Graphic representation of the percentage of methylation in normal, PIA and PC samples. PIA and PC samples were hypermethylated compared to normal samples. **(G)** graphic representation of E-cadherin protein expression by Western blotting after normalization with β-actin. It is possible to observe lack in both PIA and PC compared to normal samples. *Statistical difference between two variable comparisons.

comparison between E-cadherin expression clinical-pathological data is summarized in **Table 2**.

Comparing the E-cadherin immunoexpression between the primary tumors and its paired metastasis, no statistical difference was found ($P > 0.05$). The mean of E-cadherin negative cells was similar in primary PC and its paired metastasis (15 ± 7.09 and 16.8 ± 5.25, respectively). No correlation was found between the number of E-cadherin negative cells in the primary PC samples ($N = 11$) and its respective metastasis ($N = 11$) ($r = 0.076$, $P = 0.8223$). In addition, this comparison was no significant by regression analysis [$F (1, 9) = 0.01838$, $P = 0.08951$, $R^2 = 0.7071$]. Although in a limited number of cases, a significant difference was observed comparing E-cadherin negative cells in bone metastasis ($N = 9$; 14.77 ± 4.02) with those in soft tissues ($N = 2$; 26 ± 5.0) A positive correlation between E-cadherin negative cells ($r = 0.8565$, $P = 0.0052$) was found comparing only primary tumors with the respective paired bone metastasis. We also found a significant regression equation ($F (1, 7) = 25.08$, $P = 0.0016$, $R^2 = 0.7818$), comparing primary tumors with their respective metastasis. We observed a positive correlation between the Gleason score and the number of negative E-cadherin neoplastic cells ($R = 0.8505$ and $P < 0.0001$) and a significant regression equation [$F (1, 18) = 36.18$, $P < 0.0001$), $R^2 = 0.6678$]. Overall, prostate cancer with a high Gleason score showed a higher number of negative E-cadherin cells in comparison with those with lower Gleason scores. The linear regression graphics are shown in **Supplementary Figure 1**.

We also investigated the proliferative index in E-cadherin negative areas using E-cadherin/Ki67 double immunoexpression. All normal samples ($N = 20$) showed only membranous E-cadherin with no nuclear Ki67 expression. On the other hand, it was identified a higher number of double-stained epithelial cells in PIA samples ($N = 20$). In PC samples, areas with E-cadherin downregulation showed only scattered Ki67 expression, indicating a low proliferative index (**Supplementary Figure 2**).

Western Blotting

A strong 120 KDa band was identified in normal prostate tissues (**Figures 1D, G**). No statistical difference was observed comparing the E-cadherin expression in normal prostates with PIA samples.

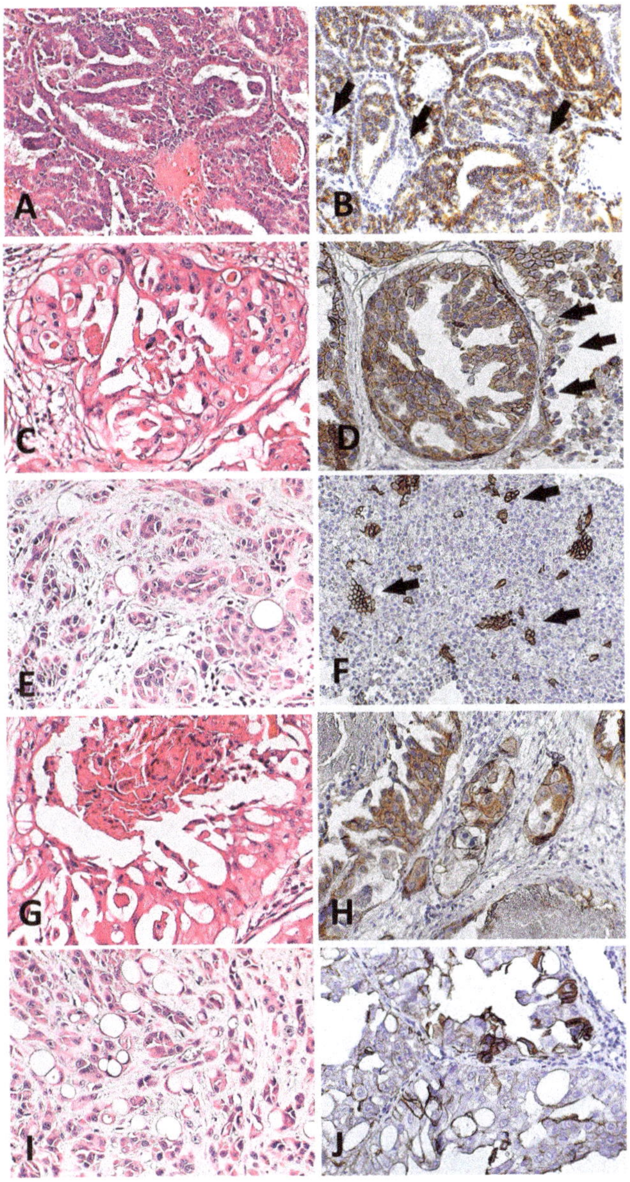

FIGURE 2 | Histological and immunohistochemical E-cadherin evaluation in canine prostate cancer (PC). **(A)** canine PC presenting a papillary pattern. It is possible to observe multifocal areas of E-cadherin loss **(B)** (arrows) in this pattern. **(C)** Canine PC with cribriform patter. Note E-cadherin membranous diffuse expression **(D)** in neoplastic cells and areas of E-cadherin loss (arrows). **(E)** Canine PC with solid pattern. **(F)** area of E-cadherin loss in canine PC with solid pattern. There are only few remaining positive cells (arrows). **(G)** Canine PC showing cribriform with central comedonecrosis pattern. **(H)** is possible to observe membranous E-cadherin expression in neoplastic cells with only few cells showing no E-cadherin expression. **(I)** Canine PC with signet ring pattern. **(J)** It is possible to observe multifocal areas with E-cadherin loss.

However, a lower E-cadherin expression was detected in PC compared to normal prostate (P = 0.0003) and PIA samples (P = 0.0001). **Supplementary Figure 3** is representative of the Western blotting assays performed in normal prostate, PIA, and PC samples.

CDH1 Gene Expression

PC samples showed lower *CDH1* transcript levels in comparison with PIA (P = 0.0038) and normal samples (P = 0.0427) (**Figure 1E**). No statistical difference was observed between the transcript levels in PIA and normal samples. Unfortunately, only five metastatic samples (5/11) were evaluated by RT-qPCR, mainly due to poor mRNA quality. The median of *CDH1* relative quantification (RQ) was 0.7 (0.2–9.5), 0.9 (0.2–5.6), 0.5 (0.02–1.7), and 3.45 (0.6–2.4) in normal, PIA, PC and metastases samples, respectively. In prostate cancer, a strong positive correlation was observed between high levels of E-cadherin protein expression and *CDH1* transcript levels (Spearman R = 0.9429; P = 0.0167) (Significant regression equation: F (1, 4) = 9.654, P= 0.036, R^2 = 0.7071). *CDH1* gene expression between the primary tumors (N = 5) and its paired metastasis (N = 5) showed no correlation (r = 0.2000, P = 0.7833) and no significant regression equation [F (1, 2) = 0.06048, P = 0.8216, R^2 = 0.01976]. A higher methylation pattern was detected in samples with lower levels of *CDH1* transcripts and a higher number of E-cadherin negative cells, which revealed a direct association of the methylation pattern with gene and protein down expression.

Quantitative Bisulfite Pyrosequencing

CDH1 promoter hypermethylation was identified in PIA and PC compared to normal samples (P < 0.0001). The median of methylation was 20.5% (7–55%), 98% (94–100%) and 95% (94–100%) in normal, PIA and PC samples, respectively (**Figure 1F**) (**Supplementary Figure 4**).

In Vitro Assays

CDH1 was hypermethylated and presented lower transcript levels (0.86±0.04) in the PC1 cell line. After the 5-Aza-dC treatment, this cell line presented an inverted methylation pattern and increased gene expression level (1.7 ±0.2).

DISCUSSION

In this study, E-cadherin gene and protein expression findings were associated with *CDH1* methylation in canine PC, which gives evidence of the regulatory mechanism of *CDH1* in canine

TABLE 2 | Mean percentage of E-cadherin negative and positive cells according to the diagnosis and Gleason score.

IHC results	Normal	PIA	PC	Metastasis	Gleason 6	Gleason 8	Gleason 10
Positive cells (%)	100±0	97.9	89.5±4.7	90.5±4.2	98.6±7.3	91%±6.9	82.6±7.1
Negative cells (%)	0±0	2.1	10.5±4.6	9.5±4.2	1.4±7.2	9±6.5	17.4±7.4

IHC' protein expression by immunohistochemistry; PIA, Proliferative inflammatory atrophy; PC, Prostate cancer.

PC. E-cadherin is a cell-to-cell adhesion molecule and its loss correlates with epithelial-mesenchymal transition, metastasis and poor prognosis (Putzke et al., 2011; Fonseca-Alves et al., 2015a). Considering the high variation among the different semi-quantitative scores for immunohistochemical evaluation, we counted the number of negative cells and provided a score. We found a higher number of negative E-cadherin cells in PC compared to PIA and normal prostate. Also, a lower number of positive cells was correlated with survival.

Similarly to our findings, Fonseca et al. (2013) and Tsui et al. (2016) reported that PIA presented a lack of E-cadherin expression compared with normal samples. Using Western blot, we confirmed these previous data. Moreover, no statistical difference was observed in PIA compared to PC in cases with a higher E-cadherin expression, which could be explained by the lack of metastatic potential and malignancy of these preneoplastic lesions. Furthermore, during cell proliferation, it is expected the presence of E-cadherin loss by epithelia cells related to cell division instead of a migration (Tsui et al., 2016). For this reason, we performed E-cadherin/Ki67 double staining and confirmed that tumor areas presented E-cadherin losses with no proliferative activity. This result strongly suggests that E-cadherin downregulation is more related to cell migration instead of proliferation. In human PC, *CDH1* hypermethylation and E-cadherin loss is more frequent in metastatic tumors with higher Gleason score (Maruyama et al., 2002). Similar results were observed in our canine PC samples. Although the Gleason score is relatively new in veterinary practice, our study is the first to associate Gleason score with overall survival and E-cadherin downregulation.

In human PC, E-cadherin downregulation is frequent in later stages of the disease and poorly differentiated tumors (Ipekci et al., 2015; Zhang et al., 2016a). Considering the dynamic process of E -cadherin expression, a group of cases with negative cells could also be associated with worse prognosis in canine PC. We showed an association between a higher number of E-cadherin negative cells with shorter survival time, suggesting that the number of E-cadherin negative cells could be used as a prognostic factor. To our knowledge, no previous studies presented the percentage of E-cadherin negative cells and their association with the prognosis in human PC (Graff et al., 1995; Yoshiura et al., 1995; Li et al., 2001; Mostafavi-Pour et al., 2015). On the other hand, in human pancreatic adenocarcinomas, Hong et al. (Hong et al., 2011) described the lowest survival time in patients with total a loss of E-cadherin compared with those with partial loss of the protein expression. The authors suggested that partial and total loss of E-cadherin are an independent negative prognostic factor. In human breast cancer, different authors associated E-cadherin decreased expression with worse prognosis, such as lower overall survival, disease-free interval, positive lymph node (Tang et al., 2012; Ricciardi et al., 2015; Wang et al., 2018), and higher proliferative rate evaluated by Ki-67 (Kashiwagi et al., 2011). In 103 prostate carcinomas, Ipekci et al. (Ipekci et al., 2015) showed E-cadherin decreased expression, but no correlation was found with disease-free survival. The authors suggested that epithelial-mesenchymal transition evaluated by E-cadherin, β-catenin, vimentin and Wnt is a late event in tumor progression. These proteins could not be detected in the primary tumor and, therefore, would not be good predictors of metastasis (Ipekci et al., 2015).

We found a strong positive correlation (r = 0.9424) between E-cadherin protein and gene expression in PC samples. Interestingly, we also found an association between the *CHD1* hypermethylation pattern with gene downregulation. The PC1 cell line was densely hypermethylated and associated with low transcript levels. After 5-Aza-dC treatment, *CDH1* hypomethylation and restoration of gene expression were detected. These results indicated an epigenetic regulation of *CDH1* in canine PC. Similar results were previously described in two prostatic cell lines, DuPro and TSUPr1 (Graff et al., 1995). Considering that DNA methylation is a reversible process, the 5-Aza-dC treatment was efficient in inducing gene demethylation, which suggested that hypermethylated tumors could be sensitive to epigenetic drugs. The hypomethylating agents have been used to treat acute myeloid leukemia (AML) with promising results (Cruijsen et al., 2014). Although our findings are preliminary, dogs could be a preclinical model in precision medicine for testing epigenetic agents in PC patients.

Although cells lacking E-cadherin expression acquire motility and show an invasive and migratory phenotype, only a few cells with no E-cadherin expression are required to develop micrometastasis (Umbas et al., 1994; Canel et al., 2013). Thus, the evaluation of this cell group is relevant for a better understanding of the metastatic process. E-cadherin downregulation occurs in most cases by posttranscriptional mechanisms (Canel et al., 2013). *CDH1* promoter hypermethylation is widely studied in many human cancers, including prostate cancer (Graff et al., 1995; Yoshiura et al., 1995; Li et al., 2001; Mostafavi-Pour et al., 2015). Interestingly, a mean of 90.5% of E-cadherin positive cells was detected in the metastasis. Our data reinforce that the modulation of the metastatic foci and adhesion molecules re-expression are pivotal for the metastasis development (Welch, 2007). A higher number of metastatic cases was observed (N = 3) in patients showing Gleason 10 (N = 8). These samples presented a mean of 17.4% of negative cells. Overall, these results suggest that a group of cells showing lack of E-cadherin expression in primary tumors would have the potential to invade and re-express E-cadherin in metastatic foci.

There is limited information regarding E-cadherin expression in human PC and its paired metastasis (Bae et al., 2011). During the invasion of an artificial basal cell membrane, prostatic cells presented loss of E-cadherin expression and re-expressed after overtaking the membrane (Bae et al., 2011). In dogs, the lack of E-cadherin expression was previously demonstrated in PCs and a complete E-cadherin loss was observed in the neoplastic emboli (Fonseca-Alves et al., 2015a). Interestingly, the paired metastasis showed E-cadherin re-expression. Thus, a dynamic E-cadherin expression occurs during the tumor progression to metastasis. Further studies to evaluate the *CDH1* methylation analysis in circulating prostate cancer cells and its prognostic value could be relevant for clinical purposes.

CONCLUSION

Our results suggested an epigenetic regulation of the E-cadherin promoter leading to E-cadherin downregulation in canine PC. The number of negative E-cadherin cells investigated by immunohistochemistry demonstrated the importance of these cells to PC prognosis. Overall, our results indicate that dogs could be a preclinical model for testing hypomethylating agents in precision medicine.

ETHICS STATEMENT

This study was approved by the Animal Ethics Committee of the University of Sao Paulo State, UNESP, Botucatu, Brazil (#107/2015).

AUTHOR CONTRIBUTIONS

CF-A wrote the first manuscript draft. CF-A performed the immunohistochemistry and qPCR experiments. CF-A, AL-F, PL, and PK performed the cell culture experiments. CF-A and RL-A conceived the project and grant funding. CF-A, SR, and HK conceived and performed the pyrosequencing experiments. VG contributed constructive comments. RL-A and SR supervised the project and revised the manuscript. All authors read and approved the final version of the manuscript.

FUNDING

This research was funded by the Sao Paulo Research Foundation (FAPESP) grant (#2012/18426-1 and 2019/24649-2). National Council for Scientific and Technological Development (CNPq) (#422139/2018-1). We also would like to thank the research grant from the National Council for Scientific and Technological Development (CNPq) (#422139/2018-1).

ACKNOWLEDGMENTS

We would like to thank Dr. Marcio Carvalho for his technical support. We also thank to the A.C. Camargo Cancer Center, SP, Brazil for allowing the access to its institutional infrastructure.

REFERENCES

Abdelrahman, A. E., Arafa, S. A., and Ahmed, R. A. (2017). Prognostic value of twist-1, E-cadherin and EZH2 in prostate cancer: an immunohistochemical study. *Turk Patoloji Derg.* 4, 198–210. doi: 10.5146/tjpath.2016.01392

Bae, K. M., Parker, N. N., Dai, Y., Vieweg, J., and Siemann, D. W. (2011). E-cadherin plasticity in prostate cancer stem cell invasion. *Am. J. Cancer Res.* 1 (1), 71–84.

Busch, E. L., Hornick, J. L., Umeton, R., Albayrak, A., Lindeman, N. I., MacConaill, L. E., et al. (2017). Somatic mutations in CDH1 and CTNNB1 in primary carcinomas at 13 anatomic sites. *Oncotarget* 8 (49), 85680–85691. doi: 10.18632/oncotarget.21115

Canel, M., Serrels, A., Frame, M. C., and Brunton, V. G. (2013). E-cadherin-integrin crosstalk incancer invasion and metastasis. *J. Cell Sci.* 126 (Pt 2), 393–401. doi: 10.1242/jcs.100115

Chao, Y. L., Shepard, C. R., and Wells, A. (2010). Breast carcinoma cells re-express E-cadherin during mesenchymal to epithelial reverting transition. *Mol. Cancer* 9, 179. doi: 10.1186/1476-4598-9-179

Cornell, K. K., Bostwick, D. G., Cooley, D. M., Hall, G., Harvey, H. J., Hendrick, M. J., et al. (2000). Clinical and pathologic aspects of spontaneous canine prostate carcinoma: a retrospective analysis of 76 cases. *Prostate* 45 (2), 173–183. doi: 10.1002/1097-0045(20001001)45:2<173::AID-PROS12>3.0.CO;2-R

Costa, C. D., Justo, A. A., Kobayashi, P. E., Story, M. M., Palmieri, C., Laufer-Amorim, R., et al. (2019). Characterization of OCT3/4, Nestin, NANOG, CD44 and CD24 as stem cell markers in canine prostate cancer. *Int. J. Biochem. Cell Biol.* 108, 21–28. doi: 10.1016/j.biocel.2019.01.002

Cruijsen, M., Lübbert, M., Wijermans, P., and Huls, G. (2014). Clinical results of hypomethylating agents in AML treatment. *J. Clin. Med.* 4 (1), 1–17. doi: 10.3390/jcm4010001

da Costa-Prando, E., Cavalli, L. R., and Rainho, C. A. (2011). Evidence of epigenetic regulation of the tumor suppressor gene cluster flanking RASSF1 in breast cancer cell lines. *Epigenetics* 6 (12), 1413–1424. doi: 10.4161/epi.6.12.18271

Debelec-Butuner, B., Alapinar, C., Ertunc, N., Gonen-Korkmaz, C., Yörükoğlu, K., and Korkmaz, K. S. (2014). TNFα-mediated loss of β-catenin/E-cadherin association and subsequent increase in cell migration is partially restored by NKX3.1 expression in prostate cells. *PloS One* 9 (10), 1–12. doi: 10.1371/journal.pone.0109868

Dhar, S., Kumar, A., Gomez, C. R., Akhtar, I., Hancock, J. C., Lage, J. M., et al. (2017). MTA1-activated Epi-microRNA-22 regulates E-cadherin and prostate cancer invasiveness. *FEBS Lett.* 591 (6), 924–933. doi: 10.1002/1873-3468.12603

Fonseca-Alves, C. E., Rodrigues, M. M., de Moura, V. M., Rogatto, S. R., and Laufer-Amorim, R. (2013). Alterations of C-MYC, NKX3.1, and E-cadherin expression in canine prostate carcinogenesis. *Microsc. Res. Tech.* 76 (12), 1250–1256. doi: 10.1002/jemt.22292

Fonseca-Alves, C. E., Kobayashi, P. E., Rivera-Calderón, L. G., and Laufer-Amorim, R. (2015a). Evidence of epithelial-mesenchymal transition in canine prostate cancer metastasis. *Res. Vet. Sci.* 100, 176–181. doi: 10.1016/j.rvsc.2015.03.001

Fonseca-Alves, C. E., Bento, D. D., Torres-Neto, R., Werner, J., Kitchell, B., and Laufer-Amorim, R. (2015b). Ki67/KIT double immunohistochemical staining in cutaneous mast cell tumors from Boxer dogs. *Res. Vet. Sci.* 102, 122–126. doi: 10.1016/j.rvsc.2015.08.007

Fonseca-Alves, C. E., Kobayashi, P. E., and Laufer-Amorim, R. (2018a). Evaluation of NKX3.1 and C-MYC expression in canine prostatic cancer. *Res. Vet. Sci.* 118, 365–370. doi: 10.1016/j.rvsc.2018.04.001

Fonseca-Alves, C. E., Kobayashi, P. E., Rivera-Calderón, L. G., Felisbino, S. L., Rinaldi, J. C., Drigo, S. A., et al. (2018b). Immunohistochemical panel to characterize canine prostate carcinomas according to aberrant p63 expression. *PloS One* 13 (6), 1–16. doi: 10.1371/journal.pone.0199173

Friedl, P., and Wolf, K. (2003). Tumour-cell invasion and migration: diversity and escapemechanisms. *Nat. Rev. Cancer.* 3 (5), 362–374. doi: 10.1038/nrc1075

Graff, J. R., Herman, J. G., Lapidus, R. G., Chopra, H., Xu, R., Jarrard, D. F., et al. (1995). E-cadherin expression is silenced by DNA hypermethylation in human breast and prostate carcinomas. *Cancer Res.* 55 (22), 5195–5199.

Hong, S. M., Li, A., Olino, K., Wolfgang, C. L., Herman, J. M., Schulick, R. D., et al. (2011). Loss of E-cadherin expression and outcome among patientswith resectable pancreatic adenocarcinomas. *Mod. Pathol.* 24 (9), 1237–1247. doi: 10.1038/modpathol.2011.74

Hoque, M. O., Topaloglu, O., Begum, S., Henrique, R., Rosenbaum, E., Van Criekinge, W., et al. (2005). Quantitative methylation-specific polymerase chain reaction gene patterns in urine sediment distinguish prostate cancer patients from control subjects. *J. Clin. Oncol.* 23 (27), 6569–6575. doi: 10.1200/JCO.2005.07.009

Humphrey, P. A., Moch, H., Cubilla, A. L., Ulbright, T. M., and Reuter, V. E. (2016). The 2016 WHO Classification of Tumours of the Urinary System and Male Genital Organs-Part B: Prostate and Bladder Tumours. *Eur. Urol.* 17, 106–119. doi: 10.1016/j.eururo.2016.02.028

Huynh, M. A., Chen, M. H., Wu, J., Braccioforte, M. H., Moran, B. J., and D'Amico, A. V. (2016). Influence of comorbidity on the risk of mortality in men with unfavorable-risk prostate cancer undergoing high-dose radiation therapy alone. *Int. J. Radiat. Oncol. Biol. Phys.* 11, 1158–1167. doi: 10.1016/j.ijrobp.2016.03.004

Ipekci, T., Ozden, F., Unal, B., Saygin, C., Uzunaslan, D., and Ates, E. (2015). Epithelial-Mesenchymal transition markers β-catenin, snail, and E-Cadherin do not predict disease free survival in prostate adenocarcinoma: a prospective study. *Pathol. Oncol. Res.* 21 (4), 1209–1216. doi: 10.1007/s12253-015-9958-z

Kashiwagi, S., Yashiro, M., Takashima, T., Aomatsu, N., Ikeda, K., Ogawa, Y., et al. (2011). Advantages of adjuvant chemotherapy for patients with triple-negativebreast cancer at Stage II: usefulness of prognostic markers E-cadherin and Ki67. *Breast Cancer Res.* 13 (6), R122. doi: 10.1186/bcr3068

Kobayashi, P. E., Fonseca-Alves, C. E., Rivera-Calderón, L. G., Carvalho, M., Kuasne, H., Rogatto, S. R., et al. (2018). Deregulation of E-cadherin, β-catenin, APC and Caveolin-1 expression occurs in canine prostate cancer and metastatic processes. *Res. Vet. Sci.* 118, 254–261. doi: 10.1016/j.rvsc.2018.03.004

Laufer-Amorim, R., Fonseca-Alves, C. E., Villacis, R. A. R., Linde, S. A. D., Carvalho, M., Larsen, S. J., et al. (2019). Comprehensive genomic profiling of androgen-receptor-negative canine prostate cancer. *Int. J. Mol. Sci.* 28, 20(7. doi: 10.3390/ijms20071555

Li, L. C., Zhao, H., Nakajima, K., Oh, B. R., Ribeiro-Filho, L. A., Carroll, P., et al. (2001). Methylation of the E-cadherin gene promoter correlates with progression of prostate cancer. *J. Urol.* 166 (2), 705–709. doi: 10.1016/S0022-5347(05)66047-8

Li, F., Pascal, L. E., Stolz, D. B., Wang, K., Zhou, Y., Chen, W., et al. (2019). E-cadherin is downregulated in benign prostatic hyperplasia and required for tight junction formation and permeability barrier in the prostatic epithelial cell monolayer. *Prostate* 79 (11), 1226–1237. doi: 10.1002/pros.23806

Livak, K. J., and Schmittgen, T. D. (2001). Analysis of relative gene expression data using real-time quantitative PCR and the 2-ΔΔCT method. *Methods* 25, 402–408. doi: 10.1006/meth.2001.1262

Maruyama, R., Toyooka, S., Toyooka, K. O., Virmani, A. K., Zöchbauer-Müller, S., Farinas, A. J., et al. (2002). Aberrant promoter methylation profile of prostate cancers and its relationship to clinicopathological features. *Clin. Cancer Res.* 8 (2), 514–519.

Mostafavi-Pour, Z., Kianpour, S., Dehghani, M., Mokarram, P., Torabinejad, S., and Monabati, A. (2015). Methylation of Integrin α4 and E-Cadherin genes in human prostate cancer. *Pathol. Oncol. Res.* 21 (4), 921–927. doi: 10.1007/s12253-015-9917-8

Palmieri, C., and Grieco, V. (2015). Proposal of Gleason-like grading system of canine prostate carcinoma in veterinary pathology practice. *Res. Vet. Sci.* 103, 11–15. doi: 10.1016/j.rvsc.2015.09.004

Putzke, A. P., Ventura, A. P., Bailey, A. M., Akture, C., Opoku-Ansah, J., Celiktaş, M., et al. (2011). Metastatic progression of prostate cancer and e-cadherin regulation by zebl and SRC family kinases. *Am. J. Pathol.* 179 (1), 400–410. doi: 10.1016/j.ajpath.2011.03.028

Ricciardi, G. R., Adamo, B., Ieni, A., Licata, L., Cardia, R., Ferraro, G., et al. (2015). Androgen Receptor (AR), E-Cadherin, and Ki-67 as emergingtargets and novel prognostic markers in triple-negative breast cancer (TNBC) patients. *PloS One* 10 (6), 1–11. doi: 10.1371/journal.pone.0128368

Rivera-Calderón, L. G., Fonseca-Alves, C. E., Kobayashi, P. E., Carvalho, M., Drigo, S. A., de Oliveira-Vasconcelos, R., et al. (2016). Alterations in PTEN, MDM2, TP53 and AR protein and gene expression are associated with canine prostate carcinogenesis. *Res. Vet. Sci.* 106, 56–61. doi: 10.1016/j.rvsc.2016.03.008

Rivera-Calderón, L. G., Fonseca-Alves, C. E., Kobayashi, P. E., Carvalho, M., Vasconcelos, R. O., and Laufer-Amorim, R. (2019). p-mTOR, p-4EBP-1 and eIF4E expression in canine prostatic carcinoma. *Res. Vet. Sci.* 122, 86–92. doi: 10.1016/j.rvsc.2018.11.006

Saramaki, O., and Visakorpi, T. (2007). Chromosomal aberrations in prostate cancer. *Front. Biosci.* 12, 3287–3301. doi: 10.2741/2312

Siegel, R. L., Miller, K. D., and Jemal, A. (2019). Cancer statistics, 2019. *CA Cancer J. Clin.* 69 (1), 7–34. doi: 10.3322/caac.21551

Singal, R., Ferdinand, L., Reis, I. M., and Schlesselman, J. J. (2004). Methylation of multiple genes in prostate cancer and the relationship with clinicopathological features of disease. *Oncol. Rep.* 12, 631–637. doi: 10.3892/or.12.3.631

Staník, M., Čapák, I., Macík, D., Vašina, J., Lžičařová, E., Jarkovský, J., et al. (2014). Sentinel lymph node dissection combined with meticuloushistology increases the detection rate of nodal metastases in prostate cancer. *Int. Urol. Nephrol.* 46 (8), 1543–1549. doi: 10.1007/s11255-014-0704-3

Tang, D., Xu, S., Zhang, Q., and Zhao, W. (2012). The expression and clinical significance of the androgen receptor and E-cadherin in triple-negative breast cancer. *Med. Oncol.* 29 (2), 526–533. doi: 10.1007/s12032-011-9948-2

Tsui, K. H., Lin, Y. H., Chung, L. C., Chuang, S. T., Feng, T. H., Chiang, K. C., et al. (2016). Prostate-derived ets factor represses tumorigenesis and modulates epithelial-to-mesenchymal transition in bladder carcinoma cells. *Cancer Lett.* 375 (1), 142–151. doi: 10.1016/j.canlet.2016.02.056

Umbas, R., Schalken, J. A., Aalders, T. W., Carter, B. S., Karthaus, H. F., Schaafsma, H. E., et al. (1992). Expression of the cellular adhesion molecule E-cadherinis reduced or absent in high-grade prostate cancer. *Cancer Res.* 52 (18), 5104–5109.

Umbas, R., Isaacs, W. B., Bringuier, P. P., Schaafsma, H. E., Karthaus, H. F., Oosterhof, G. O., et al. (1994). Decreased E-cadherin expression is associated with poor prognosis in patients with prostate cancer. *Cancer Res.* 54 (14), 3929–3933.

Wang, W., Wang, L., Mizokami, A., Shi, J., Zou, C., Dai, J., et al. (2017). Down-regulation of E-cadherin enhances prostate cancer chemoresistance via Notch signaling. *Chin. J. Cancer* 36 (1), 35. doi: 10.1186/s40880-017-0203-x

Wang, X., Dong, B., Zhang, K., Ji, Z., Cheng, C., Zhao, H., et al. (2018). E-cadherin bridges cell polarity and spindle orientation to ensure prostate epithelial integrity and prevent carcinogenesis in vivo. *PloS Genet.* 14 (8), 1–23. doi: 10.1371/journal.pgen.1007609

Welch, D. R. (2007). Do we need to redefine a cancer metastasis and staging definitions? *Breast Dis.* 26, 3–12. doi: 10.3233/BD-2007-26102

Yoshiura, K., Kanai, Y., Ochiai, A., Shimoyama, Y., Sugimura, T., and Hirohashi, S. (1995). Silencing of the E-cadherin invasion-suppressor gene by CpG methylation in human carcinomas. *Proc. Natl. Acad. Sci. U. S. A.* 92 (16), 7416–7419. doi: 10.1073/pnas.92.16.7416

Zhang, S. Q., Zhang, G. Q., and Zhang, L. (2016a). Correlation between methylation of the E-Cadherin gene and malignancy of prostate cancer. *Genet. Mol. Res.* 15 (2), 1–9. doi: 10.4238/gmr.15028046

Zhang, J., Chen, X. Y., Huang, K. J., Wu, W. D., Jiang, T., Cao, J., et al. (2016b). Expression of FoxM1 and the EMT-associated protein E-cadherin in gastric cancer and its clinical significance. *Oncol. Lett.* 12 (4), 2445–2450. doi: 10.3892/ol.2016.4917

10

The Current State of MicroRNAs as Restenosis Biomarkers

Nelson Varela[1], *Fernando Lanas*[2,3], *Luis A. Salazar*[3] *and Tomás Zambrano*[4*]

[1] Laboratory of Chemical Carcinogenesis and Pharmacogenetics, Department of Basic-Clinical Oncology, Faculty of Medicine, Universidad de Chile, Santiago, Chile, [2] Department of Internal Medicine, Faculty of Medicine, Universidad de La Frontera, Temuco, Chile, [3] Center of Molecular Biology and Pharmacogenetics, Scientific and Technological Bioresource Nucleus, Universidad de La Frontera, Temuco, Chile, [4] Department of Medical Technology, Faculty of Medicine, Universidad de Chile, Santiago, Chile

***Correspondence:**
Tomás Zambrano
tomas.zambrano@uchile.cl

In-stent restenosis corresponds to the diameter reduction of coronary vessels following percutaneous coronary intervention (PCI), an invasive procedure in which a stent is deployed into the coronary arteries, producing profuse neointimal hyperplasia. The reasons for this process to occur still lack a clear answer, which is partly why it remains as a clinically significant problem. As a consequence, there is a vigorous need to identify useful non-invasive biomarkers to differentiate and follow-up subjects at risk of developing restenosis, and due to their extraordinary stability in several bodily fluids, microRNA research has received extensive attention to accomplish this task. This review depicts the current understanding, diagnostic potential and clinical challenges of microRNA molecules as possible blood-based restenosis biomarkers.

Keywords: epigenetics, microRNAs, in-stent restenosis, biomarkers, personalized and precision medicine

INTRODUCTION

Cardiovascular disease (CVD) refers to a group of pathologies initiated by an underlying process known as atherosclerosis and ultimately affecting the heart and blood vessels. Atherosclerosis plaques build-up inside the coronary arteries, consequently limiting the blood flow and resulting in coronary artery disease (CAD). Atherosclerosis is an inflammatory disease (Ross, 1999) able to produce two morphologically opposite lesions within the coronary arteries, stenotic and non-stenotic. The last may be asymptomatic for years and clinical management is generally supported on lifestyle modifications and, eventually, pharmacological interventions in high-risk individuals. In contrast, stenotic lesions have clinical manifestations like angina pectoris, and common medical management includes revascularization procedures such as coronary artery bypass grafting (CABG) and percutaneous transluminal coronary angioplasty (PTCA), a widely performed techniques since the late 1970s to correct serious coronary atherosclerotic lesions (Gruntzig et al., 1979), restoring myocardial blood flow and reducing angina symptoms. Despite its massive use, however, elevated restenosis rates affected almost half of the patients treated (Fischman et al., 1994) and established one of the main problems of current cardiology. Restenosis is arbitrarily defined as a narrowing of vessel diameter greater than 50% to that of the reference vessel (Marx et al., 2011), and results from excessive proliferation and migration of vascular smooth muscle cells (VSMC) to the intima, eventually leading to re-narrowing of the arterial lumen (Chaabane et al., 2013). Since this problem was identified, interventional cardiology has moved from PTCA to percutaneous coronary intervention (PCI), a technique involving the placement of a stent. This procedure is the most widely performed treatment for symptomatic coronary disease patients (Serruys et al., 1994). The use of bare metal stents (BMS) has made it possible to eliminate factors that favor restenosis, such as elastic recoil and negative remodeling (Lowe et al., 2002), reducing the prevalence of restenosis from 50% to 20-30% (Kastrati et al., 1997). As the main cause of restenosis was attributed to the excessive proliferation of VSMC, the development of new technologies determined the arrival of drug-eluting stents (DES), reducing the restenosis rate below 10% (Morice et al., 2002). Despite the implementation of new stenting technologies, along with novel pharmacological or mechanical approaches to reduce restenosis incidence, this problem is still considered an important drawback, especially in high-risk patients, limiting the overall success of DES.

PATHOPHYSIOLOGY OF RESTENOSIS IN STENTED ARTERIES

Stent placement produces a mechanical vascular lesion that can be briefly divided into 3 phases:

a) Early phase: the stent produces an injury to the endothelium, damaging or totally destroying the endothelial cells (EC) that line the intimal arterial tunic, resulting in consecutive endothelial stripping, re-endothelization and subsequent generation of neo-endothelium (Grewe et al., 2000). The above is followed by an inflammatory response, including platelet activation and recruitment of circulating leukocytes, releasing cytokines and growth factors (Mitra and Agrawal, 2006).

b) Intermediate phase: characterized by the migration and proliferation of VSMC.

c) Late phase or tissue remodeling: VSMCs change from a contractile and quiescent non-proliferative G0 phase phenotype towards a highly active synthetic phenotype, with extracellular matrix (ECM) deposition in the arterial intima. Various growth factors, such as fibroblast growth factor (FGF-2), epidermal growth factor (EGF), platelet-derived growth factor (PDGF), and insulin-like growth factor (IGF) initiate VSMCs proliferation through the tyrosine kinase receptor, activating the Mitogen-activated protein kinases (MAPK) pathway. While the ECM allows the inflammatory infiltrate to adhere, the VSMC secrete hyaluronic acid and proteoglycans that interact and stabilize the fibrin-enriched ECM (Grewe et al., 2000; Mitra and Agrawal, 2006). These vascular responses, characterized by neointima proliferation and vascular remodeling, are responsible for the elevated frequency of post-PTCA restenosis. Anatomopathological studies in post-PCI restenosis demonstrated the same proliferative response of the neointima (Farb et al., 2002; Farb et al., 2004). In addition to VSMC proliferation and ECM synthesis, there is also neointima colonization by extravascular cells, e.g., endothelial progenitors or dendritic cells, together with compensatory mechanisms of apoptosis (Tuleta et al., 2008; Tuleta et al., 2010).

TYPES OF STENT: BARE METAL STENT AND DRUG-ELUTING STENT

Since the introduction of BMS in 1987 (Sigwart et al., 1987), important PTCA limitations such as restenosis and sudden narrowing of diseased arteries after angioplasty were reduced. Serruys et al. demonstrated that stent implantation reduces the need for a second coronary angioplasty compared with standard balloon angioplasty (RR 0.58, CI 0.40–0.85) mainly due to a low restenosis rate, going from 32% to 22% (Serruys et al., 1994). However, the benefit was accompanied by an increased risk of cardiovascular complications and longer hospitalization time. Stent-induced injury causes greater damage than damaged produced by standard balloon angioplasty, delineating processes of thrombosis, inflammation and proliferation (Edelman and Rogers, 1998) followed by the deposition of platelet-rich thrombi, which occur from the first days (Farb et al., 1999) until 1 month post-PCI (Komatsu et al., 1998), with additional accumulation of acute inflammatory cells such as neutrophils during the first 30 days, together with chronic inflammatory cells e.g., lymphocytes and macrophages (Farb et al., 1999). There is a correlation between the type of inflammatory reaction and the degree of injury (Rogers and Edelman, 1995), indicating that the surface of the material together with the geometric configuration of the stent contributes to neointimal hyperplasia and thrombosis. Other factors that favor restenosis development are tunica media damage, and the penetration of the stent edges into the lipid core of the atherosclerotic plaque. Both factors increase the inflammatory process within the artery and, therefore, increase intima proliferation (Farb et al., 2002). Since the introduction of combination therapy with P2Y platelet receptor antagonists (ticlopidine, clopidogrel) and acetylsalicylic acid, the incidence of post-stent thrombosis has been significantly reduced (Bertrand et al., 2000), and the majority of thrombotic events occurred within the first 10 days post-PCI. Additionally, post-stent thrombosis with BMS after the first month is considered rare (Farb et al., 2003). DES development is based on a coating containing an antiproliferative drug, so both post-PCI proliferation of the tunica intima and subsequent restenosis can be reduced (Garg and Serruys, 2010). In this way, first-generation DES devices were developed, which are

Abbreviations: AUC, area under the curve; AGO2, argonaute protein family 2; BMS, bare metal stent; CABG, coronary artery bypass grafting; CHD, coronary heart disease; CVD, cardiovascular disease; DES, drug-eluting stent; DGCR8, DiGeorge syndrome critical region 8; EC, endothelial cells; ECM, extracellular matrix; EDTA, ethylene diamine tetra-acetic acid; EGF, epidermal growth factor; FGF-2, fibroblast growth factor 2; IGF, insulin-like growth factor; ISR, in-stent restenosis; LEAOD, lower extremity arterial occlusive disease; LDL-C, low-density lipoprotein cholesterol; miRNA, micro ribonucleic acid; MAPK, mitogen-activated protein kinase; MIQE, minimum information for publication of quantitative real-time PCR experiments; mRNA, messenger ribonucleic acid; ncRNAs, non-coding RNAs; NGS, next-generation sequencing; PAD, peripheral artery disease; PCI, percutaneous coronary intervention; pre-miRNA, precursor micro ribonucleic acid; pri-miRNA, primary micro ribonucleic acid; PTCA, percutaneous transluminal coronary angioplasty; qPCR, quantitative polymerase chain reaction; RASP, rapid angiographic stenotic progression; RISC, RNA-induced silencing complex; ROC, receiver operating characteristic; Rnases, ribonucleases; snRNA, small nuclear RNAs; snoRNAs, small nucleolar RNAs; TLR, target lesion restenosis; TVR, target vessel revascularization; VSMC, vascular smooth muscle cells; XPO5, exportin 5; 3′-UTR, three prime untranslated region; 5′-UTR, five prime untranslated region.

coated with a drug-containing polymer designed to interrupt cell replication and reduce neointimal hyperplasia, markedly decreasing the occurrence of post-PCI restenosis (Herdeg et al., 2000; Curfman, 2002). However, after DES implantation, intervention centers have identified an increase in thrombosis associated with the stent placement process for up to 3 years after stent implantation, an additional complication rarely caused by the use of BMS (Luscher et al., 2007). Several reports show the occurrence of acute (<24 hours), sub-acute (<30 days), late (>30 days), and very late (>12 months) thrombosis after DES placement (McFadden et al., 2004; Pfisterer et al., 2006; Brodie et al., 2012). A large observational study revealed that from a total of 2229 consecutive patients receiving a total of 4495 DES, 29 had stent- associated thrombosis, occurring more than 30 days after stent placement, also revealing a 45% mortality rate (Iakovou et al., 2005).

MICRORNAS

In 1993, a key report involving the study of the *Caenorhabditis elegans* roundworm and showing downregulation of the LIN-14 protein by a small transcript namely lin-4 through antisense interaction between RNAs due to sequence complementarity between lin-4 and the 3'-untranslated region (3'-UTR) of the lin-14 mRNA (Lee et al., 1993) suggested a novel gene silencing mechanism affecting protein levels. Afterward, a second 21 nucleotides (nt) small RNA identified as let-7 was also implicated in the regulation of heterochronic genes related to *C. elegans* development (Reinhart et al., 2000). Moreover, the small let-7 RNA was shown to be highly conserved, indicating that its sequence is critical for functional purposes (Pasquinelli et al., 2000). These small RNAs were the 2 first of a family currently known as microRNAs (miRNAs) and further characterized as endogenous non-coding RNAs (ncRNAs) evolutionarily conserved between species with a size comprised between 20 and 23 nt, existing in both plants and animals. Their main function is to control gene expression by cleaving messenger RNA (mRNA) or through translational repression, preventing mRNA translation to its corresponding protein (Bartel, 2004). This control mechanism fine-tunes gene expression through the complementary matching of a segment comprised between nucleotides 2 to 7 of the miRNA i.e., seed region, with both the 3′- and 5′-UTR regions of target mRNAs (Lytle et al., 2007). It is estimated that miRNAs control more than 30% of the human genome (Lewis et al., 2005), through an interaction that can be reversible (Wu and Belasco, 2008). The canonical pathway of miRNA biogenesis begins with transcription from miRNA genes by RNA polymerase II, producing primary miRNAs (pri-miRNA) that undergo subsequent processing by the Drosha-DGCR8 (DiGeorge syndrome critical region 8) microprocessor complex, producing a miRNA precursor (pre-miRNA) of approximately 70 nt transported to the cytoplasm *via* exportin 5 (XPO5). Once in the cytoplasm, pre-miRNAs are further processed by RNase III (Dicer) into a double-stranded 21-23 nt miRNA. One strand of the miRNA is charged into the RNA-induced silencing complex (RISC) in conjunction with members of the Argonaute protein family (AGO2), a nuclear protein essential for miRNA maturation and functionality (Bushati and Cohen, 2007; Winter et al., 2009).

Different studies show that miRNAs orchestrate a wide network of cellular activities and are deeply involved in almost every biological pathway, regulating processes such as cell division and apoptosis (Ng et al., 2012), metabolism (Wilfred et al., 2007), intracellular signaling (Zhang et al., 2012), immune response (Taganov et al., 2006) and cell movement (Png et al., 2011). Similarly, miRNAs have been associated with restenosis-related processes, such as VSMC proliferation, migration and neointima formation (Chen et al., 2012; Yamakuchi, 2012; Gareri et al., 2016), revealing the great potential for diagnostic, prognostic, therapeutics or additional clinical manipulation. In fact, by examining the hypothesis that miRNAs produced by the placenta can be released into circulation, a set of placental miRNAs was successfully identified in maternal plasma (Chim et al., 2008), shedding light into another possible role as blood-based biomarkers, a crucial finding confirmed during the same year by a meticulous characterization of a large number of exceptionally stable miRNAs in both serum and plasma (Chen et al., 2008b). Since then, numerous reports have shown that miRNAs can be detectable in multiple fluids including urine, saliva, and cerebrospinal fluid, and even though the extracellular environment is rich in ribonucleases (RNases), miRNAs can be especially stable in serum and plasma as well, representing an enormous potential as non-invasive biomarkers for several pathologies (Gilad et al., 2008; Mitchell et al., 2008; Gupta et al., 2010). The mechanisms by which miRNAs remain particularly unaffected in circulation are due to their association with different carrier particles that confer protection against the potent blood RNases (**Figure 1**). It was first proposed that miRNAs circulate in the bloodstream by a cellular discharge mechanism through membrane-bound vesicles such as exosomes (Valadi et al., 2007; Kosaka et al., 2010), which are 50 to 100 nm vesicles released by exocytosis (Fevrier and Raposo, 2004). However, reports indicated that the abundant majority of miRNAs are exosome free and associated with Ago2 (Arroyo et al., 2011; Turchinovich et al., 2011). Importantly, as the RISC constitutes the effector component of the gene-silencing mechanism portrayed by miRNAs, it has been suggested that the miRNA-Ago2 complex is functional in circulation. Moreover, in 2011, Vickers et al. showed that miRNAs are associated with HDL in plasma not only for transport but these complexes maintain also the functional gene repression role of miRNAs directed to their cell target through delivery by a scavenger receptor BI (SR-BI)-dependent mechanism (Vickers et al., 2011). Considering that miRNAs are associated with dissimilar transport molecules, further classification of extracellular miRNAs according to their transporting molecules has been provided elsewhere (Russo et al., 2012).

BIOMARKER DISCOVERY

In general, biomarkers are classified as: (1) Diagnostic biomarkers for a specific pathology, disease or syndrome; (2) predictive biomarkers for the response to a given medication or treatment; (3) biomarkers of predictions about the probable

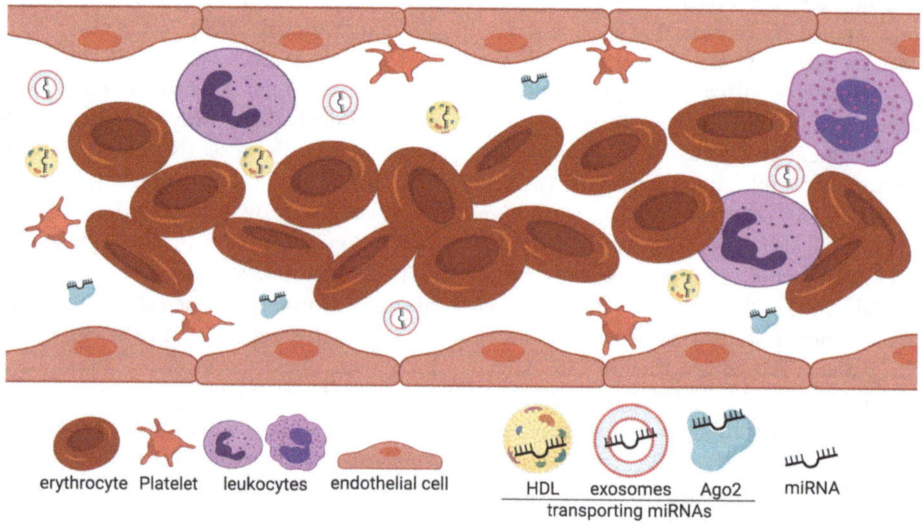

FIGURE 1 | Extracellular miRNAs are associated with different transport molecules in the bloodstream. Cell-free miRNAs are transported in the blood mainly associated with Ago2 (green) and HDL particles (yellow). To a lesser extent, miRNAs are transported *via* exosomes (light blue). Created with BioRender.

course of a disease; and (4) biomarkers of predisposition or susceptibility to a disease (Simon, 2011). According to the World Health Organization, a biomarker is "any substance, structure, process or products that can be measured in the body and influence or predict the outcome or incidence of the disease". Different study models have used cell lines, animals, patient cohorts, biopsies, biobank samples, or prospective studies as the starting point for biomarker development (Vargas and Harris, 2016). On the other hand, "omics" technologies are a particularly suitable tool for biomarkers discovery as they take advantage of the potential of the transcriptome, proteome and metabolome readings, facilitating detailed molecular characterization in a particular biological sample. Examples of these technologies are microarrays and next-generation sequencing (NGS) used for genomic and transcriptomic studies. In this sense, the usual strategy has been to describe large amounts of data from a specific molecule (e.g., miRNAs), in samples such as cell lines, animals and most importantly patients with a specific condition (McShane and Polley, 2013; Ghai and Wang, 2016) in order to generate hypotheses based on the large data available following bioinformatic analysis (Simon, 2010). Thus, new proposed biomarkers are capable, for example, of facilitating diagnosis of a certain disease or predicting the response of therapeutic interventions, such as post-stenting restenosis. Currently, a number of reasons have proposed circulating miRNAs as one of the most attractive candidates molecules to be explored as diagnosis, prognosis, and treatment biomarkers for various pathologies, mainly their extraordinary stability in blood circulation, the relative ease of extraction from the most common non-invasive matrices, and their susceptibility to sensitive detection through quantitative polymerase chain reaction (qPCR) (Gilad et al., 2008; Moldovan et al., 2014; Ghai and Wang, 2016) and rapid multiplexing platforms (Jiang et al., 2014).

CIRCULATING MIRNAS AS RESTENOSIS BIOMARKERS

Few investigations have examined the utility of cell-free miRNAs as potential in-stent restenosis (ISR) biomarkers. One of the pioneer reports was a case-control study revealing a series of 4 miRNAs -miRNA-21, miRNA-100, miRNA-143 and miRNA-145 - as candidate ISR markers, with the two latter showing the highest sensitivity and specificity according to receiver operating characteristic (ROC) curves (He et al., 2014) (**Table 1**). Consistent with their newfound role, these 4 miRNAs have been previously related to the pathogenesis of vascular diseases such as neointimal lesion formation (Ji et al., 2007), and VSMC proliferation, migration, and differentiation (Davis et al., 2008; Cordes et al., 2009; Grundmann et al., 2011; O'Sullivan et al., 2011). Interestingly, miRNA-21, miRNA-100, miRNA-143 and miRNA-145 were also able to significantly discriminate between diffuse vs. focal ISR, yet, this last finding should be interpreted with attention as it originated from additional analyses performed on a fraction of the total sample, probably introducing bias such as loss of randomization i.e. cases and controls are no longer balanced groups or lesser power related to the smaller sample. Another recent report showed that miRNA-93-5p was differentially expressed between ISR and non-ISR patients, proposing miRNA-93-5p as a robust independent ISR predictor (O'Sullivan et al., 2019). Additionally, they found

TABLE 1 | Studies reporting extracellular miRNAs as restenosis biomarkers.

miRNA	Performance	95% CI	P	Sens. (%)	Spec. (%)	Expression in restenosis patients	Groups	Grouping	Stent type	Follow-up (years)	ISR	Sample	Ethnicity	Ref
miRNA-21	AUC: 0.568	0.372-0.757	<0.05	50.1	68.6	UR	51 ISR; 130 NISR; 52 Controls	Randomization	DES	0.5 - 1	Coronary	Plasma	Chinese	He et al., 2014
miRNA-100	AUC: 0.608	0.372-0.757	<0.05	60.2	68.9	DR								
miRNA-143	AUC: 0.818	0.755-0.963	<0.001	82.1	80.1	DR								
miRNA-145	AUC: 0.880	0.791-0.987	<0.001	88.7	83.1	DR								
miRNA-93-5p	C: 0.734	not shown	0.0001	not shown	not shown	UR	39 ISR; 39 NISR	Consecutive, matched for age and diabetes	DES/ BMS	4.9	Coronary	Plasma	Caucasian	O'Sullivan et al., 2019
miRNA-93 + FHSRF + SL and SD	C: 0.769	0.00001												
miRNA-19a, miRNA-126, miRNA-210 miRNA-378	AUC: 0.776	0.722-0.831	not shown	not shown	not shown	DR	222 NISR; 64 ISR	Consecutive	DES	1	Coronary	Plasma	Chinese	Dai et al., 2019
miRNA-146a	AUC: 0674	0.567-0.781	not shown	not shown	not shown	UR	232 NISR; 23 ISR	Consecutive	DES	1	Coronary	Plasma	Chinese	Zhang et al., 2019
miRNA-146b	AUC: 0.801	0.729-0.875												
miRNA-92a (TLR)	HR: 0.55	0.34-0.88	0.013	not shown	not shown	DR	26 primary endpoint; 21 secondary endpoint; 36 controls	Consecutive	not shown	1 and 2	PAD	Serum	Caucasian	Stojkovic et al., 2018
miRNA-195 (TLR)	HR: 0.40	0.23-0.68	0.001											
miRNA-195 (TVR)	HR: 0.40	0.22-0.75	0.005											
miRNA-92a + CF (TLR)	C: 0.70	0.60-0.80	0.130											
miRNA-195 + CF (TLR)	C: 0.75	0.66-0.85	0.030											
miRNA-143	AUC: 0.866	not shown	not shown	83.7	82.6	DR	74 ISR; 91 NISR	Consecutive	BMS???	not shown	LEAOD	Serum? Plasma?	Chinese	Yu et al., 2017
miRNA-21	AUC: 0.938	0.898-0.977	not shown	83.5	98.2	DR	79 ISR; 327 NISR	Consecutive, randomly chosen	BMS	0.5	LEAOD	Plasma	Chinese	Zhang et al., 2017
miRNA-320a	AUC: 0.766	not shown	not shown	82.1	63.8	UR	78 ISR; 68 NISR; 62 controls	Consecutive	Not shown	not shown	LEAOD	Plasma	Chinese	Yuan et al., 2019
miRNA-572	AUC: 0.690	69.2	68.9											

AUC, area under the curve; BMS, bare metal stent; C, C-statistic (a comparable measure to AUC); CF, clinical factors; DR, down-regulated; DES, drug eluting stent; FHSRF, Framingham heart study risk factors; HR, hazard ratio; ISR, in-stent restenosis; LEAOD, lower extremity arterial occlusive disease; NISR, non in-stent restenosis; PAD, peripheral artery disease; Sens., sensibility; Spec., specificity; SL, stent length; SD, stent diameter; TLR, target lesion restenosis; TVR, target vessel revascularization; UR, up-regulated.

that the predictive performance of a model including main risk factors for ISR e.g., diabetes, stent length and diameter, together with common risk factors for CAD development such as age, sex, active smoking, diabetes, hypertension, and hyperlipidemia was further improved by adding miRNA-93-5p levels. Even though the results shown are encouraging, an important weakness of the study lies in the lack of additional validation in an independent cohort, restricting the extent of the results. Very recently, Dai et al. selected 14 angiogenesis-related candidate miRNAs (Dai et al., 2019) and reported 4 as independently associated with decreased restenosis risk (miRNA-19a, miRNA-126, miRNA-210, and miRNA-378). ROC curves showed that this subgroup of miRNAs had better predictive values for restenosis occurrence in Chinese population than each on its own (AUC: 0.776; 95% CI: 0.722-0.831). Moreover, they found that 2 additional miRNAs (let-7f and miR-296) correlated with a lower risk of rapid angiographic stenotic progression (RASP), and together with the previous miRNAs, the model exhibited greater performance for RASP prediction (AUC: 0.879; 95% CI: 0.841-0.917). Another similar study also performed in Chinese population recently reported that miRNA-146a and miRNA-146b were overexpressed in restenosis vs non-restenosis patients (P = 0.006), both holding prognostic value for restenosis risk in subjects with coronary heart disease (CHD) (Zhang et al., 2019). Analogously to the previous work, Zhang and colleagues also found that these miRNAs were up-regulated in RASP patients, and were both individually able to predict RASP occurrence in CHD subjects.

In the case of peripheral artery disease (PAD) ISR, the role of 11 restenosis-related circulating miRNAs (miRNA-17, miRNA-21, miRNA-92a, miRNA-126, miRNA-143, miRNA-145, miRNA-195, miRNA-221, miRNA-222, miRNA-223, and miRNA-424) was examined in a primary endpoint constituted by target lesion restenosis (TLR) and atherothrombotic events, and a secondary endpoint represented by target vessel revascularization (TVR) (Stojkovic et al., 2018). Findings showed that miRNA-92a and miRNA-195 were independent predictors of the primary endpoint, but only miRNA-195 was able to independently predict TVR. Interestingly, miRNA-143 and miRNA-145 were detected at very low expression levels and were excluded from additional analyses even though they were previously suggested as ISR markers (He et al., 2014). Nonetheless, and similarly to the report from O'Sullivan and colleagues, adding miRNA-195 to clinical factors not only improved the ability to distinguish TLR from non-TLR subjects against a model considering miRNA-92a (P = 0.012), but also proved superior to a model integrating clinical risk factors plus both miRNA-92a and miRNA-195 (Stojkovic et al., 2018) (**Table 1**).

A series of studies exploring the utility of predictive miRNAs for lower extremity arterial occlusive disease (LEAOD) restenosis have been performed. One of them identified low levels of circulating miRNA-143 in restenosis vs. non-restenosis patients, correlating this measure with smoking status, history of diabetes, glucose, and low-density lipoprotein cholesterol (LDL-C) (Yu et al., 2017). Even though a low expression of the restenosis-related miRNA-143 is consistent with the findings from He and colleagues, it is unknown if the expression pattern remains the same for the rest of the previously reported restenosis-associated miRNAs, as Yu et al. evaluated miRNA-143 only. Additionally, it is also uncertain if the analysis was performed either in serum or plasma due to authors referred to both biological fluids as interchangeable concepts, an unfortunate but substantial ambiguity hampering a clear interpretation of the results and that will be later described. Another study showed overexpression of the coronary ISR-associated miRNA-21 in LEAOD restenosis patients (Zhang et al., 2017), constituting an excellent predictor of vascular restenosis according to ROC curve analysis, with an AUC of 0.938. Moreover, miRNA-21 was correlated with age, diabetes, and hypertension, and together with diabetes, miRNA-21 represented the main risk factors for LEAOD restenosis occurrence. Lastly, a very recent report found that circulating levels of miRNA-320a and miRNA-572 were significantly overexpressed in restenosis-developing LEAOD patients (Yuan et al., 2019). ROC curves also showed that these miRNAs were capable of discerning between patients developing ISR versus patients that not, with AUC values of 0.766 and 0.690, respectively. Although the results provided are auspicious, the sample size enrolled was relatively small. Additionally, the study fails to report minimal but very relevant clinical data like the stent types used, follow-up time, and important statistical estimates (**Table 1**), however, one of the strengths lies in the inclusion of a second control group made up by healthy volunteers besides the classical non-ISR group, a similar methodological approach than the study of He et al., allowing to better discriminate miRNA behavior between these 2 conditions. In this sense, it is noteworthy that the relative expression among miRNAs evaluated by Yuan et al. was very similar between the non-ISR group and healthy volunteers. Furthermore, 2 miRNAs showed comparable levels between ISR, non-ISR and healthy volunteers, which is also consistent with previous studies, and represents an interesting outcome if we consider that current extracellular miRNA normalization is commonly based on the addition of exogenous spike-in miRNAs, a technical issue that could be more suitably replaced by analyzing endogenous miRNAs stable enough for the discovery of restenosis biomarkers. Still, additional experimentation is needed to clarify this observation.

Technical Challenges

Besides requiring a feasible and reliable analyte associated with a particular condition, miRNA routine sample analysis needs to cautiously overcome a significant amount of potentially detrimental obstacles that, if not properly managed, will not only affect miRNA analyses but most importantly, can compromise the patient's diagnosis and clinical management by inaccurate lab determinations. Consequently, before implementing miRNA measurement into day-to-day laboratory testing, a large number of technical issues must be correctly addressed. One of the very first concerns related to miRNA analysis comes from the collecting tubes employed for blood withdrawal. For instance, EDTA-collecting tubes can alter circulating miRNA detection, especially if samples are not immediately processed. Moreover, the longer it takes for sample processing, the stronger the effect on extracellular miRNA patterns (Leidinger et al., 2015). Studies show that proper attention must be paid when selecting the type of biological matrix for further miRNA analysis. For instance, serum samples were reported to contain a higher number of miRNAs than their corresponding plasma counterparts, even if analyzing the same individual, an outcome highly dependent on the measurement platforms used (Wang et al., 2012). However, various reports argue in favor of the opposing scenario, where not only plasma was reported to contain higher miRNA concentrations (McDonald et al., 2011), but miRNAs diversity was far more restricted in serum samples (Foye et al., 2017). Findings have also shown that serum- and plasma-abundant miRNAs such as miRNA-451a, miRNA-16-5p, miRNA-223-3p, and miRNA-25-3p are differentially expressed between these 2 biological fluids (Foye et al., 2017), reinforcing the idea that both fluids cannot be assumed to be interchangeable concepts regarding miRNA concentrations. Also, hemolysis affects directly the concentration of a small number of miRNAs (Kirschner et al., 2011; McDonald et al., 2011) which is consistent with reports showing particular and specific erythrocytes-derived miRNAs (Chen et al., 2008a; Kannan and Atreya, 2010). Deepening in this area, hemolysis was demonstrated to affect a far greater number of miRNAs than previously reported, compromising miRNAs previously recognized as important biomarkers for various diseases (Kirschner et al., 2013). Interestingly, the use of a ratio between the hemolysis-dependent and -independent miRNA-451 and miRNA-23a, respectively, has been proposed to better assess the degree of erythrocyte lysis and therefore, diminish the effect of hemolysis on blood-based miRNA determinations (Blondal et al., 2013).

On the other hand, important variations for biomarker discovery can be introduced at the analytical stage, which is highly dependent on the measurement platform selected. In the case of miRNAs, the most common and widely used technique corresponds to qPCR largely due to its robustness, relative ease, elevated specificity and sensitivity, broad dynamic range and high resolution, among others. However, each step required for qPCR assays can introduce a different cause of variation that can mask the biological differences we are looking to determine, and to date, several unsolved questions can affect circulating miRNA analysis when using this system. For example, to date, there is no predetermined or consensus set of extracellular miRNAs that can be used for normalization (Roberts et al., 2014), which would be the ideal scenario to allow proper comparisons between a target miRNA against a normalizer miRNA to obtain reliable miRNA expression levels. In contrast, nowadays normalization is frequently achieved by using synthetic alternatives such as exogenous miRNAs that are spiked in during RNA isolation in an attempt to avoid technical differences regarding the extraction procedure. Another different normalization strategy is the use of ncRNAs such as small nuclear RNAs (snRNA) or small nucleolar RNAs (snoRNAs), however, to select the proper normalizer, a set of these ncRNAs must be previously analyzed in each lab for validation purposes to obtain accurate results. Importantly, RNA quality is one the most fundamental determinants of reproducibility for qPCR results, and improper sample handling regarding the collection, transport or storage can affect RNA integrity and unambiguously lead to irreproducible experiments. Therefore, every RNA preparation must be meticulously assessed to ensure that nucleic acids present have not been degraded. In general, a standardized qPCR protocol should be closely followed to ensure consistency between diverse laboratories, as suggested in the MIQE guidelines (minimum information for publication of quantitative real-time PCR experiments) (Bustin et al., 2009).

Future Perspectives

miRNA research as ISR biomarkers is still at an early stage. The scarce findings reported so far include conventional flaws in study designs such as small samples, lack of proper control groups or validation cohorts, and the absence of clinical, technical and statistical data that may be crucial for a correct interpretation and reproducibility. The tolerant operative consensus at the time of reporting putative restenosis biomarkers leads to inconsistent or unreliable candidate miRNAs, and to advance the field, investigations must meet minimal and uniform conditions. Clinical outcomes should be very well defined to turn them into quantifiable events, or at least easily measurable. In this sense, large randomized, multicenter, prospective trials capable of establishing whether miRNAs can effectively predict clinical features are greatly needed.

A persistent but reasonable shortcoming regarding miRNA research as biomarkers for restenosis is represented by the candidate approach, i.e., handpicking specific RNA molecules exclusively based on previous reports. Although most of these investigations have solid grounds since they are based on the choice of miRNAs previously associated with restenosis-related mechanisms, the success rates contrast with what one might expect, since they are not even close to 100%, as the case of different studies mentioned above (Stojkovic et al., 2018; Dai et al., 2019). The candidate approach is predominantly used because is significantly less expensive than other wide-ranging strategies, such as microarray or NGS, but the loss of information can be excessive. On the contrary, using, for example, NGS allows having the clearest depiction of the total amount of miRNAs that may be relevant or even participate in the endpoint and that we could be missing when executing the candidate methodology, which ultimately points to the cost-benefit relation.

Even though important technical difficulties can further delay the arrival of miRNAs into the clinic, ongoing research in the matter has allowed the most common problems to be properly identified and therefore, prone to correction with an adequate and strictly controlled standardization of laboratory practices, including pre-analytical, analytical and post-analytical procedures, eliminating as many possible variables affecting routine miRNA determinations. But even if we carefully consider the aforementioned arguments, the complete potential of miRNAs as clinically applicable biomarkers is rather far from becoming an imminent reality, as some additional and significant questions remain poorly explored, for example, the existence of circadian oscillations of human miRNAs. A recent and very stimulating line of research has demonstrated important diurnal variations in miRNA levels (Rekker et al., 2015; Heegaard et al., 2016; Hicks et al., 2018), with important and detrimental implications for an exceedingly trivial preanalytical issue such as establishing the proper moment to collect blood samples.

AUTHOR CONTRIBUTIONS

NV wrote sections of the manuscript. TZ contributed conception, design and wrote sections of the manuscript. FL and LS contributed critical analysis and wrote sections of the manuscript. All authors contributed to manuscript revision, read and approved the submitted version.

FUNDING

This work was supported by FONDECYT-Chile (grant number 3170785).

ACKNOWLEDGMENTS

We thank Isabel Castro Massó for her collaboration in obtaining the figure.

REFERENCES

Arroyo, J. D., Chevillet, J. R., Kroh, E. M., Ruf, I. K., Pritchard, C. C., Gibson, D. F., et al. (2011). Argonaute2 complexes carry a population of circulating microRNAs independent of vesicles in human plasma. *Proc. Natl. Acad. Sci. U. S. A.* 108 (12), 5003–5008. doi: 10.1073/pnas.1019055108

Bartel, D. P. (2004). MicroRNAs: genomics, biogenesis, mechanism, and function. *Cell* 116 (2), 281–297. doi: 10.1016/s0092-8674(04)00045-5

Bertrand, M. E., Rupprecht, H. J., Urban, P., Gershlick, A. H., and Investigators, C. (2000). Double-blind study of the safety of clopidogrel with and without a loading dose in combination with aspirin compared with ticlopidine in combination with aspirin after coronary stenting: the clopidogrel aspirin stent international cooperative study (CLASSICS). *Circulation* 102 (6), 624–629. doi: 10.1161/01.cir.102.6.624

Blondal, T., Jensby Nielsen, S., Baker, A., Andreasen, D., Mouritzen, P., Wrang Teilum, M., et al. (2013). Assessing sample and miRNA profile quality in serum and plasma or other biofluids. *Methods* 59 (1), S1–S6. doi: 10.1016/j.ymeth.2012.09.015

Brodie, B., Pokharel, Y., Garg, A., Kissling, G., Hansen, C., Milks, S., et al. (2012). Predictors of early, late, and very late stent thrombosis after primary percutaneous coronary intervention with bare-metal and drug-eluting stents for ST-segment elevation myocardial infarction. *JACC Cardiovasc. Interv.* 5 (10), 1043–1051. doi: 10.1016/j.jcin.2012.06.013

Bushati, N., and Cohen, S. M. (2007). microRNA functions. *Annu. Rev. Cell Dev. Biol.* 23, 175–205. doi: 10.1146/annurev.cellbio.23.090506.123406

Bustin, S. A., Benes, V., Garson, J. A., Hellemans, J., Huggett, J., Kubista, M., et al. (2009). The MIQE guidelines: minimum information for publication of quantitative real-time PCR experiments. *Clin. Chem.* 55 (4), 611–622. doi: 10.1373/clinchem.2008.112797

Chaabane, C., Otsuka, F., Virmani, R., and Bochaton-Piallat, M. L. (2013). Biological responses in stented arteries. *Cardiovasc. Res.* 99 (2), 353–363. doi: 10.1093/cvr/cvt115

Chen, S. Y., Wang, Y., Telen, M. J., and Chi, J. T. (2008a). The genomic analysis of erythrocyte microRNA expression in sickle cell diseases. *PloS One* 3 (6), e2360. doi: 10.1371/journal.pone.0002360

Chen, X., Ba, Y., Ma, L., Cai, X., Yin, Y., Wang, K., et al. (2008b). Characterization of microRNAs in serum: a novel class of biomarkers for diagnosis of cancer and other diseases. *Cell Res.* 18 (10), 997–1006. doi: 10.1038/cr.2008.282

Chen, L. J., Lim, S. H., Yeh, Y. T., Lien, S. C., and Chiu, J. J. (2012). Roles of microRNAs in atherosclerosis and restenosis. *J. BioMed. Sci.* 19 (1), 79. doi: 10.1186/1423-0127-19-79

Chim, S. S., Shing, T. K., Hung, E. C., Leung, T. Y., Lau, T. K., Chiu, R. W., et al. (2008). Detection and characterization of placental microRNAs in maternal plasma. *Clin. Chem.* 54 (3), 482–490. doi: 10.1373/clinchem.2007.097972

Cordes, K. R., Sheehy, N. T., White, M. P., Berry, E. C., Morton, S. U., Muth, A. N., et al. (2009). miR-145 and miR-143 regulate smooth muscle cell fate and plasticity. *Nature* 460 (7256), 705–710. doi: 10.1038/nature08195

Curfman, G. D. (2002). Sirolimus-eluting coronary stents. *N. Engl. J. Med.* 346 (23), 1770–1771. doi: 10.1056/NEJM200206063462302

Dai, R., Liu, Y., Zhou, Y., Xiong, X., Zhou, W., Li, W., et al. (2019). Potential of circulating pro-angiogenic microRNA expressions as biomarkers for rapid angiographic stenotic progression and restenosis risks in coronary artery disease patients underwent percutaneous coronary intervention. *J. Clin. Lab. Anal.* e23013. doi: 10.1002/jcla.23013

Davis, B. N., Hilyard, A. C., Lagna, G., and Hata, A. (2008). SMAD proteins control DROSHA-mediated microRNA maturation. *Nature* 454 (7200), 56–61. doi: 10.1038/nature07086

Edelman, E. R., and Rogers, C. (1998). Pathobiologic responses to stenting. *Am. J. Cardiol.* 81 (7A), 4E–6E. doi: 10.1016/s0002-9149(98)00189-1

Farb, A., Sangiorgi, G., Carter, A. J., Walley, V. M., Edwards, W. D., Schwartz, R. S., et al. (1999). Pathology of acute and chronic coronary stenting in humans. *Circulation* 99 (1), 44–52. doi: 10.1161/01.cir.99.1.44

Farb, A., Weber, D. K., Kolodgie, F. D., Burke, A. P., and Virmani, R. (2002). Morphological predictors of restenosis after coronary stenting in humans. *Circulation* 105 (25), 2974–2980. doi: 10.1161/01.cir.0000019071.72887.bd

Farb, A., Burke, A. P., Kolodgie, F. D., and Virmani, R. (2003). Pathological mechanisms of fatal late coronary stent thrombosis in humans. *Circulation* 108 (14), 1701–1706. doi: 10.1161/01.CIR.0000091115.05480.B0

Farb, A., Kolodgie, F. D., Hwang, J. Y., Burke, A. P., Tefera, K., Weber, D. K., et al. (2004). Extracellular matrix changes in stented human coronary arteries. *Circulation* 110 (8), 940–947. doi: 10.1161/01.CIR.0000139337.56084.30

Fevrier, B., and Raposo, G. (2004). Exosomes: endosomal-derived vesicles shipping extracellular messages. *Curr. Opin. Cell Biol.* 16 (4), 415–421. doi: 10.1016/j.ceb.2004.06.003

Fischman, D. L., Leon, M. B., Baim, D. S., Schatz, R. A., Savage, M. P., Penn, I., et al. (1994). A randomized comparison of coronary-stent placement and balloon angioplasty in the treatment of coronary artery disease. Stent Restenosis Study Investigators. *N. Engl. J. Med.* 331 (8), 496–501. doi: 10.1056/NEJM199408253310802

Foye, C., Yan, I. K., David, W., Shukla, N., Habboush, Y., Chase, L., et al. (2017). Comparison of miRNA quantitation by Nanostring in serum and plasma samples. *PloS One* 12 (12), e0189165. doi: 10.1371/journal.pone.0189165

Gareri, C., De Rosa, S., and Indolfi, C. (2016). MicroRNAs for Restenosis and Thrombosis After Vascular Injury. *Circ. Res.* 118 (7), 1170–1184. doi: 10.1161/CIRCRESAHA.115.308237

Garg, S., and Serruys, P. W. (2010). Coronary stents: current status. *J. Am. Coll. Cardiol.* 56 (10 Suppl), S1–42. doi: 10.1016/j.jacc.2010.06.007

Ghai, V., and Wang, K. (2016). Recent progress toward the use of circulating microRNAs as clinical biomarkers. *Arch. Toxicol.* 90 (12), 2959–2978. doi: 10.1007/s00204-016-1828-2

Gilad, S., Meiri, E., Yogev, Y., Benjamin, S., Lebanony, D., Yerushalmi, N., et al. (2008). Serum microRNAs are promising novel biomarkers. *PloS One* 3 (9), e3148. doi: 10.1371/journal.pone.0003148

Grewe, P. H., Deneke, T., Machraoui, A., Barmeyer, J., and Muller, K. M. (2000). Acute and chronic tissue response to coronary stent implantation: pathologic findings in human specimen. *J. Am. Coll. Cardiol.* 35 (1), 157–163. doi: 10.1016/s0735-1097(99)00486-6

Grundmann, S., Hans, F. P., Kinniry, S., Heinke, J., Helbing, T., Bluhm, F., et al. (2011). MicroRNA-100 regulates neovascularization by suppression of mammalian target of rapamycin in endothelial and vascular smooth muscle cells. *Circulation* 123 (9), 999–1009. doi: 10.1161/CIRCULATIONAHA.110.000323

Gruntzig, A. R., Senning, A., and Siegenthaler, W. E. (1979). Nonoperative dilatation of coronary-artery stenosis: percutaneous transluminal coronary angioplasty. *N. Engl. J. Med.* 301 (2), 61–68. doi: 10.1056/NEJM197907123010201

Gupta, S. K., Bang, C., and Thum, T. (2010). Circulating microRNAs as biomarkers and potential paracrine mediators of cardiovascular disease. *Circ. Cardiovasc. Genet.* 3 (5), 484–488. doi: 10.1161/CIRCGENETICS.110.958363

He, M., Gong, Y., Shi, J., Pan, Z., Zou, H., Sun, D., et al. (2014). Plasma microRNAs as potential noninvasive biomarkers for in-stent restenosis. *PloS One* 9 (11), e112043. doi: 10.1371/journal.pone.0112043

Heegaard, N. H., Carlsen, A. L., Lilje, B., Ng, K. L., Ronne, M. E., Jorgensen, H. L., et al. (2016). Diurnal Variations of Human Circulating Cell-Free Micro-RNA. *PloS One* 11 (8), e0160577. doi: 10.1371/journal.pone.0160577

Herdeg, C., Oberhoff, M., Baumbach, A., Blattner, A., Axel, D. I., Schroder, S., et al. (2000). Local paclitaxel delivery for the prevention of restenosis: biological effects and efficacy *in vivo*. *J. Am. Coll. Cardiol.* 35 (7), 1969–1976. doi: 10.1016/s0735-1097(00)00614-8

Hicks, S. D., Khurana, N., Williams, J., Dowd Greene, C., Uhlig, R., and Middleton, F. A. (2018). Diurnal oscillations in human salivary microRNA and microbial transcription: Implications for human health and disease. *PloS One* 13 (7), e0198288. doi: 10.1371/journal.pone.0198288

Iakovou, I., Schmidt, T., Bonizzoni, E., Ge, L., Sangiorgi, G. M., Stankovic, G., et al. (2005). Incidence, predictors, and outcome of thrombosis after successful implantation of drug-eluting stents. *JAMA* 293 (17), 2126–2130. doi: 10.1001/jama.293.17.2126

Ji, R., Cheng, Y., Yue, J., Yang, J., Liu, X., Chen, H., et al. (2007). MicroRNA expression signature and antisense-mediated depletion reveal an essential role of MicroRNA in vascular neointimal lesion formation. *Circ. Res.* 100 (11), 1579–1588. doi: 10.1161/CIRCRESAHA.106.141986

Jiang, L., Shen, Y., Zheng, K., and Li, J. (2014). Rapid and multiplex microRNA detection on graphically encoded silica suspension array. *Biosens. Bioelectron* 61, 222–226. doi: 10.1016/j.bios.2014.05.020

Kannan, M., and Atreya, C. (2010). Differential profiling of human red blood cells during storage for 52 selected microRNAs. *Transfusion* 50 (7), 1581–1588. doi: 10.1111/j.1537-2995.2010.02585.x

Kastrati, A., Schomig, A., Elezi, S., Schuhlen, H., Dirschinger, J., Hadamitzky, M., et al. (1997). Predictive factors of restenosis after coronary stent placement. *J. Am. Coll. Cardiol.* 30 (6), 1428–1436. doi: 10.1016/s0735-1097(97)00334-3

Kirschner, M. B., Kao, S. C., Edelman, J. J., Armstrong, N. J., Vallely, M. P., van Zandwijk, N., et al. (2011). Haemolysis during sample preparation alters microRNA content of plasma. *PloS One* 6 (9), e24145. doi: 10.1371/journal.pone.0024145

Kirschner, M. B., Edelman, J. J., Kao, S. C., Vallely, M. P., van Zandwijk, N., and Reid, G. (2013). The Impact of Hemolysis on Cell-Free microRNA Biomarkers. *Front. Genet.* 4, 94. doi: 10.3389/fgene.2013.00094

Komatsu, R., Ueda, M., Naruko, T., Kojima, A., and Becker, A. E. (1998). Neointimal tissue response at sites of coronary stenting in humans: macroscopic, histological, and immunohistochemical analyses. *Circulation* 98 (3), 224–233. doi: 10.1161/01.cir.98.3.224

Kosaka, N., Iguchi, H., Yoshioka, Y., Takeshita, F., Matsuki, Y., and Ochiya, T. (2010). Secretory mechanisms and intercellular transfer of microRNAs in living cells. *J. Biol. Chem.* 285 (23), 17442–17452. doi: 10.1074/jbc.M110.107821

Lee, R. C., Feinbaum, R. L., and Ambros, V. (1993). The C. elegans heterochronic gene lin-4 encodes small RNAs with antisense complementarity to lin-14. *Cell* 75 (5), 843–854. doi: 10.1016/0092-8674(93)90529-y

Leidinger, P., Backes, C., Rheinheimer, S., Keller, A., and Meese, E. (2015). Towards Clinical Applications of Blood-Borne miRNA Signatures: The Influence of the Anticoagulant EDTA on miRNA Abundance. *PloS One* 10 (11), e0143321. doi: 10.1371/journal.pone.0143321

Lewis, B. P., Burge, C. B., and Bartel, D. P. (2005). Conserved seed pairing, often flanked by adenosines, indicates that thousands of human genes are microRNA targets. *Cell* 120 (1), 15–20. doi: 10.1016/j.cell.2004.12.035

Lowe, H. C., Oesterle, S. N., and Khachigian, L. M. (2002). Coronary in-stent restenosis: current status and future strategies. *J. Am. Coll. Cardiol.* 39 (2), 183–193. doi: 10.1016/s0735-1097(01)01742-9

Luscher, T. F., Steffel, J., Eberli, F. R., Joner, M., Nakazawa, G., Tanner, F. C., et al. (2007). Drug-eluting stent and coronary thrombosis: biological mechanisms and clinical implications. *Circulation* 115 (8), 1051–1058. doi: 10.1161/CIRCULATIONAHA.106.675934

Lytle, J. R., Yario, T. A., and Steitz, J. A. (2007). Target mRNAs are repressed as efficiently by microRNA-binding sites in the 5' UTR as in the 3' UTR. *Proc. Natl. Acad. Sci. U. S. A.* 104 (23), 9667–9672. doi: 10.1073/pnas.0703820104

Marx, S. O., Totary-Jain, H., and Marks, A. R. (2011). Vascular smooth muscle cell proliferation in restenosis. *Circ. Cardiovasc. Interv.* 4 (1), 104–111. doi: 10.1161/CIRCINTERVENTIONS.110.957332

McDonald, J. S., Milosevic, D., Reddi, H. V., Grebe, S. K., and Algeciras-Schimnich, A. (2011). Analysis of circulating microRNA: preanalytical and analytical challenges. *Clin. Chem.* 57 (6), 833–840. doi: 10.1373/clinchem.2010.157198

McFadden, E. P., Stabile, E., Regar, E., Cheneau, E., Ong, A. T., Kinnaird, T., et al. (2004). Late thrombosis in drug-eluting coronary stents after discontinuation of antiplatelet therapy. *Lancet* 364 (9444), 1519–1521. doi: 10.1016/S0140-6736(04)17275-9

McShane, L. M., and Polley, M. Y. (2013). Development of omics-based clinical tests for prognosis and therapy selection: the challenge of achieving statistical robustness and clinical utility. *Clin. Trials* 10 (5), 653–665. doi: 10.1177/1740774513499458

Mitchell, P. S., Parkin, R. K., Kroh, E. M., Fritz, B. R., Wyman, S. K., Pogosova-Agadjanyan, E. L., et al. (2008). Circulating microRNAs as stable blood-based markers for cancer detection. *Proc. Natl. Acad. Sci. U. S. A.* 105 (30), 10513–10518. doi: 10.1073/pnas.0804549105

Mitra, A. K., and Agrawal, D. K. (2006). In stent restenosis: bane of the stent era. *J. Clin. Pathol.* 59 (3), 232–239. doi: 10.1136/jcp.2005.025742

Moldovan, L., Batte, K. E., Trgovcich, J., Wisler, J., Marsh, C. B., and Piper, M. (2014). Methodological challenges in utilizing miRNAs as circulating biomarkers. *J. Cell Mol. Med.* 18 (3), 371–390. doi: 10.1111/jcmm.12236

Morice, M. C., Serruys, P. W., Sousa, J. E., Fajadet, J., Ban Hayashi, E., Perin, M., et al. (2002). A randomized comparison of a sirolimus-eluting stent with a standard stent for coronary revascularization. *N. Engl. J. Med.* 346 (23), 1773–1780. doi: 10.1056/NEJMoa012843

Ng, R., Song, G., Roll, G. R., Frandsen, N. M., and Willenbring, H. (2012). A microRNA-21 surge facilitates rapid cyclin D1 translation and cell cycle progression in mouse liver regeneration. *J. Clin. Invest.* 122 (3), 1097–1108. doi: 10.1172/JCI46039

O'Sullivan, J. F., Martin, K., and Caplice, N. M. (2011). Microribonucleic acids for prevention of plaque rupture and in-stent restenosis: "a finger in the dam". *J. Am. Coll. Cardiol.* 57 (4), 383–389. doi: 10.1016/j.jacc.2010.09.029

O'Sullivan, J. F., Neylon, A., Fahy, E. F., Yang, P., McGorrian, C., and Blake, G. J. (2019). MiR-93-5p is a novel predictor of coronary in-stent restenosis. *Heart Asia* 11 (1), e011134. doi: 10.1136/heartasia-2018-011134

Pasquinelli, A. E., Reinhart, B. J., Slack, F., Martindale, M. Q., Kuroda, M. I., Maller, B., et al. (2000). Conservation of the sequence and temporal expression of let-7 heterochronic regulatory RNA. *Nature* 408 (6808), 86–89. doi: 10.1038/35040556

Pfisterer, M., Brunner-La Rocca, H. P., Buser, P. T., Rickenbacher, P., Hunziker, P., Mueller, C., et al. (2006). Late clinical events after clopidogrel discontinuation may limit the benefit of drug-eluting stents: an observational study of drug-eluting versus bare-metal stents. *J. Am. Coll. Cardiol.* 48 (12), 2584–2591. doi: 10.1016/j.jacc.2006.10.026

Png, K. J., Halberg, N., Yoshida, M., and Tavazoie, S. F. (2011). A microRNA regulon that mediates endothelial recruitment and metastasis by cancer cells. *Nature* 481 (7380), 190–194. doi: 10.1038/nature10661

Reinhart, B. J., Slack, F. J., Basson, M., Pasquinelli, A. E., Bettinger, J. C., Rougvie, A. E., et al. (2000). The 21-nucleotide let-7 RNA regulates developmental timing in Caenorhabditis elegans. *Nature* 403 (6772), 901–906. doi: 10.1038/35002607

Rekker, K., Saare, M., Roost, A. M., Kaart, T., Soritsa, D., Karro, H., et al. (2015). Circulating miR-200-family micro-RNAs have altered plasma levels in patients with endometriosis and vary with blood collection time. *Fertil. Steril.* 104938-946 (4), e932. doi: 10.1016/j.fertnstert.2015.06.029

Roberts, T. C., Coenen-Stass, A. M., and Wood, M. J. (2014). Assessment of RT-qPCR normalization strategies for accurate quantification of extracellular microRNAs in murine serum. *PloS One* 9 (2), e89237. doi: 10.1371/journal.pone.0089237

Rogers, C., and Edelman, E. R. (1995). Endovascular stent design dictates experimental restenosis and thrombosis. *Circulation* 91 (12), 2995–3001. doi: 10.1161/01.cir.91.12.2995

Ross, R. (1999). Atherosclerosis–an inflammatory disease. *N. Engl. J. Med.* 340 (2), 115–126. doi: 10.1056/NEJM199901143400207

Russo, F., Di Bella, S., Nigita, G., Macca, V., Lagana, A., Giugno, R., et al. (2012). miRandola: extracellular circulating microRNAs database. *PloS One* 7 (10), e47786. doi: 10.1371/journal.pone.0047786

Serruys, P. W., de Jaegere, P., Kiemeneij, F., Macaya, C., Rutsch, W., Heyndrickx, G., et al. (1994). A comparison of balloon-expandable-stent implantation with balloon angioplasty in patients with coronary artery disease. Benestent Study Group. *N. Engl. J. Med.* 331 (8), 489–495. doi: 10.1056/NEJM199408253310801

Sigwart, U., Puel, J., Mirkovitch, V., Joffre, F., and Kappenberger, L. (1987). Intravascular stents to prevent occlusion and restenosis after transluminal angioplasty. *N. Engl. J. Med.* 316 (12), 701–706. doi: 10.1056/NEJM198703193161201

Simon, R. (2010). Clinical trials for predictive medicine: new challenges and paradigms. *Clin. Trials* 7 (5), 516–524. doi: 10.1177/1740774510366454

Simon, R. (2011). Genomic biomarkers in predictive medicine: an interim analysis. *EMBO Mol. Med.* 3 (8), 429–435. doi: 10.1002/emmm.201100153

Stojkovic, S., Jurisic, M., Kopp, C. W., Koppensteiner, R., Huber, K., Wojta, J., et al. (2018). Circulating microRNAs identify patients at increased risk of in-stent restenosis after peripheral angioplasty with stent implantation. *Atherosclerosis* 269, 197–203. doi: 10.1016/j.atherosclerosis.2018.01.020

Taganov, K. D., Boldin, M. P., Chang, K. J., and Baltimore, D. (2006). NF-kappaB-dependent induction of microRNA miR-146, an inhibitor targeted to signaling proteins of innate immune responses. *Proc. Natl. Acad. Sci. U.S.A.* 103 (33), 12481–12486. doi: 10.1073/pnas.0605298103

Tuleta, I., Skowasch, D., Peuster, M., Nickenig, G., and Bauriedel, G. (2008). Cells of primarily extravascular origin in neointima formation following stent implantation: coordinated expression of endothelial progenitor, dendritic and neural crest-derived cells. *Cardiology* 110 (3), 199–205. doi: 10.1159/000111930

Tuleta, I., Bauriedel, G., Steinmetz, M., Pabst, S., Peuster, M., Welsch, U., et al. (2010). Apoptosis-regulated survival of primarily extravascular cells in proliferative active poststent neointima. *Cardiovasc. Pathol.* 19 (6), 353–360. doi: 10.1016/j.carpath.2009.07.006

Turchinovich, A., Weiz, L., Langheinz, A., and Burwinkel, B. (2011). Characterization of extracellular circulating microRNA. *Nucleic Acids Res.* 39 (16), 7223–7233. doi: 10.1093/nar/gkr254

Valadi, H., Ekstrom, K., Bossios, A., Sjostrand, M., Lee, J. J., and Lotvall, J. O. (2007). Exosome-mediated transfer of mRNAs and microRNAs is a novel mechanism of genetic exchange between cells. *Nat. Cell Biol.* 9 (6), 654–659. doi: 10.1038/ncb1596

Vargas, A. J., and Harris, C. C. (2016). Biomarker development in the precision medicine era: lung cancer as a case study. *Nat. Rev. Cancer* 16 (8), 525–537. doi: 10.1038/nrc.2016.56

Vickers, K. C., Palmisano, B. T., Shoucri, B. M., Shamburek, R. D., and Remaley, A. T. (2011). MicroRNAs are transported in plasma and delivered to recipient cells by high-density lipoproteins. *Nat. Cell Biol.* 13 (4), 423–433. doi: 10.1038/ncb2210

Wang, K., Yuan, Y., Cho, J. H., McClarty, S., Baxter, D., and Galas, D. J. (2012). Comparing the MicroRNA spectrum between serum and plasma. *PloS One* 7 (7), e41561. doi: 10.1371/journal.pone.0041561

Wilfred, B. R., Wang, W. X., and Nelson, P. T. (2007). Energizing miRNA research: a review of the role of miRNAs in lipid metabolism, with a prediction that miR-103/107 regulates human metabolic pathways. *Mol. Genet. Metab.* 91 (3), 209 217. doi: 10.1016/j.ymgme.2007.03.011

Winter, J., Jung, S., Keller, S., Gregory, R. I., and Diederichs, S. (2009). Many roads to maturity: microRNA biogenesis pathways and their regulation. *Nat. Cell Biol.* 11 (3), 228–234. doi: 10.1038/ncb0309-228

Wu, L., and Belasco, J. G. (2008). Let me count the ways: mechanisms of gene regulation by miRNAs and siRNAs. *Mol. Cell* 29 (1), 1–7. doi: 10.1016/j.molcel.2007.12.010

Yamakuchi, M. (2012). MicroRNAs in Vascular Biology. *Int. J. Vasc. Med.* 2012, 13. doi: 10.1155/2012/794898

Yu, Z. H., Wang, H. T., and Tu, C. (2017). Diagnostic value of microRNA-143 in predicting in-stent restenosis for patients with lower extremity arterial occlusive disease. *Eur. J. Med. Res.* 22 (1), 2. doi: 10.1186/s40001-016-0240-y

Yuan, L., Dong, J., Zhu, G., Bao, J., Lu, Q., Zhou, J., et al. (2019). Diagnostic Value of Circulating microRNAs for In-Stent Restenosis in Patients with Lower Extremity Arterial Occlusive Disease. *Sci. Rep.* 9 (1), 1402. doi: 10.1038/s41598-018-36295-2

Zhang, P., Bill, K., Liu, J., Young, E., Peng, T., Bolshakov, S., et al. (2012). MiR-155 is a liposarcoma oncogene that targets casein kinase-1alpha and enhances beta-catenin signaling. *Cancer Res.* 72 (7), 1751–1762. doi: 10.1158/0008-5472.CAN-11-3027

Zhang, B., Yao, Y., Sun, Q. F., Liu, S. Q., Jing, B., Yuan, C., et al. (2017). Circulating mircoRNA-21 as a predictor for vascular restenosis after interventional therapy in patients with lower extremity arterial occlusive disease. *Biosci. Rep.* 37 (2), 1–8. doi: 10.1042/BSR20160502

Zhang, H., Zhang, Q., Liu, Y., and Xue, T. (2019). miR-146a and miR-146b predict increased restenosis and rapid angiographic stenotic progression risk in coronary heart disease patients who underwent percutaneous coronary intervention. *Ir. J. Med. Sci.* 1–8. doi: 10.1007/s11845-019-02101-9

11

Epigenetic Biomarkers in Cardiovascular Diseases

Carolina Soler-Botija[1,2*], Carolina Gálvez-Montón[1,2] and Antoni Bayés-Genís[1,2,3,4]

[1] Heart Failure and Cardiac Regeneration (ICREC) Research Program, Health Science Research Institute Germans Trias i Pujol (IGTP), Badalona, Spain, [2] CIBERCV, Instituto de Salud Carlos III, Madrid, Spain, [3] Cardiology Service, HUGTiP, Badalona, Spain, [4] Department of Medicine, Barcelona Autonomous University (UAB), Badalona, Spain

***Correspondence:**
Carolina Soler-Botija
csoler@igtp.cat

Cardiovascular diseases are the number one cause of death worldwide and greatly impact quality of life and medical costs. Enormous effort has been made in research to obtain new tools for efficient and quick diagnosis and predicting the prognosis of these diseases. Discoveries of epigenetic mechanisms have related several pathologies, including cardiovascular diseases, to epigenetic dysregulation. This has implications on disease progression and is the basis for new preventive strategies. Advances in methodology and big data analysis have identified novel mechanisms and targets involved in numerous diseases, allowing more individualized epigenetic maps for personalized diagnosis and treatment. This paves the way for what is called pharmacoepigenetics, which predicts the drug response and develops a tailored therapy based on differences in the epigenetic basis of each patient. Similarly, epigenetic biomarkers have emerged as a promising instrument for the consistent diagnosis and prognosis of cardiovascular diseases. Their good accessibility and feasible methods of detection make them suitable for use in clinical practice. However, multicenter studies with a large sample population are required to determine with certainty which epigenetic biomarkers are reliable for clinical routine. Therefore, this review focuses on current discoveries regarding epigenetic biomarkers and its controversy aiming to improve the diagnosis, prognosis, and therapy in cardiovascular patients.

Keywords: epigenetics, biomarker, microRNA, cardiovascular diseases, myocardial infarction, heart failure, atherosclerosis, hypertension

INTRODUCTION

Cardiovascular diseases (CVDs) are one of the leading causes of mortality in developed countries. Cardiovascular diseases refer to disorders affecting the structures or function of the heart and blood vessels, including hypertension, atherosclerosis, myocardial infarction (MI), ischemia/reperfusion injury, stroke, and heart failure (HF), among others (Wang et al., 2016a; Thomas et al.,

---

Abbreviations: AMI, acute myocardial infarction; ApoE, apolipoprotein E; BNP B-type natriuretic peptide; CK, creatine kinase; cTnI, cardiac troponin I; cTnT, cardiac troponin T; DOT1L, disruptor of telomeric silencing-1; ENaC, epithelial sodium channel; EZH2, enhancer of zeste homolog 2; GEO, Gene Expression Omnibus; HDAC, histone deacetylase; HF, heart failure; HFrEF, heart failure with reduced ejection fraction; HFpEF, heart failure with preserved ejection fraction; hs-cTnT, high-sensitivity cardiac troponin T; hs-CRP, high-sensitivity C-reactive protein; lncRNAs, long noncoding RNAs; LV, left ventricular; MI, myocardial infarction; miRNAs, microRNAs; ncRNAs, noncoding RNAs; NSTEMI, non- ST-segment elevation myocardial infarction; STEMI, ST-segment elevation myocardial infarction; pmiRNAs, platelet miRNAs; piRNAs, p-element-induced wimpy testis (PIWI)-interacting RNAs; tRNA, transfer RNA; ZEB1, zinc finger E-box binding homeobox 1.

2018). Mechanisms underlying the complex pathophysiology that leads to CVDs are of great interest but still far from clear. Progress in the field of epigenetics have opened a new world for the comprehension and management of human diseases, including the prevalence of CVDs, based on the role of genetics and its environmental interaction in pathological conditions (Jaenisch and Bird, 2003). Significant evidence suggests that the environment and lifestyle can define epigenetic patterns throughout life. These epigenetic patterns are a cellular memory of further environmental exposure. Epigenetic modifications are reversible, different among cell types, and can potentially lead to disease susceptibility by producing long-term changes in gene transcription (Fraga et al., 2005; Beekman et al., 2010).

Epigenetic modifications include DNA methylation and posttranslational modifications of histone tails. However, in this review, posttranscriptional regulation of gene expression by noncoding RNAs (ncRNAs) is also considered a part of the epigenetic machinery. MicroRNAs (miRNAs) are small ncRNAs that contribute to regulation of the expression of different epigenetic regulators such as DNA methyltransferases (DNMTs) and histone deacetylases (HDACs), among others. Similarly, DNA methylation and histone modifications can regulate the expression of some miRNAs, forming a feedback loop. Thus, miRNAs and epigenetic regulators cooperate to modulate the expression of mutual targets. Therefore, although miRNAs are not strictly considered epigenetic factors, they contribute to the modulation of gene expression through epigenetics. Disruption of this complex regulation may participate in the development of different diseases (Iorio et al., 2010; Hoareau-Aveilla and Meggetto, 2017; Moutinho and Esteller, 2017; Wang et al., 2017a) (**Figure 1**). DNA and histone proteins comprise the chromatin, which can be remodeled into a tightly condensed state (heterochromatin) or an open conformation (euchromatin) that would allow access to transcription factors or DNA binding proteins, allowing the regulation of gene expression (Kouzarides, 2007). Thus, epigenetics involves changes in gene expression due to chromatin adjustments that change the accessibility of DNA without changing its sequence, leading to silencing or downregulation/upregulation of gene expression (Baccarelli et al., 2010). Chromatin modifications, such as DNA methylation, consist of the transfer of a methyl group to carbon 5 of the cytosine residues [5-methylcytosine (5mC)] in CpG dinucleotides sites. CpG dinucleotides are localized throughout the genome but are more abundant in certain regions, such as gene promoters, forming so-called CpG islands. CpG methylation causes transcriptional repression by directly blocking transcription factor access to the DNA or indirectly *via* chromatin-modifying proteins (methyl-binding proteins) that recognize the methylated regions and recruit corepressors. DNA methyltransferases catalyze DNA methylation by recognizing

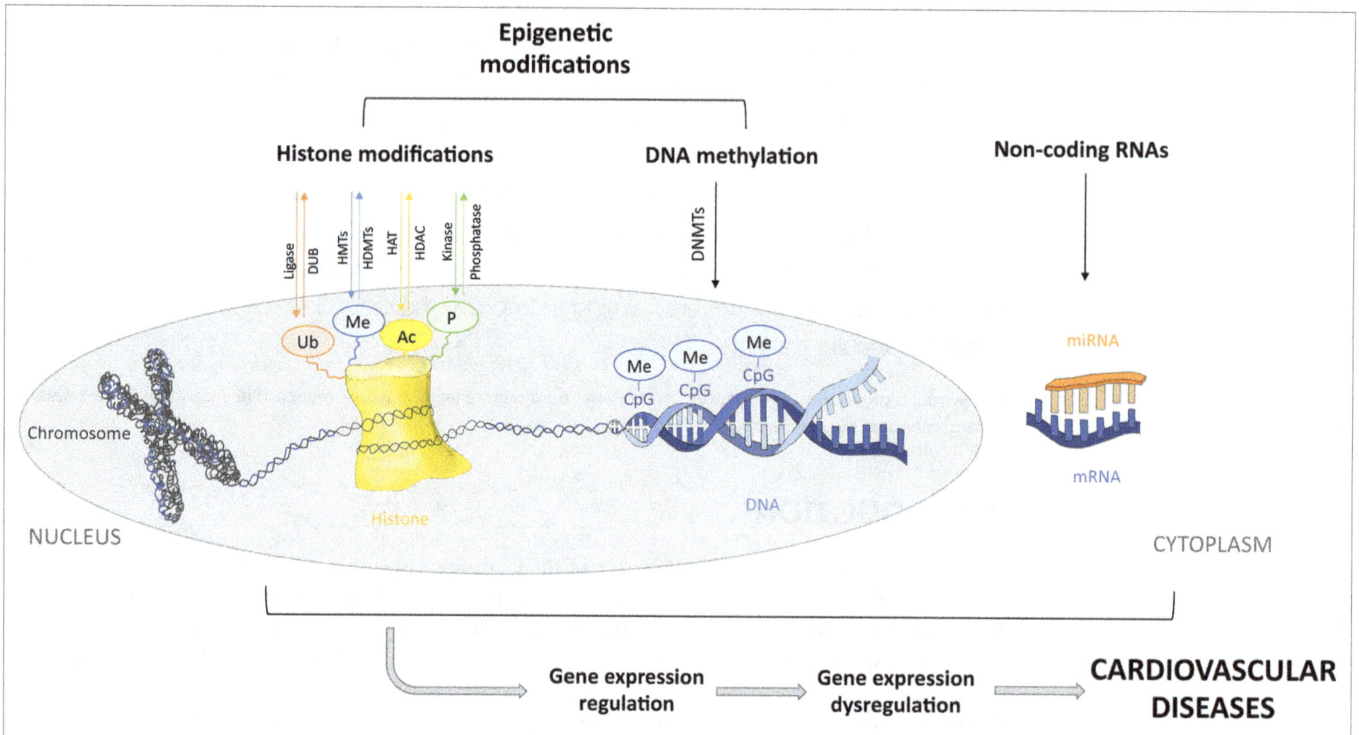

FIGURE 1 | Epigenetic regulatory mechanisms. Posttranslational modifications of histone tails by acetylation, deacetylation, ubiquitination, methylation, and phosphorylation. DNA methylation by DNA methyltransferases (DNMTs). Posttranscriptional regulation of gene expression by microRNAs. Epigenetic modifications involve silencing or downregulation/upregulation of gene expression. Dysregulation of the epigenetic machinery could lead to gene expression dysregulation and cardiovascular diseases. Ubiquitin (Ub), methionine (Me), acetyl group (Ac), phosphate (P), deubiquitinating enzyme (DUB), histone methyltransferase (HMTs), histone demethylase (HDMTs), histone acetyltransferase (HAT), histone deacetylase (HDAC), a cytosine followed by a guanine (CpG), microRNAs (miRNAs), and messenger RNA (mRNA).

and maintaining hypermethylated DNA during replication (DNMT1) or by *de novo* methylation (DNMT3a and DNMT3b). Moreover, gene bodies of actively transcribed genes normally show slightly higher DNA methylation levels as compared to gene bodies of nontranscribed genes. In contrast, hypomethylation is usually found in enhancer regions and promoters (Costantino et al., 2018). Posttranslational modification of histone tails is another epigenetic modification that regulates gene expression by chromatin remodeling. Histone acetylation, deacetylation, methylation, phosphorylation and ubiquitination change DNA accessibility, regulating gene transcription. The acetylation of histone tails is regulated by histone acetyltransferases (HATs) and HDACs. Histone acetyltransferase enzymes acetylate the lysine residues of the histones, whereas HDACs deacetylate them, promoting gene activation or silencing, respectively. Histone methylation is regulated by histone methyltransferases (HMTs) and histone demethylases (HDMT). Methylation occurs at the lysine or arginine residues and can activate or repress gene transcription depending on the degree of methylation and which residue is methylated (Li et al., 2017c; Sabia et al., 2017). The serine, threonine, and tyrosine residues of histone tails can also be phosphorylated and dephosphorylated by protein kinases and phosphatases, respectively. Histone tail phosphorylation modulates chromatin structure, taking part in transcription, DNA repair, and chromatin compaction in cell division and apoptosis (Rossetto et al., 2012). Lastly, histone tail ubiquitination is sequentially catalyzed by ligases enzymes, which attach ubiquitin to lysine residues. Ubiquitination and deubiquitination are involved in the activation of transcription and are usually associated with histone methylation. Their effect on repressing or activating transcription generally depends on what histone is modified (Cao and Yan, 2012). Finally, miRNAs regulate gene expression *via* degradation of the transcript or repression of translation when binding to the 3′-untranslated region of the target mRNA. Thus, miRNA represses mRNA translation without changing the DNA sequence of the gene. MicroRNA binding to mRNA is imperfect, so each miRNA has multiple targets. This allows the regulation of a great part of the human genome (Bartel, 2009). The miRNAs are 19-25 nucleotides in length, encoded in the genome and transcribed into primary miRNA (pri-miRNA). Pri-miRNAs derive into miRNAs precursors (pre-miRNA) by the nuclear RNase III called Dorsha and are transferred to the cytoplasm and processed by the endonuclease Dicer to generate a double-stranded miRNA duplex. This product is incorporated into an RNA-induced silencer complex (RISC)–loading complex. Then, one strand is removed from the complex, and the other strand forms a mature RISC, serving as a template for target mRNAs (Sato et al., 2011; Nishiguchi et al., 2015).

Due to this important function in gene regulation, epigenetic modifications and miRNA may play a crucial role in the development of pathological conditions, including CVDs. Understanding the epigenetic machinery underlying cardiac disorders and how these epigenetic mechanisms can be introduced into diagnostics (i.e., biomarkers) and therapies is fundamental to improving the quality of life of patients. In medicine, a biomarker is defined as a measurable characteristic that indicates a particular physiological or pathological state or a response to a therapeutic treatment (Strimbu and Tavel, 2010). Ideally, biomarkers should have easy accessibility, predictable detection, and reliability (Sun et al., 2017). It is mandatory to present a specific measurable change that clearly associates with a diagnosis or a predictable outcome. Thus, biomarkers provide information to physicians when evaluating the probability of developing a disease, making a diagnosis, evaluating the severity of a disease and its progression; during therapeutic decision making; or when monitoring a patient's response and may result in significant cost reduction (Baccarelli et al., 2010). Their classification can be based on their application (predisposition, diagnosis, monitoring, safety, prognostic, or predictive biomarkers). Predisposition biomarkers determine how likely it is for a patient to develop a certain disease and are usually utilized when there is a personal or family history that indicates a disease risk, and the results can help guide medical care. Diagnostic biomarkers are used to detect or confirm the existence of a health disorder and may assist its early detection. Monitoring biomarkers evaluate the status of a disease or determine exposure to an environmental agent or medical product. Safety biomarkers indicate the probability, presence, or extent of toxicity of a certain medical product or environmental agent. Prognostic biomarkers indicate how a disease may progress in patients who already have the particular disease. These biomarkers do not predict the treatment response but can be useful when selecting patients for treatment. Predictive biomarkers identify patients who are most likely to have a favorable or unfavorable response to a specific treatment. Thus, they can predict treatment success or undesired side effects in a particular patient. A particular disease can have different biological mechanisms in different patients. Predictive biomarkers can be associated with the specific mechanism of a health disorder. This facilitates a targeted therapy, which uses drugs specific for a particular biological mechanism associated with a disease, increasing its effectiveness (FDA-NIH Biomarker Working Group, 2016). Specifically, epigenetic biomarkers belonging to most of these classifications are discussed in this review, with a focus on CVDs. Among the epigenetic biomarkers, miRNAs are the most attractive, as they can be detected in small sample volumes, are stable, and can be obtained from plasma, serum, saliva, and urine. Interestingly, they are highly conserved, and this allows a reliable comparison between patients and animal models of disease (Matsumoto et al., 2013). Therefore, although all epigenetic mechanisms are being intensively investigated, miRNAs are evaluated the most for their use as predictive biomarkers. This review presents an overview of current research on epigenetic biomarkers in CVDs and how this knowledge can benefit the diagnosis, prognosis, and therapy for cardiovascular patients.

EPIGENETIC BIOMARKERS IN CVDS

Over the last few years, numerous studies have linked cardiovascular risk factors to epigenetic modifications in human patients. Modification of the epigenetic environment alters cardiovascular homeostasis and impacts cardiovascular disorders. The function of epigenetic mechanisms in the regulation of gene expression is well known, although the role of epigenetic marks in CVDs is not clearly understood. Thus, the exploration of epigenetic biomarkers may lead to a deep comprehension of the molecular mechanisms and pathways associated with CVDs. In this section, we focus on major CVDs, such as hypertension, atherosclerosis, MI, and HF, and the epigenetic biomarkers associated with them.

Hypertension

Arterial hypertension is a multifactorial disease with several mechanisms and metabolic systems involved in its pathogenesis. Genetic factors and environmental background may lead to alterations in multiple pathways that can eventually trigger development of the disease (Franceschini and Le, 2014). Intrauterine alterations, such as malnutrition, starvation, obesity, alcohol, drugs, nicotine, or environmental toxins, are some of the environmental factors directly related to hypertension development in the progeny (Bogdarina et al., 2007; Nuyt and Alexander, 2009). In addition, individuals who have aerobic training present with lower blood pressure than nontrained individuals (Fagard, 2006). This has an important impact on CVD risk factor control and is a nonpharmacological way to treat patients. There are also epigenetic factors that can influence the appearance of hypertension in adults, such as hypermethylation of genes, including superoxide dismutase-2 (*SOD2*) or *Granulysin*, or increased levels of histone acetylation at the promoter of the endothelial oxide synthetase gene (*eNOS*) (Wang et al., 2018b). Environmental factors are important to determining an individual's predisposition to developing major cardiovascular risk factors by means of epigenetic modifications, and identification of the epigenetic mechanisms that participate in hypertension development may help generate new treatments. This is of great interest because hypertension is a key risk factor for CVDs, including MI, HF, stroke, and end-stage renal disease (**Table 1** and **Figure 2**).

Essential hypertension is a multifactorial disease with no identifiable cause that is affected by environmental and epigenetic factors. Environmental stressors cause acetylation of histone 3 in the neurons of the area postrema, leading to an increase in pressure that results in hypertension (Irmak and Sizlan, 2006). Low activity of the 11 beta-hydroxysteroid dehydrogenase 2 (HSD11B2) induces hypertension. In a study performed in patients with essential hypertension or glucocorticoid-induced hypertension, the *HSD11B2* promoter was highly methylated. These changes may reflect a global status, with methylation of gene promoter being a potentially useful molecular biomarker to characterize hypertensive patients (Alikhani-Koopaei et al., 2004; Friso et al., 2008). Moreover, a polymorphism in the disruptor of telomeric silencing-1 gene (*DOT1L*), which encodes a methyltransferase that enhances methylation of histone 3 (H3K79) in the renal epithelial sodium channel gene (*ENaC*) promoter, is associated with blood pressure regulation (Duarte et al., 2012). It has also been reported that a *DOT1A* and *ALL1* (fused gene from chromosome 9 [Af9]) interaction is associated with H3K79 hypermethylation of the *ENaC* promoter, suppressing its transcriptional activity. This interaction is disrupted by aldosterone and causes hypomethylation of H3K79 at specific regions, disinhibiting the *ENaC* promoter and leading to hypertension. Thus, the Dot1a-Af9 pathway may also be involved in the control of genes implicated in hypertension (Zhang et al., 2009). Hypomethylation of the α-adducin gene (*ADD1*) promoter has been found to be connected to the risk of essential hypertension. However, differences between females and males have been found (Zhang et al., 2013a). Moreover, histone 3 (H3K4 or H3K9) demethylation is induced by lysine-specific demethylase-1 (LSD1), which modifies gene transcription. Hypermethylation of histone 3 has been associated with hypertension, increased vascular contraction, and decreased relaxation *via* the nitric oxide-cGMP (NO-cGMP) pathway in heterozygous *LSD1* knockout mice fed a high-salt diet (Pojoga et al., 2011). Histone deacetylation is also important in the development of pulmonary arterial hypertension. HDAC1 and HDAC5 protein levels have been demonstrated to be elevated in the lungs of patients and hypoxic rats. Inhibition of these proteins by valproic acid and suberoylanilide hydroxamic acid diminished the development of hypoxia-induced pulmonary hypertension in rats. Thus, HDAC1 and HDAC5 levels could be useful predictive biomarkers for the treatment of pulmonary hypertension in patients (Zhao et al., 2012).

In a study evaluating alterations in the global DNA methylation status of patients with essential hypertension, the level of the epigenetic marker 5mC was lower in hypertensive patients than in healthy people (Smolarek et al., 2010). In an *in vivo* model of hypertension using Dahl salt-sensitive rats, the levels of 5mC and 5-hydroxymethylcytosine (5hmC) were evaluated in the outer renal medulla. In response to salt administration, the 5mC levels were significantly higher for genes with low transcription and 5hmC levels higher in genes with higher expression. This study revealed important features of 5mC and 5hmC for understanding the role of epigenetic modifications in the regulation of hypertension (Liu et al., 2014).

Rivière et al. (2011) analyzed the regulation of somatic angiotensin-converting enzyme gene (*sACE*) expression by promoter methylation. *sACE* regulates blood pressure by catalyzing the conversion of angiotensin I into angiotensin II, a potent vasopressor. Hypermethylation of *sACE* promoter in cultures of human endothelial cells and rats was associated with transcriptional repression, suggesting an epigenetic mechanism in hypertension regulation (Rivière et al., 2011). More recently, Fan et al. (2017) demonstrated opposite results in patients with essential hypertension. The authors indicated that hypermethylation of the *ACE2* promoter may increase essential hypertension risk, with variabilities in CpG islands methylation in males and females (Fan et al., 2017).

Moreover, a genome-wide methylation study on essential hypertension revealed that changes in the DNA methylation of leukocytes are involved in the pathogenesis of hypertension. They found increased methylation in the gene encoding sulfatase 1 (*SULF1*), which is involved in apoptosis, and decreased methylation in the gene encoding prolylcarboxypeptidase (*PRCP*), a regulator of angiotensin II and III cleavage (Wang et al., 2013b). Another genome-wide study of blood pressure characteristics found new genetic variants that influence blood pressure and are

TABLE 1 | Epigenetic biomarkers in hypertension.

Epigenetic modification	Biomarker	Regulation in hypertension	Sample source	Study type	References
DNA methylation	*HSD11B2* promoter	Highly methylated	Rat's urine and tissues and human cell lines	Experimental: *in vitro* and rat model	(Alikhani-Koopaei et al., 2004)
	SERPIN3 CpG island	Hypomethylation	Placental tissue	Clinical	(Chelbi et al., 2007)
	HSD11B2 promoter	Highly methylated	Blood and urine	Clinical	(Friso et al., 2008)
	5mC	Lower levels	Blood	Clinical	(Smolarek et al., 2010)
	NKCC1 promoter	Hypomethylation	Aorta, heart and kidney	Experimental: spontaneously hypertensive rodent model	(Lee et al., 2010; Cho et al., 2011)
	sACE promoter	Hypermethylation	Blood	Clinical and experimental: *in vitro*	(Rivière et al., 2011)
	ERα promoter	Methylation	Uterine arteries	Clinical	(Dasgupta et al., 2012)
	SULF1, PRCP	*SULF1*: hypermethylation; *PRCP*: hypomethylation	Blood	Clinical	(Wang et al., 2013b)
	ADD1 promoter	Hypomethylation	Plasma	Clinical	(Zhang et al., 2013a)
	5mC, 5hmC	Higher levels	Tissue	Experimental: Dahl salt-sensitive rats	(Liu et al., 2014)
	AGT promoter	Demethylation	H295R cells and visceral adipose tissue	Experimental: *in vitro* and rat model	(Wang et al., 2014a)
	DSCR3	Hypermethylation	Maternal blood and placental tissue	Clinical	(Kim et al., 2015)
	miRNA-34a gene promoter	Hypomethylation	Placental tissue	Clinical	(Rezaei et al., 2018)
	ACE2 promoter	Hypermethylation	Plasma	Clinical	(Fan et al., 2017)
	CBS promoter	Hypermethylation	Maternal blood and placental tissue	Clinical	(Kim et al., 2015)
	MTHFD1 promoter	Hypermethylation	Plasma	Clinical	(Xu et al., 2019)
Histone modifications	H3K79	Hypermethylation	NA	Clinical	(Rodriguez-Iturbe, 2006; Duarte et al., 2012)
	Histone 3	Acetylation	Germ cells	Review	(Irmak and Sizlan, 2006)
	H3K79	DNA methylation	Bibliography	Review	(Zhang et al., 2009)
	HDAC8	Inhibition	mDCT cells and tissues	Experimental: rat models of salt-sensitive hypertension	(Mu et al., 2011)
	H3K4 or H3K9	Hypermethylation	Tissue, plasma, and urine	Experimental: LSD1 knockout mice with a high-salt diet	(Pojoga et al., 2011)
	HDAC1, HDAC5	High levels	Lung tissue and adventitial fibroblasts	Clinical and experimental: *in vitro* and hypoxic rat	(Zhao et al., 2012)
miRNA	miR-18a, miR-210, miR-152, miR-363, miR-377, miR-411, miR-518b, miR-542-3p	miR-18a, miR-363, miR-377, miR-411, miR-542-3p: underexpression; miR-210, miR-152, miR-518b: overexpression	Placental tissue	Clinical	(Zhu et al., 2009)
	22 miRNAs	15 upregulated and 7 downregulated	Serum	Clinical	(Yang et al., 2011)
	let-7b, miR-302*, miR-104, miR-128a, miR-182*, miR-133b	Overexpression	Placental tissue	Clinical	(Noack et al., 2011)
	miR-92b, miR-197, miR-342-3p, miR-296-5p, miR-26b, miR-25, miR-296-3p, miR-26a, miR-198, miR-202, miR-191, miR-95, miR-204, miR-21, miR-223	miR-92b, miR-197, miR-342-3p, miR-296-5p, miR-26b, miR-25, miR-296-3p, miR-26a, miR-198, miR-202, miR-191, miR-95, miR-204: overexpression; miR-21, miR-223: underexpression	Placental tissue	Clinical	(Choi et al., 2013)
	miR-9, miR-126	Lower levels	Peripheral blood mononuclear cells	Clinical	(Kontaraki et al., 2014)
	miR1233	Higher levels	Serum	Clinical	(Ura et al., 2014)

(Continued)

TABLE 1 | Continued

Epigenetic modification	Biomarker	Regulation in hypertension	Sample source	Study type	References
	miR-18a, miR-19b1, miR-92a1, miR-210	miR-210: upregulation; miR-18a, miR-19b1, and miR-92a1: downregulation	Plasma and placental tissue	Clinical	(Xu et al., 2014)
	miR-505	Upregulation	Plasma	Clinical	(Yang et al., 2014)
	miR-106a, miR-18b, miR-20b, miR-19b-2, miR-92a-2, miR-363	Dysregulation	Placental tissue	Clinical	(Zhang et al., 2015a)
	miR-515-5p, miR-518b, miR-518f-5p, miR-519d, miR-520h	Downregulation	Placental tissue	Clinical	(Hromadnikova et al., 2015)
	miR-335, miR-584	Upregulation	Placental tissue and HTR8/Svneo cells	Clinical and experimental: *in vitro*	(Jiang F. et al., 2015)
	miR-125b	Overexpression	Plasma and placental tissue	Clinical	(Yang et al., 2016b)
	miR-215, miR-155, miR-650, miR-210, miR-21, miR-18a, miR-19b1	MiR-215, miR-155, miR-650, miR-210, miR-21: upregulation; miR-18a, miR-19b1: downregulation	Plasma	Clinical	(Jairajpuri et al., 2017)
	miR-204-5p	Higher levels	Serum	Clinical	(Mei et al., 2017)
	let-7b*, let-7f-1*, miR-1183, miR-23c, miR-425*	miR-1183: upregulation; let-7b*, miR-23c, miR-425*, let-7f-1*: downregulation	Plasma and placental tissue	Clinical	(Gunel et al., 2017)
	miR-145	Downregulation	Placental tissue	Clinical	(Han et al., 2017)
	miR-202-3p	Upregulation	Placental tissue	Clinical	(Singh et al., 2017)
	let-7	Higher	Plasma	Clinical	(Huang et al., 2017b)
	miRNA	Dysregulation	Bibliography: Maternal serum and placental tissue	Bibliography review	(Laganà et al., 2018)
	miR-19a	Upregulation	Plasma and lung tissue	Clinical	(Chen and Li, 2017)
	miR-21	Upregulation	Peripheral blood mononuclear cells	Clinical	(Parthenakis et al., 2017)
	miR-21	Upregulation	Bibliography review	Bibliography review	(Sekar et al., 2017)
	miR-510	Upregulation	Serum	Clinical	(Krishnan et al., 2017)
	miR-206	Lower levels	Serum	Clinical	(Jin et al., 2017)
	miR-424(322)	Upregulation	Plasma	Clinical	(Baptista et al., 2018)
	miR-199a-3p, miR-208a-3p, miR-122-5p, miR-223-3p	Downregulation	Serum	Clinical	(Zhang et al., 2018c)
	miR-431-5p	Upregulation	Tissue	Experimental: mice made hypertensive and *in vitro*	(Huo et al., 2019)
	miR-143, NR_034083, NR_104181,	miR-143: upregulation; NR_034083: downregulation and NR_104181 and	Peripheral blood leucocytes	Clinical	(Chen et al., 2018b)

NA, not available.

strongly associated with local CpG island methylation. This study demonstrated the role of DNA methylation in the regulation of blood pressure (Kato et al., 2015).

The pathogenesis of hypertension is affected by alterations in ion flux mechanisms. Hypomethylation of the Na/K/2Cl cotransporter 1 gene (*NKCC1*) promoter results in overexpression in a rodent model with spontaneous hypertension (Lee et al., 2010). DNA methyltransferase activity maintained hypomethylation in the *NKCC1* promoter, playing an important role in *NKCC1* upregulation during the course of the disease. This encourages evaluation of the *NKCC1* methylation status in hypertensive patients (Cho et al., 2011). Furthermore, WNK4 is a serine-threonine kinase that negatively regulates the Na(+)-Cl(−)-cotransporter (NCC) and ENaC. This would affect the distal nephron, increasing the reabsorption of sodium. Stimulation of β(2)-adrenergic receptor (β(2)AR) in salt intake conditions would reduce *WNK4* transcription, resulting in inhibition of HDAC8 activity and increased histone acetylation. In the rat models of salt-sensitive hypertension, salt diet repressed renal WNK4 expression, activating the NCC and inducing salt-dependent hypertension. Thus, *WNK4* transcription is epigenetically modulated in the course of salt-sensitive hypertension, with the β(2)AR-WNK4 pathway as a potential therapeutic target for this disease (Mu et al., 2011).

Goyal et al. (2010) demonstrated that a low protein diet in pregnant mice leads to alterations in DNA methylation, miRNA,

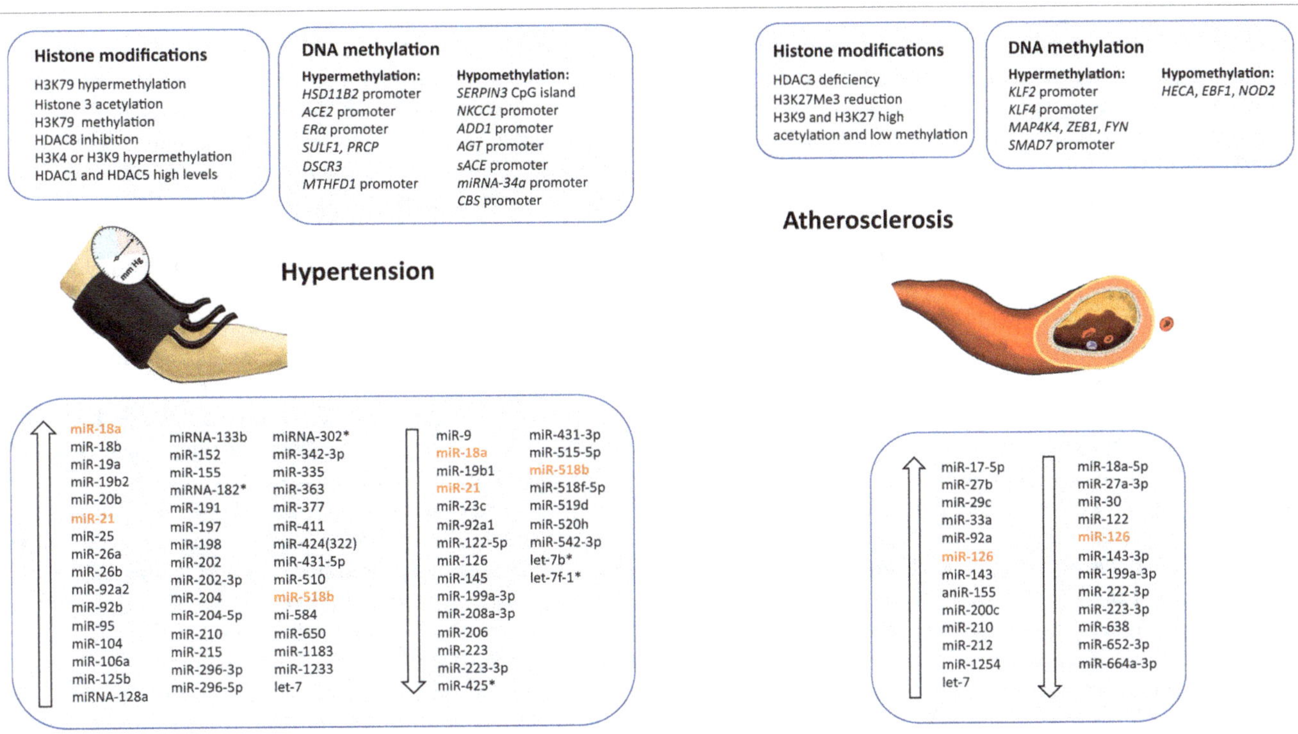

FIGURE 2 | Epigenetic modifications and microRNAs biomarkers dysregulated in atherosclerosis and hypertension. Ascending arrows indicate higher levels or upregulation, and descending arrows denote lower levels or downregulation, both compared to control conditions. Those miRNAs presenting opposite results are shown in orange.

and gene expression in the brain renin–angiotensin system, a key regulator of hypertension in adults (Goyal et al., 2010). Along the same lines, in a study carried out *in vitro* and in a rat model, DNA demethylation of the angiotensinogen gene (*AGT*) promoter activated its expression. AGT is an important substrate of the renin–angiotensin–aldosterone system and an important target in hypertension research. Elevated concentrations of circulating aldosterone and high consumption of salt stimulate the AGT gene expression in adipose-induced hypertension (Wang et al., 2014a). In addition, cystathionine β-synthase (CBS), an important enzyme in the metabolism of plasma homocysteine, is associated with hypertension and stroke. Hypermethylation of the *CBS* promoter has been demonstrated to increase the risk of both diseases, especially in male patients (Wang et al., 2019a). Similarly, hypermethylation of the methylenetetrahydrofolate dehydrogenase 1 gene (*MTHFD1*) promoter, which is also associated with homocysteine metabolism, was observed in hypertensive patients, and proposed as a potential diagnostic biomarker in patients with essential hypertension (Xu et al., 2019).

In addition to the previous classic epigenetic modifications, miRNAs often regulate hypertension and are attractive biomarkers for the disease. The miR-9 and miR-126 expression levels are significantly lower in hypertensive patients than healthy individuals and are related to hypertension prognosis and organ damage. Thus, miR-9 and miR-126 may be possible biomarkers in essential hypertension (Kontaraki et al., 2014). Moreover, ncRNAs, such as miR-143, miR-145, and NR_104181, are significantly higher in essential hypertensive patients than controls, whereas NR_027032 and NR_034083 are significantly reduced. After evaluating cardiovascular risk factors, they concluded that lower expression levels of NR_034083 and higher expression levels of NR_104181 and miR-143 were risk factors for essential hypertension (Chen et al., 2018b). Another study evaluated the correlation between miRNA let-7 expression and subclinical atherosclerosis in untreated patients with newly diagnosed essential hypertension and found increased levels in hypertensive patients, suggesting that plasma let-7 could be an indicator for monitoring end-organ damage and a biomarker for atherosclerosis in these patients (Huang et al., 2017b). Similarly, upregulation of miR-505, miR-19a, miR-21, miR-510, or miR-424(322) in blood from hypertensive patients suggests a possible use for miR-510 as a diagnostic biomarker and therapeutic target (Yang et al., 2014; Chen and Li, 2017; Krishnan et al., 2017; Parthenakis et al., 2017; Sekar et al., 2017; Baptista et al., 2018). Lower levels of the combination of miR-199a-3p, miR-208a-3p, miR-122-5p, and miR-223-3p have also been shown to be suitable for diagnosis of hypertension (Zhang et al., 2018c). Decreased miR-206 levels might also be especially useful in the detection of pulmonary hypertension in patients with left heart disease (Jin et al., 2017). Furthermore, a study in hypertensive mice produced by infusion of angiotensin II concluded that miR-431-5p knockdown delays the increase in blood pressure induced by angiotensin II and reduces vascular injury. This demonstrates its potential as a target for the treatment of hypertension and vascular injury (Huo et al., 2019).

Preeclampsia is an important pregnancy-induced syndrome characterized by hypertension and proteinuria. Chronic hypoxia is a common pregnancy stress that increases the risk of preeclampsia and is associated with changes in methylation of the estrogen receptor α gene (*ERα*) promoter. ERα is involved in adjustments to the uterine blood flow, and promoter methylation results in gene repression in uterine arteries, increasing blood pressure (Dasgupta et al., 2012). Preeclampsia also modifies the expression profile of several serine protease inhibitors (SERPINs) in the placenta. Specifically, *SERPIN3* CpG islands have a significantly low level of methylation in preeclampsia, providing a new potential marker for early diagnosis (Chelbi et al., 2007). Another study demonstrated a positive association between placenta global DNA methylation and hypertension in preeclampsia (Kulkarni et al., 2011). Next-generation sequencing technology and microarray assay analyses of the miRNA expression pattern in preeclamptic placentas versus healthy placentas have revealed that miRNAs expression is dysregulated in preeclampsia (Zhu et al., 2009; Noack et al., 2011; Yang et al., 2011; Choi et al., 2013; Xu et al., 2014; Hromadnikova et al., 2015; Zhang et al., 2015a; Gunel et al., 2017; Han et al., 2017). These results were in agreement with those found in the miRNA database from cell and tissue analyses. Thus, circulating miRNAs in the serum of pregnant women could be used as biomarkers for the diagnosis and prognosis of preeclampsia. To further demonstrate that miRNAs could be good predictors of preeclampsia, as well as its severity, circulating miRNA signatures were evaluated in women divided into groups based on preeclampsia severity. MiR-21, miR-29a, miR-125b, miR-155, miR-202-3p, miR-204-5p, miR-210, miR-215, miR-335, miR-518b, miR-584, miR-650, and miR-1233 were upregulated, whereas miR-15b, miR-18a, miR-19b1, and miR-144 were downregulated in women with severe preeclampsia compared to mild preeclampsia (Ura et al., 2014; Jiang et al., 2015; Yang et al., 2016b; Jairajpuri et al., 2017; Mei et al., 2017; Singh et al., 2017). In addition, a recent data recompilation supported a direct association between high or low expression of miRNAs in pregnancy serum and placenta in preeclamptic pregnancies (Laganà et al., 2018). Interestingly, an association has also been demonstrated between hypomethylation of the miR-34a promoter and preeclampsia severity (Rezaei et al., 2018). Another study analyzed the concentrations of Down syndrome critical region 3 (*DSCR3*), Ras association domain family 1 isoform A (*RASSF1A*), and sex-determining region Y (*SRY*) cell-free fetal DNA in maternal plasma from preeclamptic pregnancies and found that all of the markers significantly correlated with gestational age. The authors demonstrated that *DSCR3* is a novel epigenetic biomarker and an alternative to *RASSF1A* for the prediction of early-onset preeclampsia (Kim et al., 2015). However, no association was found between the methylation status of the cortisol-controlling gene (*HSD11B2*), tumor suppressor gene (*RUNX3*), or long interspersed nucleotide element-1 gene (*LINE-1*) and hypertensive disorders of pregnancy when placental DNA methylation was analyzed (Majchrzak-Celińska et al., 2017).

Atherosclerosis

Atherosclerosis is a chronic inflammatory disease characterized by the accumulation of cholesterol in the walls of large- and medium-sized arteries, the accumulation of extracellular matrix and lipids, and smooth muscle cell proliferation. This process leads to the infiltration of immune cells (mostly macrophages) and endothelial dysfunction, forming a plaque, and eventually developing into acute cardiovascular events, such as MI, peripheral vascular disease, aneurysms, and stroke (Wissler, 1991). Proatherogenic stimuli, such as low-density lipoprotein (LDL) cholesterol and oxidized LDL, have been suggested to stimulate a long-term epigenetic reprogramming of innate immune system cells. This induces a constant activation, even after the removal of atherosclerotic stimuli (Bekkering et al., 2016). Emerging evidence supports epigenetic modifications being involved in the initiation and progression of atherosclerosis, playing an important role in plaque development and vulnerability, and highlighting the importance of epigenetic biomarkers as predictors of CVDs (**Table 2** and **Figure 2**) (Xu et al., 2018).

Regarding histone modifications, HDAC3 is reported to have a protective effect in apolipoprotein E deficient (apoE−/−) mice. HDAC3 maintains the endothelial integrity, and its deficiency results in atherosclerosis (Zampetaki et al., 2010). Similarly, increased histone acetylation has been proposed to play some role in the progression of atherogenesis by modulating the expressions of proatherogenic genes (Choi et al., 2005). Histone deacetylases are upregulated in aortic smooth muscle cells when they were stimulated with mitogens. In contrast, inhibition of HDACs reduces aortic smooth muscle cell proliferation by changing cell cycle genes expression. This suggests a protective effect against atherosclerosis (Findeisen et al., 2011). Investigations of the association between changes in lysine 27 trimethylation of histone 3 (H3K27Me3), and atherosclerotic plaque development revealed a reduction in global levels of H3K27Me3 modification in vessels with advanced atherosclerotic plaques. This does not correlate with a reduction in the corresponding HMT, enhancer of zeste homolog 2 (EZH2). There was a relationship between the repression of H3K27Me3 mark in the vessels with advanced atherosclerotic plaques and the dynamic differentiation and proliferation of smooth muscle cells associated with atherosclerotic disease (Wierda et al., 2015). Histone acetylation, methylation, and the expression of their corresponding transferases in the atherosclerotic plaques of patients with carotid artery stenosis have been analyzed. Greißel et al. (2016) analyzed the expression of HATs GCN5L, P300, MYST1, and MYST2 and HMTs MLL2/4, SET7/9, hSET1A, SUV39H1, SUV39H2, ESET/SETDB1, EHMT1, EZH2, and G9a and described an enhancement in histone acetylation on H3K9 and H3K27 in the smooth muscle cells from severe atherosclerotic lesions that correlated with plaque severity. In addition, H3K9 and H3K27 methylation were significantly lower in atherosclerotic plaques and significantly associated with disease severity (Greißel et al., 2016).

DNA methylation is also involved in atherosclerosis. To identify CpG methylation profiles in the progression of atherosclerosis in the human aorta, Valencia-Morales et al. (2015) performed DNA methylation microarray analyses. They detected a correlation between histological pathology and the differential methylation of numerous autosomal genes in vascular tissue, providing potential biomarkers of damage severity and

TABLE 2 | Epigenetic biomarkers in atherosclerosis.

Epigenetic modification	Biomarker	Regulation in atherosclerosis	Sample source	Study type	References
DNA methylation	*KLF2* promoter	Methylation	HUVEC cells	Experimental: *in vitro*	(Kumar et al., 2013)
	KLF4 promoter	Methylation	HAEC cells	Experimental: *in vitro*	(Jiang et al., 2014)
	HECA, *EBF1*, *NOD2*, *MAP4K4*, *ZEB1*, *FYN*	*HECA*, *EBF1*, *NOD2*: Hypomethylated; *MAP4K4*, *ZEB1*, *FYN*: Hypermethylated	Human aortic intima and HEK293 cells	Clinical and experimental: *in vitro*	(Yamada et al., 2014)
	TIMP1, *ABCA1*, *ACAT1* promoters	Altered methylation status	Peripheral blood	Clinical	(Ma et al., 2016)
	SMAD7 promoter	Hypermethylation	Peripheral blood and atherosclerotic plaques	Clinical	(Wei et al., 2018)
	5mC, 5-hmC	Higher levels	Peripheral blood	Clinical	(Jiang et al., 2019)
Histone modifications	HDAC3	Deficiency	Aorta and HUVEC cells	Experimental: apoE−/− mice and *in vitro*	(Zampetaki et al., 2010)
	H3K27Me3	Reduction in H3K27Me3 modification	Perirenal aortic tissue patches	Clinical	(Wierda et al., 2015)
	H3K9, H3K27	Higher histone acetylation and lower histone methylation	Carotid tissue	Clinical	(Greißel et al., 2016)
miRNA	miR-130a, miR-27b, miR-210	Higher levels	Serum and intima tissue	Clinical	(Li et al., 2011)
	miR-17-5p	Higher levels	Plasma	Clinical	(Chen et al., 2015a)
	miR-143-3p, miR-222-3p	Lower levels	Microparticles	Clinical	(de Gonzalo-Calvo et al., 2016)
	miR-30	Lower levels	Plasma	Clinical	(Huang et al., 2016b)
	miR-92a	Higher levels	Plasma	Clinical	(Huang et al., 2017a)
	miR-18a-5p, miR-27a-3p, miR-199a-3p, miR-223-3p, miR-652-3p	Lower levels	Plasma	Clinical	(Vegter et al., 2017)
	miR-33a	Higher levels	Plasma	Clinical	(Kim et al., 2017)
	miR-126	Lower levels	Plasma	Experimental: apoE−/− mice	(Hao and Fan, 2017)
	miR-212	Overexpression	Serum	Clinical	(Jeong et al., 2017)
	miRNA let-7	Higher levels	Plasma	Clinical	(Huang et al., 2017b)
	miR-1254	Higher levels	Plasma	Clinical	(de Gonzalo-Calvo et al., 2018)
	miR-200c	Overexpression	Carotid plaques and plasma	Clinical	(Magenta et al., 2018)
	miR-29c	Higher levels	Plasma	Clinical	(Huang et al., 2018)
	miR-221, miR-222	Lower expression levels	Serum	Clinical	(Yilmaz et al., 2018)
	miR-638	Lower levels	Serum	Clinical	(Luque et al., 2018)
	miR-122	Higher levels	Serum	Clinical	(Wang and Yu, 2018)
	miR-221, miR-222	Higher levels in tissue samples and lower levels in whole blood	Coronary artery atherosclerotic plaques, and internal mammary arteries and whole blood	Clinical	(Bildirici et al., 2018)
	miR-664a-3p	Downregulation	Serum	Clinical	(Li et al., 2018b)
	miR-155	Higher levels	Serum	Clinical	(Qiu and Ma, 2018)
	miR-19A, miR-19B, miR-126, miR-155	Differential levels	GEO dataset	High throughput	(Mao et al., 2018)
	miR-126, miR-143	Higher levels	Plasma	Clinical	(Gao et al., 2019)

treatment targets (Valencia-Morales et al., 2015). Genes such as *Drosophila* headcase (*HECA*), early B-cell factor 1 (*EBF1*), and nucleotide-binding oligomerization domain containing 2 (*NOD2*) are significantly hypomethylated, whereas mitogen-activated protein kinase kinase kinase kinase 4 (*MAP4K4*), zinc finger E-box binding homeobox 1 (*ZEB1*), and proto-oncogene tyrosine-protein kinase (*FYN*) are hypermethylated in atheromatous plaque lesions compared to the plaque-free intima (Yamada et al., 2014). Another study described differentially methylated regions in genes associated with atherosclerosis in swine aorta endothelial cells (Jiang et al., 2015). Low-density lipoprotein cholesterol risk factor upregulates DNMT1, which methylates and represses the Krüppel-like factor 2 gene (*KLF2*) promoter. KLF2 is a transcription factor essential for endothelium homeostasis, and its repression results in endothelial dysfunction (Kumar et al., 2013). Similarly, DNMT3a upregulation in human aortic endothelial cells exposed to disturbed flow induces the methylation and repression of the Krüppel-like factor 4 gene (*KLF4*) promoter, increasing regional atherosusceptibility (Jiang et al., 2014). In an attempt to determine biomarkers of atherosclerosis in the primary stages, the DNA methylation status was determined in a selection of gene promoters associated with the disease. They analyzed the promoter methylation of ATP binding cassette subfamily A member 1 (*ABCA1*), TIMP metallopeptidase inhibitor 1 (*TIMP1*), and acetyl-CoA acetyltransferase 1 (*ACAT1*) and observed significant alterations in the peripheral blood of atherosclerosis patients (Ma et al., 2016). A recent study found that *SMAD7* expression is decreased and its promoter highly methylated in atherosclerotic plaques compared to normal artery walls. There was also increased DNA methylation of the *SMAD7* promoter in the peripheral blood of atherosclerosis patients. Thus, the *SMAD7* promoter is hypermethylated in atherosclerosis patients and their atherosclerotic plaques, with a positive association with homocysteine levels (Wei et al., 2018). Moreover, increased 5mC and 5-hmC levels, which indicate DNA methylation and hydroxymethylation, respectively, have been demonstrated in peripheral blood mononuclear cells from elderly patients with coronary heart disease. These results positively correlate with the severity of coronary atherosclerosis (Jiang et al., 2019).

MicroRNAs have also been identified as attractive epigenetic biomarkers for atherosclerosis. Li et al. (2011) examined miRNA levels in serum samples and the intima of atherosclerosis obliterans patients and compared them to controls. They observed increased levels of miR-27b, miR-130a, and miR-210 in serum and sclerotic tissue from patients, proposing these miRNAs as epigenetic biomarkers for early stages of the disease (Li et al., 2011). Later, a study with a reduced number of patients suggested that elevated levels of circulating miR-17-5p may be a useful biomarker in the diagnosis of coronary atherosclerosis (Chen et al., 2015a).

Microparticles secreted by human coronary artery smooth muscle cells are a different source of cardiovascular biomarkers. These extracellular vesicles can contain miRNAs, such as miR-21-5p, miR-143-3p, miR-145-5p, miR-221-3p, and miR-222-3p. Lower levels of miR-143-3p and miR-222-3p have been found in microparticles derived from atherosclerotic plaque areas compared to nonatherosclerotic areas (de Gonzalo-Calvo et al., 2016).

Huang et al. (2016b) evaluated the expression of miR-30 in patients with essential hypertension compared to control individuals. They observed a reduction in miR-30 levels in the hypertensive patients and in the increased carotid intima-media thickness group. Thus, the authors suggested that circulating miR-30 may be a useful noninvasive atherosclerosis biomarker for patients with essential hypertension (Huang et al., 2016b). Later, the authors also identified higher levels of miR-92a as a possible biomarker of atherosclerosis in the same type of patients (Huang et al., 2017a).With the aim of investigating correlations between circulating miRNAs specific for HF and atherosclerosis in HF patients, Vegter et al. (2017) assessed miRNAs levels and related them to biomarkers associated with atherosclerotic disease and rehospitalizations of cardiovascular patients. They demonstrated a consistent trend between a high number of atherosclerosis manifestations and lower levels of miR-18a-5p, miR-27a-3p, miR-199a-3p, miR-223-3p, and miR-652-3p. Thus, lower levels of circulating miRNAs in HF patients with atherosclerotic disease and an elevated probability of cardiovascular-related rehospitalization were described (Vegter et al., 2017). High levels of miR-33a have also been demonstrated to be a potential cause of cholesterol accumulation and to exacerbate vessel walls inflammation in atherosclerotic disease. Thus, plasma miR-33a has been proposed as a suitable biomarker in atherosclerosis (Kim et al., 2017).

In an attempt to identify more atherosclerosis biomarkers, Hao and Fan (2017) performed microarray analysis using the plasma from apoE−/− mice and discovered that a reduction in miR-126 levels is a good indicator of atherosclerotic disease. They also determined that miR-126 is involved in the mitogen-associated protein kinase (MAPK) signaling pathway, reducing cytokine release and progressing atherosclerotic pathogenesis (Hao and Fan, 2017). In contrast, Gao et al. (2019) determined that higher expression levels of miR-126 and miR-143 correlate with the presence and severity of cerebral atherosclerosis (Gao et al., 2019). In another study, the authors evaluated the synergy of circulating miRNAs with cardiovascular risk factors to estimate the presence of atherosclerosis in ischemic stroke patients. They identified miR-212 as a novel marker that enhances the estimation of atherosclerosis presence in combination with hemoglobin A_{1c}, high-density lipoprotein cholesterol, and lipoprotein(a) (Jeong et al., 2017). Another candidate biomarker for atherosclerosis is miR-200c. The authors analyzed plaque instability in the carotid arteries of patients undergoing carotid endarterectomy by examining the expression of miR-200c. Higher expression of miR-200c positively correlated with instability biomarkers, such as monocyte chemoattractant protein-1, cyclooxygenase-2, interleukin 6 (IL-6), metalloproteinases, and miR-33a/b, and negatively correlated with stability biomarkers, such as ZEB1, endothelial nitric oxide synthase, forkhead boxO1, and Sirtuin1. Thus, miR-200c could be a biomarker of atherosclerotic plaque progression and clinically useful for identifying patients at high embolic risk (Magenta et al., 2018). Along the same lines, lower serum levels of miR-638 may be a suitable biomarker of plaque vulnerability and ischemic stroke in individuals with high cardiovascular risk (Luque et al., 2018). With the intention to explore the role of miRNAs associated with carotid atherosclerosis, Mao et al. (2018) analyzed the genes differentially expressed between primary and advanced atherosclerotic plaques using two public datasets from the Gene Expression Omnibus (GEO) databases. The authors found a total of 23 miRNAs and focused on miR-19A, miR-19B, miR-126, and miR-155, which may be considered biomarkers of carotid atherosclerosis (Mao et al., 2018). In addition, Li et al. (2018b) identified downregulation of specific circulating miR-664a-3p as a biomarker of atherosclerosis in patients with obstructive sleep apnea and enlarged maximum carotid intima-media thickness (Li et al., 2018b).

Circulating miR-221 and miR-222 could also be suitable biomarkers for the diagnosis of atherosclerosis, as lower levels of these miRNAs correlate with the disease (Bildirici et al., 2018;

Yilmaz et al., 2018). However, higher levels have been found in samples from coronary atherosclerotic plaques and internal mammary arteries (Bildirici et al., 2018). On the other hand, higher circulating levels of miR-29c, miR-122, and miR-155 in coronary atherosclerosis patients might allow noninvasive detection of the disease and its severity (Huang et al., 2018; Qiu and Ma, 2018; Wang and Yu, 2018). In another interesting study that assessed whether atherosclerosis of different arterial territories, not including the coronary artery, is associated with specific circulating miRNAs, the investigators were able to identify specific miRNA profiles for each territory with atherosclerotic disease. These findings may provide a pathophysiological understanding and be useful for selecting potential biomarkers for clinical practice (Pereira-da-Silva et al., 2018).

Myocardial Infarction

Acute MI (AMI) is a threatening disease worldwide. Early and accurate differential diagnosis is critical for immediate medical intervention and improved prognosis (Reed et al., 2017). In particular, it is important to notice that patients with ST-segment elevation MI (STEMI) have different requirements than patients with non-STEMI (NSTEMI). For the first group, reperfusion therapy should be administered quickly to reduce infarct size and mortality (Authors/Task Force members et al., 2014). However, in NSTEMI patients, revascularization strategies are recommended based on individual clinical characteristics (Reed et al., 2017). Therefore, biomarkers with the capacity to diagnose and personalize a therapeutic schedule in AMI would be of great interest. Currently, the favored diagnostic biomarkers of AMI are cardiac troponin I (cTnI) and T (cTnT), both of which are released from necrotic cardiomyocytes within 2 to 4 h post-MI (Babuin and Jaffe, 2005), with maximum levels at 24 to 48 h and lasting for more than 1 week (Jaffe et al., 2006). For this reason, small repeat infarctions after the main infarction are difficult to detect. Thus, it is fundamental to identify biomarkers for very early diagnosis of STEMI and for monitoring the entire pathological process of AMI (**Table 3** and **Figure 3**).

Regarding methylation as an indicator of MI, Talens et al. (2012) investigated the association between MI and DNA methylation at six loci described to be sensitive to prenatal nutrition. As a result, the researchers demonstrated that the risk of MI in women is associated with DNA hypermethylation at *INS* and *GNASAS*-specific loci (Talens et al., 2012). Moreover, microarray analyses investigating whole-genome DNA methylation using cases from the EPICOR study and EPIC-NL cohort (Fiorito et al., 2014) identified a hypomethylated region in the zinc finger and BTB domain-containing protein 12 (*ZBTB12*) and *LINE-1*, concluding that it is possible to detect specific methylation profiles in white blood cells a few years before MI occurs. This provides a promising early biomarker of MI (Guarrera et al., 2015). Another example is the hypermethylation of the aldehyde dehydrogenase 2 gene (*ALDH2*) promoter, which is associated with myocardial injury after MI in rats. The hypermethylation downregulates *ALDH2*, inhibiting its cardioprotective role (Wang et al., 2015). Rask-Andersen et al. (2016) performed an epigenome-wide association study to identify disease-specific alterations in DNA methylation. The authors observed differential DNA methylation at 211 CpG sites in individuals with MI, and some of these sites represented genes related to cardiac function, CVD, cardiogenesis, and recovery after ischemic injury. Their results highlight genes that might be important in the pathogenesis of MI or in recovery (Rask-Andersen et al., 2016). Along the same lines, a genome-wide DNA methylation and gene ontology analysis of white blood cells from a population-based study identified four differentially methylated sites in individuals who had a previous MI. Interestingly, they found a correlation between differences in DNA methylation in blood cells and the levels of growth differentiation factor 15 (GDF-15), which was overexpressed in the myocardium of MI patients (Ek et al., 2016). Later, a genome-wide DNA methylation study of whole blood samples from MI patients and controls identified two methylated regions in zinc finger homeobox 3 (*ZFHX3*) and SWI/SNF-related, matrix-associated, actin-dependent regulator of chromatin, subfamily a, member 4 (*SMARCA4*) that were independently related to MI (Nakatochi et al., 2017).

Histone modifications are also involved in the pathological process of MI. To investigate the role of the HAT p300 in adverse left ventricular (LV) remodeling, Miyamoto et al. (2006) generated transgenic mice overexpressing wild-type p300 or its mutant in the heart. They subjected these mice to surgical MI and demonstrated that cardiac overexpression of p300 stimulated adverse LV remodeling. They concluded that the HAT activity of p300 is fundamental for the pathological course of MI (Miyamoto et al., 2006). Moreover, the class III deacetylase sirtuin 1 (SIRT1) is well known to confer a cardioprotective effect and is downregulated after cardiac injury. To understand the underlying mechanism, primary rat neonatal ventricular myocytes were exposed to ischemic or oxidative stress, leading to upregulation of the histone H3K9 methyltransferase SUV39H and downregulation of *SIRT1*. In addition, inhibition of SUV39H activity by chaetocin in wild-type mice and *SUV39H*-knockout mice protected against induced MI. SUV39H and heterochromatin protein 1 gamma cooperate to methylate the *SIRT1* promoter and repress its transcription. Thus, the authors described a role for SUV39H linking SIRT1 repression to MI (Yang et al., 2017a). To examine the role of HDAC4 in the modulation of cardiac function after an MI, Zhang et al. (2018b) generated a myocyte-specific activated HDAC4-transgenic mouse. They found that HDAC4 overexpression increases myocardial fibrosis and hypertrophy, leading to cardiac dysfunction. Furthermore, the overexpression of activated HDAC4 aggravated cardiac dysfunction and increased adverse remodeling and apoptosis in the infarcted myocardium. Thus, HDAC4 is an indicator of heart injury (Zhang et al., 2018b). More recently, the role of HDAC6 in the development of HF following MI was investigated using a rat model. The authors found that the deacetylase activity of HDAC6 is increased after MI (Nagata et al., 2019).

Abundant research has focused on miRNAs as novel biomarkers for MI. MiR-1 levels have been analyzed in plasma from patients with AMI and found to be significantly elevated, but decreased to normal levels with medication (Ai et al., 2010; Long et al., 2012a). MiR-1, miR-126, and cTnI expression levels exhibited a similar tendency. Thus, circulating miR-1 and

TABLE 3 | Epigenetic biomarkers in myocardial infarction.

Epigenetic modification	Biomarker	Regulation in myocardial infarction	Sample source	Study type	References
DNA methylation	*INS, GNASAS*	Hypermethylation	Leukocytes	Clinical	(Talens et al., 2012)
	LINE-1, ZBTB12	Hypomethylation	White blood cells	Clinical	(Guarrera et al., 2015)
	ALDH2 promoter	Hypermethylation	Experimental: rat model of MI	Experimental: rat model of MI	(Wang et al., 2015)
	ZFHX3, SMARCA4	Methylation	Whole blood	Clinical	(Nakatochi et al., 2017)
Histone modifications	p300	Overexpression	Myocardium	Experimental: mouse model of MI in HATmut p300-Tg mice	(Miyamoto et al., 2006)
	SUV39H, SIRT1	SUV39H upregulation and SIRT1 downregulation	H9C2 cells primary rat neonatal ventricular myocytes	Experimental: mouse model of MI in SUV39H−/− mice	(Yang et al., 2017a)
	HDAC4	Overexpression	Myocardium	Experimental: mouse model of MI in MHC-HDAC4-Tg mice	(Zhang et al., 2018b)
	HDAC6	Higher levels	Myocardium	Experimental: rat model of MI	(Nagata et al., 2019)
miRNA	miR-1	Higher levels	Plasma	Clinical	(Ai et al., 2010)
	miR-31, miR-126, miR-214, miR-499-5p	miR-31, miR-214: upregulation; miR-126, miR-499-5p: downregulation	Myocardium	Experimental: rat model of MI	(Shi et al., 2010)
	miR-499	Higher levels	Tissues and plasma	Clinical	(Adachi et al., 2010)
	miR-1, miR-133a, miR-133b, miR-499-5p, miR-122, miR-375	miR-1, miR-133a, miR-133b, miR-499-5p: upregulation; miR-122, miR-375: downregulation	Plasma	Clinical and experimental: mouse model of MI	(D'Alessandra et al., 2010)
	miR-1, miR-126	miR-1: increased; miR-126: decreased	Plasma	Clinical	(Long et al., 2012a)
	miR-133a	Higher levels	Plasma	Clinical	(Eitel et al., 2012)
	miR-30a, miR-195, let-7b	miR-30a, miR-195: increased; let-7: decreased	Plasma	Clinical	(Long et al., 2012b)
	miR-499-5p	Higher levels	Plasma	Clinical	(Olivieri et al., 2013)
	miR-1, miR-133a, miR-208b, miR-499	Higher levels	Plasma	Clinical	(Li et al., 2013)
	miR-150	Downregulation	plasma	Clinical	(Devaux et al., 2013)
	miR-133a	Higher levels	Plasma	Clinical	(Wang et al., 2013a)
	miR-21-5p, miR-361-5p, miR-519e-5p	miR-21-5p, miR-361-5p: increased; miR-519e-5p: reduced	Plasma	Clinical	(Wang et al., 2014b)
	miR-208a, miR-499	Higher levels in serum; miR-499: lower levels in scar, miR-208a: unchanged in scar	Serum and heart tissues	Experimental: mouse model of MI	(Xiao et al., 2014)
	miR-208b, miR-34a	Higher levels	Plasma	Clinical	(Lv et al., 2014)
	miR-328, miR-134	Higher levels	Plasma	Clinical	(He et al., 2014)
	miR-133, miR-1291, miR-663b	Higher levels	Plasma	Clinical	(Peng et al., 2014)
	miR-497	Upregulation	Plasma	Clinical	(Li et al., 2014b)
	miR-1	Higher levels	Plasma	Clinical	(Li et al., 2014a)
	miR-19a	Higher levels	Plasma	Clinical	(Zhong et al., 2014)
	miR-486-3p, miR-150-3p, miR-126-3p, miR-26a-5p, and miR-191-5p	miR-486-3p, miR-150-3p: upregulation; miR-126-3p, miR-26a-5p, miR-191-5p: downregulation	Serum	Clinical	(Hsu et al., 2014)
	miR-145	Higher levels	Serum	Clinical	(Dong et al., 2015)

(Continued)

TABLE 3 | Continued

Epigenetic modification	Biomarker	Regulation in myocardial infarction	Sample source	Study type	References
	hsa-miR-493-5p, hsa-miR-369-3p, hsa-miR-495, hsa-miR-3615, hsa-miR-433, hsa-miR-877-3p, hsa-miR-1306-3p, hsv1-miR-H2, hsa-miR-3130-5p, hcmv-miR-UL22A	hsa-miR-493-5p, hsa-miR-369-3p, hsa-miR-495, hsa-miR-3615, hsa-miR-433: upregulation, hsa-miR-877-3p, hsa-miR-1306-3p, hsv1-miR-H2, hsa-miR-3130-5p, hcmv-miR-UL22A: downregulation	Plasma	Clinical	(Liang et al., 2015)
	miR-499	Higher levels	Plasma	Clinical	(Zhang et al., 2015b)
	miR-486, miR-150	Higher levels	Plasma	Clinical	(Zhang et al., 2015c)
	miR-499	Higher levels	Plasma	Clinical	(Chen et al., 2015b)
	miR-146a, miR-21	Higher levels	Plasma	Clinical	(Liu et al., 2015a)
	miR-1, miR-208, miR-499	Higher levels	Plasma	Clinical	(Liu et al., 2015b)
	miR-208a	Higher levels	Plasma	Clinical	(Białek et al., 2015)
	miR-208	Overexpression	Plasma	Clinical	(Han et al., 2015)
	miR-122-5p	Higher levels	Plasma	Clinical	(Yao et al., 2015)
	miR-21	Higher levels	Plasma	Clinical	(Zhang et al., 2016)
	miR-99a	Downregulation	Plasma	Clinical	(Yang et al., 2016a)
	miR-19b-3p, miR-134-5p and miR-186-5p	Higher levels	Plasma	Clinical	(Wang et al., 2016b)
	miR-106a-5p, miR-424-5p, let-7g-5p, miR-144-3p, miR-660-5p	Higher levels	Blood	Clinical	(Bye et al., 2016)
	miR-19b-3p, miR-134-5p and miR-186-5p	Overexpression	Plasma	Clinical	(Wang et al., 2016b)
	miR-125b-5p, miR-30d-5p	Overexpression	Plasma	Clinical	(Jia et al., 2016)
	miR-423-5p, miR-30d	Overexpression	Plasma	Clinical	(Eryılmaz et al., 2016)
	miR-221-3p	Overexpression	Plasma	Clinical	(Coskunpinar et al., 2016)
	miR-208a	Overexpression in myocardium and high levels in serum	Myocardium and serum	Experimental: rat model of MI	(Feng et al., 2016)
	miR-133b, miR-22-5p	Upregulation	Serum/plasma	Clinical	(Maciejak et al., 2016)
	miR-103a	Higher levels in plasma	Plasma and peripheral blood mononuclear cells	Clinical and experimental: *in vitro*	(Huang et al., 2016a)
	miR-122-5p/133b	High ratio	Serum	Clinical	(Cortez-Dias et al., 2016)
	miR499a-5p	Higher levels	Plasma	Clinical	(O'Sullivan et al., 2016)
	miR-181a	Higher levels	Plasma	Clinical	(Zhu et al., 2016)
	miR-145	Decreased	Plasma	Clinical	(Zhang et al., 2017b)
	miR-133a	Higher levels	Plasma	Clinical	(Yuan et al., 2016)
	miR-208b	Higher levels	Plasma	Clinical	(Liu et al., 2017)
	miR-1, miR-92a, miR-99a, miR-143, miR-223	miR-143: increased; miR-1, miR-92a, miR-99a, miR-223: decreased	Monocytes	Clinical	(Parahuleva et al., 2017)
	miR-92a	Higher levels	Plasma	Clinical	(Zhang et al., 2017c)
	miR-208b	Overexpression	Plasma	Clinical	(Zhang and Xie, 2017)
	miR-124	Higher levels	Peripheral blood	Clinical	(Guo et al., 2017)
	miR-1, miR-21, miR-29b and miR-92a	miR-1, miR-21, miR-29b: increased	Plasma	Clinical	(Grabmaier et al., 2017)
	miR-874-3p	Downregulation	Plasma	Clinical	(Yan et al., 2017)
	pmiR-126	Lower levels	Platelet	Clinical	(Li et al., 2017b)
	miR-133a	Lower levels	Serum/Plasma	Clinical	(Zhu et al., 2018)
	miR-21	Upregulation	Serum	Clinical	(Wang et al., 2017b)
	miR-4478	Higher levels	Serum	Clinical	(Gholikhani-Darbroud et al., 2017)
	miR-23b	Higher levels	Plasma	Clinical	(Zhang et al., 2018a)
	MiR-27a, miR-31, miR-1291, miR-139-5p, miR-204, miR-375	Higher levels	GEO database	High throughput	(Wu et al., 2018a)
	miR-1, miR-133a, miR-34a	Lower levels	Myocardium	Experimental: mouse model of MI	(Qipshidze Kelm et al., 2018)

(Continued)

TABLE 3 | Continued

Epigenetic modification	Biomarker	Regulation in myocardial infarction	Sample source	Study type	References
	miR-19b, miR-223, miR-483-5p	Higher levels	Plasma	Clinical	(Li et al., 2019)
	miR-17-5p, miR-126-5p, miR-145-3p	Higher levels	Plasma	Clinical	(Xue et al., 2019)
	miR-150	Lower levels	Serum	Clinical	(Lin et al., 2019)
	miR-208b, miR-499	Higher levels	Plasma	Clinical	(Devaux et al., 2012)

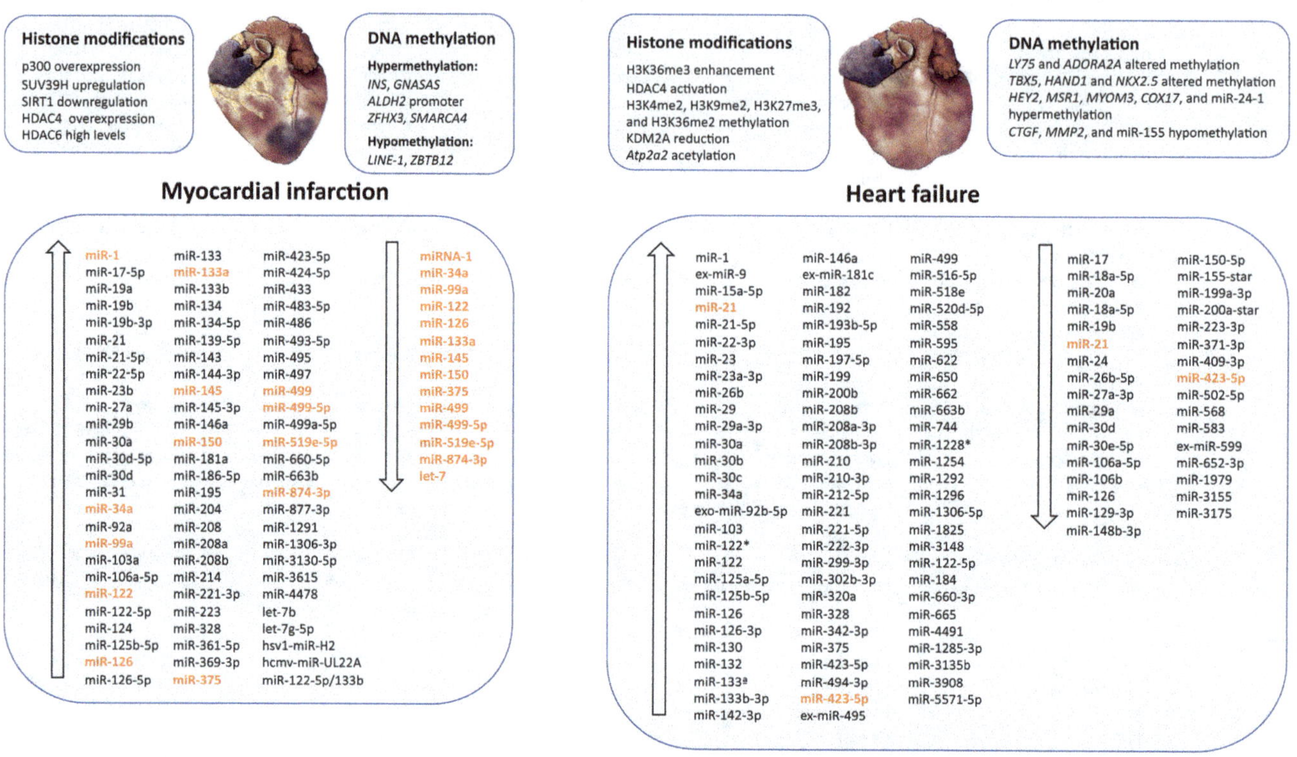

FIGURE 3 | Epigenetic modifications and microRNAs biomarkers dysregulated in myocardial infarction and heart failure. Ascending arrows indicate higher levels or upregulation, and descending arrows denote lower levels or downregulation, both compared to control conditions. Those miRNAs presenting opposite results are shown in orange.

miR-126 may be useful indicators of AMI (Long et al., 2012a). However, when miR-1 was compared to cTnT, the authors found that cTnT was more specific and sensitive than miR-1 (Li et al., 2014a). Experiments performed in a rat model of MI revealed dysregulation of several miRNAs in the myocardium. Specifically, miR-31, miR-208, and miR-214 were upregulated, and miR-126 and miR-499-5p were downregulated in infarcted rats compared to sham-operated animals (Ji et al., 2009; Shi et al., 2010). MiR-499 has been widely analyzed as a possible biomarker of MI. MiR-499 has been reported to be produced almost exclusively in the heart and plasma and is significantly increased in individuals with AMI (Adachi et al., 2010; Devaux et al., 2012). MiR-499 positively correlates with serum creatine kinase-MB (CK-MB) and cTnI increasing their diagnostic accuracy (Chen et al., 2015b; Zhang et al., 2015b). Thus, miR-499 might be a suitable biomarker for MI and a predictor of myocardial ischemia risk (Adachi et al., 2010; Chen et al., 2015b; Zhang et al., 2015b). These results were confirmed in the mouse model of MI, with elevated serum miR-208a levels. However, the expression of miR-499 was significantly reduced in the MI region, whereas miR-208a remained unchanged in the same area. One explanation is that the damaged heart might release miR-499 into the circulation (Xiao et al., 2014). Other authors observed a high correlation between circulating miRNA-208a in STEMI patients and the levels of cTnI and CK-MB mass liberated from the infarcted zone (Białek et al., 2015). Thus, cardiac miR-208 and miR-499 seemed to be better biomarkers for predicting AMI than miR-1 (Liu et al., 2015b; Liu et al., 2018a). Another study analyzed the expression of miR-208a in the myocardium and serum of infarcted rats compared to control groups, as well as the expression of cAMP-PKA to evaluate the effect of this signaling pathway in the primary stages of MI; they found increased expression of miR-208a and cAMP-PKA. Moreover, the transfection of human myocardial cells with the miR-208a analog significantly increased the amount of cAMP-PKA protein. Thus, higher expression of miR-208a in the infarcted myocardium and serum may play a role in MI by affecting the cAMP-PKA signaling pathway (Feng et al., 2016).

D'Alessandra et al. (2010) investigated plasma levels of miRNAs in acute STEMI patients and infarcted mice and found higher levels of miR-1, miR-133a, miR-133b, and miR-499-5p compared to controls, whereas miR-122 and miR-375 levels were lower only in STEMI patients. Peak miR-1, miR-133a, and miR-133b expression correlated with cTnI levels in time, whereas the time course of miR-499-5p was slower (D'Alessandra et al., 2010). This was later confirmed in an exhaustive meta-analysis of relevant publications (Cheng et al., 2014). Similarly, geriatric patients with acute NSTEMI had greater miR-499-5p levels, exhibiting greater precision in diagnosis than cTnT in patients with mild ST elevation (Olivieri et al., 2013). On the other hand, increased levels of miR-1, miR-133a, miR-208b, and miR-499 in patients with AMI have been demonstrated to not be superior to cTnT (Li et al., 2013). The use of miR-133a as a biomarker in reperfused STEMI has been evaluated and compared to cardiovascular magnetic resonance imaging; high levels of miR-133a correlated with an increased infarct scar size, worse myocardial recovery, and prominent reperfusion injury. Nevertheless, miR-133a did not add further predictive information to cardiovascular magnetic resonance and conventional markers used in clinical practice in high-risk STEMI patients (Eitel et al., 2012). Moreover, the circulating levels of miR-133a were significantly enhanced in AMI patients compared to coronary heart disease and myocardial ischemia patients, presenting a similar trend as plasma cTnI concentration. Remarkably, we found a positive correlation between circulating miR-133a levels and the severity of coronary artery stenosis. Thus, circulating miR-133a may be a suitable tool for AMI diagnosis and predicting the presence and severity of coronary damage in coronary heart disease patients (Wang et al., 2013a). These results were later confirmed (Yuan et al., 2016; Zhu et al., 2018). Nevertheless, in another study analyzing miR-133a and miR-423-5p and their relationship with cardiac biomarkers, such as B-type natriuretic peptide (BNP), C-reactive protein, and cTnI in MI patients, an increase in circulating levels of both miRNAs was observed, but these changes were not associated with LV remodeling or BNP. The authors claimed that miR-133a and miR-423-5p are not useful biomarkers of LV remodeling after MI (Bauters et al., 2013). Another controversial pair of biomarkers is miR-423-5p and miR-30d, which were found to be higher in STEMI patients without a significant correlation with cTnI (Eryılmaz et al., 2016). In addition, the analysis of circulating miR-124a and miR-133 in STEMI and cardiogenic shock patients revealed a significant upregulation of both molecules. A negative correlation was found between miR-133 and MMP-9 levels, and a relationship between miR-124 and soluble ST2 levels, a marker associated with cardiac damage. Surprisingly, this study did not connect any of the miRNAs to the extent of the injury, disease progression, or the prognosis of patient outcomes. In this case, miRNAs would not bring any benefit compared to current markers (Goldbergova et al., 2018). Moreover, elevated circulating miR-1254 was described as predicting adverse LV remodeling in STEMI patients when compared to magnetic resonance imaging. However, the diagnosis and prognosis values of miR-1254 require further research (de Gonzalo-Calvo et al., 2018). Other investigations have described miR-150-3p and miR-486-3p as being upregulated, whereas miR-26a-5p, miR-126-3p, and miR-191-5p were significantly downregulated in STEMI patients (Hsu et al., 2014). In the same manner, circulating miR-19b-3p, miR-134-5p, and miR-186-5p have been reported to be significantly elevated in the initial stages of AMI. The expression of miR-19b-3p and miR-134-5p in the plasma reached a maximum earlier than miR-186-5p. However, all three positively correlated with cTnI and achieved peak expression before cTnI, which was 8 h after admission. Interestingly, the expression of these circulating miRNAs was not altered by heparin and medications for AMI, and the combination of all three miRNAs increased their diagnostic efficacy (Wang et al., 2016b). Moreover, a higher miR-122-5p/133b ratio was found in serum from STEMI patients (Cortez-Dias et al., 2016). The NSTEMI patients presented higher serum levels of miR-4478, soluble leptin receptor, cTnI, CKMB, urea, creatinine, glucose, cholesterol, TG, and ALP but lower levels of ALT compared to healthy individuals (Gholikhani-Darbroud et al., 2017). Moreover, there was an increase in miR-143 expression in monocytes from STEMI patients, whereas miR-1, miR-92a, miR-99a, and miR-223 expression was significantly reduced. Also, monocytic expression of miR-143 positively correlated with high-sensitivity C-reactive protein (hs-CRP), but not cTnT. These findings demonstrated that circulating monocytes could also be suitable biomarkers (Parahuleva et al., 2017).

Interestingly, cell-specific miRNA patterns are able to distinguish STEMI and NSTEMI patients. A correlation was found between miRNA 30d-5p and plasma, platelets, and leukocytes in patients with STEMI and NSTEMI. Furthermore, miR-221-3p and miR-483-5p were associated with plasma and platelets, but only in NSTEMI patients (Ward et al., 2013).

High levels of plasma miR-134 and miR-328 are described as being possible AMI biomarkers, as they correlate with a superior risk of developing HF and mortality. However, the miRNA levels were not superior to high-sensitivity cTnT (hs-cTnT) concentrations (He et al., 2014). In addition, elevated levels of miR-19a, miR-22-5p, miR-27a, miR-30a, miR-30a-5p, miR-30d-5p, miR-31, miR-34a, miR-122-5p, miR-125b-5p, miR-133, miR-133b, miR-139-5p, miR-150, miR-181a, miR-195, miR-204, miR-208, miR-208b, miR-221-3p, miR-375, miR-486, miR-497, miR-499a-5p, miR-663b, miR-1291, and let-7b can be potential biomarkers for AMI, increased risk of mortality, or HF (Devaux et al., 2012; Long et al., 2012b; Devaux et al., 2013; Li et al., 2014b; Lv et al., 2014; Peng et al., 2014; Zhong et al., 2014; Han et al., 2015; Yao et al., 2015; Zhang et al., 2015c; Coskunpinar et al., 2016; Jia et al., 2016; Maciejak et al., 2016; O'Sullivan et al., 2016; Zhu et al., 2016; Liu et al., 2017; Zhang and Xie, 2017; Alavi-Moghaddam et al., 2018; Maciejak et al., 2018; Wu et al., 2018a; Wang et al., 2019b). Other potential biomarkers for AMI are downregulated in patients' plasma, such as miR-99a, miR-122-5p, and miR-874-3p (Yang et al., 2016a; Yan et al., 2017; Wang et al., 2019b). Interestingly, high levels of the combination of miR-21-5p, miR-361-5p, and miR-519e-5p or the reduction of miR-519e-5p correlates with cTnI concentrations, significantly increasing the diagnostic accuracy in AMI patients (Wang et al., 2014b; Liu et al., 2015a). Similarly, miR-21 and miR-124 have similar diagnostic ability compared to CK, CK-MB, and cTnI (Zhang et al., 2016; Guo et al., 2017).

In an attempt to predict HF and cardiovascular death after AMI, circulating miR-145, the N-terminal fragment of the precursor BNP, myocardial-band CK, and cTnI concentrations were analyzed for short- and long-term clinical outcomes. As a result, the authors concluded that miR-145 was a significant independent predictor of cardiac events, predicting long-term outcomes after AMI (Dong et al., 2015). Later, another group found that miR-145 levels were significantly lower in AMI patients and correlate with increased serum BNP and cTnT and decreased LV ejection fraction (Zhang et al., 2017b).

An miRNA array revealed differences in the miRNA expression patterns in patients with different phases of HF after MI. Specifically, human miR-369-3p, miR-433, miR-493-5p, miR-495, and miR-3615 were overexpressed, whereas miR-877-3p, miR-1306-3p, hsv1-miR-H2, miR-3130-5p, and hcmv-miR-UL22A were underexpressed in these patients. Thus, these circulating miRNAs are novel candidates as biomarkers of MI and HF (Liang et al., 2015).

An important aspect of circulating miRNAs as biomarkers is their temporal release, source, and transportation. Using the ischemia–reperfusion injury model, Deddens et al. (2016) showed that the ischemic myocardium releases extracellular vesicles. They also demonstrated that these extracellular vesicles transported specific miRNAs from the heart and muscle and were quickly detected in plasma. Interestingly, these vesicles had a high miRNAs content and rapid detection compared to traditional injury markers. This makes them a promising tool for the early detection of MI (Deddens et al., 2016). Along the same lines, microparticles and the expression levels of miR-92a were investigated in AMI and stable coronary artery disease patients and compared to cTnI. The number of microparticles and expression levels of miR-92a were higher in AMI patients than in the stable coronary artery disease patients and control groups, with a positive correlation between the levels of microparticles and cTnI. Thus, microparticles containing miR-92a may be suitable for MI diagnosis and possibly regulate dysfunctional endothelial tissue in AMI patients (Zhang et al., 2017c). However, according to Grabmaier et al. (2017), miR-92a seems to not be a good biomarker of adverse ventricular remodeling in post-AMI patients. The authors evaluated circulating miR-1, miR-21, miR-29b, and miR-92a from the SITAGRAMI trial population and found that miR-1, miR-21, and miR-29b expression was higher in AMI patients. The levels of miR-1 and miR-29b in plasma post-AMI correlated with variations in infarct volume, and the levels of miR-29b and changes in LV ejection fraction over time were also associated (Grabmaier et al., 2017).

Investigation of the expression of miR-103a in AMI patients with and without high blood pressure and the effect on endothelial cell function revealed increased levels of miR-103a in all patients but no changes in peripheral blood mononuclear cells. Moreover, miR-103a suppressed the expression of Piezo1 protein, which diminished the capacity to produce capillary tubes and the viability of human umbilical vein endothelial cells (HUVECs). Thus, miR-103a may take part in the development of high blood pressure and the initiation of AMI *via* regulation of Piezo1 expression (Huang et al., 2016a).

In a study based on samples from the HUNT study biobank, Bye et al. (2016) analyzed the utility of circulating miRNAs to predict future fatal AMI in healthy participants. MiR-424-5p and miR-26a-5p were associated exclusively with risk in men and women, respectively, suggesting a gender-specific association. They discovered that the best model for predicting future AMI consisted of miR-106a-5p, miR-424-5p, let-7g-5p, miR-144-3p, and miR-660-5p, and these miRNAs were proposed as a panel to enhance the prediction of AMI risk in healthy individuals (Bye et al., 2016).

Platelet activation is critical for AMI pathogenesis, but the role of platelet miRNAs (pmiRNAs) as biomarkers in AMI and their correlation with indices of platelet activity are unclear. Assessment of pmiR-126 expression in STEMI patients revealed reduced levels and a correlation with plasma cTnI. However, pmiR-126 expression did not correlate well with platelet activity indices, and its potential diagnostic utility is limited (Li et al., 2017b).

MiR-1, miR-133a, and miR-34a induce adverse structural remodeling to impair cardiac contractile function. Increased levels of all three miRNAs have been shown in the hearts of old MI mice compared to young MI mice, and the miR-1 increase was more prolonged and corresponded to LV wall thinning. This suggests that significantly increased levels of miR-1 in the aged post-MI heart could be a biomarker for high-risk prediction (Qipshidze Kelm et al., 2018). In addition, miRNA-21 has been reported to be overexpressed in the serum of ancient patients with AMI and to positively correlate with serum levels of CK-MB and cTnI. *In vitro* experiments with human cardiomyocytes transfected with the miR-21 mimic short hairpin RNA have shown that, following tumor necrosis factor α (TNF-α) induction, apoptosis rates are downregulated. The upregulation of miR-21 expression in the serum of elderly patients with AMI inhibited apoptosis induced by TNF-α in human cardiomyocytes *via* activation of the JNK/p38/caspase-3 signaling pathway (Wang et al., 2017b). Along the same lines, cardiomyocyte apoptosis and hypoxic reduction of cell growth can be promoted by miR-23b overexpression, suggesting that it could be a potential biomarker for STEMI (Zhang et al., 2018a).

A recent study explored the diagnostic use of circulating miRNAs in patients with acute chest pain in the emergency department. They found that higher circulating miR-19b, miR-223, and miR-483-5p levels may be clinically useful for AMI diagnosis in early phases (Li et al., 2019). Similarly, circulating miR-17-5p, miR-126-5p, and miR-145-3p levels are elevated in plasma from AMI patients. Combining these three miRNAs achieves a more precise AMI diagnosis (Xue et al., 2019). Interestingly, next-generation miRNA sequencing from whole blood samples has been useful for identifying new biomarkers of MI (Kanuri et al., 2018).

Heart Failure

Heart failure is a chronic and progressive condition that hampers the ability of the heart to pump enough blood to the body and fulfill its needs. Heart failure is caused by multiple disorders, such as hypertension, cardiomyopathy, MI, arrhythmias, or valvular diseases, among others (Khatibzadeh et al., 2013). Numerous scientific reports connect HF and epigenetic modifications (**Table 4** and **Figure 3**). High-density epigenome-wide mapping of DNA methylation in the myocardium and blood from dilated cardiomyopathy patients and healthy individuals has been analyzed. This technology has been used to find regions of epigenetic susceptibility and new biomarkers related to HF and heart dysfunction; they recognized different patterns of epigenetic methylation that were preserved through tissues—the CpGs regions identified as novel biomarkers of HF (Meder et al., 2017; Rau and Vondriska, 2017). Differentially methylated DNA regions were also identified in blood leukocytes from HF patients (Li et al., 2017a). Dilated cardiomyopathy is an important cause of HF. Genome-wide cardiac DNA methylation in idiopathic dilated cardiomyopathy patients revealed abnormal DNA methylation, which was related to important variations in the expression of lymphocyte antigen 75 (*LY75*) and adenosine receptor A2A (*ADORA2A*) mRNA (Haas et al., 2013). Similarly, genome-wide maps of DNA methylation and enrichment of histone 3 lysine-36 trimethylation (H3K36me3) in pathological and healthy hearts were analyzed. Differences in DNA methylation were found in promoter CpG islands, genes, intragenic CpG islands, and H3K36me3-rich regions of the genome. The promoters of upregulated genes had altered DNA methylation, but not the promoters of downregulated genes. In particular, an abundance of *DUX4* transcripts was associated with differences in DNA methylation and H3K36me3 enrichment. Although further studies need to be carried out, there is evidence that the expression of genes critical for the development of cardiomyopathies may be controlled by the epigenome (Movassagh et al., 2011). Moreover, in patients with dilated cardiomyopathy, there is an altered methylation pattern in the regulatory regions of cardiac development genes, such as T-box protein 5 (*TBX5*), heart and neural crest derivatives expressed 1 (*HAND1*), and NK2 homeobox 5 (*NKX2.5*) (Jo et al., 2016). Koczor et al. (2013) also studied the differential methylation patterns in patients with dilated cardiomyopathy, which is characterized by congestive HF. Computational analysis detected few differentially methylated gene promoters (*AURKB*, *BTNL9*, *CLDN5*, and *TK1*). This study provides relevant information on DNA methylation and altered expression in dilated cardiomyopathy that would help in treatment (Koczor et al., 2013).

Furthermore, epigenetic modifications have been proposed to play an important role in HF progression in the murine model of pressure overload. The researchers observed a reduction in sarcoplasmic reticulum Ca^{2+}ATPase (*Atp2a2*) levels and a significant induction of β-myosin-heavy chain (*Myh7*) mRNA levels. They also detected H3K4me2, H3K9me2, H3K27me3, and H3K36me2 and a reduction in the lysine-specific demethylase KDM2A after 8 weeks of transverse aortic constriction (Angrisano et al., 2014). *Atp2a2* is a determinant of cardiac function, and its reduced activity is a clear feature of HF. Gorski et al. (2019) investigated the role of lysine acetylation in *Atp2a2* function in HF patients and found that acetylation at lysine 492 is regulated by SIRT1 and HAT p300 and significantly reduced the gene activity (Gorski et al., 2019). All of this knowledge would be fundamental to identifying potential biomarkers and new epigenetic drugs in HF therapy. Interestingly, an association has been reported between epigenetic remodeling in the atrial natriuretic peptide (*ANP*) and *BNP* promoters and reactivation of the fetal gene program in HF. Their reported upregulation in HF patients did not respond to an increase in histone acetylation but HDAC4, which is exported from the nucleus. In contrast, demethylation of H3K9 and dissociation of heterochromatin protein 1 from gene promoters were regulated by HDAC4. Thus, HDAC4 is fundamental to histone methylation in HF caused by increased cardiac load and a potential target for treatment (Hohl et al., 2013). More recently, Glezeva et al. (2019) performed targeted DNA methylation sequencing to detect DNA methylation alterations in coding and ncRNA in cardiac interventricular septal tissue from HF patients. They found hypermethylation in *HEY2*, *MSR1*, *MYOM3*, *COX17*, and miR-24-1 and hypomethylation in *CTGF*, *MMP2*, and miR-155. Therefore, they defended a unique cohort of loci useful as diagnostic and therapeutic targets in HF (Glezeva et al., 2019).

More than 10 years ago, few reports suggested that specific miRNAs are differentially regulated in the failing heart (Divakaran and Mann, 2008; Small and Olson, 2011). Since then, an extensive evidence base has been published in the literature regarding the use of miRNAs as possible biomarkers for HF diagnosis and prognosis. In evaluating whether miRNAs can differentiate clinical HF from healthy individuals and from non-HF dyspnea, miRNA arrays have revealed miR423-5p enrichment in the blood of HF patients (Tijsen et al., 2010). However, criticisms have been raised in this study regarding age differences between groups, reduced sample size, and statistics (Kumarswamy et al., 2010). Moreover, patients with HF of different etiologies presented with different expression levels of circulating miRNAs. Ischemic HF patients were found to have a positive transcoronary gradient for miR-423-5p, miR-423, and miR-34a, but the nonischemic HF group was positive only for miR-21-3p and miR-30a. The transcoronary concentration gradient suggests that the failing heart may selectively release the miRNAs into the coronary circulation. These miRNAs could be useful for discriminating different etiologies of HF (Goldraich et al., 2014; De Rosa et al., 2018).

Circulating miRNAs have been screened in an attempt to identify any that could be used for the prognosis of ischemic HF in post-AMI patients. Knowing that p53 has been involved in HF development in mice (Sano et al., 2007), the authors took great interest in p53-responsive miRNAs. The serum levels of miR-34a, miR-192, and miR-194 were significantly and coordinately upregulated in AMI patients with ischemic HF progression, and all three were p53-responsive. Interestingly, these miRNAs were contained in extracellular vesicles, suggesting that they are circulating regulators of HF. Furthermore, there was a significant correlation between the LV end-diastolic dimension 1 year after AMI and the miR-194 and miR-34a expression levels. Thus, although further investigations are needed, these results suggest the usefulness of miR-34a, miR-192, and miR-194 in predicting the risk of HF progression after AMI (Evans and Mann, 2013; Matsumoto et al., 2013; Klenke et al., 2018).

TABLE 4 | Epigenetic biomarkers in heart failure.

Epigenetic modification	Biomarker	Regulation in heart failure	Sample source	Study type	References
DNA methylation	*LY75* and *ADORA2A*	Aberrant DNA methylation	Left ventricle myocardium and zebrafish	Clinical and experimental: zebrafish	(Haas et al., 2013)
	TBX5, *HAND1*, and *NKX2.5*	Altered DNA methylation	Myocardium	Clinical	(Jo et al., 2016)
	HEY2, *MSR1*, *MYOM3*, *COX17*, miR-24-1, *CTGF*, *MMP2*, miR-155	*HEY2*, *MSR1*, *MYOM3*, *COX17*, and miR-24-1: hypermethylation; *CTGF*, *MMP2*, and miR-155: hypomethylation	Myocardium	Clinical	(Glezeva et al., 2019)
Histone modifications	H3K36me3	H3K36me3 enhancement	Myocardium	Clinical	(Movassagh et al., 2011)
	HDAC4	HDAC4 activation	Myocardium	Clinical and experimental: mouse model of pressure overload	(Hohl et al., 2013)
	H3K4me2, H3K9me2, H3K27me3, H3K36me2, KDM2A	H3K4me2, H3K9me2, H3K27me3, and H3K36me2 methylation and KDM2A reduction	Myocardium	Experimental: mouse model of pressure overload	(Angrisano et al., 2014)
	Atp2a2	*Atp2a2* acetylation	Ventricular myocytes and myocardium	Clinical and experimental: mouse model of pressure overload in *MHC-SIRT1*−/− Tg mice and swine model of MI	(Gorski et al., 2019)
miRNA	miR423-5p	Higher levels	Plasma	Clinical	(Tijsen et al., 2010)
	miR-192	Upregulation	Serum	Clinical	(Matsumoto et al., 2013)
	miR-122*, miR-200b, miR-520d-5p, miR-622, miR-1228*, miR-558	miR-122*, miR-200b, miR-520d-5p, miR-622, miR-1228*: upregulation; miR-558: downregulation	Whole peripheral blood	Clinical	(Vogel et al., 2013)
	miR-103, miR-142-3p, miR-30b, miR-342-3p	Differentially expressed	Plasma	Clinical	(Ellis et al., 2013)
	miR-210, miR-30a	Upregulation	Serum	Clinical	(Zhao et al., 2013)
	miR-210	Higher levels	Plasma, mononuclear cells, and skeletal muscles	Clinical and experimental: Dahl salt-sensitive rats	(Endo et al., 2013)
	miR-1	Higher levels	Plasma	Clinical	(Zhang et al., 2013b)
	miR-423-5p	Positive transcoronary gradients	Transcoronary gradients	Clinical	(Goldraich et al., 2014)
	miR-423-5p	Lower levels	Plasma	Clinical	(Seronde et al., 2015)
	MiR-30c, miR-146a, miR-221, miR-328, miR-375	Downregulation	Serum	Clinical	(Watson et al., 2015)
	miR-21, miR-650, miR-744, miR-516-5p, miR-1292, miR-182, miR-1228, miR-595, miR-663b, miR-1296, miR-1825, miR-299-3p, miR-662 miR-122, miR-3148, miR-518e, miR-129-3p, miR-3155, miR-3175, miR-583, miR-568, miR-30d, miR-200a-star, miR-1979, miR-371-3p, miR-155-star, miR-502-5p	miR-21, miR-650, miR-744, miR-516-5p, miR-1292, miR-182, miR-1228, miR-595, miR-663b, miR-1296, miR-1825, miR-299-3p, miR-662 miR-122, miR-3148, miR-518e: increased; miR-129-3p, miR-3155, miR-3175, miR-583, miR-568, miR-30d, miR-200a-star, miR-1979, miR-371-3p, miR-155-star, miR-502-5p: decreased	Serum	Clinical	(Cakmak et al., 2015)
	miR-1233, miR-671-5p, miR-183-3p, miR-190a, miR-193b-3p, miR-193b-5p, miR-211-5p, miR-494	miR-1233, miR-671-5p: Upregulation; miR-183-3p, miR-190a, miR-193b-3p, miR-193b-5p, miR-211-5p, miR-494: downregulation	Whole blood and plasma	Clinical	(Wong et al., 2015)

(*Continued*)

TABLE 4 | Continued

Epigenetic modification	Biomarker	Regulation in heart failure	Sample source	Study type	References
	miR-1, miR-21	miR-1: downregulation; miR-21: upregulation	Serum	Clinical	(Sygitowicz et al., 2015)
	miR-126	Downregulation	Serum	Clinical	(Wei et al., 2015)
	miR-1, miR-21, miR-23, miR-29, miR-130, miR-195, miR-199	Upregulation	Myocardial biopsy	Clinical	(Lai et al., 2015)
	miR-106a-5p, miR-223-3p, miR-652-3p, miR-199a-3p, miR-18a-5p	Downregulation	Plasma	Clinical	(Vegter et al., 2016)
	miR-148b-3p, miR-409-3p	Downregulation	Serum and left atrial tissue	Clinical	(Chen et al., 2016)
	miR-122-5p, miR-184	Upregulation	H9C2 cells and blood and myocardium	Experimental: *in vitro* and rat model of post-MI HF	(Liu et al., 2016)
	miR-660-3p, miR-665, miR-1285-3p, miR-4491	Upregulation	Plasma and heart	Clinical	(Li et al., 2016)
	miR-18a-5p, miR-26b-5p, miR-27a-3p, miR-30e-5p, miR-106a-5p, miR-199a-3p, miR-652-3p	Lower levels	Plasma	Clinical	(Ovchinnikova et al., 2016)
	miR-19b	Lower levels	Serum and myocardial	Clinical and experimental: *in vitro*	(Beaumont et al., 2017)
	miR-30d	Lower levels	Serum	Clinical	(Xiao et al., 2017)
	miR-195-3p	Higher levels	Plasma	Clinical	(He et al., 2017)
	miR-22-3p	Higher levels	Blood	Clinical	(van Boven et al., 2017)
	miR-150-5p	Downregulation	Blood	Clinical	(Scrutinio et al., 2017)
	miR-133b-3p, miR-208b-3p, miR-125a-5p, miR-125b-5p, miR-126-3p, miR-21-5p, miR-210-3p, miR-29a-3p, miR-320a, miR-494-3p	Upregulation	Blood	Experimental: sheep model of HF	(Wong et al., 2017)
	miR-146a	Upregulation	Exosomal and total plasma	Clinical and experimental: *in vitro*	(Beg et al., 2017)
	miR-9, miR-495, miR-599, miR-181c	ex-miR-9, ex-miR-181c, ex-miR-495: increased; ex-miR-599: decreased	Exosomal and total plasma	Experimental: dogs with myxomatous mitral valve disease, mitral valve prolapse	(Yang et al., 2017b)
	miR-21-5p, miR-23a-3p, miR-222-3p	Higher levels	Plasma	Clinical and experimental: rat model of post-MI HF	(Dubois-Deruy et al., 2017)
	miRNA-21	Higher levels	Serum	Clinical	(Zhang et al., 2017a)
	miR-132	Higher levels	Plasma	Clinical	(Masson et al., 2018)
	miR-1254, miR-1306-5p	Higher levels	Blood	Clinical	(Bayés-Genis et al., 2018)
	miR-423, miR-34a, miR-21-3p, miR-30a	miR-21-3p, miR-30a: Positive transcoronary gradient in non-ischemic HF; miR-423, miR-34a: Negative transcoronary gradient in ischemic HF	Transcoronary gradients	Clinical	(De Rosa et al., 2018)
	miR-3135b, miR-3908, miR-5571-5p	Upregulation	Plasma	Clinical	(Chen et al., 2018a)
	miR-302b-3p	Higher levels	Plasma	Clinical	(Li et al., 2018a)
	exo-miR-92b-5p	increased	Serum	Clinical	(Wu et al., 2018c)
	miR-26b, miR-208b, miR-499	Higher levels	Peripheral blood mononuclear cells	Clinical	(Marketou et al., 2018)
	miR-423-5p, miR-221-5p, miR-212-5p, miR-193b-5p, miR-15a-5p, miR-208a-3p	Upregulation	Plasma, mouse myocardium and NRVMs cells	Clinical and experimental: *in vitro*, and murine model of hypertrophy and HF	(Shah et al., 2018b)
	miR-192	Upregulation	Serum	Clinical	(Klenke et al., 2018)

(Continued)

TABLE 4 | Continued

Epigenetic modification	Biomarker	Regulation in heart failure	Sample source	Study type	References
	miR-34a, miR-208b, miR-126, miR-24, miR-29a	miR-34a, miR-208b, miR-126: upregulation; miR-24, miR-29a: downregulation	Serum	Clinical	(Lakhani et al., 2018)
	miR-17, miR-20a, miR-106b	Lower levels	Plasma	Clinical	(Shah et al., 2018a)
	miR-197-5p	Upregulation	Plasma	Clinical	(Liu et al., 2018b)
	miR-133a, miR-221	Higher levels	Plasma	Clinical	(Guo et al., 2018)
	exo-miR-92b-5p	Higher levels	Serum	Clinical	(Wu et al., 2018b; Wu et al., 2018c)

Vogel et al. (2013) assessed the genome-wide miRNA expression profiles in HF patients with reduced ejection fraction (HFrEF). They demonstrated that dysregulated levels of miRNAs, such as miR-122*, miR-200b, miR-520d-5p, miR-622, miR-1228* (upregulated), or miR-558 (downregulated) significantly correlate with disease severity, as indicated by LV ejection fraction (Vogel et al., 2013). Moreover, Ellis et al. (2013) tried to find differences between HF patients and non–HF-related breathlessness, and between HFrEF and HF with preserved ejection fraction (HFpEF); although they found a differential expression of miR-103, miR-142-3p, miR-30b, and miR-342-3p in HF and breathless patients, individually, classical biomarkers such as NT-proBNP and hs-cTnT exhibited greater sensitivity and specificity. However, the combination of miRNAs with NT-proBNP significantly improved prediction performance (Ellis et al., 2013). Similarly, elevated plasma levels of miR-210 were reported in congestive HF patients, although no significant correlation was observed with BNP. However, patients with an improved BNP profile presented with low plasma miR-210 levels. MiR-210 might reflect a mismatch between heart contraction and oxygen demand in the peripheral tissues (Endo et al., 2013). Interestingly, miR-210 and miR-30a expression is upregulated in HF patients, with a tendency toward fetal values (Zhao et al., 2013). Moreover, changes in myocardial miRNA in patients with stable and end-stage HF partially resemble the fetal myocardium. Target mRNA levels negatively correlate with changes in highly expressed miRNAs in HF and fetal hearts. The circulation is dominated by miRNAs, fragments of tRNAs, and small cytoplasmic RNAs. Heart- and muscle-specific circulating miRNAs (myomirs) are also increased in advanced HF, correlating with cTnI levels. These findings support miRNA-based therapies and the use of circulating miRNAs as biomarkers for heart injury (Akat et al., 2014). Cardiac fibroblast–derived miRNAs, such as miR-660-3p, miR-665, miR-1285-3p, and miR-4491, have also been found to be significantly upregulated in heart and plasma during HF, discriminating patients from controls (Li et al., 2016). However, miRNAs in the pericardial fluid are not related to cardiovascular pathologies or clinically assessed stages of HF. MicroRNAs may be paracrine signaling factors that intervene in cardiac cells crosstalk (Kuosmanen et al., 2015).

In another study performed in patients with chronic congestive HF, microarray profiling demonstrated increased expression of miR-21, miR-122, miR-182, miR-299-3p, miR-516-5p, miR-518e, miR-595, miR-650, miR-662, miR-663b, miR-744, miR-1228, miR-1292, miR-1296, miR-1825, and miR-3148 and decreased expression of miR-30d, miR-129-3p, and miR-502-5p, miR-155-star miR-200a-star, miR-371-3p, miR-583, miR-568, miR-1979, miR-3155, and miR-3175. Among these miRNAs, miR-182 seemed to have a better prognostic value than hs-CRP (Cakmak et al., 2015). Furthermore, miR-30c, miR-146a, miR-221, miR-328, and miR-375 had different expression levels in HFrEF and HFpEF. The combination of two or more miRNAs with BNP could significantly improve the discrimination of these pathological conditions compared to BNP alone (Watson et al., 2015). Additional miRNAs have been identified as promising biomarkers to discriminate HF from healthy individuals and to differentiate HFrEF from HFpEF: miR-125a-5p, miR-183-3p, miR-190a, miR-193b-3p, miR-193b-5p, miR-211-5p, miR-494, miR-545-5p, miR-550a-5p, miR-638, miR-671-5p, miR-1233, miR-3135b, miR-3908, and miR-5571-5p. The use of a combination of miRNAs and NT-proBNP increases its discernment capacity (Schulte et al., 2015; Wong et al., 2015; Chen et al., 2018a). Similarly, increased levels of miR-133a and miR-221 can be used as suitable HF diagnostic biomarkers in elderly HF patients, and the combination of NT-proBNP and miR-133a can improve the diagnostic accuracy (Guo et al., 2018). Serum levels of miR-1, miR-21, and miR-208a have also been analyzed in symptomatic HF patients. Expression of miR-1 is reduced in symptomatic HF patients, with decreasing levels correlating with increasing severity. In contrast, miR-21 has been shown to be overexpressed with no relation to HF severity. No circulating miR-208a has been observed in symptomatic HF patients. A negative correlation between miR-1 expression and NT-proBNP has been reported in HF patients, whereas miR-21 and galectin-3 have been positively correlated. Therefore, dysregulated levels of miR-1 and miR-21 may be fundamental for HF progression (Sygitowicz et al., 2015). An inverse correlation between miR-1 levels and ejection fraction has also been reported. Thus, elevated levels of miR-1 may inhibit cardiac function and be a predictor of the onset of HF secondary to AMI (Zhang et al., 2013b).

MiR-126 has also been studied in atrial fibrillation and/or HF patients, with downregulated expression in patients and positive correlation with LV ejection fraction but a negative association with the cardiothoracic ratio and NT-proBNP. Thus, the reduction in miR-126 expression is a potential indicator of severity in atrial fibrillation and HF (Wei et al., 2015). A significant negative correlation has also been found between several miRNAs and classical clinical biomarkers indicative of a worse clinical outcome in HF patients. MiR-16-5p has been correlated to CRP, miR-106a-5p to creatinine, miR-223-3p to growth differentiation factor 15, miR-652-3p to soluble ST-2, miR-199a-3p to procalcitonin and galectin-3, and miR-18a-5p to procalcitonin (Vegter et al., 2016). Furthermore, an analysis of myocyte and fibroblast-related miRNAs and mRNAs in myocardium samples from HF patients and control individuals revealed that miR-1, miR-21, miR-23, miR-29, miR-130, miR-195, and miR-199 are significantly upregulated in HF patients, whereas miR-30, miR-133, miR-208, and miR-320 do not significantly change. Related mRNAs, such as caspase 3, collagenase I, collagenase III, and transforming growth factor (TGF), are also upregulated in HF patients. MicroRNAs involved in apoptosis, hypertrophy, and fibrosis are upregulated in the myocardium of HF patients and may be suitable biomarkers in the early stages of chronic HF and future therapeutic targets (Lai et al., 2015).

Evaluation of miR-148b-3p and miR-409-3p in mitral regurgitation patients, asymptomatic mitral regurgitation patients, and controls revealed that circulating and tissue miR-148b-3p and circulating miR-409-3p are significantly downregulated in mitral regurgitation patients with HF, and miR-148b-3p is significantly downregulated only in the mitral regurgitation patients without HF. Notably, the mRNAs of target genes of both miRNAs have been shown to be upregulated in HF patients with mitral regurgitation. Thus, circulating miR-148b-3p may be used as a biomarker of HF and miR-409-3p for incident HF in mitral regurgitation patients (Chen et al., 2016).

Specific overexpression of miR-221 in the hearts of transgenic mice has been shown to induce cardiac dysfunction and HF by impairing autophagy. In addition, *in vitro* miR-221 upregulation inhibits autophagic vesicle formation. Thus, autophagy balance and cardiac remodeling are regulated by miR-221 levels through modulation of the p27/CDK2/mTOR axis, and miR-221 might be a therapeutic target in HF (Su et al., 2015). Furthermore, high-throughput sequencing has been used to determine the differential miRNA pattern in a rat model of post-MI HF. Upregulation of miR-122-5p and miR-184 was found in HF rats, describing a proapoptotic role of both miRNAs (Liu et al., 2016). In another study using the same model, the authors identified a significant increase in miR-21-5p, miR-23a-3p, and miR-222-3p and their target *SOD2* in the plasma and myocardium of HF rats. They showed a direct interaction between miR-222-3p and *SOD2*. An inhibition or increase in *SOD2* expression was found when human cardiomyocytes were transfected with miR-222-3p mimic or inhibitor, respectively (Dubois-Deruy et al., 2017).

Myocardial fibrosis–related miRNAs, such as miR-19b, are reduced in the myocardium and serum of HF patients with aortic stenosis. Inhibition of miR-19b in cultured human fibroblasts increases the expression of connective tissue growth factor protein and the enzyme lysyl oxidase (LOX). This could lead to excessive collagen fibril cross-linking and a subsequent increase in LV stiffness in aortic stenosis patients, particularly those with HF. Thus, miR-19b could be a biomarker of alterations in the myocardial collagen network (Beaumont et al., 2017).

Numerous studies have been performed to find miRNAs with a predictive value in HF patients. Increased levels of miR-1, miR-21, miR-21-5p, miR-22-3p, miR-29a-3p, miR30d, miR-125a-5p, miR-125b-5p, miR-126-3p, miR-133b-3p, miR-195-3p, miR-197-5P, miR-208b-3p, miR-210-3p, miR-302b-3p, miR-320a, and miR-494-3p (Zhang et al., 2013b; He et al., 2017; van Boven et al., 2017; Wong et al., 2017; Xiao et al., 2017; Zhang et al., 2017a; Li et al., 2018a; Liu et al., 2018b;) or decreased levels of miR-17, miR-18a-5p, miR-20a, miR-150, miR-26b-5p, miR-27a-3p, miR-30e-5p, miR-106a-5p, miR-106b, miR-150-5p, miR-199a-3p, miR-423-5p, and miR-652-3p (Seronde et al., 2015; Ovchinnikova et al., 2016; Scrutinio et al., 2017; Shah et al., 2018a; Lin et al., 2019) have been described as potential biomarkers in HF patients. These discoveries may serve to develop miRNA-based therapies and to identify new pharmacological targets.

Beg et al. (2017) measured exosomal and total plasma miRNAs separately in HF patients to distinguish between the transfer of biological materials for signaling alteration in distant organs (exosomal) and the level of tissue damage (plasma). They found that the circulating exosomal miR-146a/miR-16 ratio was higher in HF patients, with miR-146a induced in response to inflammation. These results suggest circulating exosomal miR-146a as a biomarker of HF (Beg et al., 2017). Moreover, elevation of exosomal miRNA exo-miR-92b-5p has been suggested as a potential biomarker for the diagnosis of HF (Wu et al., 2018b; Wu et al., 2018c). In a preclinical study in dogs with myxomatous mitral valve disease, dysregulation of exosomal miR-9, miR-495, and miR-599 was observed as the dogs aged. In addition, levels of miR-9, miR-599, miR-181c, and miR-495 changed in myxomatous mitral valve disease. Thus, the exosomal miRNA expression level appears to be more specific to disease states than total plasma miRNA (Yang et al., 2017b). Furthermore, the downregulation of miR-425 and miR-744 in the plasma exosomes has been shown to induce cardiac fibrosis by suppressing TGFβ1 expression (Wang et al., 2018a).

Circulating miR-132 levels increased in chronic HF with disease severity, and lower levels improve risk prediction for HF readmission beyond traditional risk factors, but not for mortality. MiR-132 may be useful for finding strategies that would reduce rehospitalization in HF patients (Masson et al., 2018; Panico and Condorelli, 2018). Moreover, in an exhaustive analysis of two independent cohorts using a strict quality evaluation for miRNA testing, an association was found between high levels of miR-1254 and miR-1306-5p and mortality and HF hospitalization in HF patients. However, these two circulating miRNAs were not shown to improve standard predictors of prognostication, such as age, sex, hemoglobin, renal function, and NT-proBNP (Bayés-Genis et al., 2018).

MiR-26b, miR-208b, and miR-499 expression levels have been assessed in peripheral blood mononuclear cells from hypertensive HFpEF patients to evaluate their association with their exercise capacity. All three miRNAs were expressed at higher levels in the patients group, but miR-208b showed the strongest correlations with cardiopulmonary exercise test parameters, including oxygen uptake, exercise duration, and the minute ventilation–carbon dioxide production relationship (Marketou et al., 2018). In a study performed in patients and a mice model of hypertrophy and HF, miRNAs dysregulation was shown to occur during HF development in animals, with downregulation of target genes. These miRNAs were associated with adverse LV remodeling in humans, suggesting coordinated regulation of miRNA-mRNA. They also revealed target clusters of genes, such as autophagy, metabolism, and inflammation, implicated in HF mechanisms, (Shah et al., 2018b).

With the intention to establish a biomarkers panel useful for early detection of HF resulting from MI, Lakhani et al. (2018) found significant upregulation of miR-34a, miR-208b, miR-126, TGFβ-1, TNF-α, IL-6, and MMP-9 and reduced miR-24 and miR-29a levels. A positive association between IL-10 and ejection fraction in MI patients also suggested an important role of IL-10 in predicting HF (Lakhani et al., 2018).

Systems biology analyses of LV remodeling after MI allow molecular comprehensions; for example, miRNA modulation may be used as a marker of HF evolution. Two systems biology strategies were used to define an miRNA mark of LV remodeling in MI. They integrated either multiomics data (proteins and ncRNAs) produced from post-MI plasma or proteomic data generated from a rat model of MI. As a result, several miRNAs were associated with LV remodeling: miR-21-5p, miR-23a-3p, miR-222-3p, miR-17-5p, miR-21-5p, miR-26b-5p, miR-222-3p, miR-335-5p, and miR-375. These outcomes support the use of integrative systems biology analyses for the definition of miRNA marks of HF evolution (Charrier et al., 2019).

LIMITATIONS AND PERSPECTIVES OF THE EPIGENETIC BIOMARKERS

Limitations of the current field include the lack of large multicenter studies to provide convincing evidence for clinical applicability. Rather than a single ncRNA, it is likely that there will be patterns of different ncRNAs and other biomarkers (e.g., protein-based) that, together with machine-learning algorithms, will provide more sensitive and specific diagnostic and prognostic approaches to CVDs. Also, several technical challenges must be overcome before CE-marked ncRNA biomarkers will enter the clinical realm. DNA methylation and histone modifications are epigenetic mechanisms that have been reported to be sources of potential biomarkers useful in clinical practice. However, each CVD is regulated by multiple epigenetic pathways, and different CVDs are regulated by the same epigenetic mechanism, most of which are still under study. For example, hypermethylation of H3K79 (Rodriguez-Iturbe, 2006; Duarte et al., 2012) and *ACE2* promoter (Fan et al., 2017) in hypertensive patients has been described. Moreover, H3K4 and H3K9 were also hypermethylated in both mouse models of hypertension (Pojoga et al., 2011) and HF (Angrisano et al., 2014). This makes it difficult to select and implement a set of biomarkers for a particular CVD. Another potential problem is the quality of the samples, especially those obtained from collections in the pathology department. These samples are usually preserved in formaldehyde and paraffin, which highly degrades DNA. The stability, size, and integrity of a sample depend on the duration of fixation and storage (Kristensen et al., 2009). Thus, assessment of the quality of DNA is fundamental. However, the DNA methylation analysis can be performed successfully using polymerase chain reaction (PCR) methods with small amplicons in old samples (Tournier et al., 2012; Wong et al., 2014). In other cases, it is important to carefully adjust the protocol. It is also important to consider that frozen and paraffin-preserved samples may have different results, and they should not be compared without appropriate correction (García-Giménez et al., 2017).

Among the epigenetic biomarkers, miRNAs are the most promising, and numerous studies have been carried out in the last few years. The relatively easy detection and accessibility to samples in fluids, such as blood, urine, or saliva, make them very attractive. However, a few issues should be solved before their implementation in the clinical practice. The main problem is that miRNAs usually target multiple mRNAs from different genes, and one gene can be targeted by several miRNAs. This complex network should be deeply investigated before determining the use of a specific miRNA as a biomarker for the diagnosis or treatment of a particular disease (Akhtar et al., 2016). Regarding sample preparation, it is highly recommended to use plasma instead of whole blood, because if it is hemolyzed, the circulating miRNA content can be altered. Increasing the centrifugation time is also important in order to reduce platelet contamination (de Gonzalo-Calvo et al., 2017; García-Giménez et al., 2017).

Recently, great advances have been made to implement the new technology in the detection of new epigenetic biomarkers. However, a few concerns should be alleviated before their clinical implementation. Studies with big cohorts in different independent laboratories, using the same experimental design, sample preparation, methodology, and disease specifications, are necessary. Small patient cohorts should be considered as pilot studies before the validation of results in bigger sample analysis. The method of detection should be standardized for clinical application, and the clinical trials have to be randomized and prospective. It is also important to compare the new biomarkers with the classical biomarkers in order to validate them and determine their usefulness. The sensitivity and specificity for a certain disease also have to be determined for each biomarker (Engelhardt, 2012; García-Giménez et al., 2017). Regarding the method of DNA methylation detection, the luminometric methylation assay and the methylation analysis of CpG islands in repeatable elements (LINE-1) are widely used. Although there is a certain correlation with the measurements obtained with both methods, the comparison is not recommended, since a consistent bias between the results has been described (Knothe et al., 2016). Interestingly, a large multicenter study comparing DNA methylation assays compatible with routine clinical use has been performed. According to the authors, good agreement was observed between DNA methylation assays, which can be implemented in large-scale validation studies, development of new biomarkers, and clinical diagnostics (BLUEPRINT Consortium, 2016). The most used system to detect miRNAs is quantitative PCR, being the normalization protocol critical. Most laboratories use housekeeping genes or miRNAs as normalizers, changing their expression levels within serums. Another approach employs identical volumes of serum for all samples, generating different amounts of total RNA (Chen et al., 2008; Wang et al., 2009; Rockenbach et al., 2012). Both approaches include spike-in normalization, which consists of adding RNA of known sequence and quantity to calibrate measurements. However, spike-in normalization does not consider internal variation in circulating miRNA between different individuals. Thus, a combination of both methods should always be performed to guarantee results reliability (van Empel et al., 2012). Polymerase chain reaction technology has to be performed with rigorous controls to avoid artifacts in the amplification step. To overcome this problem, digital PCR based on the amplification of one single molecule per reaction constitutes a valuable option (Hindson et al., 2013). Another attractive alternative for accurate measuring RNAs is the direct nucleic acid sequencing, although it is still expensive when considering large screening analysis (Kozomara and Griffiths-Jones, 2011). Finally, it is also important to understand the processes controlling miRNAs release and stability. The correlation between circulating and tissue miRNAs is not clear, and several studies indicate that miRNA levels in blood are not a reflection of changes in the tissue of origin. The reason is that miRNAs can also be produced by immune cells (Zheng et al., 2018).

CONCLUDING REMARKS

Over the past few years, a great amount of research has focused on epigenetics and its dynamic cross-talk with genetics. Unveiling a personalized epigenetic pattern can provide a large amount of information on epigenetic machinery that could be employed to tailor diagnosis and therapeutic strategies in CVDs. Recent advances in technology and data analysis have made it possible to create detailed epigenetic maps, which may represent a new tool in the clinical practice to discern cardiovascular risk beyond traditional risk determinants. Epigenetic information can also help in predicting individual drug responses. Importantly, epigenetic biomarkers are gaining ground in the scientific community as tools for the diagnosis and prognosis of CVDs. However, discrepancies in specific diagnostic biomarkers make replication of the current results in independent laboratories, with multiple research centers and a big sample size, mandatory. All of this will lead to a standardized clinical application in the near future.

AUTHOR CONTRIBUTIONS

CS-B and AB-G conceived the idea and wrote the manuscript with support from CG-M. CG-M performed the drawings and structure of the figures. All authors contributed to manuscript revision, read and approved the submitted version.

FUNDING

This work was supported by grants from the Spanish Ministry of Economy and Competitiveness-MINECO (SAF2017-84324-C2-1-R), the Instituto de Salud Carlos III (PIC18/0014, PI18/00256), the Red de Terapia Celular–TerCel (RD16/0011/0006) and the CIBER Cardiovascular (CB16/11/00403) projects, as part of the Plan Nacional de I+D+I, and it was co-funded by ISCIII-Sudirección General de Evaluación y el Fondo Europeo de Desarrollo Regional (FEDER). This work was also funded by the Fundació La MARATÓ de TV3 (201516-10, 201502-20), the Generalitat de Catalunya (SGR2017 00483, SLT002/16/00234), the CERCA Programme/Generalitat de Catalunya, and "la Caixa" Banking Foundation.

ACKNOWLEDGMENTS

We apologize to all authors whose work could not be mentioned because of space limitations or inadvertent omissions. We are greatly grateful to Sonia V Forcales for her comments and discussion on epigenetic regulation.

REFERENCES

Adachi, T., Nakanishi, M., Otsuka, Y., Nishimura, K., Hirokawa, G., Goto, Y., et al. (2010). Plasma microRNA 499 as a biomarker of acute myocardial infarction. *Clin. Chem.* 56, 1183–1185. doi: 10.1373/clinchem.2010.144121

Ai, J., Zhang, R., Li, Y., Pu, J., Lu, Y., Jiao, J., et al. (2010). Circulating microRNA-1 as a potential novel biomarker for acute myocardial infarction. *Biochem. Biophys. Res. Commun.* 391, 73–77. doi: 10.1016/j.bbrc.2009.11.005

Akat, K. M., Moore-McGriff, D., Morozov, P., Brown, M., Gogakos, T., Correa Da Rosa, J., et al. (2014). Comparative RNA-sequencing analysis of myocardial and circulating small RNAs in human heart failure and their utility as biomarkers. *Proc. Natl. Acad. Sci. U. S. A* 111, 11151–11156. doi: 10.1073/pnas.1401724111

Akhtar, M. M., Micolucci, L., Islam, M. S., Olivieri, F., and Procopio, A. D. (2016). Bioinformatic tools for microRNA dissection. *Nucleic Acids Res.* 44, 24–44. doi: 10.1093/nar/gkv1221

Alavi-Moghaddam, M., Chehrazi, M., Alipoor, S. D., Mohammadi, M., Baratloo, A., Mahjoub, M. P., et al. (2018). A preliminary study of microRNA-208b after acute myocardial infarction: impact on 6-month survival. *Dis. Markers* 2018, 2410451-7. doi: 10.1155/2018/2410451

Alikhani-Koopaei, R., Fouladkou, F., Frey, F. J., and Frey, B. M. (2004). Epigenetic regulation of 11 beta-hydroxysteroid dehydrogenase type 2 expression. *J. Clin. Investig.* 114, 1146–1157. doi: 10.1172/JCI21647

Angrisano, T., Schiattarella, G. G., Keller, S., Pironti, G., Florio, E., Magliulo, F., et al. (2014). Epigenetic switch at atp2a2 and myh7 gene promoters in pressure overload-induced heart failure. *PLoS One* 9, e106024. doi: 10.1371/journal.pone.0106024

Authors/Task Force members, Windecker, S., Kolh, P., Alfonso, F., Collet, J.-P., Cremer, J., et al. (2014). 2014 ESC/EACTS guidelines on myocardial revascularization: the task force on myocardial revascularization of the European Society of Cardiology (ESC) and the European Association for Cardio-Thoracic Surgery (EACTS) developed with the special contribution of the European Association of Percutaneous Cardiovascular Interventions (EAPCI). *Eur. Heart J.* 35, 2541–2619. doi: 10.1093/eurheartj/ehu278

Babuin, L., and Jaffe, A. S. (2005). Troponin: the biomarker of choice for the detection of cardiac injury. *CMAJ* 173, 1191–1202. doi: 10.1503/cmaj/051291

Baccarelli, A., Rienstra, M., and Benjamin, E. J. (2010). Cardiovascular epigenetics: basic concepts and results from animal and human studies. *Circ. Cardiovasc. Genet.* 3, 567–573. doi: 10.1161/CIRCGENETICS.110.958744

Baptista, R., Marques, C., Catarino, S., Enguita, F. J., Costa, M. C., Matafome, P., et al. (2018). MicroRNA-424(322) as a new marker of disease progression in pulmonary arterial hypertension and its role in right ventricular hypertrophy by targeting SMURF1. *Cardiovasc. Res.* 114, 53–64. doi: 10.1093/cvr/cvx187

Bartel, D. P. (2009). MicroRNAs: target recognition and regulatory functions. *Cell* 136, 215–233. doi: 10.1016/j.cell.2009.01.002

Bauters, C., Kumarswamy, R., Holzmann, A., Bretthauer, J., Anker, S. D., Pinet, F., et al. (2013). Circulating miR-133a and miR-423-5p fail as biomarkers for left ventricular remodeling after myocardial infarction. *Int. J. Cardiol.* 168, 1837–1840. doi: 10.1016/j.ijcard.2012.12.074

Bayés-Genis, A., Lanfear, D. E., de Ronde, M. W. J., Lupón, J., Leenders, J. J., Liu, Z., et al. (2018). Prognostic value of circulating microRNAs on heart failure-related morbidity and mortality in two large diverse cohorts of general heart failure patients. *Eur. J. Heart Fail.* 20, 67–75. doi: 10.1002/ejhf.984

Beaumont, J., López, B., Ravassa, S., Hermida, N., José, G. S., Gallego, I., et al. (2017). MicroRNA-19b is a potential biomarker of increased myocardial collagen cross-linking in patients with aortic stenosis and heart failure. *Sci. Rep.* 7, 40696. doi: 10.1038/srep40696

Beekman, M., Nederstigt, C., Suchiman, H. E. D., Kremer, D., van der Breggen, R., Lakenberg, N., et al. (2010). Genome-wide association study (GWAS)-identified disease risk alleles do not compromise human longevity. *Proc. Natl. Acad. Sci. U. S. A* 107, 18046–18049. doi: 10.1073/pnas.1003540107

Beg, F., Wang, R., Saeed, Z., Devaraj, S., Masoor, K., and Nakshatri, H. (2017). Inflammation-associated microRNA changes in circulating exosomes of heart failure patients. *BMC Res. Notes* 10, 751. doi: 10.1186/s13104-017-3090-y

Bekkering, S., van den Munckhof, I., Nielen, T., Lamfers, E., Dinarello, C., Rutten, J., et al. (2016). Innate immune cell activation and epigenetic remodeling in symptomatic and asymptomatic atherosclerosis in humans *in vivo*. *Atherosclerosis* 254, 228–236. doi: 10.1016/j.atherosclerosis.2016.10.019

Białek, S., Górko, D., Zajkowska, A., Kołtowski, Ł., Grabowski, M., Stachurska, A., et al. (2015). Release kinetics of circulating miRNA-208a in the early phase of myocardial infarction. *Kardiologia Polska* 73, 613–619. doi: 10.5603/KP.a2015.0067

Bildirici, A. E., Arslan, S., Özbilüm Şahin, N., Berkan, Ö., Beton, O., and Yilmaz, M. B. (2018). MicroRNA-221/222 expression in atherosclerotic coronary artery plaque versus internal mammarian artery and in peripheral blood samples. *Biomarkers* 23, 670–675. doi: 10.1080/1354750X.2018.1474260

BLUEPRINT Consortium. (2016). Quantitative comparison of DNA methylation assays for biomarker development and clinical applications. *Nat. Biotechnol.* 34, 726–737. doi: 10.1038/nbt.3605

Bogdarina, I., Welham, S., King, P. J., Burns, S. P., and Clark, A. J. L. (2007). Epigenetic modification of the renin–angiotensin system in the fetal programming of hypertension. *Circ. Res.* 100, 520–526. doi: 10.1161/01.RES.0000258855.60637.58

Bye, A., Røsjø, H., Nauman, J., Silva, G. J. J., Follestad, T., Omland, T., et al. (2016). Circulating microRNAs predict future fatal myocardial infarction in healthy individuals—the HUNT study. *J. Mol. Cell Cardiol.* 97, 162–168. doi: 10.1016/j.yjmcc.2016.05.009

Cakmak, H. A., Coskunpinar, E., Ikitimur, B., Barman, H. A., Karadag, B., Tiryakioglu, N. O., et al. (2015). The prognostic value of circulating microRNAs in heart failure: preliminary results from a genome-wide expression study. *J. Cardiovasc. Med. (Hagerstown)* 16, 431–437. doi: 10.2459/JCM.0000000000000233

Cao, J., and Yan, Q. (2012). Histone ubiquitination and deubiquitination in transcription, DNA damage response, and cancer. *Front. Oncol.* 2, 26. doi: 10.3389/fonc.2012.00026

Charrier, H., Cuvelliez, M., Dubois-Deruy, E., Mulder, P., Richard, V., Bauters, C., et al. (2019). Integrative system biology analyses identify seven microRNAs to predict heart failure. *Noncoding RNA* 5, E22–E30. doi: 10.3390/ncrna5010022

Chelbi, S. T., Mondon, F., Jammes, H., Buffat, C., Mignot, T.-M., Tost, J., et al. (2007). Expressional and epigenetic alterations of placental serine protease inhibitors: SERPINA3 is a potential marker of preeclampsia. *Hypertension* 49, 76–83. doi: 10.1161/01.HYP.0000250831.52876.cb

Chen, F., Yang, J., Li, Y., and Wang, H. (2018a). Circulating microRNAs as novel biomarkers for heart failure. *Hellenic J. Cardiol.* 59, 209–214. doi: 10.1016/j.hjc.2017.10.002

Chen, J., Xu, L., Hu, Q., Yang, S., Zhang, B., and Jiang, H. (2015a). MiR-17-5p as circulating biomarkers for the severity of coronary atherosclerosis in coronary artery disease. *Int. J. Cardiol.* 197, 123–124. doi: 10.1016/j.ijcard.2015.06.037

Chen, M.-C., Chang, T.-H., Chang, J.-P., Huang, H.-D., Ho, W.-C., Lin, Y.-S., et al. (2016). Circulating miR-148b-3p and miR-409-3p as biomarkers for heart failure in patients with mitral regurgitation. *Int. J. Cardiol.* 222, 148–154. doi: 10.1016/j.ijcard.2016.07.179

Chen, S., Chen, R., Zhang, T., Lin, S., Chen, Z., Zhao, B., et al. (2018b). Relationship of cardiovascular disease risk factors and noncoding RNAs with hypertension: a case-control study. *BMC Cardiovasc. Disord.* 18, 58. doi: 10.1186/s12872-018-0795-3

Chen, W., and Li, S. (2017). Circulating microRNA as a novel biomarker for pulmonary arterial hypertension due to congenital heart disease. *Pediatr. Cardiol.* 38, 86–94. doi: 10.1007/s00246-016-1487-3

Chen, X., Ba, Y., Ma, L., Cai, X., Yin, Y., Wang, K., et al. (2008). Characterization of microRNAs in serum: a novel class of biomarkers for diagnosis of cancer and other diseases. *Cell Res.* 18, 997–1006. doi: 10.1038/cr.2008.282

Chen, X., Zhang, L., Su, T., Li, H., Huang, Q., Wu, D., et al. (2015b). Kinetics of plasma microRNA-499 expression in acute myocardial infarction. *J. Thorac. Dis.* 7, 890–896. doi: 10.3978/j.issn.2072-1439.2014.11.32

Cheng, C., Wang, Q., You, W., Chen, M., and Xia, J. (2014). MiRNAs as biomarkers of myocardial infarction: a meta-analysis. *PLoS ONE* 9, e88566. doi: 10.1371/journal.pone.0088566

Cho, H.-M., Lee, H.-A., Kim, H. Y., Han, H. S., and Kim, I. K. (2011). Expression of Na+-K+ -2Cl- cotransporter 1 is epigenetically regulated during postnatal development of hypertension. *Am. J. Hypertens.* 24, 1286–1293. doi: 10.1038/ajh.2011.136

Choi, J.-H., Nam, K.-H., Kim, J., Baek, M. W., Park, J.-E., Park, H.-Y., et al. (2005). Trichostatin A exacerbates atherosclerosis in low density lipoprotein receptor-deficient mice. *Arteriosclerosis, Thrombosis, and Vascular Biol.* 25, 2404–2409. doi: 10.1161/01.ATV.0000184758.07257.88

Choi, S. Y., Yun, J., Lee, O. J., Han, H. S., Yeo, M. K., Lee, M. A., et al. (2013). MicroRNA expression profiles in placenta with severe preeclampsia using a PNA-based microarray. *Placenta* 34, 799–804. doi: 10.1016/j.placenta.2013.06.006

Cortez-Dias, N., Costa, M. C., Carrilho-Ferreira, P., Silva, D., Jorge, C., Calisto, C., et al. (2016). Circulating miR-122-5p/miR-133b ratio is a specific early prognostic biomarker in acute myocardial infarction. *Circ. J.* 80, 2183–2191. doi: 10.1253/circj.CJ-16-0568

Coskunpinar, E., Cakmak, H. A., Kalkan, A. K., Tiryakioglu, N. O., Erturk, M., and Ongen, Z. (2016). Circulating miR-221-3p as a novel marker for early prediction of acute myocardial infarction. *Gene* 591, 90–96. doi: 10.1016/j.gene.2016.06.059

Costantino, S., Libby, P., Kishore, R., Tardif, J.-C., El-Osta, A., and Paneni, F. (2018). Epigenetics and precision medicine in cardiovascular patients: from basic concepts to the clinical arena. *Eur. Heart J.* 39, 4150–4158. doi: 10.1093/eurheartj/ehx568

D'Alessandra, Y., Devanna, P., Limana, F., Straino, S., Di Carlo, A., Brambilla, P. G., et al. (2010). Circulating microRNAs are new and sensitive biomarkers of myocardial infarction. *Eur. Heart J.* 31, 2765–2773. doi: 10.1093/eurheartj/ehq167

Dasgupta, C., Chen, M., Zhang, H., Yang, S., and Zhang, L. (2012). Chronic hypoxia during gestation causes epigenetic repression of the estrogen receptor-α gene in ovine uterine arteries *via* heightened promoter methylation. *Hypertension* 60, 697–704. doi: 10.1161/HYPERTENSIONAHA.112.198242

de Gonzalo-Calvo, D., Cediel, G., Bär, C., Núñez, J., Revuelta-Lopez, E., Gavara, J., et al. (2018). Circulating miR-1254 predicts ventricular remodeling in patients with ST-segment-elevation myocardial infarction: a cardiovascular magnetic resonance study. *Sci. Rep.* 8, 15115. doi: 10.1038/s41598-018-33491-y

de Gonzalo-Calvo, D., Cenarro, A., Civeira, F., and Llorente-Cortés, V. (2016). microRNA expression profile in human coronary smooth muscle cell-derived microparticles is a source of biomarkers. *Clin. Investig. Arterioscler.* 28, 167–177. doi: 10.1016/j.arteri.2016.05.005

de Gonzalo-Calvo, D., Iglesias-Gutiérrez, E., and Llorente-Cortés, V. (2017). Biomarcadores epigenéticos y enfermedad cardiovascular: los microARN circulantes. *Rev. Española Cardiol.* 70, 763–769. doi: 10.1016/j.recesp.2017.02.027

De Rosa, S., Eposito, F., Carella, C., Strangio, A., Ammirati, G., Sabatino, J., et al. (2018). Transcoronary concentration gradients of circulating microRNAs in heart failure. *Eur. J. Heart Fail.* 20, 1000–1010. doi: 10.1002/ejhf.1119

Deddens, J. C., Vrijsen, K. R., Colijn, J. M., Oerlemans, M. I., Metz, C. H. G., van der Vlist, E. J., et al. (2016). Circulating extracellular vesicles contain miRNAs and are released as early biomarkers for cardiac injury. *J. Cardiovasc Transl. Res.* 9, 291–301. doi: 10.1007/s12265-016-9705-1

Devaux, Y., Vausort, M., Goretti, E., Nazarov, P. V., Azuaje, F., Gilson, G., et al. (2012). Use of circulating microRNAs to diagnose acute myocardial infarction. *Clin. Chem.* 58, 559–567. doi: 10.1373/clinchem.2011.173823

Devaux, Y., Vausort, M., McCann, G. P., Zangrando, J., Kelly, D., Razvi, N., et al. (2013). MicroRNA-150: a novel marker of left ventricular remodeling after acute myocardial infarction. *Circ. Cardiovasc. Genet.* 6, 290–298. doi: 10.1161/CIRCGENETICS.113.000077

Divakaran, V., and Mann, D. L. (2008). The emerging role of microRNAs in cardiac remodeling and heart failure. *Circ. Res.* 103, 1072–1083. doi: 10.1161/CIRCRESAHA.108.183087

Dong, Y.-M., Liu, X.-X., Wei, G.-Q., Da, Y.-N., Cha, L., and Ma, C.-S. (2015). Prediction of long-term outcome after acute myocardial infarction using circulating miR-145. *Scand. J. Clin. Lab. Invest.* 75, 85–91. doi: 10.3109/00365513.2014.981855

Duarte, J. D., Zineh, I., Burkley, B., Gong, Y., Langaee, T. Y., Turner, S. T., et al. (2012). Effects of genetic variation in H3K79 methylation regulatory genes on clinical blood pressure and blood pressure response to hydrochlorothiazide. *J. Transl. Med.* 10, 56. doi: 10.1186/1479-5876-10-56

Dubois-Deruy, E., Cuvelliez, M., Fiedler, J., Charrier, H., Mulder, P., Hebbar, E., et al. (2017). MicroRNAs regulating superoxide dismutase 2 are new circulating biomarkers of heart failure. *Sci. Rep.* 7, 14747. doi: 10.1038/s41598-017-15011-6

Eitel, I., Adams, V., Dieterich, P., Fuernau, G., de Waha, S., Desch, S., et al. (2012). Relation of circulating MicroRNA-133a concentrations with myocardial damage and clinical prognosis in ST-elevation myocardial infarction. *Am. Heart J.* 164, 706–714. doi: 10.1016/j.ahj.2012.08.004

Ek, W. E., Hedman, Å. K., Enroth, S., Morris, A. P., Lindgren, C. M., Mahajan, A., et al. (2016). Genome-wide DNA methylation study identifies genes associated with the cardiovascular biomarker GDF-15. *Hum. Mol. Genet.* 25, 817–827. doi: 10.1093/hmg/ddv511

Ellis, K. L., Cameron, V. A., Troughton, R. W., Frampton, C. M., Ellmers, L. J., and Richards, A. M. (2013). Circulating microRNAs as candidate markers to distinguish heart failure in breathless patients. *Eur. J. Heart Fail.* 15, 1138–1147. doi: 10.1093/eurjhf/hft078

Endo, K., Naito, Y., Ji, X., Nakanishi, M., Noguchi, T., Goto, Y., et al. (2013). MicroRNA 210 as a biomarker for congestive heart failure. *Biol. Pharm. Bull.* 36, 48–54. doi: 10.1248/bpb.b12-00578

Engelhardt, S. (2012). Small RNA biomarkers come of age. *J. Am. Coll. Cardiol.* 60, 300–303. doi: 10.1016/j.jacc.2012.04.018

Eryılmaz, U., Akgullu, C., Beser, N., Yıldız, Ö., Kurt Ömürlü, İ., and Bozdogan, B. (2016). Circulating microRNAs in patients with ST-elevation myocardial infarction. *Anatol. J Cardiol* 16, 392–396. doi: 10.5152/AnatolJCardiol.2015.6603

Evans, S., and Mann, D. L. (2013). Circulating p53-responsive microRNAs as predictive biomarkers in heart failure after acute myocardial infarction: the long and arduous road from scientific discovery to clinical utility. *Circ. Res.* 113, 242–244. doi: 10.1161/CIRCRESAHA.113.301951

Fagard, R. H. (2006). Exercise is good for your blood pressure: effects of endurance training and resistance training. *Clin. Exp. Pharmacol. Physiol.* 33, 853–856. doi: 10.1111/j.1440-1681.2006.04453.x

Fan, R., Mao, S.-Q., Gu, T.-L., Zhong, F.-D., Gong, M.-L., Hao, L.-M., et al. (2017). Preliminary analysis of the association between methylation of the ACE2 promoter and essential hypertension. *Mol. Med. Rep.* 15, 3905–3911. doi: 10.3892/mmr.2017.6460

FDA-NIH Biomarker Working Group. (2016). BEST (Biomarkers, EndpointS, and other Tools) Resource.

Feng, G., Yan, Z., Li, C., and Hou, Y. (2016). microRNA-208a in an early stage myocardial infarction rat model and the effect on cAMP-PKA signaling pathway. *Mol. Med. Rep.* 14, 1631–1635. doi: 10.3892/mmr.2016.5402

Findeisen, H. M., Gizard, F., Zhao, Y., Qing, H., Heywood, E. B., Jones, K. L., et al. (2011). Epigenetic regulation of vascular smooth muscle cell proliferation and neointima formation by histone deacetylase inhibition. *Arteriosclerosis, Thrombosis, and Vascular Biol.* 31, 851–860. doi: 10.1161/ATVBAHA.110.221952

Fiorito, G., Guarrera, S., Valle, C., Ricceri, F., Russo, A., Grioni, S., et al. (2014). B-vitamins intake, DNA-methylation of one carbon metabolism and homocysteine pathway genes and myocardial infarction risk: the EPICOR study. *Nutr. Metab. Cardiovasc. Dis.* 24, 483–488. doi: 10.1016/j.numecd.2013.10.026

Fraga, M. F., Ballestar, E., Paz, M. F., Ropero, S., Setien, F., Ballestar, M. L., et al. (2005). Epigenetic differences arise during the lifetime of monozygotic twins. *Proc. Natl. Acad. Sci. U. S. A* 102, 10604–10609. doi: 10.1073/pnas.0500398102

Franceschini, N., and Le, T. H. (2014). Genetics of hypertension: discoveries from the bench to human populations. *Am. J. Physiol. Renal Physiol.* 306, F1–F11. doi: 10.1152/ajprenal.00334.2013

Friso, S., Pizzolo, F., Choi, S.-W., Guarini, P., Castagna, A., Ravagnani, V., et al. (2008). Epigenetic control of 11 beta-hydroxysteroid dehydrogenase 2 gene promoter is related to human hypertension. *Atherosclerosis* 199, 323–327. doi: 10.1016/j.atherosclerosis.2007.11.029

Gao, J., Yang, S., Wang, K., Zhong, Q., Ma, A., and Pan, X. (2019). Plasma miR-126 and miR-143 as potential novel biomarkers for cerebral atherosclerosis. *J. Stroke Cerebrovasc. Dis.* 28, 38–43. doi: 10.1016/j.jstrokecerebrovasdis.2018.09.008

García-Giménez, J. L., Mena-Mollá, S., Beltrán-García, J., and Sanchis-Gomar, F. (2017). Challenges in the analysis of epigenetic biomarkers in clinical samples. *Clin. Chem. Lab. Med.* 55, 1474–1477. doi: 10.1515/cclm-2016-1162

Gholikhani-Darbroud, R., Khaki-Khatibi, F., Mansouri, F., Hajahmadipoorrafsanjani, M., and Ghojazadeh, M. (2017). Decreased circulatory microRNA-4478 as a specific biomarker for diagnosing nonn–ST-segment elevation myocardial infarction (NSTEMI) and its association with soluble leptin receptor. *Bratisl. Lek. Listy* 118, 684–690. doi: 10.4149/BLL_2017_129

Glezeva, N., Moran, B., Collier, P., Moravec, C. S., Phelan, D., Donnellan, E., et al. (2019). Targeted DNA methylation profiling of human cardiac tissue reveals novel epigenetic traits and gene deregulation across different heart failure patient subtypes. *Circ. Heart Fail.* 12, e005765. doi: 10.1161/CIRCHEARTFAILURE.118.005765

Goldbergova, M. P., Lipkova, J., Fedorko, J., Sevcikova, J., Parenica, J., Spinar, J., et al. (2018). MicroRNAs in pathophysiology of acute myocardial infarction and cardiogenic shock. *Bratisl. Lek. Listy* 119, 341–347. doi: 10.4149/BLL_2018_064

Goldraich, L. A., Martinelli, N. C., Matte, U., Cohen, C., Andrades, M., Pimentel, M., et al. (2014). Transcoronary gradient of plasma microRNA 423-5p in heart failure: evidence of altered myocardial expression. *Biomarkers* 19, 135–141. doi: 10.3109/1354750X.2013.870605

Gorski, P. A., Jang, S. P., Jeong, D., Lee, A., Lee, P., Oh, J. G., et al. (2019). Role of SIRT1 in modulating acetylation of the sarco-endoplasmic reticulum Ca^{2+}-ATPase in heart failure. *Circ. Res.* 124, e63–e80. doi: 10.1161/CIRCRESAHA.118.313865

Goyal, R., Goyal, D., Leitzke, A., Gheorghe, C. P., and Longo, L. D. (2010). Brain renin–angiotensin system: fetal epigenetic programming by maternal protein restriction during pregnancy. *Reprod. Sci.* 17, 227–238. doi: 10.1177/1933719109351935

Grabmaier, U., Clauss, S., Gross, L., Klier, I., Franz, W. M., Steinbeck, G., et al. (2017). Diagnostic and prognostic value of miR-1 and miR-29b on adverse ventricular remodeling after acute myocardial infarction—the SITAGRAMI-miR analysis. *Int. J. Cardiol.* 244, 30–36. doi: 10.1016/j.ijcard.2017.06.054

Greißel, A., Culmes, M., Burgkart, R., Zimmermann, A., Eckstein, H.-H., Zernecke, A., et al. (2016). Histone acetylation and methylation significantly change with severity of atherosclerosis in human carotid plaques. *Cardiovasc. Pathol.* 25, 79–86. doi: 10.1016/j.carpath.2015.11.001

Guarrera, S., Fiorito, G., Onland-Moret, N. C., Russo, A., Agnoli, C., Allione, A., et al. (2015). Gene-specific DNA methylation profiles and LINE-1 hypomethylation are associated with myocardial infarction risk. *Clin. Epigenet.* 7, 133. doi: 10.1186/s13148-015-0164-3

Gunel, T., Hosseini, M. K., Gumusoglu, E., Kisakesen, H. I., Benian, A., and Aydinli, K. (2017). Expression profiling of maternal plasma and placenta microRNAs in preeclamptic pregnancies by microarray technology. *Placenta* 52, 77–85. doi: 10.1016/j.placenta.2017.02.019

Guo, M., Luo, J., Zhao, J., Shang, D., Lv, Q., and Zang, P. (2018). Combined use of circulating miR-133a and NT-proBNP improves heart failure diagnostic accuracy in elderly patients. *Med. Sci. Monit.* 24, 8840–8848. doi: 10.12659/MSM.911632

Guo, M.-L., Guo, L.-L., and Weng, Y.-Q. (2017). Implication of peripheral blood miRNA-124 in predicting acute myocardial infarction. *Eur. Rev. Med. Pharmacol. Sci.* 21, 1054–1059.

Haas, J., Frese, K. S., Park, Y. J., Keller, A., Vogel, B., Lindroth, A. M., et al. (2013). Alterations in cardiac DNA methylation in human dilated cardiomyopathy. *EMBO Mol. Med.* 5, 413–429. doi: 10.1002/emmm.201201553

Han, L., Zhao, Y., Luo, Q. Q., Liu, X. X., Lu, S. S., and Zou, L. (2017). The significance of miR-145 in the prediction of preeclampsia. *Bratisl. Lek. Listy* 118, 523–528. doi: 10.4149/BLL_2017_101

Han, Z., Zhang, L., Yuan, L., Liu, X., Chen, X., Ye, X., et al. (2015). Change of plasma microRNA-208 level in acute myocardial infarction patients and its clinical significance. *Ann. Transl. Med.* 3, 307. doi: 10.3978/j.issn.2305-5839.2015.10.25

Hao, X.-Z., and Fan, H.-M. (2017). Identification of miRNAs as atherosclerosis biomarkers and functional role of miR-126 in atherosclerosis progression through MAPK signalling pathway. *Eur. Rev. Med. Pharmacol. Sci.* 21, 2725–2733.

He, F., Lv, P., Zhao, X., Wang, X., Ma, X., Meng, W., et al. (2014). Predictive value of circulating miR-328 and miR-134 for acute myocardial infarction. *Mol. Cell Biochem* 394, 137–144. doi: 10.1007/s11010-014-2089-0

He, X., Ji, J., Wang, T., Wang, M.-B., and Chen, X.-L. (2017). Upregulation of circulating miR-195-3p in heart failure. *Cardiology* 138, 107–114. doi: 10.1159/000476029

Hindson, C. M., Chevillet, J. R., Briggs, H. A., Gallichotte, E. N., Ruf, I. K., Hindson, B. J., et al. (2013). Absolute quantification by droplet digital PCR versus analog real-time PCR. *Nat. Methods* 10, 1003–1005. doi: 10.1038/nmeth.2633

Hoareau-Aveilla, C., and Meggetto, F. (2017). Crosstalk between microRNA and DNA methylation offers potential biomarkers and targeted therapies in ALK-positive lymphomas. *Cancers (Basel)* 9, E100–E114. doi: 10.3390/cancers9080100

Hohl, M., Wagner, M., Reil, J.-C., Müller, S.-A., Tauchnitz, M., Zimmer, A. M., et al. (2013). HDAC4 controls histone methylation in response to elevated cardiac load. *J. Clin. Invest.* 123, 1359–1370. doi: 10.1172/JCI61084

Hromadnikova, I., Kotlabova, K., Ondrackova, M., Pirkova, P., Kestlerova, A., Novotna, V., et al. (2015). Expression profile of C19MC microRNAs in placental tissue in pregnancy-related complications. *DNA Cell Biol.* 34, 437–457. doi: 10.1089/dna.2014.2687

Hsu, A., Chen, S.-J., Chang, Y.-S., Chen, H.-C., and Chu, P.-H. (2014). Systemic approach to identify serum microRNAs as potential biomarkers for acute myocardial infarction. *Biomed. Res. Int.* 2014, 418628–418613. doi: 10.1155/2014/418628

Huang, L., Li, L., Chen, X., Zhang, H., and Shi, Z. (2016a). MiR-103a targeting Piezo1 is involved in acute myocardial infarction through regulating endothelium function. *Cardiol. J.* 23, 556–562. doi: 10.5603/CJ.a2016.0056

Huang, Y., Chen, J., Zhou, Y., Yu, X., Huang, C., Li, J., et al. (2016b). Circulating miR-30 is related to carotid artery atherosclerosis. *Clin. Exp. Hypertens.* 38, 489–494. doi: 10.3109/10641963.2016.1163370

Huang, Y., Tang, S., Ji-yan, C., Huang, C., Li, J., Cai, A.-P., et al. (2017a). Circulating miR-92a expression level in patients with essential hypertension: a potential marker of atherosclerosis. *J. Hum. Hypertens.* 31, 200–205. doi: 10.1038/jhh.2016.66

Huang, Y.-Q., Huang, C., Chen, J.-Y., Li, J., and Feng, Y.-Q. (2017b). Plasma expression level of miRNA let-7 is positively correlated with carotid intima-media thickness in patients with essential hypertension. *J. Hum. Hypertens.* 31, 843–847. doi: 10.1038/jhh.2017.52

Huang, Y.-Q., Li, J., Huang, C., and Feng, Y.-Q. (2018). Plasma microRNA-29c levels are associated with carotid intima-media thickness and is a potential biomarker for the early detection of atherosclerosis. *Cell. Physiol. Biochem.* 50, 452–459. doi: 10.1159/000494158

Huo, K.-G., Richer, C., Berillo, O., Mahjoub, N., Fraulob-Aquino, J. C., Barhoumi, T., et al. (2019). miR-431-5p knockdown protects against angiotensin II–induced hypertension and vascular injury. *Hypertension* 73, 1007–1017. doi: 10.1161/HYPERTENSIONAHA.119.12619

Iorio, M. V., Piovan, C., and Croce, C. M. (2010). Interplay between microRNAs and the epigenetic machinery: an intricate network. *Biochim. Biophys. Acta* 1799, 694–701. doi: 10.1016/j.bbagrm.2010.05.005

Irmak, M. K., and Sizlan, A. (2006). Essential hypertension seems to result from melatonin-induced epigenetic modifications in area postrema. *Med. Hypotheses* 66, 1000–1007. doi: 10.1016/j.mehy.2005.10.016

Jaenisch, R., and Bird, A. (2003). Epigenetic regulation of gene expression: how the genome integrates intrinsic and environmental signals. *Nat. Genet.* 33 Suppl, 245–254. doi: 10.1038/ng1089

Jaffe, A. S., Babuin, L., and Apple, F. S. (2006). Biomarkers in acute cardiac disease: the present and the future. *J. Am. Coll. Cardiol.* 48, 1–11. doi: 10.1016/j.jacc.2006.02.056

Jairajpuri, D. S., Malalla, Z. H., Mahmood, N., and Almawi, W. Y. (2017). Circulating microRNA expression as predictor of preeclampsia and its severity. *Gene* 627, 543–548. doi: 10.1016/j.gene.2017.07.010

Jeong, H. S., Kim, J.-Y., Lee, S. H., Hwang, J., Shin, J. W., Song, K. S., et al. (2017). Synergy of circulating miR-212 with markers for cardiovascular risks to enhance estimation of atherosclerosis presence. *PLoS One* 12, e0177809. doi: 10.1371/journal.pone.0177809

Ji, X., Takahashi, R., Hiura, Y., Hirokawa, G., Fukushima, Y., and Iwai, N. (2009). Plasma miR-208 as a biomarker of myocardial injury. *Clin. Chem.* 55, 1944–1949. doi: 10.1373/clinchem.2009.125310

Jia, K., Shi, P., Han, X., Chen, T., Tang, H., and Wang, J. (2016). Diagnostic value of miR-30d-5p and miR-125b-5p in acute myocardial infarction. *Mol. Med. Rep.* 14, 184–194. doi: 10.3892/mmr.2016.5246

Jiang, D., Sun, M., You, L., Lu, K., Gao, L., Hu, C., et al. (2019). DNA methylation and hydroxymethylation are associated with the degree of coronary atherosclerosis in elderly patients with coronary heart disease. *Life Sci.* 224, 241–248. doi: 10.1016/j.lfs.2019.03.021

Jiang, F., Li, J., Wu, G., Miao, Z., Lu, L., Ren, G., et al. (2015). Upregulation of microRNA-335 and microRNA-584 contributes to the pathogenesis of severe preeclampsia through downregulation of endothelial nitric oxide synthase. *Mol. Med. Rep.* 12, 5383–5390. doi: 10.3892/mmr.2015.4018

Jiang, Y.-Z., Jiménez, J. M., Ou, K., McCormick, M. E., Zhang, L.-D., and Davies, P. F. (2014). Hemodynamic disturbed flow induces differential DNA methylation of endothelial Kruppel-like factor 4 promoter *in vitro* and *in vivo*. *Circ. Res.* 115, 32–43. doi: 10.1161/CIRCRESAHA.115.303883

Jiang, Y.-Z., Manduchi, E., Stoeckert, C. J., and Davies, P. F. (2015). Arterial endothelial methylome: differential DNA methylation in athero-susceptible disturbed flow regions *in vivo*. *BMC Genomics* 16, 506. doi: 10.1186/s12864-015-1656-4

Jin, P., Gu, W., Lai, Y., Zheng, W., Zhou, Q., and Wu, X. (2017). The circulating microRNA-206 level predicts the severity of pulmonary hypertension in patients with left heart diseases. *Cell. Physiol. Biochem.* 41, 2150–2160. doi: 10.1159/000475569

Jo, B.-S., Koh, I.-U., Bae, J.-B., Yu, H.-Y., Jeon, E.-S., Lee, H.-Y., et al. (2016). Methylome analysis reveals alterations in DNA methylation in the regulatory regions of left ventricle development genes in human dilated cardiomyopathy. *Genomics* 108, 84–92. doi: 10.1016/j.ygeno.2016.07.001

Kanuri, S. H., Ipe, J., Kassab, K., Gao, H., Liu, Y., Skaar, T. C., et al. (2018). Next generation MicroRNA sequencing to identify coronary artery disease patients at risk of recurrent myocardial infarction. *Atherosclerosis* 278, 232–239. doi: 10.1016/j.atherosclerosis.2018.09.021

Kato, N., Loh, M., Takeuchi, F., Verweij, N., Wang, X., Zhang, W., et al. (2015). Trans-ancestry genome-wide association study identifies 12 genetic loci influencing blood pressure and implicates a role for DNA methylation. *Nat. Genet.* 47, 1282–1293. doi: 10.1038/ng.3405

Khatibzadeh, S., Farzadfar, F., Oliver, J., Ezzati, M., and Moran, A. (2013). Worldwide risk factors for heart failure: a systematic review and pooled analysis. *Int. J. Cardiol.* 168, 1186–1194. doi: 10.1016/j.ijcard.2012.11.065

Kim, H. J., Kim, S. Y., Lim, J. H., Kwak, D. W., Park, S. Y., and Ryu, H. M. (2015). Quantification and application of potential epigenetic markers in maternal plasma of pregnancies with hypertensive disorders. *IJMS* 16, 29875–29888. doi: 10.3390/ijms161226201

Kim, S. H., Kim, G. J., Umemura, T., Lee, S. G., and Cho, K. J. (2017). Aberrant expression of plasma microRNA-33a in an atherosclerosis-risk group. *Mol. Biol. Rep.* 44, 79–88. doi: 10.1007/s11033-016-4082-z

Klenke, S., Eul, S., Peters, J., Neumann, T., Adamzik, M., and Frey, U. H. (2018). Circulating miR-192 is a prognostic marker in patients with ischemic cardiomyopathy. *Future Cardiol.* 14, 283–289. doi: 10.2217/fca-2017-0108

Knothe, C., Shiratori, H., Resch, E., Ultsch, A., Geisslinger, G., Doehring, A., et al. (2016). Disagreement between two common biomarkers of global DNA methylation. *Clin. Epigenet.* 8, 60–17. doi: 10.1186/s13148-016-0227-0

Koczor, C. A., Lee, E. K., Torres, R. A., Boyd, A., Vega, J. D., Uppal, K., et al. (2013). Detection of differentially methylated gene promoters in failing and nonfailing human left ventricle myocardium using computation analysis. *Physiol. Genomics* 45, 597–605. doi: 10.1152/physiolgenomics.00013.2013

Kontaraki, J. E., Marketou, M. E., Zacharis, E. A., Parthenakis, F. I., and Vardas, P. E. (2014). MicroRNA-9 and microRNA-126 expression levels in patients with essential hypertension: potential markers of target-organ damage. *J. Am. Soc. Hypertens.* 8, 368–375. doi: 10.1016/j.jash.2014.03.324

Kouzarides, T. (2007). Chromatin modifications and their function. *Cell* 128, 693–705. doi: 10.1016/j.cell.2007.02.005

Kozomara, A., and Griffiths-Jones, S. (2011). miRBase: integrating microRNA annotation and deep-sequencing data. *Nucleic Acids Res.* 39, D152–D157. doi: 10.1093/nar/gkq1027

Krishnan, R., Mani, P., Sivakumar, P., Gopinath, V., and Sekar, D. (2017). Expression and methylation of circulating microRNA-510 in essential hypertension. *Hypertens. Res.* 40, 361–363. doi: 10.1038/hr.2016.147

Kristensen, L. S., Wojdacz, T. K., Thestrup, B. B., Wiuf, C., Hager, H., and Hansen, L. L. (2009). Quality assessment of DNA derived from up to 30 years old formalin fixed paraffin embedded (FFPE) tissue for PCR-based methylation analysis using SMART-MSP and MS-HRM. *BMC Cancer* 9, 453. doi: 10.1186/1471-2407-9-453

Kulkarni, A., Chavan-Gautam, P., Mehendale, S., Yadav, H., and Joshi, S. (2011). Global DNA methylation patterns in placenta and its association with maternal hypertension in pre-eclampsia. *DNA Cell Biol.* 30, 79–84. doi: 10.1089/dna.2010.1084

Kumar, A., Kumar, S., Vikram, A., Hoffman, T. A., Naqvi, A., Lewarchik, C. M., et al. (2013). Histone and DNA methylation–mediated epigenetic downregulation of endothelial Kruppel-like factor 2 by low-density lipoprotein cholesterol. *Arteriosclerosis, Thrombosis, and Vascular Biol.* 33, 1936–1942. doi: 10.1161/ATVBAHA.113.301765

Kumarswamy, R., Anker, S. D., and Thum, T. (2010). MicroRNAs as circulating biomarkers for heart failure: questions about MiR-423-5p. *Circ. Res.* 106, e8–author reply e9. doi: 10.1161/CIRCRESAHA.110.220616

Kuosmanen, S. M., Hartikainen, J., Hippeläinen, M., Kokki, H., Levonen, A.-L., and Tavi, P. (2015). MicroRNA profiling of pericardial fluid samples from patients with heart failure. *PLoS One* 10, e0119646. doi: 10.1371/journal.pone.0119646

Laganà, A. S., Vitale, S. G., Sapia, F., Valenti, G., Corrado, F., Padula, F., et al. (2018). miRNA expression for early diagnosis of preeclampsia onset: hope or hype? *J. Matern. Fetal. Neonatal. Med.* 31, 817–821. doi: 10.1080/14767058.2017.1296426

Lai, K.-B., Sanderson, J. E., Izzat, M. B., and Yu, C.-M. (2015). Micro-RNA and mRNA myocardial tissue expression in biopsy specimen from patients with heart failure. *Int. J. Cardiol.* 199, 79–83. doi: 10.1016/j.ijcard.2015.07.043

Lakhani, H. V., Khanal, T., Gabi, A., Yousef, G., Alam, M. B., Sharma, D., et al. (2018). Developing a panel of biomarkers and miRNA in patients with myocardial infarction for early intervention strategies of heart failure in West Virginian population. *PLoS One* 13, e0205329. doi: 10.1371/journal.pone.0205329

Lee, H.-A., Baek, I., Seok, Y. M., Yang, E., Cho, H.-M., Lee, D.-Y., et al. (2010). Promoter hypomethylation upregulates Na^{+}-K^{+}-$2Cl^{-}$ cotransporter 1 in spontaneously hypertensive rats. *Biochem. Biophys. Res. Commun.* 396, 252–257. doi: 10.1016/j.bbrc.2010.04.074

Li, B., Feng, Z.-H., Sun, H., Zhao, Z.-H., Yang, S.-B., and Yang, P. (2017a). The blood genome-wide DNA methylation analysis reveals novel epigenetic changes in human heart failure. *Eur. Rev. Med. Pharmacol. Sci.* 21, 1828–1836.

Li, G., Song, Y., Li, Y.-D., Jie, L.-J., Wu, W.-Y., Li, J.-Z., et al. (2018a). Circulating miRNA-302 family members as potential biomarkers for the diagnosis of acute heart failure. *Biomark. Med* 12, 871–880. doi: 10.2217/bmm-2018-0132

Li, H., Fan, J., Yin, Z., Wang, F., Chen, C., and Wang, D. W. (2016). Identification of cardiac-related circulating microRNA profile in human chronic heart failure. *Oncotarget* 7, 33–45. doi: 10.18632/oncotarget.6631

Li, K., Chen, Z., Qin, Y., and Wei, Y. (2018b). MiR-664a-3p expression in patients with obstructive sleep apnea: a potential marker of atherosclerosis. *Medicine (Baltimore)* 97, e9813. doi: 10.1097/MD.0000000000009813

Li, L., Li, S., Wu, M., Chi, C., Hu, D., Cui, Y., et al. (2019). Early diagnostic value of circulating microRNAs in patients with suspected acute myocardial infarction. *J. Cell Physiol.* 234, 13649–13658. doi: 10.1002/jcp.28045

Li, L.-M., Cai, W.-B., Ye, Q., Liu, J.-M., Li, X., and Liao, X.-X. (2014a). Comparison of plasma microRNA-1 and cardiac troponin T in early diagnosis of patients with acute myocardial infarction. *World. J. Emerg. Med.* 5, 182–186. doi: 10.5847/wjem.j.issn.1920-8642.2014.03.004

Li, S., Guo, L. Z., Kim, M. H., Han, J.-Y., and Serebruany, V. (2017b). Platelet microRNA for predicting acute myocardial infarction. *J. Thromb. Thrombolysis* 44, 556–564. doi: 10.1007/s11239-017-1537-6

Li, T., Cao, H., Zhuang, J., Wan, J., Guan, M., Yu, B., et al. (2011). Identification of miR-130a, miR-27b and miR-210 as serum biomarkers for atherosclerosis obliterans. *Clin. Chim. Acta* 412, 66–70. doi: 10.1016/j.cca.2010.09.029

Li, Y., Du, W., Zhao, R., Hu, J., Li, H., Han, R., et al. (2017c). New insights into epigenetic modifications in heart failure. *Front. Biosci. (Landmark Ed)* 22, 230–247. doi: 10.2741/4483

Li, Y.-Q., Zhang, M.-F., Wen, H.-Y., Hu, C.-L., Liu, R., Wei, H.-Y., et al. (2013). Comparing the diagnostic values of circulating microRNAs and cardiac troponin T in patients with acute myocardial infarction. *Clinics (Sao Paulo)* 68, 75–80. doi: 10.6061/clinics/2013(01)OA12

Li, Z., Lu, J., Luo, Y., Li, S., and Chen, M. (2014b). High association between human circulating microRNA-497 and acute myocardial infarction. *Sci. World J.* 2014, 931845–931847. doi: 10.1155/2014/931845

Liang, J., Bai, S., Su, L., Li, C., Wu, J., Xia, Z., et al. (2015). A subset of circulating microRNAs is expressed differently in patients with myocardial infarction. *Mol. Med. Rep.* 12, 243–247. doi: 10.3892/mmr.2015.3422

Lin, X., Zhang, S., and Huo, Z. (2019). Serum circulating miR-150 is a predictor of post-acute myocardial infarction heart failure. *Int. Heart J.* 60, 280–286. doi: 10.1536/ihj.18-306

Liu, G., Niu, X., Meng, X., and Zhang, Z. (2018a). Sensitive miRNA markers for the detection and management of NSTEMI acute myocardial infarction patients. *J. Thorac. Dis.* 10, 3206–3215. doi: 10.21037/jtd.2018.05.141

Liu, W., Zheng, J., Dong, J., Bai, R., Song, D., Ma, X., et al. (2018b). Association of miR-197-5p, a circulating biomarker for heart failure, with myocardial fibrosis and adverse cardiovascular events among patients with stage C or D heart failure. *Cardiology* 141, 212–225. doi: 10.1159/000493419

Liu, X., Dong, Y., Chen, S., Zhang, G., Zhang, M., Gong, Y., et al. (2015a). Circulating microRNA-146a and microRNA-21 predict left ventricular remodeling after ST-elevation myocardial infarction. *Cardiology* 132, 233–241. doi: 10.1159/000437090

Liu, X., Fan, Z., Zhao, T., Cao, W., Zhang, L., Li, H., et al. (2015b). Plasma miR-1, miR-208, miR-499 as potential predictive biomarkers for acute myocardial infarction: an independent study of Han population. *Exp. Gerontol.* 72, 230–238. doi: 10.1016/j.exger.2015.10.011

Liu, X., Meng, H., Jiang, C., Yang, S., Cui, F., and Yang, P. (2016). Differential microRNA Expression and regulation in the rat model of post-infarction heart failure. *PLoS One* 11, e0160920. doi: 10.1371/journal.pone.0160920

Liu, X., Yuan, L., Chen, F., Zhang, L., Chen, X., Yang, C., et al. (2017). Circulating miR-208b: a potentially sensitive and reliable biomarker for the diagnosis and prognosis of acute myocardial infarction. *Clin. Lab.* 63, 101–109. doi: 10.7754/Clin.Lab.2016.160632

Liu, Y., Liu, P., Yang, C., Cowley, A. W., and Liang, M. (2014). Base-resolution maps of 5-methylcytosine and 5-hydroxymethylcytosine in Dahl S rats: effect of salt and genomic sequence. *Hypertension* 63, 827–838. doi: 10.1161/HYPERTENSIONAHA.113.02637

Long, G., Wang, F., Duan, Q., Chen, F., Yang, S., Gong, W., et al. (2012a). Human circulating microRNA-1 and microRNA-126 as potential novel indicators for acute myocardial infarction. *Int. J. Biol. Sci.* 8, 811–818. doi: 10.7150/ijbs.4439

Long, G., Wang, F., Duan, Q., Yang, S., Chen, F., Gong, W., et al. (2012b). Circulating miR-30a, miR-195 and let-7b associated with acute myocardial infarction. *PLoS One* 7, e50926. doi: 10.1371/journal.pone.0050926

Luque, A., Farwati, A., Krupinski, J., and Aran, J. M. (2018). Association between low levels of serum miR-638 and atherosclerotic plaque vulnerability in patients with high-grade carotid stenosis. *J. Neurosurg.* 131, 1–8. doi: 10.3171/2018.2.JNS171899

Lv, P., Zhou, M., He, J., Meng, W., Ma, X., Dong, S., et al. (2014). Circulating miR-208b and miR-34a are associated with left ventricular remodeling after acute myocardial infarction. *IJMS* 15, 5774–5788. doi: 10.3390/ijms15045774

Ma, S.-C., Zhang, H.-P., Kong, F.-Q., Zhang, H., Yang, C., He, Y.-Y., et al. (2016). Integration of gene expression and DNA methylation profiles provides a molecular subtype for risk assessment in atherosclerosis. *Mol. Med. Rep.* 13, 4791–4799. doi: 10.3892/mmr.2016.5120

Maciejak, A., Kiliszek, M., Opolski, G., Segiet, A., Matlak, K., Dobrzycki, S., et al. (2016). miR-22-5p revealed as a potential biomarker involved in the acute phase of myocardial infarction *via* profiling of circulating microRNAs. *Mol. Med. Rep.* 14, 2867–2875. doi: 10.3892/mmr.2016.5566

Maciejak, A., Kostarska-Srokosz, E., Gierlak, W., Dluzniewski, M., Kuch, M., Marchel, M., et al. (2018). Circulating miR-30a-5p as a prognostic biomarker of left ventricular dysfunction after acute myocardial infarction. *Sci. Rep.* 8, 9883. doi: 10.1038/s41598-018-28118-1

Magenta, A., Sileno, S., D'Agostino, M., Persiani, F., Beji, S., Paolini, A., et al. (2018). Atherosclerotic plaque instability in carotid arteries: miR-200c as a promising biomarker. *Clin. Sci.* 132, 2423–2436. doi: 10.1042/CS20180684

Majchrzak-Celińska, A., Kosicka, K., Paczkowska, J., Główka, F. K., Bręborowicz, G. H., Krzyścin, M., et al. (2017). HSD11B2, RUNX3, and LINE-1 methylation in placental DNA of hypertensive disorders of pregnancy patients. *Reprod. Sci.* 24, 1520–1531. doi: 10.1177/1933719117692043

Mao, Z., Wu, F., and Shan, Y. (2018). Identification of key genes and miRNAs associated with carotid atherosclerosis based on mRNA-seq data. *Medicine (Baltimore)* 97, e9832. doi: 10.1097/MD.0000000000009832

Marketou, M. E., Kontaraki, J. E., Maragkoudakis, S., Patrianakos, A., Konstantinou, J., Nakou, H., et al. (2018). MicroRNAs in peripheral mononuclear cells as potential biomarkers in hypertensive patients with heart failure with preserved ejection fraction. *Am. J. Hypertens.* 31, 651–657. doi: 10.1093/ajh/hpy035

Masson, S., Batkai, S., Beermann, J., Bär, C., Pfanne, A., Thum, S., et al. (2018). Circulating microRNA-132 levels improve risk prediction for heart failure hospitalization in patients with chronic heart failure. *Eur. J. Heart Fail.* 20, 78–85. doi: 10.1002/ejhf.961

Matsumoto, S., Sakata, Y., Suna, S., Nakatani, D., Usami, M., Hara, M., et al. (2013). Circulating p53-responsive microRNAs are predictive indicators of heart failure after acute myocardial infarction. *Circ. Res.* 113, 322–326. doi: 10.1161/CIRCRESAHA.113.301209

Meder, B., Haas, J., Sedaghat-Hamedani, F., Kayvanpour, E., Frese, K., Lai, A., et al. (2017). Epigenome-wide association study identifies cardiac gene patterning and a novel class of biomarkers for heart failure. *Circulation* 136, 1528–1544. doi: 10.1161/CIRCULATIONAHA.117.027355

Mei, Z., Huang, B., Mo, Y., and Fan, J. (2017). An exploratory study into the role of miR-204-5p in pregnancy-induced hypertension. *Exp Ther Med* 13, 1711–1718. doi: 10.3892/etm.2017.4212

Miyamoto, S., Kawamura, T., Morimoto, T., Ono, K., Wada, H., Kawase, Y., et al. (2006). Histone acetyltransferase activity of p300 is required for the promotion of left ventricular remodeling after myocardial infarction in adult mice *in vivo*. *Circulation* 113, 679–690. doi: 10.1161/CIRCULATIONAHA.105.585182

Moutinho, C., and Esteller, M. (2017). MicroRNAs and epigenetics. *Adv. Cancer Res.* 135, 189–220. doi: 10.1016/bs.acr.2017.06.003

Movassagh, M., Choy, M.-K., Knowles, D. A., Cordeddu, L., Haider, S., Down, T., et al. (2011). Distinct epigenomic features in end-stage failing human hearts. *Circulation* 124, 2411–2422. doi: 10.1161/CIRCULATIONAHA.111.040071

Mu, S., Shimosawa, T., Ogura, S., Wang, H., Uetake, Y., Kawakami-Mori, F., et al. (2011). Epigenetic modulation of the renal β-adrenergic-WNK4 pathway in salt-sensitive hypertension. *Nat. Med.* 17, 573–580. doi: 10.1038/nm.2337

Nagata, S., Marunouchi, T., and Tanonaka, K. (2019). Histone deacetylase inhibitor SAHA treatment prevents the development of heart failure after myocardial infarction *via an* induction of heat-shock proteins in rats. *Biol. Pharm. Bull.* 42, 453–461. doi: 10.1248/bpb.b18-00785

Nakatochi, M., Ichihara, S., Yamamoto, K., Naruse, K., Yokota, S., Asano, H., et al. (2017). Epigenome-wide association of myocardial infarction with DNA methylation sites at loci related to cardiovascular disease. *Clin. Epigenet.* 9, 54. doi: 10.1186/s13148-017-0353-3

Nishiguchi, T., Imanishi, T., and Akasaka, T. (2015). MicroRNAs and cardiovascular diseases. *Biomed. Res. Int.* 2015, 682857. doi: 10.1155/2015/682857

Noack, F., Ribbat-Idel, J., Thorns, C., Chiriac, A., Axt-Fliedner, R., Diedrich, K., et al. (2011). miRNA expression profiling in formalin-fixed and paraffin-embedded placental tissue samples from pregnancies with severe preeclampsia. *J. Perinat. Med.* 39, 267–271. doi: 10.1515/jpm.2011.012

Nuyt, A. M., and Alexander, B. T. (2009). Developmental programming and hypertension. *Curr. Opin. Nephrol. Hypertens.* 18, 144–152. doi: 10.1097/MNH.0b013e328326092c

O'Sullivan, J. F., Neylon, A., McGorrian, C., and Blake, G. J. (2016). miRNA-93-5p and other miRNAs as predictors of coronary artery disease and STEMI. *Int. J. Cardiol.* 224, 310–316. doi: 10.1016/j.ijcard.2016.09.016

Olivieri, F., Antonicelli, R., Lorenzi, M., D'Alessandra, Y., Lazzarini, R., Santini, G., et al. (2013). Diagnostic potential of circulating miR-499-5p in elderly patients with acute non ST-elevation myocardial infarction. *Int. J. Cardiol.* 167, 531–536. doi: 10.1016/j.ijcard.2012.01.075

Ovchinnikova, E. S., Schmitter, D., Vegter, E. L., ter, J. M., Valente, M. A. E., Liu, L. C. Y., et al. (2016). Signature of circulating microRNAs in patients with acute heart failure. *Eur. J. Heart Fail.* 18, 414–423. doi: 10.1002/ejhf.332

Panico, C., and Condorelli, G. (2018). microRNA-132: a new biomarker of heart failure at last? *Eur. J. Heart Fail.* 20, 86–88. doi: 10.1002/ejhf.1044

Parahuleva, M. S., Euler, G., Mardini, A., Parviz, B., Schieffer, B., Schulz, R., et al. (2017). Identification of microRNAs as potential cellular monocytic biomarkers in the early phase of myocardial infarction: a pilot study. *Sci. Rep.* 7, 15974. doi: 10.1038/s41598-017-16263-y

Parthenakis, F., Marketou, M., Kontaraki, J., Patrianakos, A., Nakou, H., Touloupaki, M., et al. (2017). Low levels of microRNA-21 are a marker of reduced arterial stiffness in well-controlled hypertension. *J. Clin. Hypertens. (Greenwich)* 19, 235–240. doi: 10.1111/jch.12900

Peng, L., Chun-guang, Q., Bei-fang, L., Xue-zhi, D., Zi-hao, W., Yun-fu, L., et al. (2014). Clinical impact of circulating miR-133, miR-1291 and miR-663b in plasma of patients with acute myocardial infarction. *Diagn. Pathol.* 9, 89. doi: 10.1186/1746-1596-9-89

Pereira-da-Silva, T., Coutinho Cruz, M., Carrusca, C., Cruz Ferreira, R., Napoleão, P., and Mota Carmo, M. (2018). Circulating microRNA profiles in different arterial territories of stable atherosclerotic disease: a systematic review. *Am J Cardiovasc Dis* 8, 1–13.

Pojoga, L. H., Williams, J. S., Yao, T. M., Kumar, A., Raffetto, J. D., do Nascimento, G. R. A., et al. (2011). Histone demethylase LSD1 deficiency during high-salt diet is associated with enhanced vascular contraction, altered NO-cGMP relaxation pathway, and hypertension. *AJP: Heart Circ. Physiol.* 301, H1862–H1871. doi: 10.1152/ajpheart.00513.2011

Qipshidze Kelm, N., Piell, K. M., Wang, E., and Cole, M. P. (2018). MicroRNAs as predictive biomarkers for myocardial injury in aged mice following myocardial infarction. *J. Cell Physiol.* 233, 5214–5221. doi: 10.1002/jcp.26283

Qiu, X.-K., and Ma, J. (2018). Alteration in microRNA-155 level correspond to severity of coronary heart disease. *Scand. J. Clin. Lab. Invest.* 78, 219–223. doi: 10.1080/00365513.2018.1435904

Rask-Andersen, M., Martinsson, D., Ahsan, M., Enroth, S., Ek, W. E., Gyllensten, U., et al. (2016). Epigenome-wide association study reveals differential DNA methylation in individuals with a history of myocardial infarction. *Hum. Mol. Genet.* 25, 4739–4748. doi: 10.1093/hmg/ddw302

Rau, C. D., and Vondriska, T. M. (2017). DNA methylation and human heart failure: mechanisms or prognostics. *Circulation* 136, 1545–1547. doi: 10.1161/CIRCULATIONAHA.117.029840

Reed, G. W., Rossi, J. E., and Cannon, C. P. (2017). Acute myocardial infarction. *Lancet* 389, 197–210. doi: 10.1016/S0140-6736(16)30677-8

Rezaei, M., Eskandari, F., Mohammadpour-Gharehbagh, A., Harati-Sadegh, M., Teimoori, B., and Salimi, S. (2018). Hypomethylation of the miRNA-34a gene promoter is associated with severe preeclampsia. *Clin. Exp. Hypertens.* 41, 1–5. doi: 10.1080/10641963.2018.1451534

Rivière, G., Lienhard, D., Andrieu, T., Vieau, D., Frey, B. M., and Frey, F. J. (2011). Epigenetic regulation of somatic angiotensin-converting enzyme by DNA methylation and histone acetylation. *Epigenetics* 6, 478–489. doi: 10.4161/epi.6.4.14961

Rockenbach, G., De Melo Neto, A. J., Barcellos, N. T., and Wolff, F. H. (2012). Ethnic differences in viral dominance patterns in patients with hepatitis B virus and hepatitis C virus dual infection. *Hepatology* 55, 1640–author reply 1640. doi: 10.1002/hep.24533

Rodriguez-Iturbe, B. (2006). Arteriolar remodeling in essential hypertension: are connective tissue growth factor and transforming growth factor involved? *Kidney Int.* 69, 1104–1105. doi: 10.1038/sj.ki.5000222

Rossetto, D., Avvakumov, N., and Côté, J. (2012). Histone phosphorylation: a chromatin modification involved in diverse nuclear events. *Epigenetics* 7, 1098–1108. doi: 10.4161/epi.21975

Sabia, C., Picascia, A., Grimaldi, V., Amarelli, C., Maiello, C., and Napoli, C. (2017). The epigenetic promise to improve prognosis of heart failure and heart transplantation. *Transplant. Rev. (Orlando)* 31, 249–256. doi: 10.1016/j.trre.2017.08.004

Sano, M., Minamino, T., Toko, H., Miyauchi, H., Orimo, M., Qin, Y., et al. (2007). p53-Induced inhibition of Hif-1 causes cardiac dysfunction during pressure overload. *Nature* 446, 444–448. doi: 10.1038/nature05602

Sato, F., Tsuchiya, S., Meltzer, S. J., and Shimizu, K. (2011). MicroRNAs and epigenetics. *FEBS J.* 278, 1598–1609. doi: 10.1111/j.1742-4658.2011.08089.x

Schulte, C., Westermann, D., Blankenberg, S., and Zeller, T. (2015). Diagnostic and prognostic value of circulating microRNAs in heart failure with preserved and reduced ejection fraction. *WJC* 7, 843–860. doi: 10.4330/wjc.v7.i12.843

Scrutinio, D., Conserva, F., Passantino, A., Iacoviello, M., Lagioia, R., and Gesualdo, L. (2017). Circulating microRNA-150-5p as a novel biomarker for advanced heart failure: a genome-wide prospective study. *J. Heart Lung Transplant.* 36, 616–624. doi: 10.1016/j.healun.2017.02.008

Sekar, D., Shilpa, B. R., and Das, A. J. (2017). Relevance of microRNA 21 in different types of hypertension. *Curr. Hypertens. Rep.* 19, 57. doi: 10.1007/s11906-017-0752-z

Seronde, M.-F., Vausort, M., Gayat, E., Goretti, E., Ng, L. L., Squire, I. B., et al. (2015). Circulating microRNAs and outcome in patients with acute heart failure. *PLoS One* 10, e0142237. doi: 10.1371/journal.pone.0142237

Shah, R. V., Rong, J., Larson, M. G., Yeri, A., Ziegler, O., Tanriverdi, K., et al. (2018a). Associations of circulating extracellular RNAs with myocardial remodeling and heart failure. *JAMA Cardiol.* 3, 871–876. doi: 10.1001/jamacardio.2018.2371

Shah, R., Ziegler, O., Yeri, A., Liu, X., Murthy, V., Rabideau, D., et al. (2018b). MicroRNAs associated with reverse left ventricular remodeling in humans identify pathways of heart failure progression. *Circ. Heart Fail.* 11, e004278. doi: 10.1161/CIRCHEARTFAILURE.117.004278

Shi, B., Guo, Y., Wang, J., and Gao, W. (2010). Altered expression of microRNAs in the myocardium of rats with acute myocardial infarction. *BMC Cardiovasc. Disord.* 10, 11. doi: 10.1186/1471-2261-10-11

Singh, K., Williams, J., Brown, J., Wang, E. T., Lee, B., Gonzalez, T. L., et al. (2017). Up-regulation of microRNA-202-3p in first trimester placenta of pregnancies destined to develop severe preeclampsia, a pilot study. *Pregnancy Hypertens.* 10, 7–9. doi: 10.1016/j.preghy.2017.04.002

Small, E. M., and Olson, E. N. (2011). Pervasive roles of microRNAs in cardiovascular biology. *Nature* 469, 336–342. doi: 10.1038/nature09783

Smolarek, I., Wyszko, E., Barciszewska, A. M., Nowak, S., Gawronska, I., Jablecka, A., et al. (2010). Global DNA methylation changes in blood of patients with essential hypertension. *Med. Sci. Monit.* 16, CR149–CR155.

Strimbu, K., and Tavel, J. A. (2010). What are biomarkers? *Curr. Opin. HIV AIDS* 5, 463–466. doi: 10.1097/COH.0b013e32833ed177

Su, M., Wang, J., Wang, C., Wang, X., Dong, W., Qiu, W., et al. (2015). MicroRNA-221 inhibits autophagy and promotes heart failure by modulating the p27/CDK2/mTOR axis. *Cell Death Differ.* 22, 986–999. doi: 10.1038/cdd.2014.187

Sun, T., Dong, Y.-H., Du, W., Shi, C.-Y., Wang, K., Tariq, M.-A., et al. (2017). The role of MicroRNAs in myocardial infarction: from molecular mechanism to clinical application. *IJMS* 18, 745. doi: 10.3390/ijms18040745

Sygitowicz, G., Tomaniak, M., Błaszczyk, O., Kołtowski, Ł., Filipiak, K. J., and Sitkiewicz, D. (2015). Circulating microribonucleic acids miR-1, miR-21 and miR-208a in patients with symptomatic heart failure: preliminary results. *Arch. Cardiovasc. Dis.* 108, 634–642. doi: 10.1016/j.acvd.2015.07.003

Talens, R. P., Jukema, J. W., Trompet, S., Kremer, D., Westendorp, R. G. J., Lumey, L. H., et al. (2012). Hypermethylation at loci sensitive to the prenatal environment is associated with increased incidence of myocardial infarction. *Int. J. Epidemiol.* 41, 106–115. doi: 10.1093/ije/dyr153

Thomas, H., Diamond, J., Vieco, A., Chaudhuri, S., Shinnar, E., Cromer, S., et al. (2018). Global atlas of cardiovascular disease 2000–2016: the path to prevention and control. *Glob. Heart* 13, 143–163. doi: 10.1016/j.gheart.2018.09.511

Tijsen, A. J., Creemers, E. E., Moerland, P. D., de Windt, L. J., van der Wal, A. C., Kok, W. E., et al. (2010). MiR423-5p as a circulating biomarker for heart failure. *Circ. Res.* 106, 1035–1039. doi: 10.1161/CIRCRESAHA.110.218297

Tournier, B., Chapusot, C., Courcet, E., Martin, L., Lepage, C., Faivre, J., et al. (2012). Why do results conflict regarding the prognostic value of the methylation status in colon cancers? The role of the preservation method. *BMC Cancer* 12, 12–12. doi: 10.1186/1471-2407-12-12

Ura, B., Feriotto, G., Monasta, L., Bilel, S., Zweyer, M., and Celeghini, C. (2014). Potential role of circulating microRNAs as early markers of preeclampsia. *Taiwan J. Obstet. Gynecol.* 53, 232–234. doi: 10.1016/j.tjog.2014.03.001

Valencia-Morales, M. D. P., Zaina, S., Heyn, H., Carmona, F. J., Varol, N., Sayols, S., et al. (2015). The DNA methylation drift of the atherosclerotic aorta increases with lesion progression. *BMC Med. Genomics* 8, 7. doi: 10.1186/s12920-015-0085-1

van Boven, N., Akkerhuis, K. M., Anroedh, S. S., Rizopoulos, D., Pinto, Y., Battes, L. C., et al. (2017). Serially measured circulating miR-22-3p is a biomarker for adverse clinical outcome in patients with chronic heart failure: the Bio-SHiFT study. *Int. J. Cardiol.* 235, 124–132. doi: 10.1016/j.ijcard.2017.02.078

van Empel, V. P. M., de Windt, L. J., and da Costa Martins, P. A. (2012). Circulating miRNAs: reflecting or affecting cardiovascular disease? *Curr. Hypertens. Rep.* 14, 498–509. doi: 10.1007/s11906-012-0310-7

Vegter, E. L., Ovchinnikova, E. S., van Veldhuisen, D. J., Jaarsma, T., Berezikov, E., van der Meer, P., et al. (2017). Low circulating microRNA levels in heart failure patients are associated with atherosclerotic disease and cardiovascular-related rehospitalizations. *Clin. Res. Cardiol.* 106, 598–609. doi: 10.1007/s00392-017-1096-z

Vegter, E. L., Schmitter, D., Hagemeijer, Y., Ovchinnikova, E. S., van der Harst, P., Teerlink, J. R., et al. (2016). Use of biomarkers to establish potential role and function of circulating microRNAs in acute heart failure. *Int. J. Cardiol.* 224, 231–239. doi: 10.1016/j.ijcard.2016.09.010

Vogel, B., Keller, A., Frese, K. S., Leidinger, P., Sedaghat-Hamedani, F., Kayvanpour, E., et al. (2013). Multivariate miRNA signatures as biomarkers for non-ischaemic systolic heart failure. *Eur. Heart J.* 34, 2812–2822. doi: 10.1093/eurheartj/eht256

Wang, C., Xu, G., Wen, Q., Peng, X., Chen, H., Zhang, J., et al. (2019a). CBS promoter hypermethylation increases the risk of hypertension and stroke. *Clinics (Sao Paulo)* 74, e630. doi: 10.6061/clinics/2019/e630

Wang, F., Demura, M., Cheng, Y., Zhu, A., Karashima, S., Yoneda, T., et al. (2014a). Dynamic CCAAT/enhancer binding protein-associated changes of DNA methylation in the angiotensinogen gene. *Hypertension* 63, 281–288. doi: 10.1161/HYPERTENSIONAHA.113.02303

Wang, F., Long, G., Zhao, C., Li, H., Chaugai, S., Wang, Y., et al. (2013a). Plasma microRNA-133a is a new marker for both acute myocardial infarction and underlying coronary artery stenosis. *J. Transl. Med.* 11, 222. doi: 10.1186/1479-5876-11-222

Wang, F., Long, G., Zhao, C., Li, H., Chaugai, S., Wang, Y., et al. (2014b). Atherosclerosis-related circulating miRNAs as novel and sensitive predictors for acute myocardial infarction. *PLoS One* 9, e105734. doi: 10.1371/journal.pone.0105734

Wang, F., Ma, Y., Wang, H., and Qin, H. (2017a). Reciprocal regulation between microRNAs and epigenetic machinery in colorectal cancer. *Oncol Lett.* 13, 1048–1057. doi: 10.3892/ol.2017.5593

Wang, H., Naghavi, M., Allen, C., Barber, R. M., Bhutta, Z. A., Carter, A., et al. (2016a). Articles Global, regional, and national life expectancy, all-cause mortality, and cause-specific mortality for 249 causes of death, 1980–2015: a systematic analysis for the Global Burden of Disease Study 2015. *Lancet* 388, 1459–1544. doi: 10.1016/S0140-6736(16)31012-1

Wang, K., Zhang, S., Marzolf, B., Troisch, P., Brightman, A., Hu, Z., et al. (2009). Circulating microRNAs, potential biomarkers for drug-induced liver injury. *Proc. Natl. Acad. Sci. U. S. A* 106, 4402–4407. doi: 10.1073/pnas.0813371106

Wang, K.-J., Zhao, X., Liu, Y.-Z., Zeng, Q.-T., Mao, X.-B., Li, S.-N., et al. (2016b). Circulating MiR-19b-3p, MiR-134-5p and MiR-186-5p are promising novel biomarkers for early diagnosis of acute myocardial infarction. *Cell. Physiol. Biochem.* 38, 1015–1029. doi: 10.1159/000443053

Wang, L., Liu, J., Xu, B., Liu, Y.-L., and Liu, Z. (2018a). Reduced exosome miR-425 and miR-744 in the plasma represents the progression of fibrosis and heart failure. *Kaohsiung J. Med. Sci.* 34, 626–633. doi: 10.1016/j.kjms.2018.05.008

Wang, P., Shen, C., Diao, L., Yang, Z., Fan, F., Wang, C., et al. (2015). Aberrant hypermethylation of aldehyde dehydrogenase 2 promoter upstream sequence in rats with experimental myocardial infarction. *Biomed. Res. Int.* 2015, 503692–503613. doi: 10.1155/2015/503692

Wang, X., Falkner, B., Zhu, H., Shi, H., Su, S., Xu, X., et al. (2013b). A genome-wide methylation study on essential hypertension in young African American males. *PLoS One* 8, e53938. doi: 10.1371/journal.pone.0053938

Wang, Y., Chang, W., Zhang, Y., Zhang, L., Ding, H., Qi, H., et al. (2019b). Circulating miR-22-5p and miR-122-5p are promising novel biomarkers for diagnosis of acute myocardial infarction. *J. Cell Physiol.* 234, 4778–4786. doi: 10.1002/jcp.27274

Wang, Y., Yan, L., Zhang, Z., Prado, E., Fu, L., Xu, X., et al. (2018b). Epigenetic regulation and its therapeutic potential in pulmonary hypertension. *Front. Pharmacol.* 9, 241. doi: 10.3389/fphar.2018.00241

Wang, Y.-L., and Yu, W. (2018). Association of circulating microRNA-122 with presence and severity of atherosclerotic lesions. *PeerJ* 6, e5218. doi: 10.7717/peerj.5218

Wang, Z.-H., Sun, X.-Y., Li, C.-L., Sun, Y.-M., Li, J., Wang, L.-F., et al. (2017b). miRNA-21 expression in the serum of elderly patients with acute myocardial infarction. *Med. Sci. Monit.* 23, 5728–5734. doi: 10.12659/MSM.904933

Ward, J. A., Esa, N., Pidikiti, R., Freedman, J. E., Keaney, J. F., Tanriverdi, K., et al. (2013). Circulating cell and plasma microRNA profiles differ between non-ST-segment and ST-segment-elevation myocardial infarction. *Fam. Med. Med. Sci. Res.* 2, 108. doi: 10.4172/2327-4972.1000108

Watson, C. J., Gupta, S. K., O'Connell, E., Thum, S., Glezeva, N., Fendrich, J., et al. (2015). MicroRNA signatures differentiate preserved from reduced ejection fraction heart failure. *Eur. J. Heart Fail.* 17, 405–415. doi: 10.1002/ejhf.244

Wei, L., Zhao, S., Wang, G., Zhang, S., Luo, W., Qin, Z., et al. (2018). SMAD7 methylation as a novel marker in atherosclerosis. *Biochem. Biophys. Res. Commun.* 496, 700–705. doi: 10.1016/j.bbrc.2018.01.121

Wei, X. J., Han, M., Yang, F. Y., Wei, G. C., Liang, Z. G., Yao, H., et al. (2015). Biological significance of miR-126 expression in atrial fibrillation and heart failure. *Braz. J. Med. Biol. Res.* 48, 983–989. doi: 10.1590/1414-431x20154590

Wierda, R. J., Rietveld, I. M., van Eggermond, M. C. J. A., Belien, J. A. M., van Zwet, E. W., Lindeman, J. H. N., et al. (2015). Global histone H3 lysine 27 triple methylation levels are reduced in vessels with advanced atherosclerotic plaques. *Life Sci.* 129, 3–9. doi: 10.1016/j.lfs.2014.10.010

Wissler, R. W. (1991). Update on the pathogenesis of atherosclerosis. *Am. J. Med.* 91, 3S–9S. doi: 10.1016/0002-9343(91)90050-8

Wong, L. L., Armugam, A., Sepramaniam, S., Karolina, D. S., Lim, K. Y., Lim, J. Y., et al. (2015). Circulating microRNAs in heart failure with reduced and preserved left ventricular ejection fraction. *Eur. J. Heart Fail.* 17, 393–404. doi: 10.1002/ejhf.223

Wong, L. L., Rademaker, M. T., Saw, E. L., Lew, K. S., Ellmers, L. J., Charles, C. J., et al. (2017). Identification of novel microRNAs in the sheep heart and their regulation in heart failure. *Sci. Rep.* 7, 8250. doi: 10.1038/s41598-017-08574-x

Wong, S. Q., Li, J., Tan, A. Y.-C., Vedururu, R., Pang, J.-M. B., Do, H., et al. (2014). Sequence artefacts in a prospective series of formalin-fixed tumours tested for mutations in hotspot regions by massively parallel sequencing. *BMC Med. Genomics* 7, 23–10. doi: 10.1186/1755-8794-7-23

Wu, K., Zhao, Q., Li, Z., Li, N., Xiao, Q., Li, X., et al. (2018a). Bioinformatic screening for key miRNAs and genes associated with myocardial infarction. *FEBS Open Bio.* 8, 897–913. doi: 10.1002/2211-5463.12423

Wu, T., Chen, Y., Du, Y., Tao, J., Li, W., Zhou, Z., et al. (2018b). Circulating exosomal miR-92b-5p is a promising diagnostic biomarker of heart failure with reduced ejection fraction patients hospitalized for acute heart failure. *J. Thorac. Dis.* 10, 6211–6220. doi: 10.21037/jtd.2018.10.52

Wu, T., Chen, Y., Du, Y., Tao, J., Zhou, Z., and Yang, Z. (2018c). Serum exosomal MiR-92b-5p as a potential biomarker for acute heart failure caused by dilated cardiomyopathy. *Cell. Physiol. Biochem.* 46, 1939–1950. doi: 10.1159/000489383

Xiao, J., Gao, R., Bei, Y., Zhou, Q., Zhou, Y., Zhang, H., et al. (2017). Circulating miR-30d predicts survival in patients with acute heart failure. *Cell. Physiol. Biochem.* 41, 865–874. doi: 10.1159/000459899

Xiao, J., Shen, B., Li, J., Lv, D., Zhao, Y., Wang, F., et al. (2014). Serum microRNA-499 and microRNA-208a as biomarkers of acute myocardial infarction. *Int. J. Clin. Exp. Med.* 7, 136–141.

Xu, M., Li, J., Chen, X., Han, L., Li, L., and Liu, Y. (2019). MTHFD1 promoter hypermethylation increases the risk of hypertension. *Clin. Exp. Hypertens.* 41, 422–427. doi: 10.1080/10641963.2018.1501057

Xu, P., Zhao, Y., Liu, M., Wang, Y., Wang, H., Li, Y.-X., et al. (2014). Variations of microRNAs in human placentas and plasma from preeclamptic pregnancy. *Hypertension* 63, 1276–1284. doi: 10.1161/HYPERTENSIONAHA.113.02647

Xu, S., Pelisek, J., and Jin, Z. G. (2018). Atherosclerosis is an epigenetic disease. *Trends Endocrinol. Metab.* 29, 739–742. doi: 10.1016/j.tem.2018.04.007

Xue, S., Liu, D., Zhu, W., Su, Z., Zhang, L., Zhou, C., et al. (2019). Circulating MiR-17-5p, MiR-126-5p and MiR-145-3p are novel biomarkers for diagnosis of acute myocardial infarction. *Front. Physiol.* 10, 123. doi: 10.3389/fphys.2019.00123

Yamada, Y., Nishida, T., Horibe, H., Oguri, M., Kato, K., and Sawabe, M. (2014). Identification of hypo- and hypermethylated genes related to atherosclerosis by a genome-wide analysis of DNA methylation. *Int. J. Mol. Med.* 33, 1355–1363. doi: 10.3892/ijmm.2014.1692

Yan, Y., Song, X., Li, Z., Zhang, J., Ren, J., Wu, J., et al. (2017). Elevated levels of granzyme B correlated with miR-874-3p downregulation in patients with acute myocardial infarction. *Biomark. Med.* 11, 761–767. doi: 10.2217/bmm-2017-0144

Yang, G., Weng, X., Zhao, Y., Zhang, X., Hu, Y., Dai, X., et al. (2017a). The histone H3K9 methyltransferase SUV39H links SIRT1 repression to myocardial infarction. *Nat. Commun.* 8, 14941. doi: 10.1038/ncomms14941

Yang, Q., Jia, C., Wang, P., Xiong, M., Cui, J., Li, L., et al. (2014). MicroRNA-505 identified from patients with essential hypertension impairs endothelial cell migration and tube formation. *Int. J. Cardiol.* 177, 925–934. doi: 10.1016/j.ijcard.2014.09.204

Yang, Q., Lu, J., Wang, S., Li, H., Ge, Q., and Lu, Z. (2011). Application of next-generation sequencing technology to profile the circulating microRNAs in the serum of preeclampsia versus normal pregnant women. *Clin. Chim. Acta* 412, 2167–2173. doi: 10.1016/j.cca.2011.07.029

Yang, S.-Y., Wang, Y.-Q., Gao, H.-M., Wang, B., and He, Q. (2016a). The clinical value of circulating miR-99a in plasma of patients with acute myocardial infarction. *Eur. Rev. Med. Pharmacol. Sci.* 20, 5193–5197.

Yang, V. K., Loughran, K. A., Meola, D. M., Juhr, C. M., Thane, K. E., Davis, A. M., et al. (2017b). Circulating exosome microRNA associated with heart failure secondary to myxomatous mitral valve disease in a naturally occurring canine model. *J. Extracell Vesicles* 6, 1350088. doi: 10.1080/20013078.2017.1350088

Yang, W., Wang, A., Zhao, C., Li, Q., Pan, Z., Han, X., et al. (2016b). miR-125b enhances IL-8 production in early-onset severe preeclampsia by targeting sphingosine-1-phosphate lyase 1. *PLoS One* 11, e0166940. doi: 10.1371/journal.pone.0166940

Yao, X.-L., Lu, X.-L., Yan, C.-Y., Wan, Q.-L., Cheng, G.-C., and Li, Y.-M. (2015). Circulating miR-122-5p as a potential novel biomarker for diagnosis of acute myocardial infarction. *Int. J. Clin. Exp. Pathol.* 8, 16014–16019.

Yilmaz, S. G., Isbir, S., Kunt, A. T., and Isbir, T. (2018). Circulating microRNAs as novel biomarkers for atherosclerosis. *In Vivo* 32, 561–565. doi: 10.21873/invivo.11276

Yuan, L., Liu, X., Chen, F., Zhang, L., Chen, X., Huang, Q., et al. (2016). Diagnostic and prognostic value of circulating microRNA-133a in patients with acute myocardial infarction. *Clin. Lab.* 62, 1233–1241. doi: 10.7754/Clin.Lab.2015.151023

Zampetaki, A., Zeng, L., Margariti, A., Xiao, Q., Li, H., Zhang, Z., et al. (2010). Histone deacetylase 3 is critical in endothelial survival and atherosclerosis development in response to disturbed flow. *Circulation* 121, 132–142. doi: 10.1161/CIRCULATIONAHA.109.890491

Zhang, C., Li, Q., Ren, N., Li, C., Wang, X., Xie, M., et al. (2015a). Placental miR-106a~363 cluster is dysregulated in preeclamptic placenta. *Placenta* 36, 250–252. doi: 10.1016/j.placenta.2014.11.020

Zhang, D., Yu, Z.-Y., Cruz, P., Kong, Q., Li, S., and Kone, B. C. (2009). Epigenetics and the control of epithelial sodium channel expression in collecting duct. *Kidney Int.* 75, 260–267. doi: 10.1038/ki.2008.475

Zhang, J., Li, Y., and Zhao, Q. (2018a). Circulating miR-23b as a novel biomarker for early risk stratification after ST-elevation myocardial infarction. *Med. Sci. Monit.* 24, 1517–1523. doi: 10.12659/MSM.908060

Zhang, J., Xing, Q., Zhou, X., Li, J., Li, Y., Zhang, L., et al. (2017a). Circulating miRNA-21 is a promising biomarker for heart failure. *Mol. Med. Rep.* 16, 7766–7774. doi: 10.3892/mmr.2017.7575

Zhang, L. X., Du, J., Zhao, Y. T., Wang, J., Zhang, S., Dubielecka, P. M., et al. (2018b). Transgenic overexpression of active HDAC4 in the heart attenuates cardiac function and exacerbates remodeling in infarcted myocardium. *J. Appl. Physiol.* 125, 1968–1978. doi: 10.1152/japplphysiol.00006.2018

Zhang, L., Chen, X., Su, T., Li, H., Huang, Q., Wu, D., et al. (2015b). Circulating miR-499 are novel and sensitive biomarker of acute myocardial infarction. *J. Thorac. Dis.* 7, 303–308. doi: 10.3978/j.issn.2072-1439.2015.02.05

Zhang, L.-N., Liu, P.-P., Wang, L., Yuan, F., Xu, L., Xin, Y., et al. (2013a). Lower ADD1 gene promoter DNA methylation increases the risk of essential hypertension. *PLoS ONE* 8, e63455. doi: 10.1371/journal.pone.0063455

Zhang, M., Cheng, Y.-J., Sara, J. D., Liu, L.-J., Liu, L.-P., Zhao, X., et al. (2017b). Circulating microRNA-145 is associated with acute myocardial infarction and heart failure. *Chin. Med. J.* 130, 51–56. doi: 10.4103/0366-6999.196573

Zhang, R., Lan, C., Pei, H., Duan, G., Huang, L., and Li, L. (2015c). Expression of circulating miR-486 and miR-150 in patients with acute myocardial infarction. *BMC Cardiovasc. Disord.* 15, 51. doi: 10.1186/s12872-015-0042-0

Zhang, R., Niu, H., Ban, T., Xu, L., Li, Y., Wang, N., et al. (2013b). Elevated plasma microRNA-1 predicts heart failure after acute myocardial infarction. *Int. J. Cardiol.* 166, 259–260. doi: 10.1016/j.ijcard.2012.09.108

Zhang, W.-Q., and Xie, B.-Q. (2017). A meta-analysis of the relations between blood microRNA-208b detection and acute myocardial infarction. *Eur. Rev. Med. Pharmacol. Sci.* 21, 848–854.

Zhang, X., Wang, X., Wu, J., Peng, J., Deng, X., Shen, Y., et al. (2018c). The diagnostic values of circulating miRNAs for hypertension and bioinformatics analysis. *Biosci. Rep.* 38, BSR20180525. doi: 10.1042/BSR20180525

Zhang, Y., Cheng, J., Chen, F., Wu, C., Zhang, J., Ren, X., et al. (2017c). Circulating endothelial microparticles and miR-92a in acute myocardial infarction. *Biosci. Rep.* 37, BSR20170047. doi: 10.1042/BSR20170047

Zhang, Y., Liu, Y.-J., Liu, T., Zhang, H., and Yang, S.-J. (2016). Plasma microRNA-21 is a potential diagnostic biomarker of acute myocardial infarction. *Eur. Rev. Med. Pharmacol. Sci.* 20, 323–329.

Zhao, D.-S., Chen, Y., Jiang, H., Lu, J.-P., Zhang, G., Geng, J., et al. (2013). Serum miR-210 and miR-30a expressions tend to revert to fetal levels in Chinese adult patients with chronic heart failure. *Cardiovasc. Pathol.* 22, 444–450. doi: 10.1016/j.carpath.2013.04.001

Zhao, L., Chen, C.-N., Hajji, N., Oliver, E., Cotroneo, E., Wharton, J., et al. (2012). Histone deacetylation inhibition in pulmonary hypertension: therapeutic potential of valproic acid and suberoylanilide hydroxamic acid. *Circulation* 126, 455–467. doi: 10.1161/CIRCULATIONAHA.112.103176

Zheng, B., Xi, Z., Liu, R., Yin, W., Sui, Z., Ren, B., et al. (2018). The function of microRNAs in B-cell development, lymphoma, and their potential in clinical practice. *Front. Immunol.* 9, 936. doi: 10.3389/fimmu.2018.00936

Zhong, J., He, Y., Chen, W., Shui, X., Chen, C., and Lei, W. (2014). Circulating microRNA-19a as a potential novel biomarker for diagnosis of acute myocardial infarction. *IJMS* 15, 20355–20364. doi: 10.3390/ijms151120355

Zhu, J., Yao, K., Wang, Q., Guo, J., Shi, H., Ma, L., et al. (2016). Circulating miR-181a as a potential novel biomarker for diagnosis of acute myocardial infarction. *Cell. Physiol. Biochem.* 40, 1591–1602. doi: 10.1159/000453209

Zhu, L., Liu, F., Xie, H., and Feng, J. (2018). Diagnostic performance of microRNA-133a in acute myocardial infarction: a meta-analysis. *Cardiol. J.* 25, 260–267. doi: 10.5603/CJ.a2017.0126

Zhu, X.-M., Han, T., Sargent, I. L., Yin, G.-W., and Yao, Y.-Q. (2009). Differential expression profile of microRNAs in human placentas from preeclamptic pregnancies vs normal pregnancies. *Am. J. Obstet. Gynecol.* 200, 661.e1–661.e7. doi: 10.1016/j.ajog.2008.12.045

12

Circulating Serum MicroRNAs as Potential Diagnostic Biomarkers of Posttraumatic Stress Disorder

Clara Snijders[1], Julian Krauskopf[2], Ehsan Pishva[1,3], Lars Eijssen[1,4], Barbie Machiels[1], Jos Kleinjans[2], Gunter Kenis[1], Daniel van den Hove[1], Myeong Ok Kim[5], Marco P. M. Boks[6], Christiaan H. Vinkers[7,8], Eric Vermetten[9,10,11,12], Elbert Geuze[6,11], Bart P. F. Rutten[1†] and Laurence de Nijs[1†*]

[1] Department of Psychiatry and Neuropsychology, School for Mental Health and Neuroscience, Maastricht University, Maastricht, Netherlands, [2] Department of Toxicogenomics, Maastricht University, Maastricht, Netherlands, [3] College of Medicine and Health, University of Exeter Medical School, Exeter, United Kingdom, [4] Department of Bioinformatics (BiGCaT), NUTRIM School of Nutrition and Translational Research in Metabolism, Maastricht University, Maastricht, Netherlands, [5] Division of Applied Life Science (BK 21), College of Natural Sciences, Gyeongsang National University, Jinju, South Korea, [6] UMC Utrecht Brain Center, Department of Psychiatry, Utrecht, Netherlands, [7] Amsterdam UMC (location VUmc), Department of Anatomy and Neurosciences, Amsterdam, Netherlands, [8] Amsterdam UMC (location VUmc), Department of Psychiatry, Amsterdam, Netherlands, [9] Arq, Psychotrauma Research Expert Group, Diemen, Netherlands, [10] Department of Psychiatry, Leiden University Medical Center, Leiden, Netherlands, [11] Military Mental Healthcare, Netherlands Ministry of Defense, Utrecht, Netherlands, [12] Department of Psychiatry, New York University School of Medicine, New York, United States

***Correspondence:**
Laurence de Nijs
Laurence.denijs@maastrichtuniversity.nl

†These authors share senior authorship

Posttraumatic stress disorder (PTSD) is a psychiatric disorder that can develop upon exposure to a traumatic event. While most people are able to recover promptly, others are at increased risk of developing PTSD. However, the exact underlying biological mechanisms of differential susceptibility are unknown. Identifying biomarkers of PTSD could assist in its diagnosis and facilitate treatment planning. Here, we identified serum microRNAs (miRNAs) of subjects that underwent a traumatic event and aimed to assess their potential to serve as diagnostic biomarkers of PTSD. Next-generation sequencing was performed to examine circulating miRNA profiles of 24 members belonging to the Dutch military cohort Prospective Research in Stress-Related Military Operations (PRISMO). Three groups were selected: "susceptible" subjects who developed PTSD after combat exposure, "resilient" subjects without PTSD, and nonexposed control subjects ($N = 8$ per group). Differential expression analysis revealed 22 differentially expressed miRNAs in PTSD subjects compared to controls and 1 in PTSD subjects compared to resilient individuals (after multiple testing correction and a log2 fold-change cutoff of $\geq|1|$). Weighted Gene Coexpression Network Analysis (WGCNA) identified a module of coexpressed miRNAs which could distinguish between the three groups. In addition, receiver operating characteristic curve analyses suggest that the miRNAs with the highest module memberships could have a strong diagnostic accuracy as reflected by high areas under the curves. Overall, the results of our pilot study suggest that serum miRNAs could potentially serve as diagnostic biomarkers of PTSD, both individually or grouped within a cluster of coexpressed miRNAs. Larger studies are now needed to validate and build upon these preliminary findings.

Keywords: posttraumatic stress disorder, circulating miRNAs, diagnostic biomarker, trauma, susceptibility

BACKGROUND

Posttraumatic stress disorder (PTSD) is a psychiatric disorder that can develop upon exposure to a life-threatening traumatic event, i.e., an event capable of producing intense feelings of fear, helplessness, and horror (Association, 2013). Symptoms associated with PTSD include re-experiencing of the traumatic event, avoidance behavior, overall negative mood, and hyperarousal (Association, 2013). The economic burden associated with PTSD is substantial, and patients with PTSD are at increased risk of committing suicide and having familial issues such as marital problems (Fontana and Rosenheck, 1994; Tarrier and Gregg, 2004; Nock and Kessler, 2006; Ferry et al., 2015). Although ~60% of individuals within Western Europe will one day be exposed to a traumatic event, only ~6% of these individuals develop PTSD while others show a positive psychological adaptation process denoted as resilience (Kalisch et al., 2017; Koenen et al., 2017). However, some populations such as military soldiers are at elevated risk for trauma exposure, making PTSD a relatively common chronic disorder in the combat Veteran population (Thomas et al., 2017). Currently, a variety of treatment options exist for PTSD, without one being clearly superior to another (Yehuda et al., 2014). Moreover, pharmacological treatment options for PTSD are at best moderately effective and only work for a subset of patients (Richter-Levin et al., 2018). Therefore, increasing efforts are being made to unravel the biological underpinnings of PTSD in order to develop more efficient therapeutic strategies. It is now becoming clear that epigenetic mechanisms are involved in the lasting behavioral and molecular effects of trauma exposure (Schmidt et al., 2011; Snijders et al., 2018a).

Epigenetics refers to a variety of processes that are triggered by environmental factors and cause lasting but reversible alterations in gene expression (Goldberg et al., 2007). Among epigenetic mechanisms, noncoding RNA molecules such as microRNAs (miRNAs) are involved in the posttranscriptional regulation of gene expression by binding to specific messenger RNAs (Peschansky and Wahlestedt, 2014). Several miRNAs have been found implicated in PTSD, shedding much needed light on the underlying pathophysiological underpinnings of this disorder (Wingo et al., 2015; Bam et al., 2016a, Bam et al., 2016b; Martin et al., 2017). Such findings emphasize the notion that expression profiles of miRNAs could one day serve as relatively easily accessible biomarkers or be embedded within a network of several relevant biological processes that together could more accurately reflect the complexity of PTSD. For those individuals who have difficulties recognizing or properly describing their symptoms, identifying such markers could be of use in clinical contexts in order to objectively confirm the presence of the disorder and establish appropriate treatment plans when needed (Lehrner and Yehuda, 2014). Using these markers could be equally relevant during postdeployment medical screenings since military service members may have secondary reasons to not fully disclose their symptoms (Yehuda et al., 2013).

Here, we aimed to identify serum miRNAs that could one day serve as diagnostic biomarkers of PTSD. We further aimed to gain insights in the coexpression patterns of these miRNAs, their predicted gene targets and underlying biological pathways, along with their diagnostic accuracy. We hypothesized that specific miRNAs are differentially expressed between subjects with PTSD, trauma-exposed healthy individuals (referred to as "resilient" subjects in this paper), and nonexposed healthy controls. For this, we performed next-generation sequencing (NGS) on serum samples of 24 military members belonging to a Dutch military cohort, and we compared miRNA profiles between the three groups. Our findings suggest that miRNAs could potentially serve as biomarkers of PTSD, both individually or grouped within a cluster of coexpressed miRNAs. Larger studies are now needed in order to further validate and build upon these preliminary findings.

MATERIALS AND METHODS

Participants

A subset of military personnel (24 males) was selected from the larger Prospective Research in Stress-Related Military Operations (PRISMO) study, a prospective cohort of Dutch military members deployed to Afghanistan for 4 months (Reijnen et al., 2015; Eekhout et al., 2016). Based on the level of combat exposure during deployment and the severity of postdeployment PTSD symptoms, three subgroups were identified: 1) susceptible individuals, i.e., trauma-exposed subjects with deployment-related PTSD symptoms at 6 months follow-up; 2) resilient individuals, i.e., trauma-exposed soldiers with no PTSD diagnosis at follow-up; and 3) controls, i.e., deployed, but nonexposed and mentally healthy military members. Blood samples were collected at the Utrecht University Medical Center at 6 months postdeployment. Trauma exposure was assessed using a 19-item deployment experiences checklist (van Zuiden et al., 2011). The severity of PTSD symptoms was established using the 22-item Self-Rating Inventory for PTSD (SRIP) (Hovens et al., 2002). Information on smoking and alcohol was collected using self-report measures. This study was approved by the ethical committee of University Medical Center Utrecht (01-333/0) and conducted in accordance with the Declaration of Helsinki. All participants gave written informed consent.

RNA Isolation

Total RNA was isolated from 300μl human serum using the *mir*Vana PARIS kit (Ambion) according to the manufacturer's instructions. Briefly, the samples were incubated with an equal volume of denaturing solution, acid-phenol/chloroform was added, and the samples spun for 5min at 10,000×*g*. The aqueous phase was recovered and passed through a filter which was washed three times with the provided wash solutions. Final RNA was eluted in 100μl nuclease-free water. The concentrations and quality of the recovered RNA were measured using the Agilent Bioanalyzer 2100 (Agilent Technologies, Inc., CA, USA). All eluates were stored at −80°C until further use.

Small RNA Library Preparation and Next-Generation Sequencing

Barcoded libraries ($N = 24$, 8 per group) were prepared with an input of 25ng total RNA using the Illumina Small RNA TruSeq kit (Illumina, CA, USA). Briefly, 3′ and 5′ RNA adapters were added, the samples were reverse transcribed and amplified using 11 PCR cycles. All samples were processed in parallel and received a unique barcode. The complementary DNA constructs were gel purified and concentrated by ethanol precipitation. The quality control was performed using Agilent's 2100 Bioanalyzer with a High-Sensitivity DNA Chip. The 24 samples were pooled ($N = 8$ per group) and sequenced in duplicate using the Illumina HiSeq 2000 DNA sequence platform according to the manufacturer's protocol (GEO accession: GSE137624).

Small RNA Sequencing Data Analysis

Quality control of the raw sequences was done using FastQC (v. 0.11.3), and reads were preprocessed and mapped to the latest release of miRBase (v. 21) (Baras et al., 2015) utilizing miRge with default settings (Kozomara and Griffiths-Jones, 2014). In order to compensate for bias introduced by very low abundant sequences, only those miRNAs with an average of 50 counts (or more) across samples were considered for further analyses.

Differential Expression Analysis

Data normalization and differential expression analysis was conducted with the DESeq2 package in R (v. 3.5.2) (Love et al., 2014) thereby correcting for age, alcohol use, and smoking status. Resulting p-values were controlled by the false discovery rate (FDR) at 5% (Benjamini and Hochberg, 1995).

Weighted Gene Coexpression Network Construction and Module Detection

The identified miRNAs were used to construct coexpression networks using the Weighted Gene Coexpression Network Analysis (WGCNA) R package (Langfelder and Horvath, 2008). Normalized miRNA data was used as input. An adjacency matrix was generated by calculating Pearson's correlations between all miRNAs. Next, topological overlap between miRNAs was calculated using a power of 9. We performed 200 rounds of bootstrapping in order to construct a network that is robust to outliers. The cutreeDynamic function in the dynamicTreeCut R package was then used to identify coexpression modules of positively correlated miRNAs with high topological overlap. Modules with at least 30 miRNAs were assigned a color. Modules with highly correlated eigengenes were merged using the mergeCloseModules function in R. Pearson correlations between module eigengenes, age, smoking status, and alcohol were calculated. Welch's t-tests were performed in order to detect differences between module eigengenes of the control subjects and the trauma-exposed individuals. One-way ANOVAs were performed to detect differences between the three groups. When significant, the post-hoc Tukey HSD test was used to detect pairwise group differences.

Target Gene Pathway and Enrichment Analyses

The experimentally validated miRNA–target interactions database miRTarBase 6.0 (Chou et al., 2018) was used to identify gene targets of miRNAs. In order to narrow down the amount of target genes for further analyses, one-sided Fisher tests (with FDR multiple correction) were performed to evaluate whether the amount of miRNAs targeting a specific gene was significantly higher than expected by chance. Those genes were then analyzed for enriched Kyoto Encyclopedia of Genes and Genomes (KEGG) pathways and Gene Ontology terms (GO terms) using the online Database for Annotation, Visualization and Integrated Discovery (DAVID) v6.8 (Huang da et al., 2009; Huang da et al., 2009).

Statistical Analyses

To detect differences in age, number of previous deployments, cigarette smoking, alcohol use, trauma exposure scores, and SRIP scores between the groups, the Welch ANOVA with Games–Howell post-hoc test was applied. Since data on alcohol use at the 6 months follow-up time point was not available for all subjects, predeployment values were used instead. For each individual, smoking status was estimated based on their unique methylation patterns in 183CpGs, as previously described (Zeilinger et al., 2013). Finally, the classification accuracy of specific miRNAs was determined by calculating the area under the receiver operating characteristic (ROC) curve (AUC) in R.

RESULTS

Demographic Characteristics

A total of 24 subjects were included in the present study, of which 8 developed PTSD following deployment, 8 were resilient, and 8 were nonexposed controls (**Supplementary Table 1**). Based on the sequencing results, four subjects were excluded due to having a distinctively lower amount of reads causing great variation in expression data between samples. The three groups did not differ in terms of age, number of previous deployments, smoking status, and alcohol use (**Table 1**). On average, subjects with PTSD and resilient individuals were exposed to a similar amount of traumatic events, which was significantly more than the nonexposed controls [$F(2, 8.8) = 54.67$, $p < 0.001$. Games–Howell post-hoc showed $p < 0.001$ for PTSD versus control, and resilient versus control]. Finally, resilient and control subjects had similar postdeployment PTSD scores as measured by the SRIP, which were significantly lower than the average score of the PTSD group [$F(2, 11.15) = 25.23$, $p < 0.001$. Games–Howell post-hoc showed $p < 0.001$ for PTSD versus resilient, and PTSD versus control].

miRNAs Sequencing and Differential Expression Analysis

Small RNA sequencing yielded an average of 9.5 million unfiltered sequencing reads across all samples. After adaptor trimming and

TABLE 1 | Demographic characteristics of the 20 subjects remaining after outlier exclusion.

	Susceptible (*N* = 8)	Resilient (*N* = 6)	Control (*N* = 6)	*p*-value
Age when deployed	22.13 (0.61)	34.17 (4.88)	27.50 (3.62)	0.083
Number of previous deployments	0.29 (0.18)	0.83 (0.48)	0.17 (0.17)	0.465
Cigarette smoking	2.79 (1.65)	−1.43 (1.30)	−0.15 (1.89)	0.194
Alcohol use	2.86 (0.67)	1.17 (0.40)	1.83 (0.60)	0.155
Trauma exposure score	7.75 (0.98)	7.17 (0.75)	0.5 (0.22)	<0.001
SRIP PTSD score	55.25 (4.01)	25.50 (1.63)	24.50 (1.46)	<0.001

Data are presented as mean (SE). SRIP, self-rating inventory for posttraumatic stress disorder.

size selection, 1.9 million high-quality reads remained, which were aligned to miRNA sequences from miRBase (release 21). As mentioned earlier, principal component analysis revealed the presence of four outliers, which were excluded from further analysis. The count data were then filtered for miRNAs that showed an average of 50 reads or more across all samples. This resulted in the identification of 306 different miRNAs. Differential expression analysis in DESeq2 revealed that a total of 123 miRNAs showed differential expression between PTSD cases and nonexposed controls, while 4 were downregulated in PTSD cases compared to resilient individuals (**Supplementary Table 2**). Selecting those miRNAs with a log2 fold-change (FC) value$\geq|1.0|$ and FDR adjusted $p < 0.05$ revealed that one miRNA, miR-1246, was downregulated in PTSD subjects compared to resilient subjects and 22 were differentially expressed between PTSD subjects and nonexposed controls (**Table 2, Figure 1**). Of these, 4 were downregulated and 18 were upregulated. We used the Venn tool to identify those differentially expressed miRNAs that are specific for PTSD only (**Figure 2**). Two miRNAs were identified at the intersection of the blue and yellow circles, i.e., miR-4454 and miR-210-3p. Both miRNAs were significantly downregulated in PTSD subjects compared to resilient subjects and controls and not differentially expressed between resilient subjects and controls, suggesting that these could be more specific to PTSD (**Supplementary Table 2**). However, both miRNAs had log2 FC values of −0.61 and −0.54, which does not pass our threshold of $\geq|1.0|$.

Weighted Gene Coexpression Network Analysis

WGCNA was applied using the 306 identified miRNAs in order to detect clusters of coexpressed miRNAs. Based on the sample dendrogram, one outlier was removed from further analyses (**Supplementary Figure 1**). We identified three miRNA modules (**Figure 3**). The turquoise, blue, and brown modules each had

TABLE 2 | Differentially expressed microRNAs (miRNAs) between posttraumatic stress disorder (PTSD) cases versus controls and PTSD cases versus resilient individuals with a log2 fold-change value$\geq|1.0|$ and FDR adjusted $p < 0.05$.

Nr	PTSD vs. control				PTSD vs. resilient			
	miRNA	*Log2 FC*	*p-value*	*FDR adj p-value*	*miRNA*	*Log2 FC*	*p-value*	*FDR adj p-value*
1	hsa-miR-218-2-3p	3.22	1.65E−02	4.20E−02	hsa-miR-1246	−1.06	3.54E−04	3.05E−02
2	hsa-miR-3609	3.05	8.22E−06	6.62E−05				
3	hsa-miR-432-5p	2.37	8.44E−04	3.31E−03				
4	hsa-miR-138-5p	2.29	2.18E−16	9.54E−15				
5	hsa-miR-221-5p	2.06	6.11E−13	1.34E−11				
6	hsa-miR-4485-3p	1.98	3.45E−15	9.59E−14				
7	hsa-miR-31-5p	1.92	2.16E−15	7.35E−14				
8	hsa-miR-146b-5p	1.67	1.86E−25	2.85E−23				
9	hsa-miR-5096	1.62	1.81E−06	1.84E−05				
10	hsa-miR-222-3p	1.56	2.81E−15	8.61E−14				
11	hsa-miR-1273g-3p	1.55	7.23E−05	3.75E−04				
12	hsa-miR-302a-5p	1.49	6.61E−09	1.06E−07				
13	hsa-miR-221-3p	1.45	1.03E−14	2.62E−13				
14	hsa-miR-619-5p	1.40	1.74E−04	8.31E−04				
15	hsa-miR-335-5p	1.28	7.18E−28	2.20E−25				
16	hsa-miR-146b-3p	1.25	6.30E−11	1.13E−09				
17	hsa-miR-3175	1.17	1.95E−04	9.20E−04				
18	hsa-miR-3656	1.00	1.07E−02	2.86E−02				
19	hsa-miR-184	−1.20	1.58E−05	1.01E−04				
20	hsa-let-7d-5p	−1.27	1.22E−18	9.33E−17				
21	hsa-miR-98-5p	−1.33	1.57E−22	1.60E−20				
22	hsa-miR-146a-5p	−2.04	1.52E−08	2.22E−07				

The table is organized based on decreasing log2 fold-change values. miRNA, microRNA; log2 FC, log2 fold-change.

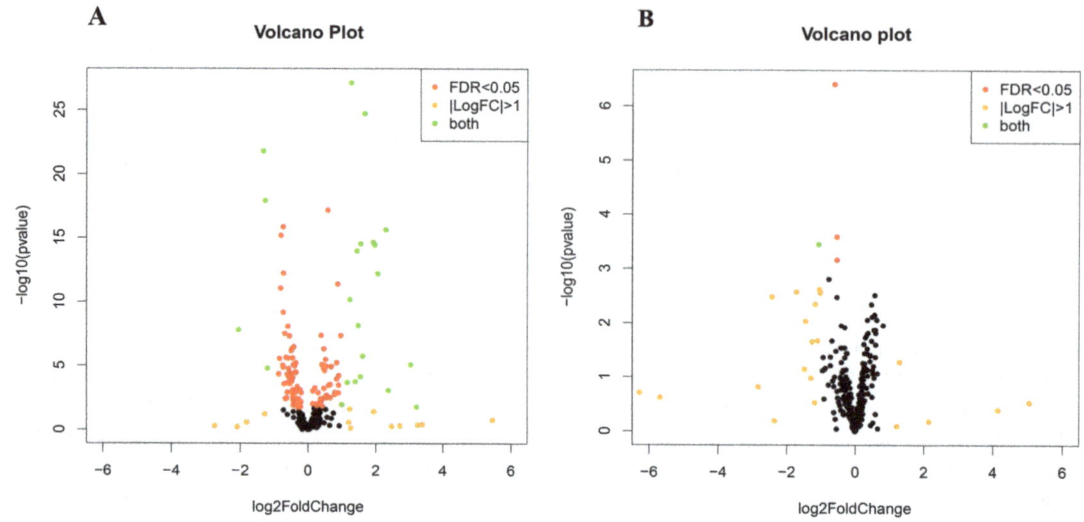

FIGURE 1 | Volcano plots of differentially expressed microRNAs (miRNAs) between posttraumatic stress disorder (PTSD) cases and controls **(A)** and PTSD cases and resilient subjects **(B)**. Black dots represent nonsignificantly differentially expressed miRNAs, red dots represent significant miRNAs with a log2 FC<|1|, orange dots represent nonsignificant miRNAs with a log2 FC≥|1|, and green dots represent significantly differentially expressed miRNAs with a log2 FC≥|1|. Significance is declared when adjusted $p<0.05$.

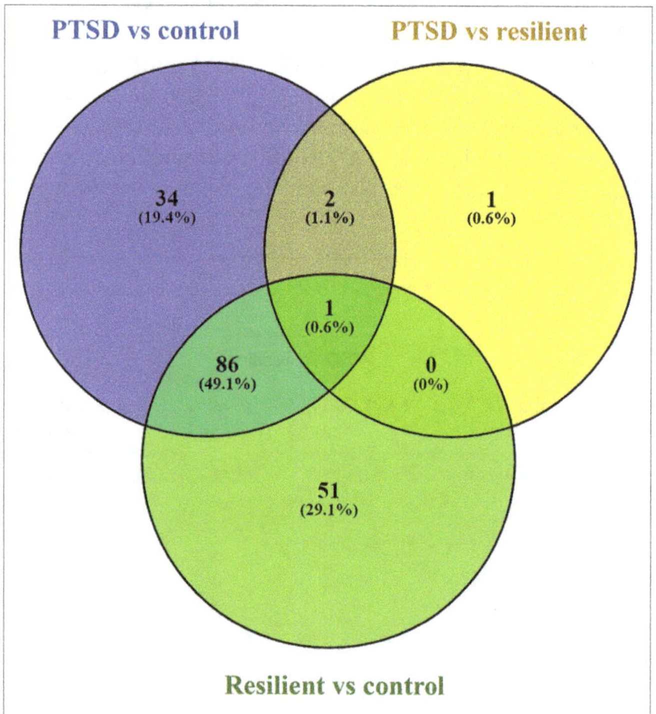

FIGURE 2 | Venn diagram showing overlapping microRNAs (miRNAs). Of particular interest here are the two miRNAs at the intersection of the blue and yellow circle (but not the green), i.e., miR-4454 and miR-210-3p. Obtained using https://bioinfogp.cnb.csic.es/tools/venny/index.html

84, 79, and 65 miRNAs, respectively. None of the modules were associated with the potential covariates age, smoking status, or alcohol use (**Supplementary Figure 2**). Within each module, the module eigengenes were significantly different between trauma-exposed individuals and nonexposed controls for the turquoise and blue modules (p = 2.67×10^{-04}, p = 2.51×10^{-06}, respectively) but not for the brown module (p = 0.196; **Figure 3A**). When stratifying the trauma-exposed individuals into PTSD subjects and resilient subjects, the individual eigengenes of the blue module were significantly different between PTSD subjects and resilient individuals (p = 1.46×10^{-03}; **Figure 3B**), which was not the case for the other modules. We therefore focused on the blue module for further analyses.

Out of the 79 miRNAs belonging to this module, 67 were differentially expressed between PTSD subjects and controls (**Table 1**), including miR-138-5p, the hub miRNA (**Table 3**). In order to evaluate the diagnostic accuracy of some of these miRNAs, we performed ROC analysis for those miRNAs with the highest absolute module memberships. The five most contributing miRNAs, i.e., miR-221-3p, miR-335-5p, miR-138-5p, miR-222-3p, and miR-146-5p (**Table 3**), could perfectly distinguish PTSD subjects and controls (AUC of 1 for all miRNAs; **Supplementary Figure 3** A.1 and A.2 for miR-221-3p). These miRNAs could equally well differentiate PTSD subjects from resilient subjects, except for miR-221-3p and miR-222-3p (AUC of 0.95 and 0.98, respectively). When obtaining ROC curves using miRNA expression levels adjusted for confounders (i.e., age, smoking, and alcohol use), all miRNAs could still distinguish PTSD subjects from controls (**Supplementary Figure 3** B.1 and B.2 for miR-221-3p). However, differentiating PTSD from resilience was less accurate as reflected by AUCs of 0.625, 0.775, 0.725, 0.675, and 0.775 for miR-221-3p, miR-335-5p, miR-138-5p, miR-222-3p, and miR-146-5p, respectively (**Supplementary Figure 3** B.1 and B.2 for miR-221-3p).

Target Gene Pathway and GO Enrichment Analyses

Validated gene targets of the 79 miRNAs comprised within the blue module were obtained from the online database miRTarBase

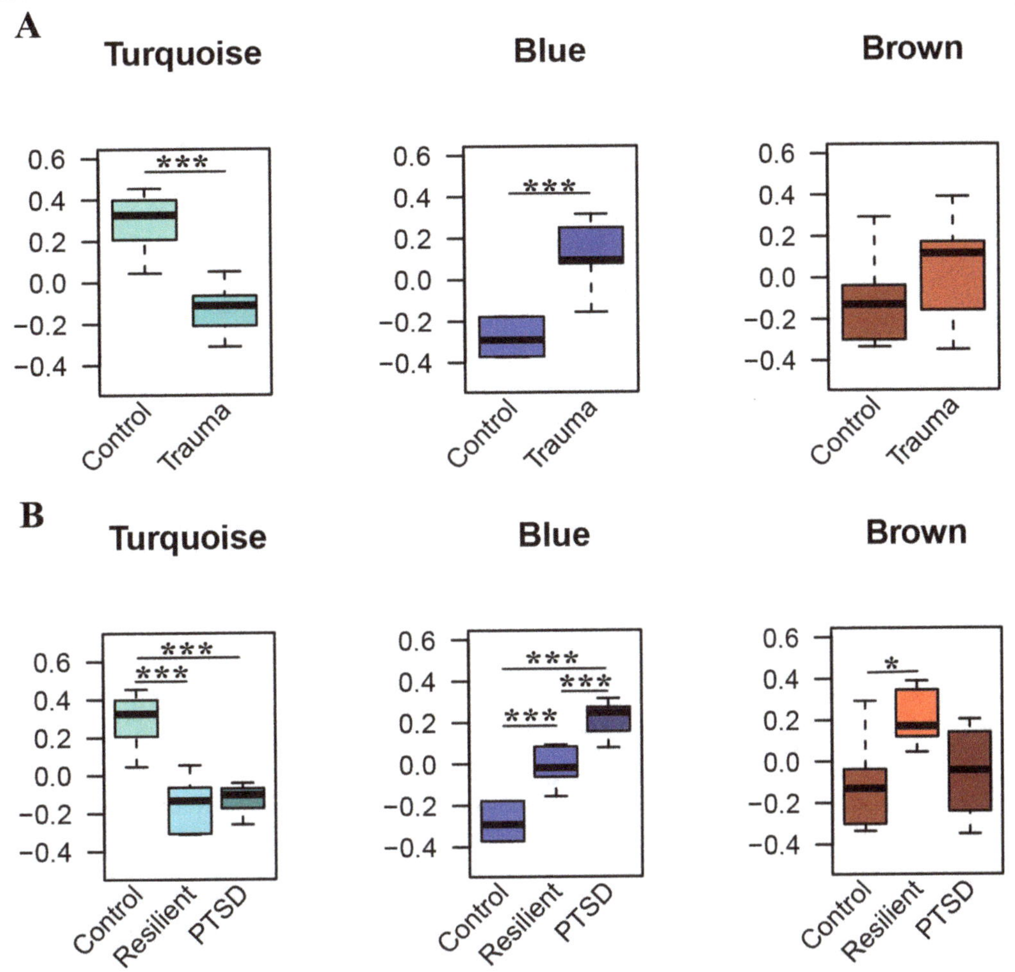

FIGURE 3 | Significant modules of coexpressed miRNAs. The y-axis displays the module eigengene values. Groups are stratified by trauma exposure **(A)**, and trauma exposure and PTSD status **(B)**. Significances were detected using Welch tests **(A)** or one-way ANOVAs **(B)** $^{*}p < 0.05$, $^{***}p < 0.001$.

(Chou et al., 2018). In order to narrow down this extensive set of target genes (N = 9270), Fisher tests were performed to select only those genes that were targeted by significantly more miRNAs than expected by chance. This revealed a set of 146 genes, which were considered for pathway and enrichment analyses (**Supplementary Table 3**). After FDR adjustment, 15 significantly enriched KEGG pathways were identified of which most were cancer-related (**Table 4**). GO enrichment analyses of these target genes further identified eight significant biological processes, five molecular functions, and six cellular components (**Table 5**). The most enriched GO terms were related to apoptotic processes, protein binding, and intracellular compartments, respectively (**Table 5**).

DISCUSSION

In this study, we aimed to identify the diagnostic biomarker potential of circulating miRNAs for PTSD using serum samples from Dutch military subjects. We further aimed to gain insights in the coexpression patterns of these miRNAs, their predicted gene targets, and underlying biological pathways. Our preliminary findings suggest that 1) certain miRNAs could potentially serve as individual biomarkers of susceptibility, and 2) the coexpression of a specific set of miRNAs could accurately distinguish between subjects with PTSD, resilient individuals, and nonexposed controls. Such markers could be useful in clinical settings for accurate diagnosis and treatment planning, which is especially relevant for individuals who have that have difficulties associating their symptoms to a traumatic event, are unable to describe their symptoms, or are unwilling to fully disclose them (Yehuda et al., 2013).

Differential expression analysis identified 1 differentially expressed miRNA between subjects with PTSD and resilient individuals and 22 between subjects with PTSD and nonexposed controls (after multiple testing correction and a log2 FC cutoff of ≥|1|). Of these, miR-138-5p was significantly overexpressed in subjects with PTSD as compared to controls, and WGCNA revealed that this was the hub miRNA of the blue module. Serum levels of this miRNA were previously found altered in a rat model

TABLE 3 | MicroRNAs (miRNAs) belonging to the Weighted Gene Coexpression Network Analysis (WGCNA) blue module.

Nr	miRNA	Nr	miRNA
1	hsa-miR-221-3p	41	hsa-miR-641
2	hsa-miR-335-5p	42	hsa-miR-208a-3p
3	hsa-miR-138-5p	43	hsa-miR-18a-3p
4	hsa-miR-222-3p	44	hsa-miR-193a-5p
5	hsa-miR-146b-5p	45	hsa-miR-411-5p*
6	hsa-miR-31-5p	46	hsa-miR-148a-5p
7	hsa-miR-340-5p	47	hsa-miR-505-3p
8	hsa-miR-210-3p	48	hsa-miR-214-3p
9	hsa-miR-208b-3p	49	hsa-miR-335-3p
10	hsa-miR-302a-5p	50	hsa-miR-4485-3p
11	hsa-let-7i-5p	51	hsa-miR-10a-5p
12	hsa-miR-4454	52	hsa-miR-212-3p
13	hsa-miR-146b-3p	53	hsa-miR-331-3p
14	hsa-miR-99b-3p	54	hsa-miR-490-3p*
15	hsa-let-7a-3p	55	hsa-miR-20a-5p
16	hsa-miR-221-5p	56	hsa-miR-455-5p
17	hsa-miR-27a-3p/27b-3p	57	hsa-miR-874-5p
18	hsa-miR-127-3p	58	hsa-miR-675-5p
19	hsa-miR-3200-3p	59	hsa-miR-504-5p
20	hsa-miR-128-3p	60	hsa-miR-654-3p*
21	hsa-miR-20b-5p	61	hsa-miR-30a-3p*
22	hsa-miR-199a-3p	62	hsa-miR-425-3p
23	hsa-miR-181c-5p	63	hsa-miR-183-5p
24	hsa-miR-652-3p	64	hsa-miR-532-3p*
25	hsa-miR-4662a-5p	65	hsa-miR-193b-3p*
26	hsa-miR-17-5p/106a-5p	66	hsa-miR-130a-3p
27	hsa-miR-146a-5p	67	hsa-miR-7151-5p*
28	hsa-miR-148a-3p	68	hsa-miR-23a-3p
29	hsa-miR-708-5p	69	hsa-miR-877-3p*
30	hsa-miR-34a-5p	70	hsa-miR-424-3p
31	hsa-miR-574-3p	71	hsa-miR-151a-3p
32	hsa-miR-145-3p	72	hsa-miR-3175
33	hsa-miR-490-5p	73	hsa-miR-361-3p
34	hsa-miR-148b-5p	74	hsa-miR-92b-5p
35	hsa-miR-143-3p	75	hsa-miR-181a-3p
36	hsa-miR-184	76	hsa-miR-328-3p*
37	hsa-miR-199b-3p	77	hsa-miR-423-3p*
38	hsa-miR-628-5p	78	hsa-miR-139-5p*
39	hsa-miR-132-3p	79	hsa-miR-339-3p*
40	hsa-miR-181c-3p		

miRNAs with a star were not differentially expressed in PTSD cases versus controls or versus resilient subjects. The miRNAs are ranked based on their absolute module membership (highest to lowest).

of restraint stress (Balakathiresan et al., 2014), while hippocampal miR-138-5p levels were associated with the formation of fear memories in mice (Li et al., 2018). Another miRNA, miR-1246, was the only significant miRNA that was downregulated in PTSD cases compared to resilient subjects and had a log2 FC>|1|. This miRNA was previously found downregulated in peripheral blood mononuclear cells of war veterans suffering from PTSD as compared to healthy nontrauma-exposed controls (Bam et al., 2016b). Such findings suggest that these miRNAs could be implicated in PTSD and potentially aid in diagnosing this disorder.

The three modules of coexpressed miRNAs identified by WGCNA revealed that most of the detected miRNAs could be clustered based on similarities in their expression patterns. The blue module contained 79 miRNAs which could significantly

TABLE 4 | Significant Kyoto Encyclopedia of Genes and Genomes (KEGG) pathways.

Nr	Term	*p* value	FDR adj *p* value
1	Pathways in cancer	2.94E−10	3.66E−07
2	Pancreatic cancer	6.27E−09	7.79E−06
3	HTLV-I infection	1.26E−08	1.56E−05
4	Small cell lung cancer	8.93E−08	1.11E−04
5	Melanoma	2.14E−07	2.65E−04
6	Hepatitis B	2.23E−07	2.77E−04
7	FoxO signaling pathway	8.06E−07	1.00E−03
8	Colorectal cancer	9.16E−07	1.14E−03
9	Prostate cancer	1.38E−06	1.71E−03
10	MicroRNAs in cancer	2.34E−06	2.91E−03
11	Chronic myeloid leukemia	2.93E−06	3.63E−03
12	Apoptosis	1.14E−05	1.41E−02
13	Central carbon metabolism in cancer	1.41E−05	1.75E−02
14	MAPK signaling pathway	1.49E−05	1.85E−02
15	Glioma	1.56E−05	1.94E−02

These pathways were identified using the online Database for Annotation, Visualization and Integrated Discovery (DAVID) v6.8.

differentiate between trauma-exposed individuals and nonexposed controls. Interestingly, within the trauma-exposed individuals, the expression profiles of these miRNAs were significantly different between individuals with and without PTSD. This highlights the importance of including and studying not only non-trauma exposed controls but also trauma-exposed healthy individuals in order to disentangle PTSD effects from trauma-related effects. Moreover, 67 of the miRNAs of the blue module, including its hub miRNA, were significantly differentially expressed between PTSD cases and controls, which enhances the notion that these miRNAs could be relevant for PTSD.

Of the five miRNAs with the highest module membership, we calculated the AUCs to assess their diagnostic accuracy (Grund and Sabin, 2010). In order to determine the biomarker potential of these miRNAs, i.e., their potential to reflect PTSD regardless of any other confounding condition, we used uncorrected miRNA expression values. Interestingly, the results suggest that these miRNAs could almost perfectly distinguish PTSD subjects from resilient individuals and controls. However, these results were not reflected by the DESeq2 analyses in which the expression levels of these miRNAs were not different between PTSD cases and resilient individuals. Part of this discrepancy can most likely be attributed to confounding effects, as DESeq2 analyses were corrected for age, alcohol, and smoking status. When obtaining the ROC curves using confounder-adjusted miRNA expression values, the AUCs more accurately corresponded to the DESeq2 results. Although these results suggest that the expression of our selected miRNAs fluctuates with confounders, they mostly strengthen the need of replication in larger cohorts. This will further be valuable in determining whether these miRNAs could be specific for PTSD only as opposed to trauma more broadly.

Enrichment of GO terms indicated that target genes of the coexpressed miRNAs in the blue module are enriched in several KEGG pathways of which most were cancer-related. This suggests that these miRNAs could be implicated in cancer pathways that are also involved in signaling cascades possibly related to PTSD.

TABLE 5 | Significant gene ontology (GO) terms enriched for a subset of target genes (N = 218) of the coexpressed microRNAs (miRNAs) from the blue module (N = 70).

Nr	GO ID	GO term	*p*-value	FDR adj *p*-value
	Biological process			
1	GO:0008630	Intrinsic apoptotic signaling pathway in response to DNA damage	5.11E−09	8.60E−06
2	GO:0071456	Cellular response to hypoxia	1.19E−07	2.00E−04
3	GO:0071260	Cellular response to mechanical stimulus	1.46E−07	2.45E−04
4	GO:0006919	Activation of cysteine-type endopeptidase activity involved in apoptotic process	4.96E−07	8.35E−04
5	GO:0043066	Negative regulation of apoptotic process	1.54E−06	2.59E−03
6	GO:0045944	Positive regulation of transcription from RNA polymerase II promoter	2.35E−06	3.95E−03
7	GO:0030308	Negative regulation of cell growth	8.64E−06	1.45E−02
8	GO:0097192	Extrinsic apoptotic signaling pathway in absence of ligand	9.20E−06	1.55E−02
	Molecular function			
1	GO:0005515	Protein binding	8.15E−13	1.13E−09
2	GO:0044822	Poly(A) RNA binding	3.81E−07	5.29E−04
3	GO:0008134	Transcription factor binding	3.77E−06	5.23E−03
4	GO:0042802	Identical protein binding	1.11E−05	1.54E−02
5	GO:0031625	Ubiquitin protein ligase binding	2.41E−05	3.34E−02
	Cellular component			
1	GO:0005829	Cytosol	6.27E−12	8.32E−09
2	GO:0005654	Nucleoplasm	8.76E−08	1.16E−04
3	GO:0005741	Mitochondrial outer membrane	2.53E−06	3.36E−03
4	GO:0005634	Nucleus	1.73E−05	2.29E−02
5	GO:0016020	Membrane	2.49E−05	3.31E−02
6	GO:0005739	Mitochondrion	3.34E−05	4.43E−02

Identified using the online Database for Annotation, Visualization, and Integrated Discovery (DAVID) v6.8.

The target genes were also involved in several biological processes of which most were involved in apoptotic processes. Previous studies found reduced level of apoptotic markers in the serum of subjects with PTSD (Mkrtchian et al., 2013) and abnormal apoptosis in specific brain regions of animals undergoing single prolonged stress as a model for PTSD (Han et al., 2013; Li et al., 2013; Jia et al., 2018). These findings indicate a potential apoptosis dysfunction that could contribute to the inflammation pattern frequently observed within PTSD (Mkrtchian et al., 2013). Furthermore, the involvement of the identified genes in cellular responses after mechanical stimuli could indicate the need to correct for traumatic brain injuries, which are not uncommon among military members. Unfortunately, this information was not available for the present study. Finally, enriched molecular function GO terms suggest their involvement in the binding of proteins and RNA, while the significant cellular component GO terms show involvement of intracellular compartments such as the cytosol and the nucleoplasm.

Of note, the present paper refers to trauma-exposed healthy individuals as being "resilient" in order to create a clear differentiation between trauma-exposed healthy subjects and nonexposed control subjects. However, we do acknowledge and emphasize that resilience is more than just the reverse side of PTSD or the absence of symptomatology (Kalisch et al., 2017; Snijders et al., 2018b). Instead, resilience is an active and dynamic process that needs to remain separated from the multifaceted and complex nature of PTSD. This complexity further suggests that identifying one true and valid biomarker of susceptibility is likely not realistic. We therefore urge future studies to combine findings such as the ones presented in this paper with several other biological networks and phenotypic profiles in order to develop a cross-dimensional, global understanding of PTSD.

The main strength of this study lies in the inclusion of three different groups, i.e., PTSD subjects, resilient subjects, and nonexposed healthy controls, which allows us to disentangle PTSD- from trauma-related effects. However, the study is mainly limited by its relatively small sample size consisting of male subjects only. Given the existence of female- and male-biased miRNAs as recently reported by Cui, Yang et al. (2018) (Cui et al., 2018), these findings may not be applicable to the female population. This study population may also differ from other cohorts such as civilians in terms of demographics, psychological characteristics, and type of experienced trauma, which limits the extrapolation potential. Next, one could question the validity of self-report PTSD measures and whether the observed markers are specific to PTSD since certain comorbidities such as (history of) traumatic brain injuries were not available and thus not accounted for.

In conclusion, this paper presents preliminary evidence for using specific miRNAs as diagnostic biomarkers of PTSD, either individually or grouped within coexpressed clusters. Identifying reliable biomarkers of PTSD is essential for accurate diagnosis and treatment planning. We therefore encourage future studies to build upon these findings by aiming to replicate these in larger cohorts and thus pave the way for functional studies to gain insights into the precise roles of these miRNAs in stress susceptibility.

ETHICS STATEMENT

The studies involving human participants were reviewed and approved by The ethical committee of University Medical Center Utrecht (01-333/0). The patients/participants provided their written informed consent to participate in this study.

AUTHOR CONTRIBUTIONS

LN, BR, GK, DH, JKl, and MK participated in the conception and the design of the study. MB, CV, EV, and EG recruited the participants and collected the blood samples. CS and BM performed the experiments. CS, JKr, EP, and LE performed the bioinformatics analysis. CS wrote the manuscript. LN, BR, and MK provided the necessary fundings. All authors critically read, commented, provided scientific content and approved the final manuscript.

FUNDING

This work has been funded by the European Union's Horizon 2020 research and innovation program under the Marie Sklodowska-Curie grant agreement N0. 707362 (LN) and by a VIDI award number 91718336 from the Netherlands Scientific Organization (BR).

SUPPLEMENTARY MATERIAL

SUPPLEMENTARY FIGURE S1 | Sample dendrogram to detect outliers. Clustering was based on miRNA expression data. Sample names were relabeled as 1-20.

SUPPLEMENTARY FIGURE S2 | Correlations of modules detected by WGCNA and the following potential covariates: age, smoking status and alcohol use. P-values are presented between brackets. ME: module eigengene.

SUPPLEMENTARY FIGURE S3 | Receiver operating characteristic (ROC) curve for the miRNA with the highest module membership in the blue module, i.e. miR-221-3p. The graphs represent PTSD vs control without confounders (A.1) or with confounders (B.1), and PTSD vs resilient without confounders (A.2) or with confounders (B.2).

REFERENCES

American Psychiatric Association. (2013). *Diagnostic and Statistical Manual of Mental Disorders* (5th ed.). Arlington, VA: American Psychiatric Association.

Balakathiresan, N. S., Chandran, R., Bhomia M., Jia M., Li H., Maheshwari, R. K., et al. (2014). Serum and amygdala microRNA signatures of posttraumatic stress: fear correlation and biomarker potential. *J. Psychiatric Res.* 57, 65–73. doi: 10.1016/j.jpsychires.2014.05.020

Bam, M., Yang. X., Zumbrun, EE., Zhong, Y., Zhou, J., Ginsberg, J. P., et al. (2016).Dysregulated immune system networks in war veterans with PTSD is an outcome of altered miRNA expression and DNA methylation. *Sci. Rep.* 6, 31209. doi: 10.1038/srep31209

Bam, M., Yang, X., Zhou, J., Ginsberg, J. P., Leyden, Q., Nagarkatti, P. S., et al. (2016). Evidence for epigenetic regulation of pro-inflammatory cytokines, interleukin-12 and interferon gamma, in peripheral blood mononuclear cells from PTSD patients. *J. Neuroimmune Pharmacol.* 11 (1), 168–181. doi: 10.1007/s11481-015-9643-8

Baras, A. S., Mitchell, C. J., Myers, J. R., Gupta, S., Weng, L. C., Ashton, J. M., et al. (2015). miRge - A Multiplexed Method of Processing Small RNA-Seq Data to Determine MicroRNA Entropy. *PLoS One* 10p (11), e0143066. doi: 10.1371/journal.pone.0143066

Benjamini, Y., and Hochberg, Y. (1995). Controlling the false discovery rate: a practical and powerful approach to multiple testing. *J. R. Stat. Soc.* 57, 289–300. doi: 10.1111/j.2517-6161.1995.tb02031.x

Chou, C. H., Shrestha, S., Yang, C. D., Chang, N. W., Lin, Y. L., Liao, K. W., et al. (2018). miRTarBase update 2018: a resource for experimentally validated microRNA-target interactions. *Nucleic Acids Res.* 46, D296–D302. doi: 10.1093/nar/gkx1067

Cui, C., Yang, W., Shi, J., Zhou, Y., Yang, J., Cui, Q., et al. (2018). Identification and analysis of human sex-biased MicroRNAs. *Genomics Proteomics Bioinf.* 16 (3), 200–211. doi: 10.1016/j.gpb.2018.03.004

Eekhout, I., Reijnen, A., Vermetten, E., and Geuze, E., (2016). Post-traumatic stress symptoms 5 years after military deployment to Afghanistan: an observational cohort study. *Lancet Psychiatry* 3 (1), 58–64. doi: 10.1016/S2215-0366(15)00368-5

Ferry, F. R., Brady, S. E., Bunting, B. P., Murphy, S. D., Bolton, D., O'Neill, S. M., et al. (2015). The economic burden of PTSD in Northern Ireland. *J Trauma Stress* 28 (3), 191–197. doi: 10.1002/jts.22008

Fontana, A., and Rosenheck, R. (1994). Traumatic war stressors and psychiatric symptoms among World War II, Korean, and Vietnam War veterans. *Psychology Aging* 9 (1), 27–33. doi: 10.1037/0882-7974.9.1.27

Goldberg, A. D., Allis, C. D., and Bernstein, E. (2007). Epigenetics: a landscape takes shape. *Cell* 128 (4), 635–638. doi: 10.1016/j.cell.2007.02.006

Grund, B., and Sabin, C. (2010). Analysis of biomarker data: logs, odds ratios, and receiver operating characteristic curves. *Curr. Opin. HIV AIDS* 5 (6), 473–479. doi: 10.1097/COH.0b013e32833ed742

Han, F., Yan, S., and Shi, Y. (2013). Single-prolonged stress induces endoplasmic reticulum-dependent apoptosis in the hippocampus in a rat model of post-traumatic stress disorder. *PLoS One* 8 (7), e69340. doi: 10.1371/journal.pone.0069340

Hovens, J. E., Bramsen, I., and van der Ploeg, H. M. (2002). Self-rating inventory for posttraumatic stress disorder: review of the psychometric properties of a new brief Dutch screening instrument. *Percept. Motor Skills* 94 (3), 996–1008. doi: 10.2466/pms.2002.94.3.996

Huang da, W., Sherman, B. T., and Lempicki, R. A. (2009). Systematic and integrative analysis of large gene lists using DAVID bioinformatics resources. *Nat. Protoc.* 4 (1), 44–57. doi: 10.1038/nprot.2008.211

Huang da, W., Sherman, B. T., and Lempicki, R. A. (2009). Bioinformatics enrichment tools: paths toward the comprehensive functional analysis of large gene lists. *Nucleic Acids Res.* 37 (1), 1–13. doi: 10.1093/nar/gkn923

Jia, Y., Han, Y., Wang, X., and Han, F. (2018). Role of apoptosis in the post-traumatic stress disorder model-single prolonged stressed rats. *Psychoneuroendocrinology* 95, 97–105. doi: 10.1016/j.psyneuen.2018.05.015

Kalisch, R., Baker, D. G., Basten, U., Boks, M. P., Bonanno, G. A., Brummelman, E., et al. (2017). The resilience framework as a strategy to combat stress-related disorders. *Nat. Hum. Behav.* 1 (11), 784–790. doi: 10.1038/s41562-017-0200-8

Koenen, K. C., Ratanatharathorn, A., Ng, L., McLaughlin, K. A., Bromet, E. J., Stein, D. J., et al. (2017). Posttraumatic stress disorder in the world mental health surveys. *Psychol. Med.* 47 (13), 2260–2274. doi: 10.1017/S0033291717000708

Kozomara, A., and Griffiths-Jones, S. (2014). miRBase: annotating high confidence microRNAs using deep sequencing data. *Nucleic Acids Res.* 42, D68–D73. doi: 10.1093/nar/gkt1181

Langfelder, P., and Horvath, S. (2008). WGCNA: an R package for weighted correlation network analysis. *BMC Bioinformatics* 9, 559. doi: 10.1186/1471-2105-9-559

Lehrner, A., and Yehuda, R. (2014). Biomarkers of PTSD: military applications and considerations. *Eur. J. Psychotraumatol.* 5, 10.3402/ejpt.v5.23797. doi: 10.3402/ejpt.v5.23797

Li, Y., Han, F., and Shi, Y. (2013). Increased neuronal apoptosis in medial prefrontal cortex is accompanied with changes of Bcl-2 and bax in a rat model of post-traumatic stress disorder. *J. Mol. Neurosci.* 51 (1), 127–137. doi: 10.1007/s12031-013-9965-z

Li, D. W., Liu, J. Z., Li, S. C., Yang, J. B., Sun, H. H., Wang, A. H., et al. (2018). Fear conditioning downregulates miR-138 expression in the hippocampus to facilitate the formation of fear memory. *Neuroreport* 29 (16), 1418–1424. doi: 10.1097/WNR.0000000000001129

Love, M. I., Huber, W., and Anders, S. (2014). Moderated estimation of fold change and dispersion for RNA-seq data with DESeq2. *Genome Biol.* 15 (12), 550. doi: 10.1186/s13059-014-0550-8

Martin, C. G., Kim, H., Yun, S., Livingston, W., Fetta, J., Mysliwiec, V., et al. (2017). Circulating miRNA associated with posttraumatic stress disorder in a cohort of military combat veterans. *Psychiatry Res.* 251, 261–265. doi: 10.1016/j.psychres.2017.01.081

Mkrtchyan, G. M., Boyadzhyan, A. S., Avetyan, D. G., and Sukiasyan, S. G., (2014). The involvement of abnormal apoptosis in the disturbance of synaptic plasticity in posttraumatic stress disorder. *Neurosci. Behav. Physiol.* 44 (4), 26–29.

Nock, M. K., and Kessler, R. C. (2006). Prevalence of and risk factors for suicide attempts versus suicide gestures: analysis of the national comorbidity survey. *J. Abnorm. Psychol.* 115 (3), 616–623. doi: 10.1037/0021-843X.115.3.616

Peschansky, V. J., and Wahlestedt, C. (2014). Non-coding RNAs as direct and indirect modulators of epigenetic regulation. *Epigenetics* 9 (1), 3–12. doi: 10.4161/epi.27473

Reijnen, A., Rademaker, A. R., Vermetten, E., and Geuze, E. (2015). Prevalence of mental health symptoms in Dutch military personnel returning from deployment to Afghanistan: a 2-year longitudinal analysis. *Eur. Psychiatry* 30 (2), 341–346. doi: 10.1016/j.eurpsy.2014.05.003

Richter-Levin, G., Stork, O., and Schmidt, M. V. (2018). Animal models of PTSD: a challenge to be met. *Mol. Psychiatry* 24, 1135–1156. doi: 10.1038/s41380-018-0272-5

Schmidt, U., Holsboer, F., and Rein, T. (2011). Epigenetic aspects of posttraumatic stress disorder. *Dis. Markers* 30 (2-3), 77–87. doi: 10.1155/2011/343616

Snijders, C., de Nijs, L., Baker, D. G., Hauger, R. L., van den Hove, D., Kenis, G., et al. (2018a). MicroRNAs in post-traumatic stress disorder. *Curr. Top Behav. Neurosci.* 38, 23–46. doi: 10.1007/7854_2017_32

Snijders, C., Pries, L. K., Sgammeglia, N., Al Jowf, G., Youssef, N. A., de Nijs, L., et al. (2018b). Resilience against traumatic stress: current developments and future directions. *Front. Psychiatry* 9, 676. doi: 10.3389/fpsyt.2018.00676

Tarrier, N., and Gregg, L. (2004). Suicide risk in civilian PTSD patients–predictors of suicidal ideation, planning and attempts. *Soc. Psychiatry Psychiatr. Epidemiol.* 39 (8), 655–661. doi: 10.1007/s00127-004-0799-4

Thomas, M. M., Harpaz-Rotem, I., Tsai, J., Southwick, S. M., and Pietrzak, R.H. (2017). Mental and physical health conditions in us combat veterans: results from the national health and resilience in veterans study. *Prim. Care Companion CNS Disord.* 19 (3). doi: 10.4088/PCC.17m02118

van Zuiden, M., Geuze, E., Willemen, H. L., Vermetten, E., Maas, M., Heijnen, C. J., et al. (2011). Pre-existing high glucocorticoid receptor number predicting development of posttraumatic stress symptoms after military deployment. *Am. J. Psychiatry* 168 (1), 89–96. doi: 10.1176/appi.ajp.2010.10050706

Wingo, A. P., Almli, L. M., Stevens, J. S., Klengel. T., Uddin, M., Li, Y., et al. (2015). DICER1 and microRNA regulation in post-traumatic stress disorder with comorbid depression. *Nat. Commun.* 6, 10106. doi: 10.1038/ncomms10106

Yehuda, R., Neylan, T. C., Flory, J. D., and McFarlane, A. C. (2013). The use of biomarkers in the military: from theory to practice. *Psychoneuroendocrinology* 38 (9), 1912–1922. doi: 10.1016/j.psyneuen.2013.06.009

Yehuda, R., Vermetten, E., McFarlane, A. C., and Lehrner, A. (2014). PTSD in the military: special considerations for understanding prevalence, pathophysiology and treatment following deployment. *Eur. J. Psychotraumatol.* 5. doi: 10.3402/ejpt.v5.25322

Zeilinger, S., Kühnel, B., Klopp, N., Baurecht, H., Kleinschmidt, A., Gieger, C., et al. (2013). Tobacco smoking leads to extensive genome-wide changes in DNA methylation. *PLoS One* 8 (5), e63812. doi: 10.1371/journal.pone.0063812

Zhou, J., Nagarkatti, P., Zhong, Y., Ginsberg, J. P., Singh, N. P., Zhang, J., et al. (2014). Dysregulation in microRNA expression is associated with alterations in immune functions in combat veterans with post-traumatic stress disorder. *PLoS One* 9 (4), e94075. doi: 10.1371/journal.pone.0094075

13

Epigenetics of Bladder Cancer: Where Biomarkers and Therapeutic Targets Meet

*Victor G. Martinez[1,2], Ester Munera-Maravilla[1,2,3], Alejandra Bernardini[1,2,3], Carolina Rubio[1,2,3], Cristian Suarez-Cabrera[1,2], Cristina Segovia[1,2], Iris Lodewijk[1,2], Marta Dueñas[1,2,3], Mónica Martínez-Fernández[4] and Jesus Maria Paramio[1,2,3]**

[1] Biomedical Research Institute I+12, University Hospital 12 de Octubre, Madrid, Spain, [2] Molecular Oncology Unit, CIEMAT (Centro de Investigaciones Energéticas, Medioambientales y Tecnológicas), Madrid, Spain, [3] Centro de Investigación Biomédica en Red de Cáncer (CIBERONC), Madrid, Spain, [4] Genomes & Disease Lab, CiMUS (Center for Research in Molecular Medicine and Chronic Diseases), Universidade de Santiago de Compostela, Santiago de Compostela, Spain

***Correspondence:**
Jesus Maria Paramio
jesusm.paramio@ciemat.es

Bladder cancer (BC) is the most common neoplasia of the urothelial tract. Due to its high incidence, prevalence, recurrence and mortality, it remains an unsolved clinical and social problem. The treatment of BC is challenging and, although immunotherapies have revealed potential benefit in a percentage of patients, it remains mostly an incurable disease at its advanced state. Epigenetic alterations, including aberrant DNA methylation, altered chromatin remodeling and deregulated expression of non-coding RNAs are common events in BC and can be driver events in BC pathogenesis. Accordingly, these epigenetic alterations are now being used as potential biomarkers for these disorders and are being envisioned as potential therapeutic targets for the future management of BC. In this review, we summarize the recent findings in these emerging and exciting new aspects paving the way for future clinical treatment of this disease.

Keywords: Epigenetic, chromatin remodelling, bladder cancer, biomarkers, therapeutic target

INTRODUCTION

BC is a common urogenital cancer which represents a current clinical and social problem. At diagnosis, two thirds of patients present a non-muscle invasive bladder cancer (NMIBC), a relatively limited aggressive disease confined to the bladder and without signs of invasion of the underlying muscle layer. The remaining patients display muscle-invasive bladder cancer (MIBC) (Knowles and Hurst, 2015). This pathological classification also defines clinical management. NMIBC is treated by transurethral resection, which can be followed by intravesical instillation with Bacillus Calmette-Guérin (BCG) or mitomycin (Babjuk et al., 2017). However, a large proportion (60–75%) of NMIBC patients relapse and, in some cases (15–25%), the recurrent tumor shows signs of MIBC indicating tumor progression (van Rhijn et al., 2009). The current therapeutic options for MIBC include radical cystectomy and platin-based chemotherapy in adjuvant or neoadjuvant settings (Stenzl et al., 2011). However, in a high proportion of cases, the disease progresses showing metastatic spread, which is associated with extremely low survival rates (Stenzl et al., 2011; Pal et al., 2013; Witjes et al., 2014a). No major improvement in MIBC management occurred during the last decades, until recent years, in which immunotherapy has been shown to increase survival with responses in 20–30% of the patients presenting advanced and metastatic BC (Powles et al., 2014; Rosenberg et al., 2016; Balar et al., 2017; Bellmunt et al., 2017; Plimack et al., 2017). As in other cancers, immunotherapy in BC is mainly based on the use of antibodies that prevent PD-1/PD-L1 interaction, the so called immune checkpoint, leading to immune killing of tumor cells (Pardoll, 2012). The limited activity of immune checkpoint inhibitors in the clinics has led to the consideration of possible combinations of different immune and non-immune therapies (Gotwals et al., 2017). Moreover, in the case of BC patients, it is unclear which patients are more likely to benefit from this treatment (Powles et al., 2014; Rosenberg et al., 2016; Balar et al., 2017; Bellmunt et al., 2017; Plimack et al., 2017). Thus, there is a need not only for more effective therapies in patients with advanced BC, but also for new biomarkers that will help to define which patients may benefit from immunotherapy (Havel et al., 2019).

Epigenetics are heritable but reversible modifications that alter gene expression without changing primary DNA sequences. Epigenome functions are fundamental for the normal status of gene expression and their alterations affect basic cellular processes such as proliferation, differentiation and apoptosis, which may lead to important diseases including cancer (Liep et al., 2012; Baylin and Jones, 2016). Therefore, epigenetic-based cancer biomarkers are promising tools for detection, diagnosis, assessment of prognosis, and prediction of response to therapy (Esteller, 2008; Jerónimo and Henrique, 2014). An extraordinary number of alterations in epigenetic machinery have been observed in BC, affecting DNA methylation (Marques-Magalhaes et al., 2018), chromatin organization, histone modifications (Weinstein et al., 2014; Robertson et al., 2018) and non-coding RNAs expression (Pop-Bica et al., 2017; Taheri et al., 2018). This has produced a large body of evidence indicating that epigenetic machinery could represent a putative target for BC management, a source of valuable biomarkers for diagnostic, prognostic and response prediction, and also a novel research field with amazing new insights into the molecular mechanisms of cancer biology governing cell autonomous cancer processes as well as the intricate cross talk between cancer cells and their niche.

CHROMATIN REMODELERS IN BC

The epigenome is defined by changes that do not involve alterations in the DNA nucleotide sequence. These changes are broadly divided into DNA methylation and modifications of the histone tails that allow the opening or closing of the chromatin. The functions of the epigenome are fundamental for normal gene expression, and its alterations affect basic cellular processes (Tsai and Baylin, 2011;Liep et al., 2012). The aberrant epigenetic landscape is a hallmark of human cancer (Han et al., 2012; Mio et al., 2019; Zhao et al., 2019) and, in particular, characterizes BC as an epigenome disease, as studies of complete exome sequencing have shown that it presents frequent alterations in the genes that govern the organization of chromatin and histone modifications, either by mutation or by its expression/altered function (Gui et al., 2011; Weinstein et al., 2014).

Nevertheless, the mechanisms for epigenetic regulation of gene expression are not limited to chromatin modifiers or DNA methylation changes, as non-coding RNAs are also involved (Fabbri and Calin, 2010; Gupta et al., 2010; Kogo et al., 2011) (**Figure 1**).

DNA Methylation in BC

Methylation of DNA is the process by which a methyl group is added by a covalent bound to the 5' position of a cytosine ring of the DNA molecule. The methylation event is a frequent epigenetic episode and usually occurs on a cytosine followed by a guanine (CpG dinucleotide). There are regions of the genome, termed CpG islands, which contain a higher density of the CpG dinucleotide than the rest of the genome (Li et al., 2016a). These CpG islands are located in sites that normally overlap with gene regulatory regions (Baylln et al., 1997). Thereupon, there are CpG islands at promoter/5' regions of 50% of all known genes and they are normally unmethylated (Reinert, 2012) which is associated with (potentially) active transcription (Jones and Liang, 2009). CpG islands are also found in gene bodies and their methylation status positively correlates with gene expression (Yang et al., 2014). DNA methylation is a key process in mammalian development, and its alterations are hallmarks of diseases, including cancer. Changes in normal DNA methylation status exist in approximately 50–90% of BCs, including DNA hypermethylation of promoter sites of *A3BP1*, *NPTX2*, *ZIC4*, *PAX5A*, *MGMT*, *IGSF4*, *GDF15*, *SOX11*, *HOXA9*, *MEIS1*, *VIM*, *STK11*, *MSH6*, *BRCA1*, *TBX2*, *TBX3*, *TERT*, *GATA2*, *DAPK1*, *CDH4*, *CCND2*, *GSTP1*, *CDKN2A*, *CDKN2B*, *WIF1*, *RASSF1A*, among others (Porten, 2018). These genes are mainly tumor suppressors that belong to biological pathways such as DNA repair, cell cycle control, cell invasion and apoptosis (Reinert et al., 2011; Sánchez-Carbayo, 2012). DNA methylation of promoter regions typically negatively affects gene expression, which can promote the development (Costa et al., 2010; Chung et al., 2011) and progression of BC (Yates et al., 2007; Kandimalla et al., 2012; Casadevall et al., 2017), and can predict therapy outcomes (Agundez et al., 2011; Xylinas et al., 2016).

First studies of DNA methylation in BC focused on potential genes which methylated status might correlate with stage, grade and recurrence. More recently, the development of modern whole-genome DNA methylation assays has allowed to analyze in depth the BC methylome. Wolff et al. stablished that most DNA methylation changes happen in early BC and are conserved in carcinoma *in situ*, non-invasive as well as invasive tumors, and are located in CpG islands (Wolff et al., 2010). Furthermore, the degree and extent of hypermethylation correlates with grade and stage since low-grade tumors have less altered methylation loci compared to high-grade and invasive tumors (Catto et al., 2005; Yates et al., 2007; Wolff et al., 2010). DNA methylation also separates mutation status of *FGFR3*. NMIBC *FGFR3* wild-type tumors, which have a poorer prognosis compared to *FGFR3* mutant NMIBC (Van Rhijn et al., 2012), were more methylated than *FGFR3*-mutant tumors (Serizawa et al., 2011; Kandimalla et al., 2012). Besides, in low-grade non-invasive tumors, DNA hypomethylation was more frequent than in invasive tumors (Wolff et al., 2010). Hypermethylation of *ZO2*, *MYOD* and *CDH13* was also detected in normal-appearing urothelium from bladder with cancer compared to urothelium from healthy

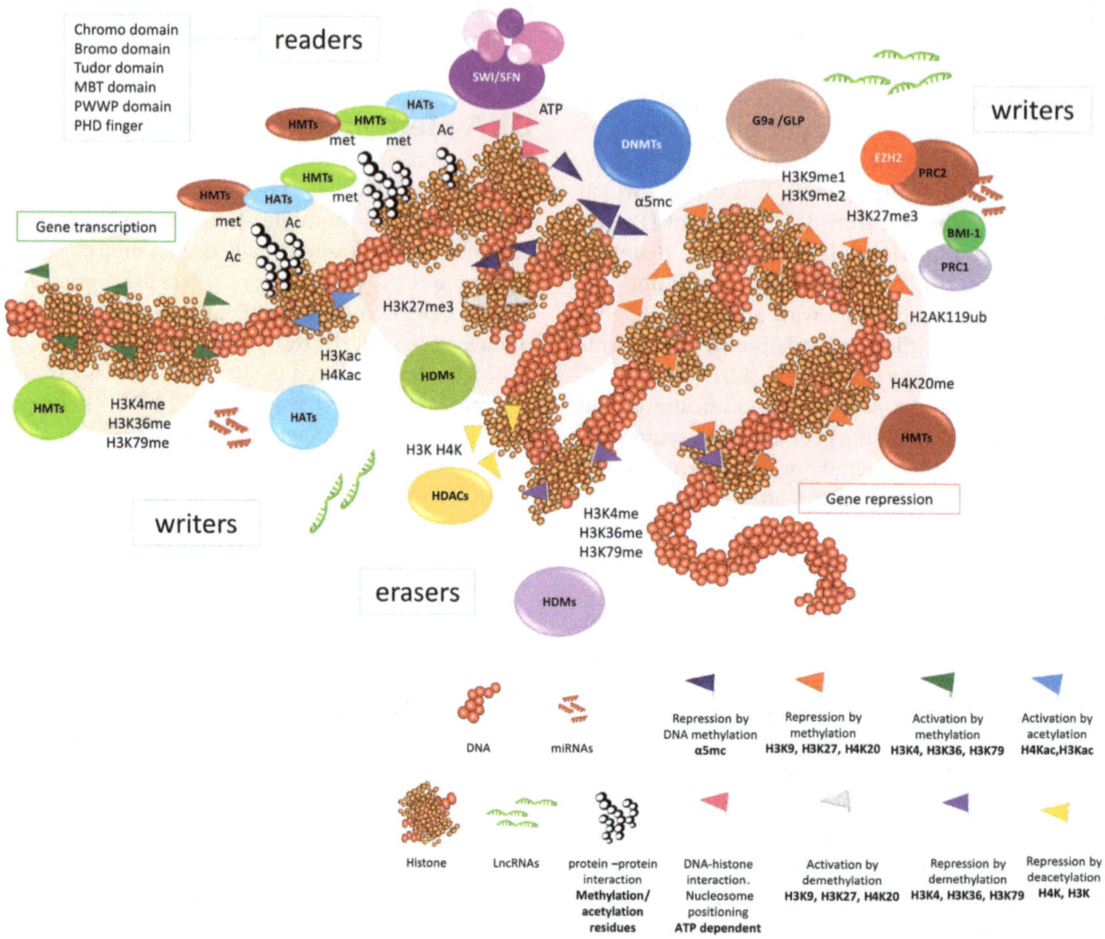

FIGURE 1 | Epigenetic regulation in cancer cells. General scheme of the dynamic interaction of DNA methylation, histone modifications, positioning of nucleosomes, among other factors, that participate in the mechanisms of the epigenome to regulate gene expression. Thus, the tumor cell acquires a particular identity. DNA methylation is present throughout the genome, however we can find aberrant DNA methylations or alterations in the DNMTs enzymes (methyltranferases of DNA nucleotides) in the tumor. The methylation mark H3K27 is the main brand that controls the gene repression in euchromatin. The remodeling enzymes called *writers* (HMT, histone methyltransferase, HAT, histone acetyltransferase), *erasers* (HDM, histone demethylase; HDAC, histone deacetylase) and *readers* (specialized interaction motif containing proteins that recognize post-translational modifications, mostly acetylation and methylation) of the main histone modifications work in a coordinated manner for the regulation of gene transcription. Depending on the genes they regulate, they are recruited to the same place to function together. Therefore, all these molecules are subject of study as possible therapeutic targets.

bladder, indicating an epigenetic 'field defect' and a possible contribution to a loss of epithelial integrity, likely generating a permissive environment for tumor recurrences (Wolff et al., 2010; Majewski et al., 2019).

Since several genes were identified as frequently hypermethylated in primary BC, diagnosis could be performed based on the methylated status of a gene set. For instance, methylation of *IPF1*, *GALR1*, *TAL1*, *PENK* and *TJP2* was found to be higher in MIBC tumors than in NMIBC (Wolff et al., 2010). Sacristan et al. indicated that methylation of *RARB*, *CD44*, *GSTP1*, *IGSF4*, *CHFR*, *PYCARD*, *TP53*, *STK11* and *GATA5* distinguished low-grade versus high-grade tumors, whereas Olkhov-Mitsel et al. stablished that the inclusion of *GP5* and *ZSCAN12* in a methylation panel could feasibly distinguish high-grade and low-grade BC (Olkhov-Mitsel et al., 2017). Unluckily, the overlap between genes found in different studies is limited.

Since 20% of BC patients recur, finding epigenetic markers of progression would be useful to predict recurrence. A wide study reviewed 87 articles reporting the association of epigenetic markers with prognostic outcomes (Casadevall et al., 2017). However, the prognostic influence of epigenetic alterations in BC remains unclear. *CACNA1G* (García-Baquero et al., 2014) and *TBX3* (Kandimalla et al., 2012) were associated with progression and *SFRP5* correlated with recurrence (García-Baquero et al., 2014). *CDNK2A* is methylated in 64% of BCs, however, inconsistent results were found in prognosis (Casadevall et al., 2017). Based on TCGA data, methylation and expression levels of *SOWAHC* were found to be correlated with prognosis (Yang et al., 2019). *HOX* genes appear hypermethylated in almost all aggressive tumors (Reinert et al., 2011; Kandimalla et al., 2012), and *HOXA9* promoter methylation correlated with higher recurrence, progression, and death by cancer in NMIBC and

MIBC (Kitchen et al., 2015) and was associated with cisplatin resistance in BC cell lines (Xylinas et al., 2016). High-risk NMIBC manifest higher rates of progression to invasive tumors than low- and intermediate-risk bladder tumors, which in many cases do not recur or progress. Recently, some investigations proposed multiple CpG sites differentially methylated between high-risk recurrence/progression tumors and less aggressive low-risk no-recurrence tumors (Kitchen et al., 2018; Peng et al., 2018).

A three-gene methylation panel which differentiates between patients with metastatic and free of cancer lymph nodes might also be predictive of metastasis development, and enable the selection of patients that would benefit from lymph node resection and neoadjuvant chemotherapy (Stubendorff et al., 2019). In patients undergoing BCG treatment, methylation status of *MSH6* and *THBS1* may help to distinguish responders to therapy, and methylation of *GATA5* associated with survival (Agundez et al., 2011), allowing the possible identification of patients requiring a more aggressive therapy. After chemotherapeutic treatment, the *MDR1* gene was found to be overexpressed in BC compared with untreated tumors, and in tumors from patients that eventually recurred. This overexpression correlated negatively with methylation of CpG sites in the promoter region (Tada et al., 2000). An interesting study tested gene methylation in second recurrences in bladder of primary upper-tract urothelial carcinomas, and stablished that the methylation rate in certain genes tend to increase with the number of recurrences, which may be a predictive factor for recurrences after surgery (Guan et al., 2018). Nevertheless, the existence of inconsistent results and lack of validation studies hampers at present relevance of these findings (Casadevall et al., 2017; Porten, 2018).

Less data is reported about hypomethylation status in BC. In 1983, a pioneer study reported that hypomethylation could distinguish genes of cancer cells compared with their normal counterparts (Feinberg and Vogelstein, 1983). In normal cells, certain CpG rich satellite repeats are strongly methylated, such as LINE-1 (Schulz, 2006). Interestingly, these regions are strongly hypomethylated in all types of BC (Kreimer et al., 2013) and could translate in genomic instability (Wolff et al., 2010). Besides, as a tissue-fingerprint, the hypomethylation pattern of LINE-1 seems to be specific for each tumor type and tissue (Sharma et al., 2019). Furthermore, a different type of study analyzed global methylation in DNA from blood cells and found that leukocyte DNA hypomethylation is a risk factor for BC (Moore et al., 2008).

DNA methylation is catalyzed by three DNA methyltransferases (DNMT): DNMT1, DNMT3A and DNMT3B. DNMT1 is the keeper of the regular methylation status of the genome after cell replication (Goll and Bestor, 2005), whereas DNMT3a and DNMT3b are *de novo* methyltransferases (Okano et al., 1999). Mutations in chromatin regulatory genes are present in around 76% of BC (Robertson et al., 2018) and are more frequently found in BC than in any other solid tumor (Weinstein et al., 2014). However, the alterations regarding DNMTs in BC are mainly found to be an increase in their expression (Li et al., 2016a). Several genes that are methylated in BC are repressed by polycomb complexes (Wolff et al., 2010; Kandimalla et al., 2012). These complexes composed of EZH2 recruit DNMTs required for DNA methylation (Viré et al., 2006), which suggests an upstream regulation of methylation in BC.

Chromatin Remodeling and Histone Modification in BC

Mutations in chromatin remodeling genes are very frequent in BC (Robertson et al., 2018), affecting 89% of histone remodelers and 64% of nucleosome positioning genes in MIBC (Weinstein et al., 2014; Robertson et al., 2018). The post-translational modifications of histones, such as acetylation, methylation, phosphorylation or ubiquination in specific residues of lysines, arginines and serines (Allis et al., 2007; Rothbart and Strahl, 2014), modulate the dynamic and reversible changes in chromatin structural changes. This "histone code" can be written, erased and read by different molecules modulating transcription (Gillette and Hill, 2015). Therefore, chromatin remodelers can be classified as writers (methyltransferases (HMTs) or acetylases (HATs)), erasers (demethylases (HDMs) and deacetylases (HDACs)) and readers, which are further divided in proteins or effector complexes that interact with specific domains (Gillette and Hill, 2015; Hyun et al., 2017), and nucleosome remodeling multiprotein complexes that are able to alter DNA-histone contacts. The main marks of gene transcription are acetylation of histone 3 and histone 4 (H3Kac, H4Kac) and methylation of histone 3 on lysine 4, 36 and 79 (H3K4me, H3K36me, H3K79me), while methylation of histone 3 on lysine 9 and 27 and histone 4 on lysine 20 (H3K9me, H3K27me, H4K20me) represent important marks for gene repression (Bernstein et al., 2007) (**Figure 1**).

Writers

Histone methyltransferase EZH2 catalyzes H3K27me2 and H3K27me3 marks to regulate the repression of gene expression (Deb et al., 2014), and compacts chromatin with other molecules like BMI-1 (Cao et al., 2005) (**Figure 1**). Its involvement in tumor development and progression is a common characteristic of several human tumors, including BC (Yamaguchi and Hung, 2014). It has been demonstrated that the existence of the oncogenic axis Rb-E2F-EZH2 predicts recurrence and progression in NMIBC (Santos et al., 2014) and promotes global changes in gene expression, including the aberrant expression of lncRNAs such as *HOTAIR* (Martínez-Fernández et al., 2015b), and the silencing of several microRNAs, such as mir-200 family (Martínez-Fernández et al., 2015a). Several studies have shown that EZH2 also interacts with other modifiers such as DNMTs, HDAC or G9a, that could explain some oncological properties of EZH2. The importance of these non-canonical functions of EZH2 in BC is still not well understood, although it could favor intratumoral heterogeneity (Gupta et al., 2011).

Histone methyltransferase G9a (EHMT2) is considered an oncogenic epigenetic factor (Lee et al., 2015), which can be involved in urothelial tumors (Shankar et al., 2013; Cho et al., 2015). This enzyme binds GLP (EHMT1) and catalyzes H3K9me2 leading to gene silencing through physical interaction with cofactors (Bian et al., 2015; Maier et al., 2015; Simon et al., 2015; Hu et al., 2018) and/or non-coding RNAs (Nagano et al., 2008). Additionally, G9a may interact with EZH2 allowing the silencing of specific loci in a cooperative way (Mozzetta et al., 2014; Mozzetta et al., 2015) becoming a possible target for advanced metastatic BC (Segovia et al., 2019).

Methyltransferase KMT2D (MLL2), which catalyzes H3K4me1 and H3K4me2 (Lee et al., 2013), displays the highest mutation rate among all HMTs in BC (Weinstein et al., 2014) in close association with tumor development, recurrence (Wu et al., 2016a) and resistance to therapy (Lu et al., 2017). *KMT2C* (MLL3) is also commonly mutated in high grade NMIBC (Weinstein et al., 2014; Hurst et al., 2017) and in luminal papillary and basal squamous MIBC subtypes (Robertson et al., 2018), and its silencing affects DNA damage response genes (Rampias et al., 2019). Additionally, somatic mutations of 13 HMT genes, including *NSD1* and *NSD3*, are present in a high proportion of BC tumors (Ding et al., 2019). Moreover, the genes encoding acetyltransferases EP300 and CREBBP are among the genes most frequently inactivated by mutation in human BC (Gui et al., 2011; Duex et al., 2018b).

Erasers

The gene encoding histone demethylase KDM6A (UTX), located on the X chromosome, is one of the genes most frequently mutated in BC (Gui et al., 2011; Nickerson et al., 2014). This demethylase can specifically erase the marks written by EZH2 (Agger et al., 2007; Lee et al., 2007). Mutations in *KDM6A* are more common in NIMBC and in women (Hurst et al., 2017), and tend to be mutually exclusive with *MLL2* alterations (Kim et al., 2015a) suggesting a predominant silenced chromatin during bladder carcinogenesis (Casadevall et al., 2017). In some cases, it has been associated with *RB1* mutation in high grade urothelial tumors (Balbás-Martínez et al., 2013; Ross et al., 2014).

Acetylation of lysine residues in histone tails results in a more open state of the chromatin (Roger et al., 2011) and histone acetylation levels decrease during progression towards MIBC (Ellinger et al., 2016). Furthermore, the deregulated expression of various HDACs, like HDAC1, 2, 3 and 6, has been described in urothelial tumors in close association with malignancy (Chen et al., 2011; Li et al., 2016b; Niegisch et al., 2013; Poyet et al., 2014; Lee and Song, 2017).

Readers

The effects of epigenetic marks are mediated through effector complexes which "read" marks and facilitate the DNA–histone and protein–protein interactions. This provides recruitment platforms for other epigenetic regulators to specific DNA loci (Dawson and Kouzarides, 2012) (**Figure 1**). The methylation and acetylation writers usually have reader domains (predominantly bromodomain (BRD) and plant homeodomain (PHD) finger) that allow recognition of the histone methylation/acetylation status (Dawson and Kouzarides, 2012; Biswas and Rao, 2018).

Methyl CpG sites are recognized by proteins that contain conserved binding domains such as methyl CpG binding domain (MBD), SRA domain and zinc finger (ZnF). These proteins work together with other factors to alter the transcriptional status of DNA (Biswas and Rao, 2018). The histone methylated residues are recognized by conserved binding domains such as PHD finger, Tudor domain, PWWP (Pro-Trp-Trp-Pro) domain, chromodomain, malignant brain tumor domain (MBT), ankyrin repeats (present in G9a and GLP1), ZnFs and WD40 domain, among others. Furthermore, BRDs, double PHD finger and Yeats domains bind specifically to acetylated residues of histones (Dhalluin et al., 1999; Fischle, 2003; Kouzarides, 2007; Taverna et al., 2007; Dawson and Kouzarides, 2012; Biswas and Rao, 2018). BRDs are present in the acetylation writers CBP and p300 along with several protein interaction motifs, both closely related proteins have been deeply investigated since they are able to acetylate the four histones (Dawson and Kouzarides, 2012). Additionally, BRDs of chromatin remodeling enzymes BRM (*SMARCA2*) and BRG1 (*SMARCA4*) recognize multiple acetylation sites at H3 and H4. In BC, the BRD4 histone acetylation reader is overexpressed and can upregulate C-MYC, which controls the expression of cell cycle progression genes, enhancing the recruitment of this factor to the EZH2 promoter and subsequently upregulating EZH2 expression, which has a significant relevance on tumor growth (Wu et al., 2016b). Consequently, EZH2 promotes growth of BC by chromatin modification (Wu et al., 2016b), especially in tumors with loss of *KDM6A* (Ler et al., 2017). Some susceptibilities to EZH2 inhibitors have been found in relation to mutations in components of SWI/SNF complexes such as *ARID1B* (12%), *SMARCA4* (15%) *SMARCA2* (16%) (Helming et al., 2014; Bitler et al., 2015; Kim et al., 2015b). This is relevant in the context of BC, since components of the SWI/SNF complexes are also frequently altered in BC patients (Knowles and Hurst, 2015; Robertson et al., 2018). Other remodelers such as the SWI/SNF nucleosomal complex component, *ARID1A*, often show inactivating mutations or deep eliminations in both MIBC (Weinstein et al., 2014; Robertson et al., 2018) and NIMBC (Hurst et al., 2017).

An additional complexity of chromatin remodeling lies in the fact that many chromatin regulators have more than one type of reader domain, and their binding to chromatin can be further influenced by histone modifications (Ruthenburg et al., 2007). The understanding of the dynamic plasticity of DNA and histone modifications will allow us to open new venues to the management and treatment of BC.

Non-Coding RNAs in BC Etiology and Progression

Non-coding RNAs (ncRNA) represent an important role in the epigenetic changes leading to BC development and progression. Additional to transfer RNA and ribosomal RNA molecules, which represent the most abundant ncRNAs (3–10 × 10^7 and 3–10 × 10^6 molecules per cell, respectively), several ncRNA classes can be distinguished, including long non-coding RNA (lncRNA), transcribed ultraconserved region (T-UCR), circular RNA (circRNA), small interfering RNA (siRNA), Y RNA (Y RNA), micro-RNA (miRNA; miR), piwi-interacting RNA (piRNA), small nucleolar RNAs and small nuclear ribonucleic acid (Palazzo and Lee, 2015; Anastasiadou et al., 2017; Gulìa et al., 2017)

NcRNA molecules are specific RNAs which are not translated into proteins, and represent essential regulatory roles in practically every aspect of cellular function. They have been suggested to exert an essential function in the maintenance of genomic stability, mainly through adjusting DNA expression and complex formation with other ncRNA molecules as well as proteins. Consequently, the description of ncRNA function in isolation is very complicated. Several ncRNAs (like miRNAs) are able to target the messenger RNAs (mRNAs) of multiple other genes, whereas the mRNA of one gene can also be targeted by numerous miRNAs. Furthermore, miRNAs can interact with other ncRNA molecules, like lncRNAs and circRNAs, in order to control their stability, while lncRNAs and circRNAs are able to regulate the abundance of miRNAs. Besides, ncRNAs can interact with individual proteins and protein complexes which might facilitate specific protein targeting or the assembly of protein complexes by providing a scaffold (Anastasiadou et al., 2017; Gulìa et al., 2017).

LncRNAs and miRNAs represent the two main classes of ncRNA involved in BC epigenetic etiology as well as progression, and will be discussed in detail below. Additionally, some other ncRNA molecules associated to this pathology will be briefly described.

Long Non-Coding RNAs

LncRNAs consist of more than 200 nucleotides, and are involved in several essential biochemical processes (Wang and Chang, 2011). Clark et al. examined about 7,200 lncRNA molecules and described a wide variation in stability, ranging from half-lives of less than 30 min for unstable molecules to half-lives of more than 48 h for extremely stable lncRNAs, with a median lncRNA half-life of 3.5 h (Clark et al., 2012). Besides, these lncRNA molecules have been found to be significantly less abundant than, for example, total mRNA (3–50 × 10^3 versus 3–10 × 10^5 molecules per cell, respectively) (Palazzo and Lee, 2015). Many lncRNAs were found to be differentially expressed in a wide range of tumor tissues compared to corresponding healthy control tissues, suggesting an important role in carcinogenesis (Martens-Uzunova et al., 2014; Bhan et al., 2017). In BC, deregulation of lncRNAs has been found to contribute to carcinogenesis in several ways including sustained proliferative signaling and induction of invasion as well as metastasis (Bhan et al., 2017).

LncRNA expression in BC has been extensively reviewed (Gulìa et al., 2017; Taheri et al., 2018). Based on their expression patterns and functions in BC tissue compared to healthy control tissue, lncRNA molecules can be classified in two groups, either showing increased (oncogenic lncRNAs) or decreased (tumor suppressor lncRNAs) expression in tumor tissue. For example, oncogenic lncRNA-*UCA1* has been reported to induce epithelial-mesenchymal transition (EMT) and promote BC cell migration and invasion through the miR-145–ZEB1/2–FSCN1 pathway, as well as by targeting miR-582-5p or modulation of the miR-143/HMGBG1 signaling pathway (Xue et al., 2016; Luo et al., 2017; Wu et al., 2019a). Overexpression of *UCA1* has been associated with high risk of poor outcome in BC. Accordingly, the use of *UCA1* as potential biomarker is subject of ongoing research (Wang et al., 2006; Cui et al., 2017). LncRNA-*H19* has been found to be abundantly expressed in BC leading to increased miR-675 expression, thus inhibiting TP53 activation (Ariel et al., 2000; Liu et al., 2016). LncRNA-*H19* has further been described to promote metastasis and EMT through E-cadherin inhibition as well as by targeting miR-29b-3p (Lv et al., 2017; Zhu et al., 2018). Other well-described oncogenic lncRNAs involved in BC include *MALAT1*, *HOTAIR*, *TUG1*, *ANRIL* and *PVT1*, whereas well-known lncRNAs-*MEG3* and *GAS5* represent tumor suppressor lncRNA molecules (Sun et al., 2015; Gulìa et al., 2017; Guo et al., 2018; Liu et al., 2017b; Xie et al., 2017a; Yang et al., 2017; Yu et al., 2019; Jiao et al., 2018; Liu et al., 2018a; Wang et al., 2018b; Huang et al., 2019a; Tian et al., 2019). Even though many other oncogenic and tumor suppressor lncRNAs have recently been identified in BC, they need further investigation to validate their relevance in this disease. Additionally, the use of specific lncRNA as biomarkers or therapeutic targets is subject of ongoing research and will be further discussed below.

Micro-RNAs

As abovementioned, lncRNAs extensively interact with miRNA in the regulation of oncogenic pathways. MiRNAs consist of 21–24 nucleotides and play important roles in the regulation of gene expression (Sohel, 2016). Mature miRNAs have shown high stability reflecting half-lives of approximately 8 hours in the cell, which is reflected in a relatively high abundance of miRNA molecules (1–3 × 10^5 molecules per cell) (Palazzo and Lee, 2015).

Aberrantly expressed miRNAs have been found in BC tissues causing an altered expression of target genes, resulting in BC development and progression (Zhu et al., 2011). As for lncRNAs, miRNA expression in BC has been extensively reviewed (Enokida et al., 2016; Gulìa et al., 2017). The aberrant expression of several miRNAs has been found to alter two main genetic pathways predisposing to BC. Some miRNAs target the FGFR3 pathway (including miR-99a, miR-100, miR-101, and miR-145), while other miRNA molecules modify the TP53 pathway (such as miR-21 and miR-373) (Homami and Ghazi, 2016). Like lncRNAs, miRNA molecules can be divided in oncogenic miRNAs or tumor suppressor miRNAs. For example, the decreased expression of miR-34a in BC has an anti-metastatic function through the CD44/EMT signaling pathway (Yu et al., 2014) and through targeting NOTCH1 and HNF4G also negatively modulates BC cell proliferation and invasion (Zhang et al., 2012; Sun et al., 2015). Accordingly, low expression of miR-34 has been found to be correlated with unfavorable prognosis (Xie et al., 2017b). Besides, downregulation of the tumor suppressor miR-200 family has been proposed to be associated with poor prognosis in BC, and the use of this family as prognostic marker has been indicated (Wiklund et al., 2011; Martínez-Fernández et al., 2015a). The miR-200 family consists of five different members, namely miR-200a, miR-200b, miR-200c, miR-429 and miR-141, and has been suggested to play an essential role in the inhibition of the EMT process by regulation of ZEB1 and ZEB2 transcription factors (Korpal et al., 2008; Park et al., 2008).

Many other tumor suppressor and oncogenic miRNAs have been extensively described or recently discovered as particular players in BC (Enokida et al., 2016; Gulìa et al., 2017). For example, low expression of miR-100, miR-101 and miR-214, as well as high expression of miR-452, miR-21, miR-222, miR-182, miR-133b, miR-155, miR-145, and miR-152 has been correlated with unfavorable prognosis(Xie et al., 2017b).

Given their deregulated expression, the miRNAs have been widely studied as therapeutic target and biomarkers in different pathologies, including several types of cancers (Romero-Cordoba et al., 2014; Shah and Calin, 2014; Chan et al., 2015). Accordingly, the study of miRNAs in liquid biopsy offers great perspective for diagnostic and prognostic purposes. These objectives will be further discussed below.

Other ncRNA

CircRNA molecules represent a type of ncRNA that are covalently closed in a loop at the 3′ and 5′ ends. The lack of free 3′ or 5′ ends provides increased resistance of circRNAs to exoribonuclease-dependent RNA degradation, which results in a prolonged half-life of over 48 h (Jeck and Sharpless, 2014). Even though their cellular functions are still largely unknown, various circRNAs have shown relevance in multiple cancer types (Zhang et al., 2017; Kristensen et al., 2018). Although circRNA research in BC is still scarce, several circRNAs have been shown to be highly expressed in human BC. These endogenous circRNAs competitively target specific miRNAs, thereby suppressing miRNA activity by acting as a miRNA sponge. For example, circTCF25 has been demonstrated to promote cell proliferation and metastasis by acting as a RNA sponge for miR-103a-3p and miR-107, resulting in increased CDK6 levels (Zhong et al., 2016). Besides, circRNA-MYLK and circRNA-CTDP1 competitively bind miR-29a-3p leading to enhanced expression of its target genes *DNMT3B*, *VEGFA*, *HAS3* and *ITGB1*, resulting in angiogenesis, EMT and metastasis (Huang et al., 2016; Zhong et al., 2017). Recently, additional circRNA molecules representing an oncogenic role in BC tumorigenesis and progression have been discovered, including circCEP128, circRNA-VANGL1, circPRMT5 and circRNA-cTFRC (Chen et al., 2018; Wu et al., 2018; Zeng et al., 2019; Su et al., 2019).

Contrarily to the oncogenic role of several circRNAs, some circRNAs act as tumor suppressors and have been shown to be downregulated in human BC. For example, circRNA-ITCH has been shown to suppress the aggressive biological behavior of BC through increased expression of p21 and PTEN by sponging miR-17 and miR-224, whereas circRNA-BCRC-3 has been found to act as a sponge of miR-182-5p resulting in enhanced expression of p27 (Xie et al., 2018; Yang et al., 2018a). Other circRNA molecules which have recently been discovered to mediate anti-oncogenic functions include circRNA-BCRC4, circRNA-Cdr1as and circMTO1 (Li et al., 2017; Li et al., 2018a; Liu et al., 2018b).

Their extensive abundance, stability and tissue-specific expression make circRNAs attractive molecules for clinical research (Barrett and Salzman, 2016). Further research into their regulatory mechanisms on miRNA expression will help us to improve our knowledge regarding their function in carcinogenesis and may provide insights in the use of circRNA molecules as predictive and diagnostic biomarkers as well as novel therapeutic targets (Kulcheski et al., 2016; Han et al., 2017).

Y RNA molecules are small ncRNAs (21–24 nucleotides) necessary for DNA replication through interactions with chromatin and initiation proteins. Four Y RNAs have been identified and found to be highly evolutionary conserved, namely Y1, Y3, Y4 and Y5 (Christov et al., 2006). These ncRNAs are protected from degradation by its interaction with Ro, a ribonucleoprotein particle that provides stability to these molecules, and their abundance has been found to be relatively high (about 1×10^5 molecules per cell) (Christov et al., 2006; Chen et al., 2007). Even though a role for Y RNAs in BC has been indicated by various studies, contradicting observations have been published (Christov et al., 2008; Tolkach et al., 2017). Christov et al. described the significant overexpression of two Y RNAs, Y1 and Y3, whereas Tolkach et al. published the significant downregulation of all four Y RNAs in BC tissue compared to tissue of healthy controls. Accordingly, this emphasizes the need for further studies to clarify the possible role of Y RNA in BC etiology and progression.

PiRNA molecules are short single strands non-coding RNAs (26–31 nucleotides) mediating epigenetic and post-transcriptional gene silencing through interactions with PIWI proteins (Siomi et al., 2011). Their small size suggests particular resistance to degradation, which can result in the presence of relatively high levels of piRNA molecules (Palazzo and Lee, 2015; Pardini and Naccarati, 2017). Deregulated expression of some piRNAs has been found in different cancer types (Chalbatani et al., 2019). In BC, Martinez et al. described the association of high levels of piRNA FR004819 with poorer survival, whereas Taubert et al. defined a significant association between diminished *PIWIL2* expression and poor prognosis (Martinez et al., 2015; Taubert et al., 2015). Additionally, piRABC has been observed to be downregulated in BC tissue and has been identified as an important piRNA in the development and progression of this pathology. Besides, it has been proposed that piRABC may promote cell apoptosis in BC by upregulation of the TNFSF4 protein (Chu et al., 2015; Chalbatani et al., 2019).

EPIGENETIC REGULATION OF THE BC MICROENVIRONMENT

Immune Cell Compartment

Cancer initiation and tumor progression are often associated with the inhibition of anticancer immune response and dysregulation of inflammatory activity (Berraondo et al., 2016; Sukari et al., 2016). Different solid tumors are characterized by the presence of immune cells, such as T and B lymphocytes, natural killer (NK) cells, macrophages, and antigen-presenting cells in the tissue microenvironment (TME). These immune cells exhibit different behaviors and morphologies as a result of aberrant differentiation (Olivieri et al., 2016), sometimes driven by epigenetically regulated lineage-specific changes influencing the expression of genes crucial for the identity of immune cells and promoting cellular responses to stimuli (Herold et al., 2012; Smith and Meissner, 2013; Luperchio et al., 2014) (**Figure 2**).

Recently, some studies have shown that post-translational modification of histones may regulate the behavior of cells involved in the immune response, including tumor associated macrophages (TAMs), regulatory T cells (Tregs), dendritic cells (DCs), NK cells, myeloid-derived suppressor cells (MDSCs), effector T cells (Teffs), and others (Liu et al., 2017a). Based on whole-genome bisulfite sequencing datasets from

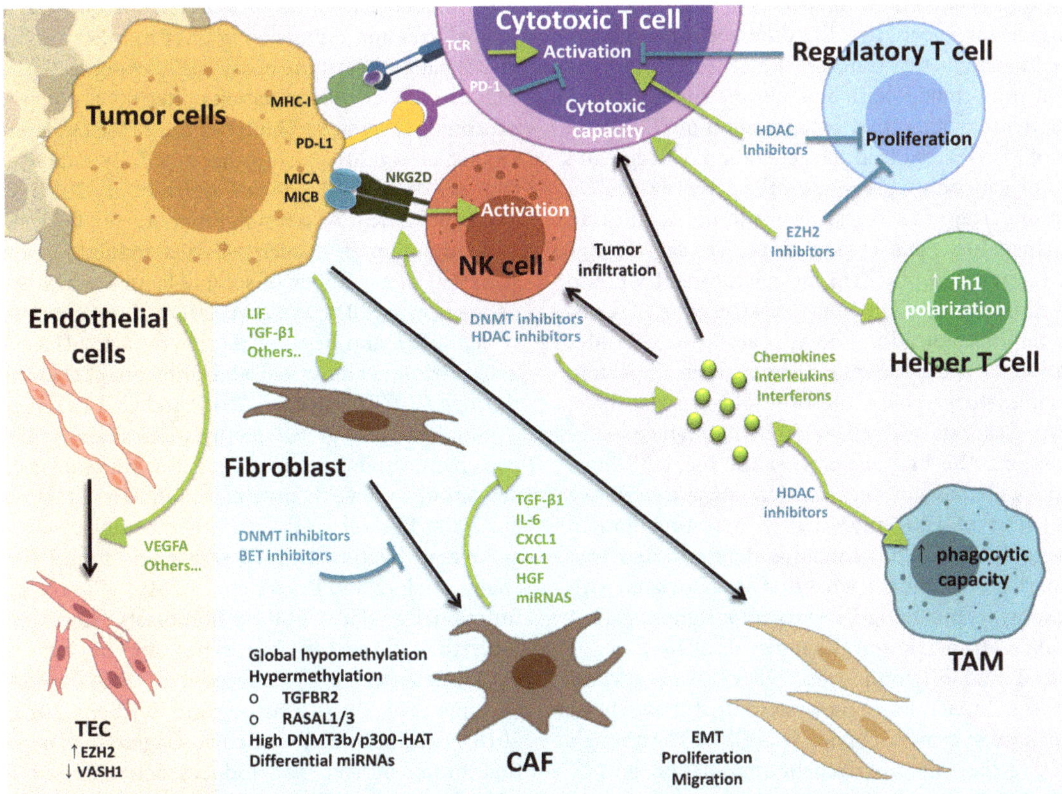

FIGURE 2 | Epigenetic landscape of the tumor microenvironment. Tumor cells can influence the stroma through different factors, being soluble factors the most characterized. Tumor-derived VEGFA induces EZH2 in TEC, which drives hypermethylation of anti-angiogenic Vash1. Also induced by tumor cells, CAF differentiation is associated with several epigenetic features and can be blocked by a number of chromatin remodelers inhibitors. In turn, CAFs promote tumor growth and metastasis *via* secretion of soluble factors and matrix remodeling. On the immune side, cytotoxic T cells and natural killer cells are the main effectors of the anti-cancer immune response. Balance between activating and inhibiting signals coming from tumor targeted cells determines cytotoxic activity of these cells. Other immune cells such as regulatory T cells and macrophages are key in the anti-cancer immune response. Of note, myeloid and lymphoid lineages present inverse methylation patterns in cancer tissues, contributing to aberrant functionality. Inhibition of epigenetic writers can block regulatory T cell differentiation and function, while promoting anti-tumor activity in effector cells. Reverting tumor-driven epigenetic modifications imprinted in the TME may condition the tumor stroma for effective elimination of malignant cells in combination with existing treatments such as immunotherapy. TEC, tumor endothelial cells; CAF, cancer-associated fibroblasts; EMT, epithelial–mesechymal transition; TAM, tumor-associated macrophage.

the BLUEPRINT Epigenome Project (http://www.blueprint-epigenome.eu), Schuyler et al. identified inverse methylation patterns in the myeloid and lymphoid lineages in cancer tissues, where lymphoid-derived neoplasms lose CpG methylation patterns whereas myeloid malignancies significantly increase levels of DNA methylation (Schuyler et al., 2016). These observations have been reproduced by other authors showing that different methylation patterns contribute to the activation of myeloid and lymphoid cancer cells (Bröske et al., 2009; Bock et al., 2012).

The main component of the immune infiltrates present in solid tumors are TAMs, which have been frequently associated with worse prognosis. Compared to the binary M1/M2 classification, TAMs include multiple populations sharing features of both M1 and M2 phenotypes that in many cases do not fit the M1/M2 classification. Nonetheless, it offers a useful working frame for the study of TAMs, in which the overall consensus is that M1 macrophages are anti-tumorigenic, while M2 macrophages can promote tumor growth. M2-macrophage marker genes are epigenetically regulated by reciprocal changes in histone H3 lysine-4 (H3K4) and histone H3 lysine-27 (H3K27) methylation. After IL-4 stimulation, a decrease of H3K27 dimethylation and trimethylation (H3K27me2/3) marks occur as well as the transcriptional activation of specific M2 marker genes. Additionally to methylation, during monocyte to macrophage differentiation, there is a massive reconfiguration of lysine acetylation patterns at gene regulatory elements with a positive correlation between transcriptionally permissive H3 histone acetylation and the activity of regulatory elements (Bistoni et al., 1986).

When analyzing the activation/polarization status of tumor infiltrating lymphocytes (TILs), TAMs and DCs, several studies have shown that the methylation status of immune genes in these cells influences the tumor immune response in the TME, and correlates with the density of TILs and tumor progression. For example, in naïve $CD4^+$ T cells the interferon-γ (*IFN-γ*) gene promoter and upstream enhancer is methylated. However, in Th1 lymphocytes, where the expression of *IFN-γ* is induced, the *IFN-γ* gene promoter and enhancer are demethylated, suggesting an important role in Th1/Th2 differentiation (Janson et al., 2008). The histone methyl transferase EZH2 has also been shown to play an important role in shaping the function of T cells. Wang et al. demonstrated that accumulation of H3K4me3 in the promoter of *FOXP3* results in the generation of Tregs, and pharmacological or genetic suppression of the activity of EZH2 on tumor-infiltrating Tregs (TI-Tregs) results in the acquisition of pro-inflammatory functions (Wang et al., 2018a) (**Figure 2**). In addition, suppression of EZH2 modulates the TME and enhances the infiltration of $CD8^+$ and $CD4^+$ effector T cells, which can favor tumor eradication (Wang et al., 2018a). Besides H3K27 methylation, G9a-dependent H3K9me2 is an important regulator of inflammatory gene expression and has also been implicated in several aspects of T cell biology. Although genome-wide studies mapping the binding of G9a (or the H3K9me2 mark) in immune cells has not been carried out, a descriptive genome-wide analysis of H3K9me2 marks in resting human lymphocytes using ChIP-on-chip methods demonstrated that this epigenetic mark is enriched on genes that are associated with several specific pathways including T cell receptor signaling, IL-4 signaling, and GATA3 transcription (Zhang et al., 2018a).

In addition to T and B lymphocytes, NK cells are effector lymphocytes of the innate immune system that have been shown to control tumor growth (Vivier et al., 2008). Although studies investigating the role of epigenetic modulation on NK cell activation and cytotoxicity are still scarce, some reports indicate that histone acetylation is involved in the regulation of NK cell activation and effector functions (Schenk et al., 2016; Raulet et al., 2017). Particularly in cancer, HDAC inhibitors have been shown to modulate the expression of NK ligands on the surface of neuroblastoma, melanoma, osteosarcoma, colon and Merkel cell (Zhu et al., 2015; Kiany et al., 2017) (**Figure 2**). Besides, Hicks et al. shows that HDAC inhibitors, in addition to significantly enhancing the expression of multiple NK ligands and death receptors resulting in enhanced NK cell-mediated lysis, also increases tumor cell PD-L1 expression both *in vitro* and in carcinoma xenografts (Hicks et al., 2018). This data offers a rationale for combining HDAC inhibitors with inhibitors of the PD-1/PD-L1 axis, including for patients who are refractory or expected not to respond to these therapies alone due to absent or low PD-L1 tumor expression.

Cancer-Associated Fibroblasts

The tumor stroma is defined as the non-malignant cells and extracellular components that surround tumors, with a fundamental role in growth and progression. Fibroblasts in the tumor microenvironment differentiate into cancer-associated fibroblasts (CAFs), being one of the main components in the tumor stroma (**Figure 2**). CAFs play key roles in all cancerous stages, the vast majority of the studies demonstrating pro-tumoral functions that include extracellular matrix remodeling, angiogenesis, immune suppression and drug resistance (Kalluri, 2016; Tao et al., 2017; Ziani et al., 2018).

The current knowledge on CAF biology in BC is scarce and mostly coming from *in vitro* experiments. Nonetheless, it has been shown that there is a positive correlation between the presence of active CAFs and expression of EMT markers and worse prognosis in BC patients (Schulte et al., 2012; Wu et al., 2017). *In vitro*, BC cells can induce differentiation of healthy fibroblast into CAFs *via* exosomes (Ringuette Goulet et al., 2018; De Palma et al., 2019; Goulet et al., 2019) and other not fully characterized secreted factors (Wang et al., 2007; Grimm et al., 2015; Shi et al., 2015; Yeh et al., 2015). As a result, differentiated CAFs induce motility and migration in cancer cells *via* induction of EMT through secretion of a number of soluble factors which include TGF-β1 (Zhuang et al., 2015; Wu et al., 2017), IL-6 (Yeh et al., 2015; Goulet et al., 2019), and hepatocyte growth factor (HGF) (Wang et al., 2007; Grimm et al., 2015), and/or by direct chemokine attraction through CXCL1 (Shi et al., 2015) and CCL1 (Yeh et al., 2015).

Studies using global methylation analysis have shown that epigenetic modification plays a fundamental role in fibroblast activation and CAF differentiation (Hu et al., 2005; Jiang et al., 2008; Bechtel et al., 2010; Lamprecht et al., 2018). Indeed, an overall hypomethylated status was found in human CAFs (Jiang et al., 2008; Eckert et al., 2019) (**Figure 2**), as well as in functionally related fibrotic fibroblasts (Komatsu et al., 2012). Nevertheless, certain key genes appear hypermethylated in CAFs such as *Tgfbr2* (Banerjee et al., 2014), *RASAL1* and others (Bechtel et al., 2010; Zeisberg and Zeisberg, 2013; Mishra et al., 2018). Seminal work by Cedric Gaggioli's group demonstrated that tumor-derived LIF induces activation of DNMT3b and p300-HAT in CAFs, which sustain JAK1/STAT3 signaling, necessary to maintain a pro-invasive activity (Albrengues et al., 2015). More recently, the nicotinamide N-methyltransferase has been shown as fundamental for CAF´s protumoral behavior *in vitro* and *in vivo*, directly affecting DNA and histone methylation (Eckert et al., 2019). CAF differentiation and activity *in vivo* can be blocked by treating with the DNMT inhibitor 5′-Aza-2′-deoxycytidine (Albrengues et al., 2015; Eckert et al., 2019), acting specifically in pancreatic CAFs compared to normal fibroblasts (Yu et al., 2012). Relevant results when DNMT inhibitors are considered for therapy, which will be further discussed below.

Interestingly, the RasGTP *RASAL3*, negative regulator of the Ras signaling pathway, was also found hypermethylated in prostate cancer (PCa) CAFs (Mishra et al., 2018), increasing Ras signaling in these cells, which drives support of tumor growth and neuroendocrine differentiation. Noteworthy, switch in CAFs towards a Warburg metabolism has been implicated in tumor immune evasion in PCa (Comito et al., 2019), which adds further clinical relevance of epigenetic-mediated changes in CAFs metabolism. Indeed, an *in vitro* 3D-microfluidoc system has shown that CAFs provide metabolic support to proliferation and invasion of BC cells (Shi et al., 2015). The role of epigenetic modifications in this phenomenon and its relevance *in vivo* will require further investigation.

Besides DNA methylation, other epigenetic modifications have been observed in the tumor stroma (Li et al., 2015; Du and Che, 2017; Schoepp et al., 2017; Vafaee et al., 2017; Zhao et al., 2017; Kim et al., 2018). In a proof-of-concept study, Zong et al. showed that overexpression of the non-histone chromosomal high-mobility group protein family member Hmga2 in urogenital sinus mesenchymal cells drives tumorigenesis in a model for prostatic intraepithelial neoplasia (Zong et al., 2012). In models for pancreatic cancer and *in situ* skin squamous cell carcinomas, an inhibitor of the BRD and extraterminal domain (BET) family proteins decreases tumor growth affecting specifically CAF´s secretome (Yamamoto et al., 2016; Kim et al., 2017). Since targeting histone acetylation has been proposed for combined therapy in BC (Yoon et al., 2011), it would be necessary to characterize the histone acetylation status of stromal cells in BC patients.

Many studies show that miRNAs play fundamental roles in CAF differentiation and function, a subject that has been extensively reviewed (Chou et al., 2013; Kohlhapp et al., 2015; Kuninty et al., 2016; Marks et al., 2016). MiRNAs can be expressed by CAFs or incorporated from other sources, mainly cancer cells *via* exosomes (Pang et al., 2015). The opposite is also possible, when CAFs modulate cancer cell behavior *via* transfer of miRNAs (Josson et al., 2015; Shah et al., 2015). In BC, a study compared miRNA expression between fibroblasts from healthy and tumoral human bladder, finding higher expression of miR-16 and miR-320 (Enkelmann et al., 2011). Which functions are these miRNAs regulating in CAFs and whether they can be used as surrogate markers for stroma abundance would require further investigations.

Tumor Endothelial Cells

In solid cancers, increased *de novo* formation of blood vasculature, known as angiogenesis, is normally observed and provides adequate nourishment for the growing tumor (**Figure 2**). The link between vasculature density and worse prognosis in BC is well documented (Bochner et al., 1995). Indeed, targeting angiogenesis *via* disruption of vascular endothelial growth factor (VEGF) signaling is being considered for treating BC in combination with existing therapies (Petrylak et al., 2016; Sonpavde and Bellmunt, 2016).

Tumor endothelial cells (TECs) display a number of characteristics compared to normal endothelium (Hashizume et al., 2000; Hida et al., 2004). In BC, exacerbated proliferation and sprouting of TECs has been linked to staging and lower survival in patients (Roudnicky et al., 2013; Roudnicky et al., 2017). Invasive BC cell lines show increased adhesion to endothelial cells *via* MUC1 and CD43 binding to ICAM-1, which could be linked to metastatic potential (Laurent et al., 2014; Sundar Rajan et al., 2017). Besides, an *in vitro* study shows that TECs may promote BC cell growth through a paracrine loop involving secretion of epidermal growth factor by TECs in response to tumor-derived VEGFs (Huang et al., 2019b). Finally, TECs have been found in MIBC with aberrant expression of a non-anti-angiogenic thrombospondin-2 variant, also responsible for uncontrolled angiogenesis in these tumors (Roudnicky et al., 2018).

It is well known that epigenetic modifications play a role in endothelial cell (ECs) proliferation, differentiation and pathogenesis (Hulshoff et al., 2018; Nagai et al., 2018; Schlereth et al., 2018; Stone et al., 2018; Nicorescu et al., 2019). In fact, recent work by Wang S. and colleagues shows that response to VEGFA, a master regulator of EC biology, strongly relies on epigenetic mechanisms (Wang et al., 2019). Although less explored, several studies have addressed the role of epigenetic modifications in TECs (Marks et al., 2016). Chromatin remodeling inhibitors reduce tumor growth and angiogenesis by acting on both tumor cells (Kim et al., 2001) and ECs (Deroanne et al., 2002; Hellebrekers et al., 2006). More specifically, high expression of EZH2 in ECs is associated with high-stage and grade, and decreased overall survival in epithelial ovarian cancers (Lu et al., 2010). The authors showed that tumor-derived VEGFs induce expression of EZH2 in ECs, which in turn drives hypermethylation of the anti-angiogenic gene, *Vash1* (Lu et al., 2010) (**Figure 2**). Of note, EZH2 expression in ECs is also under control of the vascular endothelial cadherin, which appears reduced in ovarian TECs (Morini et al., 2018). As new anti-cancer therapies targeting both DNMTs and methylation readers evolve, it is necessary to evaluate their effect in TECs.

Importantly, CAF and TEC biology has a meeting point in what is known as endothelial-to-mesenchymal transition (EndMT) in cancer (Zeisberg et al., 2007). By ChIP-seq, Nagai N. and collaborators found that the transcription factor ERG/FLI1 associates with H3K27ac marks at enhancer/promoter regions of various EC-specific genes, inducing expression of miR-126, which represses EndMT genes. Using available data, the authors also found that lower expression of ERG was significantly related to poor prognosis (Nagai et al., 2018).

NEW THERAPIES IN EPIGENETICS

Epigenetic changes have been suggested as essential for tumor development (Biswas and Rao, 2017). As discussed before, aberrant DNA methylation, histone modifications and chromatin states, as well as aberrant expression of ncRNAs can be used as potential targets by specific drugs and combined with existing therapies. Several molecules targeting epigenetic alterations have been developed and used in different cancers. In the following section, we describe the most recent cancer drugs targeting some epigenetic enzymes. Although in most cases their applications in BC are still in its very early days, we will focus on how they are currently studied in this context.

Drugs Targeting Writers

DNA Methyltransferase Inhibitors

DNMTs inhibitors (DNTMi) are classified in two major subtypes: nucleoside and non-nucleoside inhibitors. Decitabine (5-aza-2'-deoxycytidine) and Azacytidine (5-azacytidine) are cytosine analogues and the best known nucleoside DNMTi. Decitabine and Azacytidine are currently approved by FDA for the treatment of specific forms of myelodysplastic syndromes, chronic myelomonocytic leukemia and acute myeloid leukemia (Lu et al., 2011; Giagounidis et al., 2014). Regarding BC, *in vitro* experiments have demonstrated that Decitabine enhances cisplatin susceptibility, suggesting that combination of both drugs could improve clinical responses (Shang et al., 2008; Wu et al., 2019b). Moreover, Decitabine has completed phase II trials for treatment of BC and phase I trials in combination with tetrahydrouridine (Shang et al., 2008; Bertino and Otterson, 2011).

Second generation nucleoside DNMTi, such as Guadecitabine (SGI-110) or 4'-thio-2'- deoxycytidine, have been developed in order to reduce high toxicity without reducing the therapeutic dose needed. Clinical trials for 4'-thio-2'- deoxycytidine are currently recruiting patients for the treatment of advanced solid tumors (NCT03366116). On the other hand, SGI-110 is in clinical stage for various cancers such as acute myeloid leukemia and myeloidDdysplastic syndrome (NCT03603964), and for different solid tumors like advanced hepatocellular carcinomas (NCT01752933). Also, it has been tested in combination with other therapies such as Ipilimumab in metastatic melanoma (NCT02608437) or with carboplatin in ovarian cancer (NCT01696032), among others. As immune checkpoint inhibitors are currently used in BC, their combination with these second generation DNMTi could represent an attractive scenario to improve the therapeutic response or to expand the number of patients that benfit from immunotherapy. Some others like SGI-1027, a quinoline derivative, and Nanaomycin A, a quinone antibiotic, which are reported to inhibit all three DNMTs or only DNMT3a, respectively, are in preclinical stages for colorectal cancer (Datta et al., 2009; Kuck et al., 2010) (**Figure 3** and **Table 1**).

Apart from these inhibitors, various non-nucleoside DNMTi have been developed and suggested to minimize the direct effect on DNA (Villar-garea et al., 2003). Non-nucleoside analogues, such as Procainamide and MG98, inhibit methylation by binding to the CpG regions of DNA and blocking the activity of DNMTs. MG98, for example, was tested against metastatic renal cell carcinoma but the clinical trial was stopped due to its toxicity (Winquist et al., 2006). However, it has also been evaluated in combination with interferon and results are promising at a specific dose (Amato et al., 2012). Moreover, MG98 was tested in BC patients but the researchers did not find response to the treatment (Plummer et al., 2009).

Histone Lysine Methyltransferase Inhibitors

As it was previously described in this review, HMTs such as G9a and EZH2 are considered oncogenic epigenetic factors in BC (Cho et al., 2015). One of the first histone lysine methyltransferase inhibitors (HKMTi), specific against G9a (EHMT2), was BIX-01294 (Kubicek et al., 2007), which has been shown to inhibit cell proliferation in BC cell lines and induce apoptosis in neuroblastoma cells (Cui et al., 2015). Since then, numerous and improved inhibitors related to G9a blocking have been developed. Various studies have been carried out in molecules like A-366, BRD4770 or UNC0638, in different types of cancer such as neuroblastoma, breast or leukemias (Vedadi et al., 2012; Yuan et al., 2012; Pappano et al., 2015).

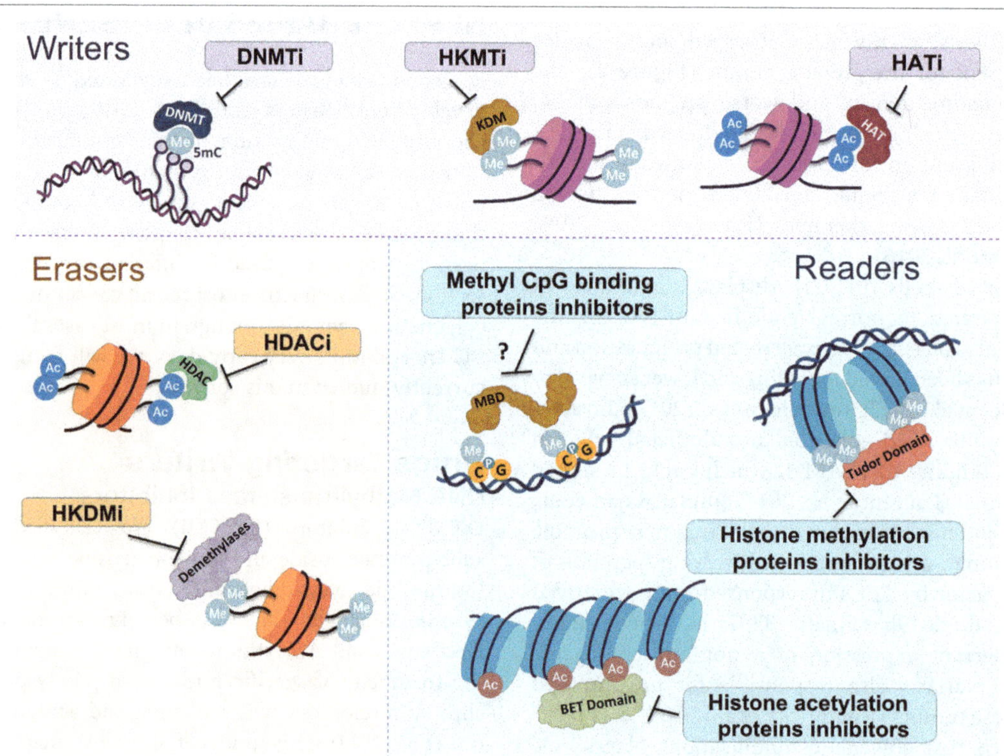

FIGURE 3 | Most representative epigenetic inhibitors targeting writers, readers and erasers. Epigenetic alterations are considered to be reversible and, therefore, all these molecules are subject of study as promising therapeutic targets for cancer treatment. Three main groups of epigenetic drugs can be distinguished according to their targets. The group of compounds targeting epigenetic writers consists mainly of DNMT, HKMT and HAT inhibitors. The second group is directed against epigenetic erasers, which includes HDAC and HKDM inhibitors. Finally, inhibitors of methyl CpG binding proteins, histone methylation and acetylation proteins form the third group targeting epigenetic readers. DNMTi, methyltranferases of DNA inhibitor; HKMTi, histone lysine methyltransferase inhibitor; HATi, histone acetyltransferase inhibitor; HDACi, histone deacetylase inhibitor; HKDMi, histone lysine demethylase inhibitor.

TABLE 1 | A representation of experimental epigenetic drugs targeting writers, readers and erasers.

Category	Compound Name	Development Stage	Cancer Type	References
Drugs Targeting Epigenetic Writers				
DNA Methyltransferase inhibitors (DNMTi)				
Nucleoside analogue	Decitabine	Approved	MDS	Giagounidis et al., 2014; Lu et al., 2011
	Azacytidine	Approved	MDS	Giagounidis et al., 2014; Lu et al., 2011
	Guadecitabine	Clinical	MDS, AML	NCT03603964
Non-nucleoside analogue	MG98	Clinical	MRCC	Winquist et al., 2006
	SGI-1027	Preclinical	Colorectal	Datta et al., 2009
	Nanaomycin A	Preclinical	Colorectal	Kuck et al., 2010
Histone Lysine Methyltransferase inhibitors (HKMTi)				
G9a	A-366	Preclinical	Neuroblastoma	Pappano et al., 2015
	BRD4770	Preclinical	Breast	Vedadi et al., 2012
	UNC0638	Preclinical	Leukemia	Yuan et al., 2012
EZH2	UNC1999	Preclinical	Large B-cell lymphoma	Konze et al., 2014
	GSK343	Preclinical	Glioblastoma	Yu et al., 2017
	GSK126	Clinical	Large B-cell lymphomas	NCT02082977
	EPZ6438	Clinical	B-cell Lymphomas	NCT03010982
Histone Acetyltransferase inhibitors (HATi)				
p300	C646	Preclinical	Gastric	Gajer et al., 2015
	PU141	Preclinical	Neuroblastoma	Wang et al., 2017
Drugs Targeting Epigenetic Readers				
Histone Methylation Proteins				
PHD Finger Domain (JARID1A)	Amiodarone	Preclinical	AML	Wagner et al., 2012
MBT Domain	UNC926	Preclinical	Target domain inhibition	Herold et al., 2012
Chromodomain (CBX7)	MS37452	Preclinical	Target domain inhibition	Ren et al., 2015
Histone Acetylation Proteins				
Bet Bromodomain	(+) - JQ1	Preclinical	Colorectal	Zhang et al., 2018b
	OTX015	Clinical	Advanced Solid tumors	NCT02698176
Drugs Targeting Epigenetic Erasers				
Histone Lysine demethylase inhibitors (HKDMi)				
LSD1 Inhibitors	Pargyline	Preclinical	Target domain inhibition	Yang et al., 2018b
	HCl-2509	Preclinical	Neuroblastoma	Gupta et al., 2018
JmjC Domain inhibitors	IOX1	Preclinical	Target domain inhibition	Hopkinson et al., 2013
Histone Deacetylase inhibitors (HDACi)				
Hydroxamic Acid Derivates	Vorinostat	Approved	CTCL	Mann et al., 2007
	Panobinostat	Approved	Blood neoplasias	Eckschlager et al., 2017
	Reminostat	Clinical	Hodgkin's lymphoma	NCT01037478
	Quisinostat	Clinical	Ovarian cancer	NCT02948075

MDS, Myelodysplastic syndromes; MRCC, Metastasic renal cell carcinoma; AML, Acute Myeloid Leukaemia; CTCL, Cutaneous T cell-lymphoma.

Recently, CM272 was described as a novel G9a/DNMT1 dual inhibitor with remarkable antitumor effect in BC *in vitro* and *in vivo* (José-Enériz et al., 2017; Segovia et al., 2019). On the same line, the catalytic subunits of PRC2, EZH1 and EZH2, which catalyze the methylation of H3K27, have been well described in cancer. Some inhibitors of this complex have been studied and they are classified into three groups: (i) pyridone-indazole scaffold like UNC1999 or GSK343 (Konze et al., 2014; Yu et al., 2017) which has been demonstrated to inhibit BC cell lines growth and metastasis (Chen et al., 2019), (ii) pyridone-indole scaffold such as GSK126 (NCT02082977) and (iii) pyridone-phenyl scaffold including EPZ6438 (Brach et al., 2017), known also as Tazemetostat, which has achieved phase I/II trial (NCT03854474) for the treatment of patients with locally advanced or metastatic urothelial carcinoma in combination with pembrolizumab. The potential use of EZH2 in the BC context has been recently reviewed and discussed (Martínez-Fernández et al., 2015c; Segovia and Paramio, 2017).

Histone Acetyltransferase Inhibitors

HATs are typically grouped into three broad families, namely the p300/CBP, the Gcn5 related N-acetyl-transferase and the MYST family. Among them, p300/CBP seems to be frequently mutated in BC (Duex et al., 2018a) and was reported to be associated with doxorubicin resistance (Takeuchi et al., 2012), so it could be a promising molecular therapeutic target for this disease. Accordingly, C646 and PU141 have been demonstrated to be promising in gastric cancer and neuroblastoma, respectively (Gajer et al., 2015; Wang et al., 2017). However, there is very little evidence for useful histone acetyltransferase inhibitors (HATi) being developed and tested (Baell and Miao, 2016), even though the search for new small-molecule HATi has been intense in the last decades (**Figure 3**). Although, to our knowledge no HATi are being tested in BC, it is important to consider that HAT gene deficiencies may confer susceptibilities to other inhibitors, opening new possible therapeutic approaches for various tumors, including BC (Ogiwara et al., 2016).

Drugs Targeting Readers

Methyl CpG Binding Proteins

Sites of DNA methylation recruit two important protein families: MBD and ZnF proteins. The MBD protein family uses its DNA binding domains and other protein-protein domains to alter the transcriptional state of the DNA (Ginder and Williams, 2018). However, the MBD family is not the only protein family that allows the recognition of methylated DNA; for example, the Kaiso protein family (Kaiso/ZBTB33, ZBTB4 and ZBTB38) uses a three-finger zinc motif to bind methylated CGCG (Hendrich and Bird, 2015). Additionally, it has been demonstrated that ZBTB38 promotes cell migration, invasive growth and EMT in BC cell lines (Jing et al., 2018), whereas high MBD2 expression was significantly associated with reduced bladder carcinoma risk (Zhu et al., 2004). Even though different experimental approaches have identified these proteins as good therapeutic targets, inhibitors have not yet been developed to slow down their action (**Figure 3**).

Histone Methylation Proteins

The histone methyl protein family is a large family of proteins that binds differently to methylated lysine and arginine residues and can be divided into several subfamilies: Tudor domain, PHD finger, MBT, chromodomain and BRD. The most studied family among them is the PHD family, which comprises a group of versatile readers of the epigenome that can recognize both methylation and acetylation marks and has been involved in cancer progression (Hayami et al., 2010). Recently, Wagner et al. discovered various compounds that inhibit the PHD of this protein (Wagner et al., 2012). Among them, Amiodarone is able to induce apoptosis in the T24 BC cell line (Bognar et al., 2017). Upregulated UHRF1 (E3 ubiquitin-protein ligase 1), which contains PHDs, has also been shown to promote BC cell invasion *in vitro* and *in vivo* by epigenetic silencing of KiSS1 (Zhang et al., 2014).

Histone Acetylation Proteins

In general, histone acetylation is related to transcriptional activation. Different protein domains that bind specifically to acetylated histones have been identified so far, including the BRD, double PHD finger and Yeats domains. The BRD family identifies acetylated lysine residues, such as those on the *N*-terminal tails of histones, and has been proposed as an attractive therapeutic target due to its involvement in various cancer types. The BET family has been thoroughly investigated (Biswas and Rao, 2018). The first inhibitors of the BET family, I-BET762 (GSK525762) and (+)-JQ1, were reported in 2010 (Filippakopoulos et al., 2010). The inhibitor I-BET762 has recently been studied for dose escalation clinical studies to investigate the safety, pharmacokinetics, pharmacodynamics, and clinical activity in various tumors (NCT01587703), but BC patients were not included in this study. (+)-JQ1 interferes with BRD4 function, blocking the formation of the NUT-BRD4 oncoprotein, and various studies have shown its efficacy in hematological and solid malignancies (Abedin et al., 2016; Ocaña et al., 2017; Gao et al., 2018; Sakaguchi et al., 2018; Tan et al., 2018; Zhang et al., 2018b). Regarding BC, the (+)-JQ1 inhibitor induces autophagy through activation of the LKB1/AMPK pathway, contributing to the inhibition of proliferation of BC cell lines *in vitro* (Li et al., 2019). In combination with Mitomicyn C, (+)-JQ1 enhances cell death, which offers the possibility of a dose reduction of the chemotherapeutic agent (Simm et al., 2018). Hölscher et al. had also shown significant synergistic effects on the induction of apoptosis in urothelial cancer cells by treatment with (+)-JQ1 and Romidepsin, an HDAC inhibitor (HDACi), thus suggesting a promising new combination therapy approach for urothelial cancer (Hölscher et al., 2018).

Even though BRD3 inhibitors have not been studied as much as those of the BRD2/4, it has been observed that I-BET151, a pan-BET inhibitor that targets BRD3 (Picaud et al., 2013), halts the progression of the cell cycle and decreases cell proliferation *in vitro* and *in vivo* by targeting lncRNA *HOTAIR* in glioblastoma (Pastori et al., 2014). Remarkably, *HOTAIR* increased expression is also associated with poor clinical outcome in BC (Martínez-Fernández et al., 2015b), thereby indicating the possible relevance of studying I-BET151 inhibitor in this type of cancer.

Drugs Targeting Erasers

Epigenetic marks can be 'erased', depending on the requirement of the cell, by a group of enzymes that oppose to the writers. Since they also modulate gene expression affecting tumor suppressor genes or oncogenes, they can be considered potential targets.

Histone Lysine Demethylase Inhibitors

Researchers have been exploring inhibitory molecules for the HKDMs KDM1 (LSD1) and KDM2-8 for years (Højfeldt et al., 2013). Early compounds were developed based on the structural characteristics of LSD1 (Yang et al., 2018b). Treatment with LSD1 inhibitor supressed BC cell proliferation and androgen-induced transcription, supporting a novel role for the androgen receptor-KDM (lysine demethylases) complex in BC initiation and progression (Kauffman et al., 2012). Even though numerous LSD1 inhibitors have been reported in the literature, they are in the initial phase of development and there are still many problems that have to be overcome before histone lysine demethylase inhibitors (HKDMi) can reach the clinic (**Figure 3**).

Histone Deacetylase Inhibitors

Various reports have shown that HDACs could be involved in regulating protein function and tumorigenesis. In this line, the use of HDACi has been clinically validated in cancer treatment and, so far, four drugs have been approved by the FDA: Vorinostat, Romidepsin, Panobinostat and Belinostat (**Figure 3**). Vorinostat was the first pan-HDACi approved by the FDA for the treatment of advanced primary cutaneous T-cell lymphoma (Mann et al., 2007). Next, various pharmaceutical companies developed other molecules such as Panobinostat or Belinostat (Eckschlager et al., 2017), all of them intended initially for blood neoplasias.

Moreover, HDACi are being studied for BC therapy (Kaletsch et al., 2018). Romidepsin and Vorinostat have been tested in a phase II trial as monotherapy, and Vorinostat has also completed phase I trials as a combination therapy with docetaxel, but it was surprisingly toxic and had limited efficacy (Cheung et al., 2008). Additionally, Belinostat has obtained positive responses in BC cells through decreasing cell proliferation *in vitro* and *in vivo* (Buckley et al., 2007) and is being tested in clinical trials against various solid tumors including BC (NCT00413322, NCT00413075).

Apart from the hydroxamic acid derivates, which are approved for the clinic, other molecules are in different phases of study. Some of them are Reminostat (4SC-201) evaluated for Hodgkin's lymphoma (NCT01037478), Quisinostat (JNJ-26481585) for the treatment of ovarian cancer (NCT02948075), or Abexinostat (PCI-24781) which is being evaluated for sarcoma in combination with Doxorubicin (NCT01027910). **Table 1** summarizes HDACi approved and some experimental HDACi in different stages of clinical development.

Epigenetic drugs, as seen previously, have been approved as monotherapy for the treatment of different types of cancer. In addition, the combination of epigenetic drugs with standard chemotherapy or immunotherapy has been explored in recent years with promising results. The basis for this approach comes from results showing that epigenetic drugs reduce the apoptotic threshold, reverse drug resistance and/or induce immune response. Regarding BC, a large proportion of patients are not candidates to chemotherapy due to comorbidities. The use of epigenetic drugs could bring the possibility of a dose reduction, which makes these compounds attractive candidates for combination therapy for these BC patients (Witjes et al., 2014b; Fardi et al., 2018).

Drugs Targeting ncRNAs

LncRNAs

Even though no lncRNA-based targeted BC treatment has been developed so far, modulation of lncRNA expression as a therapy seems promising and has already been described for other cancer types (Bhan et al., 2017). Methods described for the modulation of lncRNA expression include the use of antisense oligonucleotide (ASO) or lncRNA-specific siRNAs for transcript destabilization or degradation, as well as transcript alteration by modulation of lncRNA-encoded promotor activity. Additionally, functional disruption of lncRNAs through aptamers antagonizing the interaction with their binding partners, or the production of synthetic molecules interfering with the association between lncRNAs and regulatory factors, are possible mechanisms to modulate lncRNA expression (Bhan et al., 2017). Finally, these ncRNAs might be valuable in combination therapy and augmentation of therapeutic efficacy since modulation of their expression can enhance the therapeutic sensitivity of tumors (Bhan et al., 2017).

MiRNAs

There are many approaches that have been employed to silence miRNAs in cancer. These include anti-miRNA oligonucleotides (AMOs), miRNA-masking antisense oligonucleotides, peptide nucleic acids and miRNA sponges (Garzon et al., 2010). AMOs mechanism relies on the complementary base pairing of the oligonucleotide sequence to its target miRNA. Therefore, these molecules can repress cellular mRNAs involved in tumor progression and proliferation, and they can also act as competitive inhibitors of miRNAs and impair their interaction with other molecules (Lima et al., 2018b). Joana Filipa and colleagues showed that, using AMOs, they were able to silence the expression of upregulated miR-9 in a cancer cell model of gastric cancer (Lima et al., 2018a).

For BC treatment, there are some indirect therapeutic approaches that affect miRNA expression. For instance, some EZH2 inhibitors act in BC cells modulating the expression of miR-101 (Wang et al., 2014) or miR-143 (Zhang et al., 2015). However, some of these miRNAs are also induced by specific oncogenic insults in BC, indicating the potential problems of considering them as possible targets for treatment (Segovia et al., 2017).

Remarkably, a miRNA-based drug mimicking miR-34a has reached a phase I clinical trial (NCT01829971). MiRNA-34a significance in various human cancers, including BC, is increasingly recognized nowadays (Bader, 2012; Misso et al., 2014), hence the expectation in this new approach.

Other nCRNAs

CircRNAs and piRNAs have been described as a promising therapeutic target in multiple cancer types, including BC (see corresponding section). Potential strategies for the modulation of circRNA expression include the use of ASOs or siRNAs in order to antagonize these ncRNAs, as well as the application of the CRISPR/Cas system to partially or completely remove oncogenic circRNAs (Zhang and Xin, 2018). Regarding the modulation of piRNA expression, possible strategies include the use of synthetic piRNAs at the transcriptional and posttranscriptional level, while antibodies against PIWI proteins might be effective as a posttranscriptional approach (Assumpção et al., 2015). Nonetheless, none of these approaches are being tested in BC therapy so far.

EPIGENETIC ALTERATIONS AS BIOMARKERS IN BC: THE POTENTIAL USE OF LIQUID BIOPSY

Regarding diagnosis and surveillance of BC, a combination of cystoscopy and urine cytology is the most widely used methodology nowadays. Currently, cystoscopy is the gold standard method in clinical practice for detection and follow-up of this disease, with a sensitivity of 85–90% to detect exophytic tumors. However, this technique is highly invasive, showing a big inter-observer and intra-observer variation. On the other hand, BC urinary cytology shows a specificity of approximately 98% but a low sensitivity of 38%. The high rates of recurrence and progression of BC require continuous follow-up of patients by cystoscopy (every 3–6 months during the next 5 years) and urine cytology, making BC one of the most costly malignancies for the National Health systems of developed countries (Lodewijk et al., 2018).

For these reasons, there is a clear need to improve the current systems of diagnosis, prognosis and surveillance of BC patients. Based on the important role of epigenetic modifications in this disease, status evaluation of the involved molecules could contribute to improve these available systems. In this context, liquid biopsy has emerged as a non-invasive way to determine the genomic landscape of cancer patients, as well as to monitor treatment response, quantify minimal residual disease, and assess therapy resistance (Bardelli and Pantel, 2017; Di Meo et al., 2017; Heitzer et al., 2017; Khetrapal et al., 2018). Liquid biopsy makes reference to the sampling and assessment of biological fluids. In genitourinary cancer, due to the proximity of tumors, urine has been considered a bona fide liquid biopsy sample, being one of the most interesting samples for its easy access and collection. However, in MIBC patients after cystectomy, serum and plasma could be the most appropriate liquid biopsy samples given its invasive and metastatic character (Lodewijk et al., 2018). Currently, there are several systems to detect and follow-up BC using liquid biopsy biomarkers (including sediment cells in urine samples, CTCs in blood samples as well as RNAs and proteins in both cases), which present sensitivity and specificity values within a range of 38–98% and 65–98%, respectively (Lodewijk et al., 2018). The determination of epigenetic alterations in liquid biopsy samples, such as variation in expression levels of ncRNAs or changes in DNA methylation profiles, could improve the predictive values of the current systems of BC diagnosis, prognosis and monitoring. Next, some of the most relevant studies of epigenetic biomarkers in urine and serum/plasma samples are discussed.

Non-Coding RNAs as Epigenetic Biomarkers in Liquid Biopsy of BC Patients

Among the different ncRNAs previously described, miRNAs have been the most widely studied molecules in liquid biopsies so far. MiRNA molecules have several characteristics which make them potential candidates as good biomarkers in liquid biopsy samples: i) they show very homogeneous expression levels among individuals and specific expression profiles in different types of tissue (Liang et al., 2007); ii) they are included in a protein complex and, usually, in exosomes, which confers them high stability, preserving their integrity and preventing their degradation (Weber et al., 2010; Ge et al., 2014; Martínez-Fernández et al., 2016); iii) there are several systems designed to determinate ncRNA expression using RT-qPCR, which allow evaluating a large number of miRNAs from very small amounts of total RNA and at a low cost.

Given the potential of miRNAs, many studies have evaluated their predictive properties, individually or in combination, in the urine of BC patients. In this context, high expression levels of miR-146a-5p and miR-106b have been related with invasion and high grade and stage BC (Zhou et al., 2014; Sasaki et al., 2016). NMIBC patients present high levels of miR-214 in urine samples and, curiously, expression of this miRNA was inversely correlated with risk of recurrence of BC patients (Kim et al., 2013). Besides, some miRNAs such as miR-92a-3p and miR-140-5p have been associated with progression after recurrence (Ingelmo-Torres et al., 2017). Yun and collaborators have demonstrated that urine miR-145 expression levels decrease in BC patients with respect to healthy controls, both in non-invasive and invasive tumors (77.8% and 84.1% sensitivity, respectively, and 61.1% specificity in both cases). They observed an association between downregulation of miR-200a and high risk of recurrence in patients with invasive tumors (Yun et al., 2012). Besides, miR-155 has proved to be a good biomarker in urine samples, distinguishing non-invasive tumors, inflammation and healthy controls with a sensitivity of 80.2% and a specificity of 84.6% (Zhang et al., 2016).

As previously mentioned, detection of miRNA deregulation in serum or plasma may have special relevance in invasive and metastatic tumors. Yang and colleagues observed miR-210 increased expression levels in serum samples of BC patients, being associated with tumor stage, grade, and useful to predict tumor progression (AUC = 0.898) (Yang et al., 2015). Moreover, some studies using plasma have found a positive correlation between upregulation of miR-19a and miR-200b with tumor grade and stage respectively, whereas miR-92 and miR-33 presented inverse association with tumor stage (Adam et al., 2013; Feng et al., 2014).

In recent years, several panels of miRNAs (encompassing profiles from 6 to 25 miRNAs) have been developed in both urine and serum for BC diagnosis, prognosis and monitoring of recurrence. In this context, we have recently gathered some of the main miRNA profiles in BC liquid biopsies which can be consulted in Table 2 at Lodewijk et al. (2018).

Although variation in lncRNA expression levels has not been studied as widely as miRNAs in liquid biopsy samples, altered levels of expression of these molecules have been found in urine and blood samples of BC patients. Increased expression levels of *UCA1* in urine samples has been associated with the presence of high-grade NMIBC, and an integrative meta-analysis including more than 500 BC patients and healthy donors determined that its upregulation may predict BC (81% sensitivity and 86% specificity, AUC = 0.88) (Wang et al., 2006; Cui et al., 2017). In addition, other lncRNAs such as *HOTAIR*, *MALAT1*, *HOX-AS-2*, *OTX2-AS1*, *HYMAI*, *LINC00477* and *LOC100506688*, have shown upregulation in urine exosomes of MIBC patients (Berrondo et al., 2016). In addition, *H19* gene expression is significantly higher in BC patients, and its presence has been detected in the urine of 90.5% of patients *versus* 25.9% of healthy controls (AUC = 0.933) (Gielchinsky et al., 2017).

Additionally, other ncRNAs such as piRNAs and circRNA have been evaluated in biofluids. Both molecules have shown a particular resistance to degradation by exoribonuclease, making them ideal candidates for biomarker development (Pardini and Naccarati, 2017; Vo et al., 2019). Several studies have reported that piRNAs are widely detected in liquid biopsy samples, being especially abundant in urine samples and, therefore, good candidates as new biomarkers for BC. Although no deregulated piRNAs have been found in urine or blood of BC patients so far, expression level alterations of some of these molecules have been shown in liquid biopsy samples of other tumor types (Freedman et al., 2016; Iliev et al., 2016; Yuan et al., 2016; Pardini and Naccarati, 2017). Regarding circRNA, Vo and collaborators have recently developed MiOncoCirc, a technology based on exome capture RNA-seq, which stands as the first cancer-focused circRNA resource to facilitate the study of circRNAs as new biological markers of cancer (Vo et al., 2019). They were able to identify candidate circRNAs which could serve as biomarkers for prostate cancer, detecting circRNAs in urine (Vo et al., 2019). This technology could open new possibilities to find new biomarkers with predictive values in liquid biopsy samples of BC patients. Nevertheless, even though circRNAs show great potential as valuable biomarker in urine, these RNAs seem to be highly susceptible to circulating RNA endonucleases showing a half-life of only 15 seconds in human serum, which limits their use as a biomarker in this biological fluid (Jeck and Sharpless, 2014).

DNA Methylation Profiles as Epigenetic Biomarkers in Liquid Biopsy of BC Patients.

As mentioned above, changes in methylation are chemically stable and have been broadly reported in BC. Therefore, they are an interesting source of candidate biomarkers to be detected in biofluids including both blood and urine. Currently, there are multiple methods for detecting changes in methylation comprising global genome methylation and specific genes of interest assays. The majority of methods to evaluate specific genes are based on bisulfite conversion followed by PCR and sequencing, pyrosequencing or methylation-specific PCR, among others, which generally show a high sensitivity and specificity and low assay-to-assay variability (Kurdyukov and Bullock, 2016). Already in 2002, Valenzuela and collaborators found that methylation in *p16(lNK4a)* promoter in serum could be useful as diagnostic biomarker with 22% of sensitivity, 95% of specificity and a positive predictive value of 0.98 (Valenzuela et al., 2002). Also in serum, both the methylation in promoters of protocadherin 17 (*PCDH17*) and protocadherin-10 (*PCDH10*) showed an association with BC poor prognosis (Lin et al., 2012; Luo et al., 2014). A slight association between hypermethylation in *p16(lNK4a)* and *DAPK* promoter regions and NMIBC has been also described (Jabłonowski et al., 2011). Finally, the presence of hypermethylated DNA in *APC*, *GSTP1* or *TIG1* in the serum of BC patients was associated with a worse outcome showing 80% sensitivity and 93% specificity for BC detection (Ellinger et al., 2015).

Important for BC, alterations in DNA methylation can be also assessed both in circulating cell-free DNA and in cells shed into urine. In general, it seems that a prevalence of hypermethylated genes is found in urine from BC patients. For instance, the evaluation of methylation in *TWIST1* and *NID2* in urine sediment has shown 90% sensitivity and 93% specificity (Renard et al., 2010; Fantony et al., 2017; van der Heijden et al., 2018). Other studies showed promising results using methylation of *CFTR*, *SALL3* and *TWIST1* genes in urine cell pellets in combination with cytology (van der Heijden et al., 2018). Interestingly, *SOX-1*, *IRAK3*, and *Li-MET* genes methylation status has showed better recurrence predictivity than urine cytology and cystoscopy (80 vs. 35 vs. 15%) (Su et al., 2014). Also in urine sediments, methylation in *p14ARF*, *p16INK4A*, *RASSF1A*, *DAPK*, and *APC* showed a correlation with BC grade and stage (Pietrusiński et al., 2017). Guo et al. used the methylation status for *VIM*, *RASSF1A*, *GDF15*, and *TMEFF2* to identify BC with 82% sensitivity and 53% specificity (Li et al., 2018b). *RBBP8* has been identified as almost exclusively hypermethylated in BC (Mijnes et al., 2018), while Chen et al. showed *CDH13* methylation as a biomarker with prognostic value for BC screening in urine samples (Ren et al., 2016). Using quantitative methylation-specific PCR, a novel two-gene panel with high accuracy in an urine-based test has just been described (Bosschieter et al., 2019). When stratifying in low- or high-risk NMIBC patients, 97.6% sensitivity and 84.8% specificity were obtained using promoter hypermethylation of *HS3ST2*, *SEPTIN9* and *SLIT2* genes in combination with *FGFR3* mutation (Roperch et al., 2016). Interestingly, Patchsung et al. obtained a sensitivity and specificity of 96% for BC screening using a combination of the urinary hypomethylated *LINE-1* loci and the plasma protein carbonyl content (Patchsung et al., 2012). But methylation value has not only been studied in genes and their promoters: for example, last year Shindo et al. reported a study using the methylation of four miRNAs (miR-9-3, miR-124-2, miR-124-3, and miR-137) in voided urine samples, finding an association with recurrence and radical cystectomy (Kitajima et al., 2017).

As a consequence of these new results, there are currently several clinical trials using promising urine-based tests. Among them, Bladder EpiCheck™ (based on the use of methylation-sensitive restriction enzymes followed by RT-PCR) includes a panel of 15 DNA methylation patterns for the identification of recurrent BC from urine samples. First validation results with data from 357 patients showed 88% specificity and a negative predictive value (NPV) of 94.4% for the detection of any cancer, and a NPV of 99.3% for the detection of high-grade cancer (D'Andrea et al., 2019). Another test is AssureMDx, which uses methylation of *OTX1*, *ONECUT2* and *TWIST1* in addition to mutational load of *FGFR3*, *TERT* and *HRAS* in cell pellets from urine samples, showing a sensitivity of 93–97% and a specificity around 81.7–86% (van Kessel et al., 2017). Finally, Uromark was described 2 years ago as a targeted bisulfite next-generation sequencing assay based on 150 CpG loci to diagnose BC from urine with a sensitivity of 98%, specificity of 97% and NPV of 97% for the detection of primary BC (Feber et al., 2017). Following these results, DETECT I and DETECT II are two multi-centre prospective observational studies designed to conduct a robust validation of the UroMark assay. DETECT I will recruit patients having diagnostic investigations for haematuria, while DETECT II will recruit patients with new or recurrent BC to determine respectively the NPV and the sensitivity of UroMark.

As a conclusion, although validation studies are still ongoing, the recent and promising results prompt us to be optimistic and have confidence in a near clinical implementation of a urine methylation test for BC diagnosis and prognosis.

FUTURE PROSPECTS

It is clear that epigenetics has reshaped most of our concepts of biology and, undoubtedly, molecular biology understanding of human pathologies. From the point of view of those researchers interested in BC, or even in cancer in general, it is almost impossible to predict what the future will bring us in this field, but there are two clear emerging facets at our hands. On the one hand, the use of compounds interfering with many epigenetic processes combined with other therapies currently in the clinics and, on the other hand, the use of these therapies directed not only towards the tumor cells, but also the tumor niche. Obviously, from our current knowledge of immunotherapies, there is a faint border between these two concepts.

Epigenetic drugs, as seen in the previous sections, have been approved as monotherapy for the treatment of different types of cancer. Additionally, they have been shown to synergize with other epigenetic substances or anticancer therapies. The first preclinical investigations focused on the combination of DNMTi and HDACi (Cameron et al., 1999). After a while and due to the development of new epigenetic agents directed to other targets such as HMTs, HDMs or BRDs, new synergistic combinations with DNMTi and/or HDACi are being explored. In addition, due to the importance of immunotherapy in cancer, the combination of epigenetic drugs with standard chemotherapy or immunotherapy has also increased in recent years (Dunn and Rao, 2017). This is based on the theory of using epigenetic drugs to reduce the apoptotic threshold, reverse drug resistance or induce immune responses for further treatment such as chemotherapy or immunotherapy. The concept of partnering epigenetic therapy with reshaping stromal component strategies has generated a wave of translational research that highlights the potential for this approach in many different cancer types. Epigenetic drugs such as DMNTi and HDACi can reverse immune suppression, and modulate stromal cells and extracellular matrix *via* several mechanisms such as enhancing expression of tumor-associated antigens, components of the antigen processing and presenting machinery pathways, immune checkpoint inhibitors, chemokines, and other immune-related genes, as well as changing the CAFs secretomes that will favor or impede the tumor growth. But deep studies of each component interaction are still in their early days. The discoveries in these areas have established a highly promising basis for studies using combined epigenetic and immunotherapeutic agents as anti-cancer therapies with expected long lasting antitumor responses.

Finally, new areas of research such as the use of new gene targeting strategies as therapeutic tools or the potential role of epigenetic mechanisms leading to altered glycosylation, which may clearly impact the liquid biopsy and immunotherapy fields (Dall'Olio and Trinchera, 2017), may represent new horizons in BC management and detection.

AUTHOR CONTRIBUTIONS

All authors contributed equally to review the current literature and write specific sections. The whole work was coordinated by JP. All the authors agreed with the final version.

FUNDING

This study was funded by the following: FEDER cofounded MINECO grant SAF2015-66015-R, grant ISCIII-RETIC RD12/0036/0009, PIE 15/00076 and CB/16/00228 to JP. VM is funded by Consejería de investigación e Innovación, Comunidad de Madrid (ref 2018-T2/BMD-10342).

REFERENCES

Abedin, S. M., Boddy, C. S., and Munshi, H. G. (2016). BET inhibitors in the treatment of hematologic malignancies: current insights and future prospects. *Oncol. Targets Ther.* 9, 5943–5953. doi: 10.2147/OTT.S100515

Adam, L., Wszolek, M. F., Liu, C.-G., Jing, W., Diao, L., Zien, A., et al. (2013). Plasma microRNA profiles for bladder cancer detection. *Urol. Oncol. Semin. Orig. Investig.* 31, 1701–1708. doi: 10.1016/j.urolonc.2012.06.010

Agger, K., Cloos, P. A. C., Christensen, J., Pasini, D., Rose, S., Rappsilber, J., et al. (2007). UTX and JMJD3 are histone H3K27 demethylases involved in HOX gene regulation and development. *Nature* 449, 731–734. doi: 10.1038/nature06145

Agundez, M., Grau, L., Palou, J., Algaba, F., Villavicencio, H., and Sanchez-Carbayo, M. (2011). Evaluation of the Methylation Status of Tumour Suppressor Genes for Predicting Bacillus Calmette-Guérin Response in Patients With T1G3 High-Risk Bladder Tumours. *Eur. Urol.* 60, 131–140. doi: 10.1016/j.eururo.2011.04.020

Albrengues, J., Bertero, T., Grasset, E., Bonan, S., Maiel, M., Bourget, I., et al. (2015). Epigenetic switch drives the conversion of fibroblasts into proinvasive cancer-associated fibroblasts. *Nat. Commun.* 6, 10204. doi: 10.1038/ncomms10204

Allis, C. D., Berger, S. L., Cote, J., Dent, S., Jenuwien, T., Kouzarides, T., et al. (2007). New Nomenclature for Chromatin-Modifying Enzymes. *Cell* 131, 633–636. doi: 10.1016/j.cell.2007.10.039

Amato, R. J., Stephenson, J., Hotte, S., Nemunaitis, J., Karl, B., Reid, G., et al., (2012). MG98, a Second-Generation DNMT1 Inhibitor, in the Treatment of Advanced Renal Cell Carcinoma. *Cancer Invest.* 2, 415–421. doi: 10.3109/07357907.2012.675381.

Anastasiadou, E., Jacob, L. S., and Slack, F. J. (2017). Non-coding RNA networks in cancer. *Nat. Rev. Cancer* 18, 5–18. doi: 10.1038/nrc.2017.99

Ariel, I., de Groot, N., and Hochberg, A. (2000). Imprinted H19 gene expression in embryogenesis and human cancer: the oncofetal connection. *Am. J. Med. Genet.* 91, 46–50. doi: 10.1002/(sici)1096-8628(20000306)91:1<46::aid-ajmg8>3.0.co;2-i

Assumpção, C. B., Calcagno, D. Q., Araújo, T. M. T., Santos, S. E. B., dos, Santos, Â. K. C. R., dos, Riggins, G. J., et al. (2015). The role of piRNA and its potential clinical implications in cancer. *Epigenomics* 7, 975–984. doi: 10.2217/epi.15.37

Babjuk, M., Böhle, A., Burger, M., Capoun, O., Cohen, D., Compérat, E. M., et al. (2017). EAU Guidelines on Non–Muscle-invasive Urothelial Carcinoma of the Bladder: Update 2016. *Eur. Urol.* 71, 447–461. doi: 10.1016/j.eururo.2016.05.041

Bader, A. G. (2012). MiR-34 - a microRNA replacement therapy is headed to the clinic. *Front. Genet.* 3, 1–9. doi: 10.3389/fgene.2012.00120

Baell, J. B., and Miao, W. (2016). Histone acetyltransferase inhibitors: where art thou? *Futur. Med. Chem.* 8, 1525–1528. doi: 10.4155/fmc-2016-0151

Balar, A. V., Galsky, M. D., Rosenberg, J. E., Powles, T., Petrylak, D. P., Bellmunt, J., et al. (2017). Atezolizumab as first-line treatment in cisplatin-ineligible patients with locally advanced and metastatic urothelial carcinoma: a single-arm, multicentre, phase 2 trial. *Lancet* 389, 67–76. doi: 10.1016/S0140-6736(16)32455-2

Balbás-Martínez, C., Sagrera, A., Carrillo-de-Santa-Pau, E., Earl, J., Márquez, M., Vazquez, M., et al. (2013). Recurrent inactivation of STAG2 in bladder cancer is not associated with aneuploidy. *Nat. Genet.* 45, 1464–1469. doi: 10.1038/ng.2799

Banerjee, J., Mishra, R., Li, X., Jackson, R. S., Sharma, A., and Bhowmick, N. A. (2014). A reciprocal role of prostate cancer on stromal DNA damage. *Oncogene* 33, 4924–4931. doi: 10.1038/onc.2013.431

Bardelli, A., and Pantel, K. (2017). Liquid Biopsies, What We Do Not Know (Yet). *Cancer Cell* 31, 172–179. doi: 10.1016/j.ccell.2017.01.002

Barrett, S. P., and Salzman, J., (2016). Circular RNAs: analysis, expression and potential functions. *Development*. 143, 1838–1847. doi: 10.1242/dev.128074

Baylin, S. B., and Jones, P. A. (2016). Epigenetic Determinants of Cancer. *Cold Spring Harb. Perspect. Biol.* 8, a019505. doi: 10.1101/cshperspect.a019505

Baylln, S. B., Herman, J. G., Graff, J. R., Vertino, P. M., and Issa, J.-P. (1997). Alterations in DNA Methylation: A Fundamental Aspect of Neoplasia. *Adv. Cancer Res.* 72, 141–196. doi: 10.1016/S0065-230X(08)60702-2

Bechtel, W., McGoohan, S., Zeisberg, E. M., Müller, G. A., Kalbacher, H., Salant, D. J., et al. (2010). Methylation determines fibroblast activation and fibrogenesis in the kidney. *Nat. Med.* 16, 544–550. doi: 10.1038/nm.2135

Bellmunt, J., de Wit, R., Vaughn, D. J., Fradet, Y., Lee, J. L., Fong, L., et al. (2017). Pembrolizumab as Second-Line Therapy for Advanced Urothelial Carcinoma. *N. Engl. J. Med.* 376, 1015–1026. doi: 10.1056/NEJMoa1613683

Bernstein, B. E., Meissner, A., and Lander, E. S. (2007). The mammalian epigenome. *Cell* 128, 669–681. doi: 10.1016/j.cell.2007.01.033

Berraondo, P., Minute, L., Ajona, D., Corrales, L., Melero, I., and Pio, R. (2016). Innate immune mediators in cancer: between defense and resistance. *Immunol. Rev.* 274, 290–306. doi: 10.1111/imr.12464

Berrondo, C., Flax, J., Kucherov, V., Siebert, A., Osinski, T., Rosenberg, A., et al. (2016). Expression of the long non-coding RNA HOTAIR correlates with disease progression in Bladder Cancer and Is Contained in Bladder Cancer Patient Urinary Exosomes. *PloS One* 11, e0147236. doi: 10.1371/journal.pone.0147236

Bertino, E. M., and Otterson, G. A. (2011). Romidepsin: a novel histone deacetylase inhibitor for cancer. *Expert Opin. Investig. Drugs* 20, 1151–1158. doi: 10.1517/13543784.2011.594437

Bhan, A., Soleimani, M., and Mandal, S. S. (2017). Long noncoding RNA and cancer: A new paradigm. *Cancer Res.* 77, 3965–3981. doi: 10.1158/0008-5472.CAN-16-2634

Bian, C., Chen, Q., and Yu, X. (2015). The zinc finger proteins ZNF644 and WIZ regulate the G9a/GLP complex for gene repression. *ELife* 4(e05606). doi: 10.7554/elife.05606

Bistoni, F., Vecchiarelli, A., Cenci, E., Puccetti, P., Marconi, P., and Cassone, A. (1986). Evidence for macrophage-mediated protection against lethal Candida albicans infection. *Infect. Immun.* 51, 668–674.

Biswas, S., and Rao, C. M. (2017). Epigenetics in cancer: Fundamentals and Beyond. *Pharmacol. Ther.* 173, 118–134. doi: 10.1016/j.pharmthera.2017.02.011

Biswas, S., and Rao, C. M. (2018). Epigenetic tools (The Writers, The Readers and The Erasers) and their implications in cancer therapy. *Eur. J. Pharmacol.* 837, 8–24. doi: 10.1016/j.ejphar.2018.08.021

Bitler, B. G., Aird, K. M., Garipov, A., Li, H., Amatangelo, M., Kossenkov, A. V., et al. (2015). Synthetic lethality by targeting EZH2 methyltransferase activity in ARID1A-mutated cancers. *Nat. Med.* 21, 231–238. doi: 10.1038/nm.3799

Bochner, B. H., Cote, R. J., Weidner, N., Groshen, S., Chen, S.-C., Skinner, D. G., et al. (1995).). Angiogenesis in Bladder Cancer: Relationship Between Microvessel Density and Tumor Prognosis. *JNCI J. Natl. Cancer Inst.* 87, 1603–1612. doi: 10.1093/jnci/87.21.1603

Bock, C., Beerman, I., Lien, W.-H., Smith, Z. D., Gu, H., Boyle, P., et al. (2012). DNA methylation dynamics during *in vivo* differentiation of blood and skin stem cells. *Mol. Cell* 47, 633–647. doi: 10.1016/j.molcel.2012.06.019

Bognar, Z., Fekete, K., Antus, C., Hocsak, E., Bognar, R., Tapodi, A., et al. (2017). Desethylamiodarone—A metabolite of amiodarone—Induces apoptosis on T24 human bladder cancer cells *via* multiple pathways. *PloS One* 12, 1–18. doi: 10.1371/journal.pone.0189470

Bosschieter, J., Nieuwenhuijzen, J. A., Hentschel, A., van Splunter, A. P., Segerink, L. I., Vis, A. N., et al. (2019). A two-gene methylation signature for the diagnosis of bladder cancer in urine. *Epigenomics* 11, 337–347. doi: 10.2217/epi-2018-0094

Brach, D., Johnston-blackwell, D., Drew, A., Lingaraj, T., Motwani, V., Warholic, N. M., et al. (2017). EZH2 Inhibition by Tazemetostat Results in Altered Dependency on B-cell Activation Signaling in DLBCL. *Mol. Cancer Ther.* 16 (11). doi: 10.1158/1535-7163.MCT-16-0840

Bröske, A.-M., Vockentanz, L., Kharazi, S., Huska, M. R., Mancini, E., Scheller, M., et al. (2009). DNA methylation protects hematopoietic stem cell multipotency from myeloerythroid restriction. *Nat. Genet.* 41, 1207–1215. doi: 10.1038/ng.463

Buckley, M. T., Yoon, J., Yee, H., Chiriboga, L., Liebes, L., Ara, G., et al. (2007). The histone deacetylase inhibitor belinostat (PXD101) suppresses bladder cancer cell growth *in vitro* and *in vivo*. *J. Transl. Med.* 5, 1–12. doi: 10.1186/1479-5876-5-49

Cameron, E. E., Bachman, K. E., Myöhänen, S., Herman, J. G., and Baylin, S. B. (1999). Synergy of demethylation and histone deacetylase inhibition in the re-expression of genes silenced in cancer. *Nat. Genet.* 21, 103–107. doi: 10.1038/5047

Cao, R., Tsukada, Y., and Zhang, Y. (2005). Role of Bmi-1 and Ring1A in H2A Ubiquitylation and Hox Gene Silencing. *Mol. Cell* 20, 845–854. doi: 10.1016/J.MOLCEL.2005.12.002

Casadevall, D., Kilian, A. Y., and Bellmunt, J. (2017). The prognostic role of epigenetic dysregulation in bladder cancer: A systematic review. *Cancer Treat. Rev.* 61, 82–93. doi: 10.1016/j.ctrv.2017.10.004

Catto, J. W. F., Azzouzi, A.-R., Rehman, I., Feeley, K. M., Cross, S. S., Amira, N., et al. (2005). Promoter hypermethylation is associated with tumor location, stage, and subsequent progression in transitional cell carcinoma. *J. Clin. Oncol.* 23, 2903–2910. doi: 10.1200/JCO.2005.03.163

Chalbatani, G. M., Dana, H., Memari, F., Gharagozlou, E., Ashjaei, S., Kheirandish, P., et al. (2019). Biological function and molecular mechanism of piRNA in cancer. *Pract. Lab. Med.* 13, 1–6. doi: 10.1016/j.plabm.2018.e00113

Chan, B., Manley, J., Lee, J., and Singh, S. R. (2015). The emerging roles of microRNAs in cancer metabolism. *Cancer Lett.* 356, 301–308. doi: 10.1016/j.canlet.2014.10.011

Chen, W., Wu, W., Li, X., Zhao, L., and Chen, W. (2011). HDAC6 and SIRT2 promote bladder cancer cell migration and invasion by targeting cortactin. *Oncol. Rep.* 27, 819–824. doi: 10.3892/or.2011.1553

Chen, X., Chen, R.-X., Wei, W.-S., Li, Y.-H., Feng, Z.-H., Tan, L., et al. (2018). PRMT5 Circular RNA Promotes Metastasis of Urothelial Carcinoma of the Bladder through Sponging miR-30c to Induce Epithelial–Mesenchymal Transition. *Clin. Cancer Res.* 24, 6319–6330. doi: 10.1158/1078-0432.CCR-18-1270

Chen, X., Wurtmann, E. J., Van Batavia, J., Zybailov, B., Washburn, M. P., and Wolin, S. L. (2007). An ortholog of the Ro autoantigen functions in 23S rRNA maturation in D. radiodurans. *Genes Dev.* 21, 1328–1339. doi: 10.1101/gad.1548207

Chen, Z., Du, Y., Liu, X., Chen, H., Weng, X., Guo, J., et al. (2019). EZH2 inhibition suppresses bladder cancer cell growth and metastasis *via the* JAK2/STAT3 signaling pathway. *Oncol. Lett.* 18, 907–915. doi: 10.3892/ol.2019.10359

Cheung, E. M., Quinn, D. I., Tsao-Wei, D. D., Groshen, S. G., Aparicio, A. M., Twardowski, P., et al. (2008). Phase II study of vorinostat (Suberoylanilide Hydroxamic Acid, SAHA) in patients with advanced transitional cell urothelial cancer (TCC) after platinum-based therapy—California Cancer Consortium/University of Pittsburgh NCI/CTEP-sponsored trial. *J. Clin. Oncol.* 26, 16058–16058. doi: 10.1200/jco.2008.26.15_suppl.16058

Cho, H.-S., Kelly, J. D., Hayami, S., Toyokawa, G., Takawa, M., Yoshimatsu, M., et al. (2015). Enhanced Expression of EHMT2 Is Involved in the Proliferation of Cancer Cells through Negative Regulation of SIAH1. *Neoplasia* 13, 676–IN10. doi: 10.1593/neo.11512

Chou, J., Shahi, P., and Werb, Z. (2013). microRNA-mediated regulation of the tumor microenvironment. *Cell Cycle* 12, 3262–3271. doi: 10.4161/cc.26087

Christov, C. P., Gardiner, T. J., Szuts, D., and Krude, T. (2006). Functional Requirement of Noncoding Y RNAs for Human Chromosomal DNA Replication. *Mol. Cell. Biol.* 26, 6993–7004. doi: 10.1128/mcb.01060-06

Christov, C. P., Trivier, E., and Krude, T. (2008). Noncoding human Y RNAs are overexpressed in tumours and required for cell proliferation. *Br. J. Cancer* 98, 981–988. doi: 10.1038/sj.bjc.6604254

Chu, H., Hui, G., Yuan, L., Shi, D., Wang, Y., Du, M., et al. (2015). Identification of novel piRNAs in bladder cancer. *Cancer Lett.* 356, 561–567. doi: 10.1016/j.canlet.2014.10.004

Chung, W., Bondaruk, J., Jelinek, J., Lotan, Y., Liang, S., Czerniak, B., et al. (2011). Detection of bladder cancer using novel DNA methylation biomarkers in urine sediments. *Cancer Epidemiol. Biomarkers Prev.* 20, 1483–1491. doi: 10.1158/1055-9965.EPI-11-0067

Clark, M. B., Johnston, R. L., Inostroza-Ponta, M., Fox, A. H., Fortini, E., Moscato, P., et al. (2012). Genome-wide analysis of long noncoding RNA stability. *Genome Res.* 22, 885–898. doi: 10.1101/gr.131037.111

Comito, G., Iscaro, A., Bacci, M., Morandi, A., Ippolito, L., Parri, M., et al. (2019). Lactate modulates CD4+ T-cell polarization and induces an immunosuppressive environment, which sustains prostate carcinoma progression *via* TLR8/miR21 axis. *Oncogene* 38, 3681–3695. doi: 10.1038/s41388-019-0688-7

Costa, V. L., Henrique, R., Danielsen, S. A., Duarte-Pereira, S., Eknaes, M., Skotheim, R. I., et al. (2010). Three epigenetic biomarkers, GDF15, TMEFF2, and VIM, accurately predict bladder cancer from DNA-based analyses of urine samples. *Clin. Cancer Res.* 16, 5842–5851. doi: 10.1158/1078-0432.CCR-10-1312

Cui, J., Sun, W., Hao, X., Wei, M., Su, X., Zhang, Y., et al. (2015). EHMT2 inhibitor BIX-01294 induces apoptosis through PMAIP1-USP9X-MCL1 axis in human bladder cancer cells. *Cancer Cell Int.* 15, 1–9. doi: 10.1186/s12935-014-0149-x

Cui, X., Jing, X., Long, C., Yi, Q., Tian, J., and Zhu, J. (2017). Accuracy of the urine UCA1 for diagnosis of bladder cancer: a meta-analysis. *Oncotarget* 8, 35222–35233. doi: 10.18632/oncotarget.16473

D'Andrea, D., Soria, F., Zehetmayer, S., Gust, K. M., Korn, S., Witjes, J. A., et al. (2019). Diagnostic accuracy, clinical utility and influence on decision-making of a methylation urine biomarker test in the surveillance of non-muscle-invasive bladder cancer. *BJU Int.* 123, 959–967. doi: 10.1111/bju.14673

Dall'Olio, F., and Trinchera, M. (2017). Epigenetic Bases of Aberrant Glycosylation in Cancer. *Int. J. Mol. Sci.* 18(5), 998. doi: 10.3390/ijms18050998

Datta, J., Ghoshal, K., Denny, W. A., Gamage, S. A., Darby, G., Phiasivongsa, P., et al. (2009). A New Class of Quinoline-Based DNA Hypomethylating Agents Reactivates Tumor Suppressor Genes by Blocking DNA Methyltransferase 1 Activity and Inducing Its Degradation. *Cancer Res.* 69 (10), 4277–4285. doi: 10.1158/0008-5472.CAN-08-3669

Dawson, M. A., and Kouzarides, T. (2012). Cancer epigenetics: from mechanism to therapy. *Cell* 150, 12–27. doi: 10.1016/j.cell.2012.06.013

De Palma, G., Di Lorenzo, V. F., Krol, S., and Paradiso, A. V. (2019). Urinary exosomal shuttle RNA: Promising cancer diagnosis biomarkers of lower urinary tract. *Int. J. Biol. Markers*, 34 (2), 101–107. doi: 10.1177/1724600819827023

Deb, G., Singh, A. K., and Gupta, S. (2014). EZH2: Not EZHY (Easy) to Deal. *Mol. Cancer Res.* 12, 639–653. doi: 10.1158/1541-7786.MCR-13-0546

Deroanne, C. F., Bonjean, K., Servotte, S., Devy, L., Colige, A., Clausse, N., et al. (2002). Histone deacetylases inhibitors as anti-angiogenic agents altering vascular endothelial growth factor signaling. *Oncogene* 21, 427–436. doi: 10.1038/sj.onc.1205108

Dhalluin, C., Carlson, J. E., Zeng, L., He, C., Aggarwal, A. K., Zhou, M.-M., et al. (1999). Structure and ligand of a histone acetyltransferase bromodomain. *Nature* 399, 491–496. doi: 10.1038/20974

Di Meo, A., Bartlett, J., Cheng, Y., Pasic, M. D., and Yousef, G. M. (2017). Liquid biopsy: A step forward towards precision medicine in urologic malignancies. *Mol. Cancer* 16, 1–14. doi: 10.1186/s12943-017-0644-5

Ding, B., Yan, L., Zhang, Y., Wang, Z., Zhang, Y., Xia, D., et al. (2019). Analysis of the role of mutations in the KMT2D histone lysine methyltransferase in bladder cancer. *FEBS Open Bio* 9, 693–706. doi: 10.1002/2211-5463.12600

Du, H., and Che, G. (2017). Genetic alterations and epigenetic alterations of cancer-associated fibroblasts. *Oncol. Lett.* 13, 3–12. doi: 10.3892/ol.2016.5451

Duex, J. E., Swain, K. E., Dancik, G. M., Paucek, R. D., Owens, C., Churchill, M. E. A., et al. (2018a). Functional Impact of Chromatin Remodeling Gene Mutations and Predictive Signature for Therapeutic Response in Bladder Cancer. *Mol. Cancer Res.* 16, 69–77. doi: 10.1158/1541-7786.MCR-17-0260

Duex, J. E., Swain, K. E., Dancik, G. M., Paucek, R. D., Owens, C., Churchill, M. E. A., et al. (2018b). Functional Impact of Chromatin Remodeling Gene Mutations and Predictive Signature for Therapeutic Response in Bladder Cancer. *Mol. Cancer Res.* 16, 69–77. doi: 10.1158/1541-7786.MCR-17-0260

Dunn, J., and Rao, S. (2017). Epigenetics and immunotherapy: The current state of play. *Mol. Immunol.* 87, 227–239. doi: 10.1016/j.molimm.2017.04.012

Eckert, M. A., Coscia, F., Chryplewicz, A., Chang, J. W., Hernandez, K. M., Pan, S., et al. (2019). Proteomics reveals NNMT as a master metabolic regulator of cancer-associated fibroblasts. *Nature* 569, 723–728. doi: 10.1038/s41586-019-1173-8

Eckschlager, T., Plch, J., Stiborova, M., and Hrabeta, J. (2017). Histone Deacetylase Inhibitors as Anticancer Drugs. *Int. J. Mol. Sci.* 18(7), 1414. doi: 10.3390/ijms18071414

Ellinger, J., Müller, S. C., and Dietrich, D. (2015). Epigenetic biomarkers in the blood of patients with urological malignancies. *Expert Rev. Mol. Diagn.* 15, 505–516. doi: 10.1586/14737159.2015.1019477

Ellinger, J., Schneider, A.-C., Bachmann, A., Kristiansen, G., Müller, S. C., and Rogenhofer, S. (2016). Evaluation of Global Histone Acetylation Levels in Bladder Cancer Patients. *Anticancer Res.* 36, 3961–3964.

Enkelmann, A., Heinzelmann, J., von Eggeling, F., Walter, M., Berndt, A., Wunderlich, H., et al. (2011). Specific protein and miRNA patterns characterise tumour-associated fibroblasts in bladder cancer. *J. Cancer Res. Clin. Oncol.* 137, 751–759. doi: 10.1007/s00432-010-0932-6

Enokida, H., Yoshino, H., Matsushita, R., and Nakagawa, M. (2016). The role of microRNAs in bladder cancer. *Investig. Clin. Urol.* 57, S60. doi: 10.4111/icu.2016.57.s1.s60

Esteller, M. (2008). Epigenetics in Cancer. *N. Engl. J. Med.* 358, 1148–1159. doi: 10.1056/NEJMra072067

Fabbri, M., and Calin, G. A. (2010). Epigenetics and miRNAs in Human Cancer. *Adv. Genet.* 70, 87–99. doi: 10.1016/B978-0-12-380866-0.60004-6

Fantony, J. J., Longo, T. A., Gopalakrishna, A., Owusu, R., Lance, R. S., Foo, W.-C., et al. (2017). Urinary NID2 and TWIST1 methylation to augment conventional urine cytology for the detection of bladder cancer. *Cancer Biomark.* 18, 381–387. doi: 10.3233/CBM-160261

Fardi, M., Solali, S., and Farshdousti Hagh, M. (2018). Epigenetic mechanisms as a new approach in cancer treatment: An updated review. *Genes Dis.* 5, 304–311. doi: 10.1016/j.gendis.2018.06.003

Feber, A., Dhami, P., Dong, L., de Winter, P., Tan, W. S., Martínez-Fernández, M., et al. (2017). UroMark—a urinary biomarker assay for the detection of bladder cancer. *Clin. Epigenet.* 9(1), 1–10. doi: 10.1186/s13148-016-0303-5

Feinberg, A. P., and Vogelstein, B. (1983). Hypomethylation distinguishes genes of some human cancers from their normal counterparts. *Nature* 301, 89–92. doi: 10.1038/301089a0

Feng, Y., Liu, J., Kang, Y., He, Y., Liang, B., Yang, P., et al. (2014). miR-19a acts as an oncogenic microRNA and is up-regulated in bladder cancer. *J. Exp. Clin. Cancer Res.* 33, 67. doi: 10.1186/PREACCEPT-9242556491295527

Fischle, W. (2003). Molecular basis for the discrimination of repressive methyl-lysine marks in histone H3 by Polycomb and HP1 chromodomains. *Genes Dev.* 17, 1870–1881. doi: 10.1101/gad.1110503

Freedman, J. E., Gerstein, M., Mick, E., Rozowsky, J., Levy, D., Kitchen, R., et al. (2016). Diverse human extracellular RNAs are widely detected in human plasma. *Nat. Commun.* 7, 11106. doi: 10.1038/ncomms11106

Gajer, J. M., Furdas, S. D., Gründer, A., Gothwal, M., Heinicke, U., Keller, K., et al. (2015). Histone acetyltransferase inhibitors block neuroblastoma cell growth *in vivo*. *Oncogenesis* 4, e137. doi: 10.1038/oncsis.2014.51

Gao, Z., Yuan, T., Zhou, X., Ni, P., Sun, G., Li, P., et al. (2018). Targeting BRD4 proteins suppresses the growth of NSCLC through downregulation of eIF4E expression. *Cancer Biol. Ther.* 19, 407–415. doi: 10.1080/15384047.2018.1423923

García-Baquero, R., Puerta, P., Beltran, M., Alvarez-Mújica, M., Alvarez-Ossorio, J. L., and Sánchez-Carbayo, M. (2014). Methylation of tumor suppressor genes in a novel panel predicts clinical outcome in paraffin-embedded bladder tumors. *Tumor Biol.* 35, 5777–5786. doi: 10.1007/s13277-014-1767-6

Garzon, R., Marcucci, G., and Croce, C. M. (2010). Targeting microRNAs in cancer: rationale, strategies and challenges. *Nat. Rev. Drug Discovery* 9, 775–789. doi: 10.1038/nrd3179

Ge, Q., Zhou, Y., Lu, J., Bai, Y., Xie, X., and Lu, Z. (2014). miRNA in Plasma Exosome is Stable under Different Storage Conditions. *Molecules* 19, 1568–1575. doi: 10.3390/molecules19021568

Giagounidis, A., Schoch, R., Gattermann, N., Sanz, G., List, A., Gore, S. D., et al. (2014). Efficacy of azacitidine compared with that of conventional care regimens in the treatment of higher-risk myelodysplastic syndromes: a randomised, open-label, phase III study. *Lancet Oncol.* 10, 223–232. doi: 10.1016/S1470-2045(09)70003-8.Efficacy

Gielchinsky, I., Gilon, M., Abu-lail, R., Matouk, I., Hochberg, A., Gofrit, O. N., et al. (2017). *H19* non-coding RNA in urine cells detects urothelial carcinoma: a pilot study. *Biomarkers* 22, 1–6. doi: 10.1080/1354750X.2016.1276625

Gillette, T. G., and Hill, J. A. (2015). Readers, writers, and erasers: chromatin as the whiteboard of heart disease. *Circ. Res.* 116, 1245–1253. doi: 10.1161/CIRCRESAHA.116.303630

Ginder, G. D., and Williams, D. C. (2018). Readers of DNA methylation, the MBD family as potential therapeutic targets. *Pharmacol. Ther.* 184, 98–111. doi: 10.1016/j.pharmthera.2017.11.002

Goll, M. G., and Bestor, T. H. (2005). Eukaryotic cytosine methyltransferases. *Annu. Rev. Biochem.* 74, 481–514. doi: 10.1146/annurev.biochem.74.010904.153721

Gotwals, P., Cameron, S., Cipolletta, D., Cremasco, V., Crystal, A., Hewes, B., et al. (2017). Prospects for combining targeted and conventional cancer therapy with immunotherapy. *Nat. Rev. Cancer* 17, 286–301. doi: 10.1038/nrc.2017.17

Goulet, C. R., Champagne, A., Bernard, G., Vandal, D., Chabaud, S., Pouliot, F., et al. (2019). Cancer-associated fibroblasts induce epithelial-mesenchymal transition of bladder cancer cells through paracrine IL-6 signalling. *BMC Cancer* 19, 137. doi: 10.1186/s12885-019-5353-6

Grimm, S., Jennek, S., Singh, R., Enkelmann, A., Junker, K., Rippaus, N., et al. (2015). Malignancy of bladder cancer cells is enhanced by tumor-associated fibroblasts through a multifaceted cytokine-chemokine loop. *Exp. Cell Res.* 335, 1–11. doi: 10.1016/j.yexcr.2015.04.001

Guan, B., Xing, Y., Xiong, G., Cao, Z., Fang, D., Li, Y., et al. (2018). Predictive value of gene methylation for second recurrence following surgical treatment of first bladder recurrence of a primary upper-tract urothelial carcinoma. *Oncol. Lett.* 15, 9397–9405. doi: 10.3892/ol.2018.8498

Gui, Y., Guo, G., Huang, Y., Hu, X., Tang, A., Gao, S., et al. (2011). Frequent mutations of chromatin remodeling genes in transitional cell carcinoma of the bladder. *Nat. Genet.* 43, 875–878. doi: 10.1038/ng.907

Gulìa, C., Baldassarra, S., Signore, F., Rigon, G., Pizzuti, V., Gaffi, M., et al. (2017). Role of Non-Coding RNAs in the Etiology of Bladder Cancer. *Genes (Basel)* 8, 339. doi: 10.3390/genes8110339

Guo, P., Zhang, G., Meng, J., He, Q., Li, Z., and Guan, Y. (2018). Upregulation of Long Noncoding RNA TUG1 Promotes Bladder Cancer Cell Proliferation, Migration, and Invasion by Inhibiting miR-29c. *Oncol. Res. Featur. Preclin. Clin. Cancer Ther.* 26, 1083–1091. doi: 10.3727/096504018X15152085755247

Gupta, P. B., Fillmore, C. M., Jiang, G., Shapira, S. D., Tao, K., Kuperwasser, C., et al. (2011). Stochastic State Transitions Give Rise to Phenotypic Equilibrium in Populations of Cancer Cells. *Cell* 146, 633–644. doi: 10.1016/j.cell.2011.07.026

Gupta, S., Doyle, K., Mosbruger, T. L., Butterfield, A., Ast, A., Kaadige, M., et al. (2018). Reversible LSD1 inhibition with HCI-2509 induces the p53 gene expression signature and disrupts the MYCN signature in high- risk neuroblastoma cells. *Oncotarget* 9 (11), 9907–9924.

Gupta, R. A., Shah, N., Wang, K. C., Kim, J., Horlings, H. M., Wong, D. J., et al. (2010). Long non-coding RNA HOTAIR reprograms chromatin state to promote cancer metastasis. *Nature* 464, 1071–1076. doi: 10.1038/nature08975

Han, C., Seebacher, N. A., Hornicek, F. J., Kan, Q., and Duan, Z. (2017). Regulation of microRNAs function by circular RNAs in human cancer. *Oncotarget* 8, 64622–64637. doi: 10.18632/oncotarget.19930

Han, H., Wolff, E. M., and Liang, G. (2012). Epigenetic Alterations in Bladder Cancer and Their Potential Clinical Implications. *Adv. Urol.* 2012, 1–11. doi: 10.1155/2012/546917

Hashizume, H., Baluk, P., Morikawa, S., McLean, J. W., Thurston, G., Roberge, S., et. al (2000). Openings between Defective Endothelial Cells Explain Tumor Vessel Leakiness. *Am. J. Pathol.* 156, 1363–1380. doi: 10.1016/S0002-9440(10)65006-7

Havel, J. J., Chowell, D., and Chan, T. A. (2019). The evolving landscape of biomarkers for checkpoint inhibitor immunotherapy. *Nat. Rev. Cancer* 19, 133–150. doi: 10.1038/s41568-019-0116-x

Hayami, S., Yoshimatsu, M., Veerakumarasivam, A., Unoki, M., Iwai, Y., Tsunoda, T., et al. (2010). Overexpression of the JmjC histone demethylase KDM5B in human carcinogenesis: Involvement in the proliferation of cancer cells through the E2F/RB pathway. *Mol. Cancer* 9, 1–14. doi: 10.1186/1476-4598-9-59

Heitzer, E., Perakis, S., Geigl, J. B., and Speicher, M. R. (2017). The potential of liquid biopsies for the early detection of cancer. *NPJ Precis. Oncol.* 1 (36). doi: 10.1038/s41698-017-0039-5

Hellebrekers, D. M. E. I., Jair, K.-W., Viré, E., Eguchi, S., Hoebers, N. T. H., Fraga, M. F., et al. (2006). Angiostatic activity of DNA methyltransferase inhibitors. *Mol. Cancer Ther.* 5, 467–475. doi: 10.1158/1535-7163.MCT-05-0417

Helming, K. C., Wang, X., Wilson, B. G., Vazquez, F., Haswell, J. R., Manchester, H. E., et al. (2014). ARID1B is a specific vulnerability in ARID1A-mutant cancers. *Nat. Med.* 20, 251–254. doi: 10.1038/nm.3480

Hendrich, B., and Bird, A. (2015). Identification and Characterization of a Family of Mammalian Methyl-CpG Binding Proteins. *Mol. Cell. Biol.* 18, 6538–6547. doi: 10.1128/mcb.18.11.6538

Herold, J. M., James, L. I., Korboukh, V. K., Gao, C., Coil, K. E., Bua, D. J., et al. (2012). Structure–activity relationships of methyl-lysine reader antagonists. *Med. Chem. Commun.* 3, 45–51. doi: 10.1039/C1MD00195G

Hicks, K. C., Fantini, M., Donahue, R. N., Schwab, A., Knudson, K. M., Tritsch, S. R., et al. (2018). Epigenetic priming of both tumor and NK cells augments antibody-dependent cellular cytotoxicity elicited by the anti-PD-L1 antibody avelumab against multiple carcinoma cell types. *Oncoimmunology* 7, e1466018. doi: 10.1080/2162402X.2018.1466018

Hida, K., Hida, Y., Amin, D. N., Flint, A. F., Panigrahy, D., Morton, C. C., et al. (2004). Tumor-Associated Endothelial Cells with Cytogenetic Abnormalities. *Cancer Res.* 64, 8249–8255. doi: 10.1158/0008-5472.CAN-04-1567

Højfeldt, J. W., Agger, K., and Helin, K. (2013). Histone lysine demethylases as targets. *Nat. Publ. Gr.* 12, 917–930. doi: 10.1038/nrd4154

Hölscher, A. S., Schulz, W. A., Pinkerneil, M., Niegisch, G., and Hoffmann, M. J. (2018). Combined inhibition of BET proteins and class I HDACs synergistically induces apoptosis in urothelial carcinoma cell lines. *Clin. Epigenet.* 10, 1–14. doi: 10.1186/s13148-017-0434-3

Homami, A., and Ghazi, F. (2016). MicroRNAs as biomarkers associated with bladder cancer. *Med. J. Islam. Repub. Iran* 30.

Hopkinson, R.J., Tumber, A., Yapp, C., Chowdhury, R., Aik, W.S., Che, K.H., et al. (2013). 5-Carboxy-8-hydroxyquinoline is a broad spectrum 2-oxoglutarate oxygenase inhibitor which causes iron translocation. *Chem Sci.* 4 (8), 3110–3117. doi: 10.1039/C3SC51122G

Hu, L., Zang, M., Wang, H.-X., Zhang, B.-G., Wang, Z.-Q., Fan, Z.-Y., et al. (2018). G9A promotes gastric cancer metastasis by upregulating ITGB3 in a SET domain-independent manner. *Cell Death Dis.* 9, 278. doi: 10.1038/s41419-018-0322-6

Hu, M., Yao, J., Cai, L., Bachman, K. E., van den Brûle, F., Velculescu, V., et al. (2005). Distinct epigenetic changes in the stromal cells of breast cancers. *Nat. Genet.* 37, 899–905. doi: 10.1038/ng1596

Huang, C., Liao, X., Jin, H., Xie, F., Zheng, F., Li, J., et al. (2019a). MEG3, as a Competing Endogenous RNA, Binds with miR-27a to Promote PHLPP2 Protein Translation and Impairs Bladder Cancer Invasion. *Mol. Ther. Nucleic Acids* 16, 51–62. doi: 10.1016/j.omtn.2019.01.014

Huang, M., Zhong, Z., Lv, M., Shu, J., Tian, Q., and Chen, J. (2016). Comprehensive analysis of differentially expressed profiles of lncRNAs and circRNAs with associated co-expression and ceRNA networks in bladder carcinoma. *Oncotarget* 7, 47186–47200. doi: 10.18632/oncotarget.9706

Huang, Z., Zhang, M., Chen, G., Wang, W., Zhang, P., Yue, Y., et al. (2019b). Bladder cancer cells interact with vascular endothelial cells triggering EGFR signals to promote tumor progression. *Int. J. Oncol.* 54, 1555–1566. doi: 10.3892/ijo.2019.4729

Hulshoff, M. S., Xu, X., Krenning, G., and Zeisberg, E. M. (2018). Epigenetic Regulation of Endothelial-to-Mesenchymal Transition in Chronic Heart Disease. *Arterioscler. Thromb. Vasc. Biol.* 38, 1986–1996. doi: 10.1161/ATVBAHA.118.311276

Hurst, C. D., Alder, O., Platt, F. M., Droop, A., Stead, L. F., Burns, J. E., et al. (2017). Genomic Subtypes of Non-invasive Bladder Cancer with Distinct Metabolic Profile and Female Gender Bias in KDM6A Mutation Frequency. *Cancer Cell* 32, 701–715.e7. doi: 10.1016/j.ccell.2017.08.005

Hyun, K., Jeon, J., Park, K., and Kim, J. (2017). Writing, erasing and reading histone lysine methylations. *Exp. Mol. Med.* 49, e324–e324. doi: 10.1038/emm.2017.11

Iliev, R., Fedorko, M., Machackova, T., Mlcochova, H., Svoboda, M., Pacik, D., et al. (2016). Expression Levels of PIWI-interacting RNA, piR-823, Are Deregulated in Tumor Tissue, Blood Serum and Urine of Patients with Renal Cell Carcinoma. *Anticancer Res.* 36, 6419–6423. doi: 10.21873/anticanres.11239

Ingelmo-Torres, M., Lozano, J. J., Izquierdo, L., Carrion, A., Costa, M., Gomez, L., et al. (2017). Urinary cell microRNA-based prognostic classifier for non-muscle invasive bladder cancer. *Oncotarget* 8, 18238–18247. doi: 10.18632/oncotarget.15315

Jabłonowski, Z., Reszka, E., Gromadzińska, J., Wąsowicz, W., and Sosnowski, M. (2011). Hypermethylation of p16 and DAPK promoter gene regions in patients with non-invasive urinary bladder cancer. *Arch. Med. Sci.* 3, 512–516. doi: 10.5114/aoms.2011.23421

Janson, P. C. J., Marits, P., Thörn, M., Ohlsson, R., Winqvist, O., Gerard, J. R., et al. (2008). CpG methylation of the IFNG gene as a mechanism to induce immunosuppression [correction of immunosupression] in tumor-infiltrating lymphocytes. *J. Immunol.* 181, 2878–2886. doi: 10.4049/jimmunol.181.4.2878

Jeck, W. R., and Sharpless, N. E. (2014). Detecting and characterizing circular RNAs. *Nat. Biotechnol.* 32, 453–461. doi: 10.1038/nbt.2890

Jerónimo, C., and Henrique, R. (2014). Epigenetic biomarkers in urological tumors: A systematic review. *Cancer Lett.* 342, 264–274. doi: 10.1016/j.canlet.2011.12.026

Jiang, L., Gonda, T. A., Gamble, M. V., Salas, M., Seshan, V., Tu, S., et al. (2008). Global Hypomethylation of Genomic DNA in Cancer-Associated

Myofibroblasts. *Cancer Res.* 68, 9900–9908. doi: 10.1158/0008-5472.CAN-08-1319

Jiao, D., Li, Z., Zhu, M., Wang, Y., Wu, G., and Han, X. (2018). LncRNA MALAT1 promotes tumor growth and metastasis by targeting miR-124/foxq1 in bladder transitional cell carcinoma (BTCC). *Am. J. Cancer Res.* 8, 748–760.

Jing, J., Liu, J., Wang, Y., Zhang, M., Yang, L., Shi, F., et al. (2018). The role of ZBTB38 in promoting migration and invasive growth of bladder cancer cells. *Oncol. Rep.* 41 (3), 1980–1990. doi: 10.3892/or.2018.6937

Jones, P. A., and Liang, G. (2009). Rethinking how DNA methylation patterns are maintained. *Nat. Rev. Genet.* 10, 805–811. doi: 10.1038/nrg2651

José-Enériz, E. S., Agirre, X., Rabal, O., Vilas-Zornoza, A., Sanchez-Arias, J. A., Miranda, E., et al. (2017). Discovery of first-in-class reversible dual small molecule inhibitors against G9a and DNMTs in hematological malignancies. *Nat. Commun.* 8, 15424. doi: 10.1038/ncomms15424

Josson, S., Gururajan, M., Sung, S. Y., Hu, P., Shao, C., Zhau, H. E., et al. (2015). Stromal fibroblast-derived miR-409 promotes epithelial-to-mesenchymal transition and prostate tumorigenesis. *Oncogene* 34, 2690–2699. doi: 10.1038/onc.2014.212

Kaletsch, A., Pinkerneil, M., Hoffmann, M. J., Jaguva Vasudevan, A. A., Wang, C., Hansen, F. K., et al. (2018). Effects of novel HDAC inhibitors on urothelial carcinoma cells. *Clin. Epigenet.* 10, 1–18. doi: 10.1186/s13148-018-0531-y

Kalluri, R. (2016). The biology and function of fibroblasts in cancer. *Nat. Rev. Cancer* 16, 582–598. doi: 10.1038/nrc.2016.73

Kandimalla, R., van Tilborg, A. A. G., Kompier, L. C., Stumpel, D. J. P. M., Stam, R. W., Bangma, C. H., et al. (2012). Genome-wide analysis of CpG island methylation in bladder cancer identified TBX2, TBX3, GATA2, and ZIC4 as pTa-specific prognostic markers. *Eur. Urol.* 61, 1245–1256. doi: 10.1016/j.eururo.2012.01.011

Kauffman, E. C., Robinson, B. D., Downes, M., Powell, L. G., Ming, M., Scherr, D. S., et al. (2012). Role of androgen receptor and associated lysine-demethylase coregulators, LSD1 and JMJD2A, in localized and advanced human bladder cancer. *Mol. Carcinog.* 50, 931–944. doi: 10.1002/mc.20758.Role

Khetrapal, P., Lee, M. W. L., Tan, W. S., Dong, L., de Winter, P., Feber, A., et al. (2018). The role of circulating tumour cells and nucleic acids in blood for the detection of bladder cancer: A systematic review. *Cancer Treat. Rev.* 66, 56–63. doi: 10.1016/J.CTRV.2018.03.007

Kiany, S., Huang, G., and Kleinerman, E. S. (2017). Effect of entinostat on NK cell-mediated cytotoxicity against osteosarcoma cells and osteosarcoma lung metastasis. *Oncoimmunology* 6, e1333214. doi: 10.1080/2162402X.2017.1333214

Kim, D. E., Procopio, M.-G., Ghosh, S., Jo, S.-H., Goruppi, S., Magliozzi, F., et al. (2017). Convergent roles of ATF3 and CSL in chromatin control of cancer-associated fibroblast activation. *J. Exp. Med.* 214, 2349–2368. doi: 10.1084/jem.20170724

Kim, D. J., Dunleavey, J. M., Xiao, L., Ollila, D. W., Troester, M. A., Otey, C. A., et. al (2018). Suppression of TGFβ-mediated conversion of endothelial cells and fibroblasts into cancer associated (myo)fibroblasts *via* HDAC inhibition. *Br. J. Cancer* 118, 1359–1368. doi: 10.1038/s41416-018-0072-3

Kim, J., Akbani, R., Creighton, C. J., Lerner, S. P., Weinstein, J. N., Getz, G., et al. (2015a). Invasive Bladder Cancer: Genomic Insights and Therapeutic Promise. *Clin. Cancer Res.* 21, 4514–4524. doi: 10.1158/1078-0432.CCR-14-1215

Kim, K. H., Kim, W., Howard, T. P., Vazquez, F., Tsherniak, A., Wu, J. N., et al. (2015b). SWI/SNF-mutant cancers depend on catalytic and non-catalytic activity of EZH2. *Nat. Med.* 21, 1491–1496. doi: 10.1038/nm.3968

Kim, M. S., Kwon, H. J., Lee, Y. M., Baek, J. H., Jang, J.-E., Lee, S.-W., et al. (2001). Histone deacetylases induce angiogenesis by negative regulation of tumor suppressor genes. *Nat. Med.* 7, 437–443. doi: 10.1038/86507

Kim, S. M., Kang, H. W., Kim, W. T., Kim, Y.-J., Yun, S. J., Lee, S.-C., et al. (2013). Cell-Free microRNA-214 From Urine as a Biomarker for Non-Muscle-Invasive Bladder Cancer. *Korean J. Urol.* 54, 791. doi: 10.4111/kju.2013.54.11.791

Kitajima, H., Itoh, N., Shindo, T., Maruyama, R., Nojima, M., Suzuki, H., et al. (2017). Evaluation of Urinary DNA Methylation as a Marker for Recurrent Bladder Cancer: A 2-Center Prospective Study. *Urology* 113, 71–78. doi: 10.1016/j.urology.2017.11.025

Kitchen, M. O., Bryan, R. T., Emes, R. D., Luscombe, C. J., Cheng, K., Zeegers, M. P., et al. (2018). HumanMethylation450K Array–Identified Biomarkers Predict Tumour Recurrence/Progression at Initial Diagnosis of High-risk Non-muscle Invasive Bladder Cancer. *Biomark. Cancer* 10, 1179299X1775192. doi: 10.1177/1179299x17751920

Kitchen, M. O., Bryan, R. T., Haworth, K. E., Emes, R. D., Luscombe, C., Gommersall, L., et al. (2015). Methylation of HOXA9 and ISL1 Predicts Patient Outcome in High-Grade Non-Invasive Bladder Cancer. *PloS One* 10, e0137003. doi: 10.1371/journal.pone.0137003

Knowles, M. A., and Hurst, C. D. (2015). Molecular biology of bladder cancer: New insights into pathogenesis and clinical diversity. *Nat. Rev. Cancer* 15, 25–41. doi: 10.1038/nrc3817

Kogo, R., Shimamura, T., Mimori, K., Kawahara, K., Imoto, S., Sudo, T., et al. (2011). Long noncoding RNA HOTAIR regulates polycomb-dependent chromatin modification and is associated with poor prognosis in colorectal cancers. *Cancer Res.* 71, 6320–6326. doi: 10.1158/0008-5472.CAN-11-1021

Kohlhapp, F. J., Mitra, A. K., Lengyel, E., and Peter, M. E. (2015). MicroRNAs as mediators and communicators between cancer cells and the tumor microenvironment. *Oncogene* 34, 5857–5868. doi: 10.1038/onc.2015.89

Komatsu, Y., Waku, T., Iwasaki, N., Ono, W., Yamaguchi, C., and Yanagisawa, J. (2012). Global analysis of DNA methylation in early-stage liver fibrosis. *BMC Med. Genomics* 5, 5. doi: 10.1186/1755-8794-5-5

Konze, K. D., Macnevin, C. J., Liu, F., Gao, C., Huang, X., Kuznetsova, E., et al. (2014). An orally bioavailable chemical probe of the lysine methyltransferase ezh2 and ezh1. *ACS Chemical Biology* 8 (6), 1324–1334. doi: 10.1021/cb400133j

Korpal, M., Lee, E. S., Hu, G., and Kang, Y. (2008). The miR-200 family inhibits epithelial-mesenchymal transition and cancer cell migration by direct targeting of E-cadherin transcriptional repressors ZEB1 and ZEB2. *J. Biol. Chem.* 283, 14910–14914. doi: 10.1074/jbc.C800074200

Kouzarides, T. (2007). Chromatin Modifications and Their Function. *Cell* 128, 693–705. doi: 10.1016/j.cell.2007.02.005

Kreimer, U., Schulz, W. A., Koch, A., Niegisch, G., and Goering, W. (2013). HERV-K and LINE-1 DNA Methylation and Reexpression in Urothelial Carcinoma. *Front. Oncol.* 3, 255. doi: 10.3389/fonc.2013.00255

Kristensen, L. S., Hansen, T. B., Venø, M. T., and Kjems, J. (2018). Circular RNAs in cancer: Opportunities and challenges in the field. *Oncogene* 37, 555–565. doi: 10.1038/onc.2017.361

Kubicek, S., Sullivan, R. J. O., August, E. M., Hickey, E. R., Zhang, Q., Teodoro, M. L., et al., (2007). Technique Reversal of H3K9me2 by a Small-Molecule Inhibitor for the G9a Histone Methyltransferase. *Mol. Cell* 1, 473–481. doi: 10.1016/j.molcel.2007.01.017

Kuck, D., Caulfield, T., Lyko, F., and Medina-franco, J. L., (2010). Nanaomycin A Selectively Inhibits DNMT3B and Reactivates Silenced Tumor Suppressor Genes in Human Cancer Cells. *Mol. Cancer Ther.* 9 (11), 3015–3024. doi: 10.1158/1535-7163.MCT-10-0609

Kulcheski, F. R., Christoff, A. P., and Margis, R. (2016). Circular RNAs are miRNA sponges and can be used as a new class of biomarker. *J. Biotechnol.* 238, 42–51. doi: 10.1016/j.jbiotec.2016.09.011

Kuninty, P. R., Schnittert, J., Storm, G., and Prakash, J. (2016). MicroRNA Targeting to Modulate Tumor Microenvironment. *Front. Oncol.* 6, 3. doi: 10.3389/fonc.2016.00003

Kurdyukov, S., and Bullock, M. (2016). DNA methylation analysis: Choosing the right method. *Biology (Basel)* 5 (1), 3. doi: 10.3390/biology5010003

Lamprecht, S., Sigal-Batikoff, I., Shany, S., Abu-Freha, N., Ling, E., Delinasios, G. J., et al. (2018). Teaming up for trouble: Cancer cells, transforming growth factor-β1 signaling and the epigenetic corruption of stromal naïve fibroblasts. *Cancers* 10(61). doi: 10.3390/cancers10030061

Laurent, V. M., Duperray, A., Sundar Rajan, V., and Verdier, C. (2014). Atomic Force Microscopy Reveals a Role for Endothelial Cell ICAM-1 Expression in Bladder Cancer Cell Adherence. *PloS One* 9, e98034. doi: 10.1371/journal.pone.0098034

Lee, J.-E., Wang, C., Xu, S., Cho, Y.-W., Wang, L., Feng, X., et al. (2013). H3K4 mono- and di-methyltransferase MLL4 is required for enhancer activation during cell differentiation. *Elife* 2, e01503. doi: 10.7554/eLife.01503

Lee, J.-Y., Lee, S.-H., Heo, S.-H., Kim, K.-S., Kim, C., Kim, D.-K., et al. (2015). Novel Function of Lysine Methyltransferase G9a in the Regulation of Sox2 Protein Stability. *PloS One* 10, e0141118. doi: 10.1371/journal.pone.0141118

Lee, K.-H., and Song, C. G. (2017). Epigenetic regulation in bladder cancer: development of new prognostic targets and therapeutic implications. *Transl. Cancer Res.* 6, S677–S688. doi: 10.21037/14111

Lee, M. G., Villa, R., Trojer, P., Norman, J., Yan, K.-P., Reinberg, D., et al. (2007). Demethylation of H3K27 regulates polycomb recruitment and H2A ubiquitination. *Science* 318, 447–450. doi: 10.1126/science.1149042

Ler, L. D., Ghosh, S., Chai, X., Thike, A. A., Heng, H. L., Siew, E. Y., et al. (2017). Loss of tumor suppressor KDM6A amplifies PRC2-regulated transcriptional repression in bladder cancer and can be targeted through inhibition of EZH2. *Sci. Transl. Med.* 9, eaai8312. doi: 10.1126/scitranslmed.aai8312

Li, B., Xie, F., Zheng, F., Jiang, G., Zeng, F., and Xiao, X. (2017). Overexpression of CircRNA BCRC4 regulates cell apoptosis and MicroRNA-101/EZH2 signaling in bladder cancer. *Curr. Med. Sci.* 37, 886–890. doi: 10.1007/s11596-017-1822-9

Li, F., Yang, C., Zhang, H.-B., Ma, J., Jia, J., Tang, X., et al. (2019). BET inhibitor JQ1 suppresses cell proliferation *via* inducing autophagy and activating LKB1/AMPK in bladder cancer cells. *Cancer Med.* 8 (10) 1–14. doi: 10.1002/cam4.2385

Li, H.-T., Duymich, C. E., Weisenberger, D. J., and Liang, G. (2016a). Genetic and Epigenetic Alterations in Bladder Cancer. *Int. Neurourol. J.* 20, S84–S94. doi: 10.5213/inj.1632752.376

Li, P., Shan, J.-X., Chen, X.-H., Zhang, D., Su, L.-P., Huang, X.-Y., et al. (2015). Epigenetic silencing of microRNA-149 in cancer-associated fibroblasts mediates prostaglandin E2/interleukin-6 signaling in the tumor microenvironment. *Cell Res.* 25, 588–603. doi: 10.1038/cr.2015.51

Li, P., Yang, X., Yuan, W., Yang, C., Zhang, X., Han, J., et al. (2018a). CircRNA-Cdr1as Exerts Anti-Oncogenic Functions in Bladder Cancer by Sponging MicroRNA-135a. *Cell. Physiol. Biochem.* 46, 1606–1616. doi: 10.1159/000489208

Li, Q. Q., Hao, J. J., Zhang, Z., Hsu, I., Liu, Y., Tao, Z., et al. (2016b). Histone deacetylase inhibitor-induced cell death in bladder cancer is associated with chromatin modification and modifying protein expression: A proteomic approach. *Int. J. Oncol.* 48, 2591–2607. doi: 10.3892/ijo.2016.3478

Li, X.-Y., Zhang, K., Li, X.-S., Xiong, G.-Y., He, Q., Yang, K.-W., et al. (2018b). Detection of urothelial carcinoma, upper tract urothelial carcinoma, bladder carcinoma, and urothelial carcinoma with gross hematuria using selected urine-DNA methylation biomarkers: A prospective, single-center study. *Urol. Oncol. Semin. Orig. Investig.* 36, 342.e15–342.e23. doi: 10.1016/j.urolonc.2018.04.001

Liang, Y., Ridzon, D., Wong, L., and Chen, C. (2007). Characterization of microRNA expression profiles in normal human tissues. *BMC Genomics* 8, 166. doi: 10.1186/1471-2164-8-166

Liep, J., Rabien, A., and Jung, K. (2012). Feedback networks between microRNAs and epigenetic modifications in urological tumors. *Epigenetics* 7, 315–325. doi: 10.4161/epi.19464

Lima, J. F., Carvalho, J., Pinto-Ribeiro, I., Almeida, C., Wengel, J., Cerqueira, L., et al. (2018a). Targeting miR-9 in gastric cancer cells using locked nucleic acid oligonucleotides. *BMC Mol. Biol.* 19, 1–13. doi: 10.1186/s12867-018-0107-6

Lima, J. F., Cerqueira, L., Figueiredo, C., Oliveira, C., and Azevedo, N. F. (2018b). Anti-miRNA oligonucleotides: A comprehensive guide for design. *RNA Biol.* 15, 338–352. doi: 10.1080/15476286.2018.1445959

Lin, Y., Li, Z., He, Z., Guan, T., and Ma, J. (2012). Clinical and Prognostic Significance of Protocadherin-10 (PCDH10) Promoter Methylation in Bladder Cancer. *J. Int. Med. Res.* 40, 2117–2123. doi: 10.1177/030006051204000609

Liu, C., Chen, Z., Fang, J., Xu, A., Zhang, W., and Wang, Z. (2016). H19-derived miR-675 contributes to bladder cancer cell proliferation by regulating p53 activation. *Tumour Biol.* 37, 263–270. doi: 10.1007/s13277-015-3779-2

Liu, G., Zhao, X., Zhou, J., Cheng, X., Ye, Z., and Ji, Z. (2018a). Long non-coding RNA MEG3 suppresses the development of bladder urothelial carcinoma by regulating miR-96 and TPM1. *Cancer Biol. Ther.* 19, 1039–1056. doi: 10.1080/15384047.2018.1480279

Liu, H., Bi, J., Dong, W., Yang, M., Shi, J., Jiang, N., et al. (2018b). Invasion-related circular RNA circFNDC3B inhibits bladder cancer progression through the miR-1178-3p/G3BP2/SRC/FAK axis. *Mol. Cancer* 17, 161. doi: 10.1186/s12943-018-0908-8

Liu, M., Zhou, J., Chen, Z., and Cheng, A. S.-L. (2017a). Understanding the epigenetic regulation of tumours and their microenvironments: opportunities and problems for epigenetic therapy. *J. Pathol.* 241, 10–24. doi: 10.1002/path.4832

Liu, Q., Liu, H., Cheng, H., Li, Y., Li, X., and Zhu, C. (2017b). Downregulation of long noncoding RNA TUG1 inhibits proliferation and induces apoptosis through the TUG1/miR-142/ZEB2 axis in bladder cancer cells. *Oncol. Targets Ther.* 10, 2461–2471. doi: 10.2147/OTT.S124595

Lodewijk, I., Dueñas, M., Rubio, C., Munera-Maravilla, E., Segovia, C., Bernardini, A., et al. (2018). Liquid Biopsy Biomarkers in Bladder Cancer: A Current Need for Patient Diagnosis and Monitoring. *Int. J. Mol. Sci.* 19, 2514. doi: 10.3390/ijms19092514

Lu, C., Han, H. D., Mangala, L. S., Ali-Fehmi, R., Newton, C. S., Ozbun, L., et al. (2010). Regulation of Tumor Angiogenesis by EZH2. *Cancer Cell* 18, 185–197. doi: 10.1016/j.ccr.2010.06.016

Lu, C., Paschall, A. V., Shi, H., Savage, N., Waller, J. L., Sabbatini, M. E., et al. (2017). The MLL1-H3K4me3 axis-mediated PD-L1 expression and pancreatic cancer immune evasion. *J. Natl. Cancer Inst.* 109, djw283. doi: 10.1093/jnci/djw283

Lu, M., Selleslag, D., Labar, B., Germing, U., Salih, H. R., Beeldens, F., et al., (2011). Low-Dose Decitabine Versus Best Supportive Care in Elderly Patients With Intermediate- or High-Risk Myelodysplastic Syndrome (MDS) Ineligible for Intensive Chemotherapy : Final Results of the Randomized Phase III Study of the European Organisation for R. *J. Clin. Oncol.* 29, 1987–1996. doi: 10.1200/JCO.2010.30.9245

Luo, J., Chen, J., Li, H., Yang, Y., Yun, H., Yang, S., et al. (2017). LncRNA UCA1 promotes the invasion and EMT of bladder cancer cells by regulating the miR-143/HMGB1 pathway. *Oncol. Lett.* 14, 5556–5562. doi: 10.3892/ol.2017.6886

Luo, Z.-G., Li, Z.-G., Gui, S.-L., Chi, B.-J., and Ma, J.-G. (2014). Protocadherin-17 promoter methylation in serum-derived DNA is associated with poor prognosis of bladder cancer. *J. Int. Med. Res.* 42, 35–41. doi: 10.1177/0300060513504705

Luperchio, T. R., Wong, X., and Reddy, K. L. (2014). Genome regulation at the peripheral zone: lamina associated domains in development and disease. *Curr. Opin. Genet. Dev.* 25, 50–61. doi: 10.1016/J.GDE.2013.11.021

Maier, V. K., Feeney, C. M., Taylor, J. E., Creech, A. L., Qiao, J. W., Szanto, A., et al. (2015). Functional Proteomic Analysis of Repressive Histone Methyltransferase Complexes Reveals ZNF518B as a G9A Regulator. *Mol. Cell. Proteomics* 14, 1435–1446. doi: 10.1074/mcp.M114.044586

Majewski, T., Yao, H., Bondaruk, J., Chung, W., Lee, S., Lee, J. G., et al. (2019). Whole-Organ Genomic Characterization of Mucosal Field Effects Initiating Bladder Carcinogenesis. *Cell Rep.* 26, 2241–2256.e4. doi: 10.1016/j.celrep.2019.01.095

Mann, B. S., Johnson, J. R., Cohen, M. H., Justice, R., and Pazdur, R. (2007). FDA Approval Summary: Vorinostat for Treatment of Advanced Primary Cutaneous T-Cell Lymphoma. *Oncologist* 12 (10), 1247–1252. doi: 10.1634/theoncologist.12-10-1247

Marks, D. L., Olson, R. L., and Fernandez-Zapico, M. E. (2016). Epigenetic control of the tumor microenvironment. *Epigenomics* 8, 1671–1687. doi: 10.2217/epi-2016-0110

Marques-Magalhaes, A., Graca, I., Henrique, R., and Jeronimo, C. (2018). Targeting DNA Methyltranferases in Urological Tumors. *Front. Pharmacol.* 9, 366. doi: 10.3389/fphar.2018.00366

Martens-Uzunova, E. S., Böttcher, R., Croce, C. M., Jenster, G., Visakorpi, T., and Calin, G. A. (2014). Long noncoding RNA in prostate, bladder, and kidney cancer. *Eur. Urol.* 65, 1140–1151. doi: 10.1016/j.eururo.2013.12.003

Martínez-Fernández, M., Dueñas, M., Feber, A., Segovia, C., García-Escudero, R., Rubio, C., et al. (2015a). A Polycomb-mir200 loop regulates clinical outcome in bladder cancer. *Oncotarget* 6, 42258–42275. doi: 10.18632/oncotarget.5546

Martínez-Fernández, M., Feber, A., Dueñas, M., Segovia, C., Rubio, C., Fernandez, M., et al. (2015b). Analysis of the Polycomb-related lncRNAs HOTAIR and ANRIL in bladder cancer. *Clin. Epigenet.* 7, 109. doi: 10.1186/s13148-015-0141-x

Martínez-Fernández, M., Paramio, J. M., and Dueñas, M. (2016). RNA Detection in Urine. *J. Mol. Diagnostics* 18, 15–22. doi: 10.1016/j.jmoldx.2015.07.008

Martínez-Fernández, M., Rubio, C., Segovia, C., López-Calderón, F. F., Dueñas, M., and Paramio, J. M. (2015c). EZH2 in bladder cancer, a promising therapeutic target. *Int. J. Mol. Sci.* 16, 27107–27132. doi: 10.3390/ijms161126000

Martinez, V. D., Vucic, E. A., Thu, K. L., Hubaux, R., Enfield, K. S. S., Pikor, L. A., et al. (2015). Unique somatic and malignant expression patterns implicate PIWI-interacting RNAs in cancer-type specific biology. *Sci. Rep.* 5, 10423. doi: 10.1038/srep10423

Mijnes, J., Veeck, J., Gaisa, N. T., Burghardt, E., de Ruijter, T. C., Gostek, S., et al. (2018). Promoter methylation of DNA damage repair (DDR) genes in human tumor entities: RBBP8/CtIP is almost exclusively methylated in bladder cancer. *Clin. Epigenet.* 10, 1–20. doi: 10.1186/s13148-018-0447-6

Mio, C., Bulotta, S., Russo, D., and Damante, G. (2019). Reading Cancer: Chromatin Readers as Druggable Targets for Cancer Treatment. *Cancers (Basel)* 11, 61. doi: 10.3390/cancers11010061

Mishra, R., Haldar, S., Placencio, V., Madhav, A., Rohena-Rivera, K., Agarwal, P., et al. (2018). Stromal epigenetic alterations drive metabolic and neuroendocrine prostate cancer reprogramming. *J. Clin. Invest.* 128, 4472–4484. doi: 10.1172/JCI99397

Misso, G., Di Martino, M. T., De Rosa, G., Farooqi, A. A., Lombardi, A., Campani, V., et al. (2014). Mir-34: A new weapon against cancer? *Mol. Ther. Nucleic Acids* 3, e195. doi: 10.1038/mtna.2014.47

Moore, L. E., Pfeiffer, R. M., Poscablo, C., Real, F. X., Kogevinas, M., Silverman, D., et al. (2008). Genomic DNA hypomethylation as a biomarker for bladder cancer susceptibility in the Spanish Bladder Cancer Study: a case-control study. *Lancet Oncol.* 9, 359–366. doi: 10.1016/S1470-2045(08)70038-X

Morini, M. F., Giampietro, C., Corada, M., Pisati, F., Lavarone, E., Cunha, S. I., et al (2018). VE-Cadherin–Mediated Epigenetic Regulation of Endothelial Gene Expression. *Circ. Res.* 122, 231–245. doi: 10.1161/CIRCRESAHA.117.312392

Mozzetta, C., Pontis, J., and Ait-Si-Ali, S. (2015). Functional Crosstalk Between Lysine Methyltransferases on Histone Substrates: The Case of G9A/GLP and Polycomb Repressive Complex 2. *Antioxid. Redox Signal.* 22, 1365–1381. doi: 10.1089/ars.2014.6116

Mozzetta, C., Pontis, J., Fritsch, L., Robin, P., Portoso, M., Proux, C., et al. (2014). The histone H3 lysine 9 methyltransferases G9a and GLP regulate polycomb repressive complex 2-mediated gene silencing. *Mol. Cell* 53, 277–289. doi: 10.1016/j.molcel.2013.12.005

Nagai, N., Ohguchi, H., Nakaki, R., Matsumura, Y., Kanki, Y., Sakai, J., et al. (2018). Downregulation of ERG and FLI1 expression in endothelial cells triggers endothelial-to-mesenchymal transition. *PloS Genet.* 14, e1007826. doi: 10.1371/journal.pgen.1007826

Nagano, T., Mitchell, J. A., Sanz, L. A., Pauler, F. M., Ferguson-Smith, A. C., Feil, R., et al. (2008). The Air noncoding RNA epigenetically silences transcription by targeting G9a to chromatin. *Science* 322, 1717–1720. doi: 10.1126/science.1163802

Nickerson, M. L., Dancik, G. M., Im, K. M., Edwards, M. G., Turan, S., Brown, J., et al. (2014). Concurrent alterations in TERT, KDM6A, and the BRCA pathway in bladder cancer. *Clin. Cancer Res.* 20, 4935–4948. doi: 10.1158/1078-0432.CCR-14-0330

Nicorescu, I., Dallinga, G. M., de Winther, M. P. J., Stroes, E. S. G., and Bahjat, M. (2019). Potential epigenetic therapeutics for atherosclerosis treatment. *Atherosclerosis* 281, 189–197. doi: 10.1016/j.atherosclerosis.2018.10.006

Niegisch, G., Knievel, J., Koch, A., Hader, C., Fischer, U., Albers, P., et al. (2013). Changes in histone deacetylase (HDAC) expression patterns and activity of HDAC inhibitors in urothelial cancers. *Urol. Oncol. Semin. Orig. Investig.* 31, 1770–1779. doi: 10.1016/j.urolonc.2012.06.015

Ocaña, A., Nieto-Jiménez, C., and Pandiella, A. (2017). BET inhibitors as novel therapeutic agents in breast cancer. *Oncotarget* 8, 71285–71291. doi: 10.18632/oncotarget.19744

Ogiwara, H., Sasaki, M., Mitachi, T., Oike, T., Higuchi, S., Tominaga, Y., et al. (2016). Targeting p300 addiction in cbp-deficient cancers causes synthetic lethality by apoptotic cell death due to abrogation of MYC expression. *Cancer Discovery* 6, 430–445. doi: 10.1158/2159-8290.CD-15-0754

Okano, M., Bell, D. W., Haber, D. A., and Li, E. (1999). DNA methyltransferases Dnmt3a and Dnmt3b are essential for *de novo* methylation and mammalian development. *Cell* 99, 247–257. doi: 10.1016/S0092-8674(00)81656-6

Olivieri, M., Ferro, M., Terreri, S., Durso, M., Romanelli, A., Avitabile, C., et al. (2016). Long non-coding RNA containing ultraconserved genomic region 8 promotes bladder cancer tumorigenesis. *Oncotarget* 7(15), 20636–20654. doi: 10.18632/oncotarget.7833

Olkhov-Mitsel, E., Savio, A. J., Kron, K. J., Pethe, V. V., Hermanns, T., Fleshner, N. E., et al. (2017). Epigenome-wide DNA methylation profiling identifies differential methylation biomarkers in high-grade bladder cancer. *Transl. Oncol.* 10, 168–177. doi: 10.1016/j.tranon.2017.01.001

Pal, S. K., Milowsky, M. I., and Plimack, E. R. (2013). Optimizing systemic therapy for bladder cancer. *JNCCN J. Natl. Compr. Cancer Netw.* 11, 793–804. doi: 10.6004/jnccn.2013.0101

Palazzo, A. F., and Lee, E. S. (2015). Non-coding RNA: what is functional and what is junk? *Front. Genet.* 6, 2. doi: 10.3389/fgene.2015.00002

Pang, W., Su, J., Wang, Y., Feng, H., Dai, X., Yuan, Y., et al. (2015). Pancreatic cancer-secreted miR-155 implicates in the conversion from normal fibroblasts to cancer-associated fibroblasts. *Cancer Sci.* 106, 1362–1369. doi: 10.1111/cas.12747

Pappano, W. N., Guo, J., He, Y., Ferguson, D., Jagadeeswaran, S., Osterling, D. J., et al. (2015). The histone methyltransferase inhibitor A-366 uncovers a role for G9a/GLP in the epigenetics of leukemia. *PloS One* 10, 1–13. doi: 10.1371/journal.pone.0131716

Pardini, B., and Naccarati, A. (2017). Altered piRNA Profiles in bladder cancer: a new challenge in the next- generation sequencing era? *J. Genet. Genomes* 1 (2), 1000110.

Pardoll, D. M. (2012). The blockade of immune checkpoints in cancer immunotherapy. *Nat. Rev. Cancer* 12, 252–264. doi: 10.1038/nrc3239

Park, S. M., Gaur, A. B., Lengyel, E., and Peter, M. E. (2008). The miR-200 family determines the epithelial phenotype of cancer cells by targeting the E-cadherin repressors ZEB1 and ZEB2. *Genes Dev.* 22, 894–907. doi: 10.1101/gad.1640608

Pastori, C., Daniel, M., Penas, C., Volmar, C.-H., Johnstone, A. L., Brothers, S. P., et al. (2014). BET bromodomain proteins are required for glioblastoma cell proliferation. *Epigenetics* 9, 611–620. doi: 10.4161/epi.27906

Patchsung, M., Boonla, C., Amnattrakul, P., Dissayabutra, T., Mutirangura, A., and Tosukhowong, P. (2012). Long interspersed nuclear element-1 hypomethylation and oxidative stress: correlation and bladder cancer diagnostic potential. *PloS One* 7, e37009. doi: 10.1371/journal.pone.0037009

Peng, D., Ge, G., Xu, Z., Ma, Q., Shi, Y., Zhou, Y., et al. (2018). Diagnostic and prognostic biomarkers of common urological cancers based on aberrant DNA methylation. *Epigenomics* 10, 1189–1199. doi: 10.2217/epi-2018-0017

Petrylak, D. P., Tagawa, S. T., Kohli, M., Eisen, A., Canil, C., Sridhar, S. S., et al. (2016). Docetaxel as monotherapy or combined with ramucirumab or icrucumab in second-line treatment for locally advanced or metastatic urothelial carcinoma: an open-label, three-arm, randomized controlled phase II Trial. *J. Clin. Oncol.* 34, 1500–1509. doi: 10.1200/JCO.2015.65.0218

Picaud, S., Wells, C., Felletar, I., Brotherton, D., Martin, S., Savitsky, P., et al. (2013). RVX-208, an inhibitor of BET transcriptional regulators with selectivity for the second bromodomain. *Proc. Natl. Acad. Sci. U. S. A.* 110, 19754–19759. doi: 10.1073/pnas.1310658110

Pietrusiński, M., Kępczyński, Ł, Jędrzejczyk, A., Borkowska, E., Traczyk-Borszyńska, M., Constantinou, M., et al. (2017). Detection of bladder cancer in urine sediments by a hypermethylation panel of selected tumor suppressor genes. *Cancer Biomark.* 18, 47–59. doi: 10.3233/CBM-160673

Plimack, E. R., Bellmunt, J., Gupta, S., Berger, R., Chow, L. Q., Juco, J., et al. (2017). Safety and activity of pembrolizumab in patients with locally advanced or metastatic urothelial cancer (KEYNOTE-012): a non-randomised, open-label, phase 1b study. *Lancet Oncol.* 18, 212–220. doi: 10.1016/S1470-2045(17)30007-4

Plummer, R., Vidal, L., Griffin, M., Lesley, M., De Bono, J., Coulthard, S., et al. (2009). Phase I study of MG98, an oligonucleotide antisense inhibitor of human DNA methyltransferase 1, given as a 7-day infusion in patients with advanced solid tumors. *Clin. Cancer Res.* 15, 3177–3183. doi: 10.1158/1078-0432.CCR-08-2859

Pop-Bica, C., Gulei, D., Cojocneanu-Petric, R., Braicu, C., Petrut, B., and Berindan-Neagoe, I. (2017). Understanding the role of non-coding rnas in bladder cancer: from dark matter to valuable therapeutic targets. *Int. J. Mol. Sci.* 18(7), 1514. doi: 10.3390/ijms18071514

Porten, S. P. (2018). Epigenetic alterations in bladder cancer. *Curr. Urol. Rep.* 19. doi: 10.1007/s11934-018-0861-5

Powles, T., Eder, J. P., Fine, G. D., Braiteh, F. S., Loriot, Y., Cruz, C., et al. (2014). MPDL3280A (anti-PD-L1) treatment leads to clinical activity in metastatic bladder cancer. *Nature* 515, 558–562. doi: 10.1038/nature13904

Poyet, C., Jentsch, B., Hermanns, T., Schweckendiek, D., Seifert, H.-H., Schmidtpeter, M., et al. (2014). Expression of histone deacetylases 1, 2 and 3 in urothelial bladder cancer. *BMC Clin. Pathol.* 14, 10. doi: 10.1186/1472-6890-14-10

Rampias, T., Karagiannis, D., Avgeris, M., Polyzos, A., Kokkalis, A., Kanaki, Z., et al. (2019). The lysine-specific methyltransferase KMT2C/MLL3 regulates DNA repair components in cancer. *EMBO Rep.* 20, e46821. doi: 10.15252/embr.201846821

Raulet, D. H., Marcus, A., and Coscoy, L. (2017). Dysregulated cellular functions and cell stress pathways provide critical cues for activating and targeting natural killer cells to transformed and infected cells. *Immunol. Rev.* 280, 93–101. doi: 10.1111/imr.12600

Reinert, T. (2012). Methylation markers for urine-based detection of bladder cancer: the next generation of urinary markers for diagnosis and surveillance of bladder cancer. *Adv. Urol.* 2012, 503271. doi: 10.1155/2012/503271

Reinert, T., Modin, C., Castano, F. M., Lamy, P., Wojdacz, T. K., Hansen, L. L., et al. (2011). Comprehensive genome methylation analysis in bladder cancer: identification and validation of novel methylated genes and application of these as urinary tumor markers. *Clin. Cancer Res.* 17, 5582–5592. doi: 10.1158/1078-0432.CCR-10-2659

Ren, C., Morohashi, K., Plotnikov, A. N., Jakoncic, J., Smith, S. G., Li, J., et al. (2015). Small-molecule modulators of methyl-lysine binding for the CBX7 chromodomain. *Chem. Biol.* 22 (2), 161–168. doi: 10.1016/j.chembiol.2014.11.021

Ren, Y., Huang, T., Lou, Z., Weng, G., Chen, F., Fan, X., et al. (2016). Clinical significance of CDH13 promoter methylation as a biomarker for bladder cancer: a meta-analysis. *BMC Urol.* 16, 1–9. doi: 10.1186/s12894-016-0171-5

Renard, I., Joniau, S., van Cleynenbreugel, B., Collette, C., Naômé, C., Vlassenbroeck, I., et al. (2010). Identification and validation of the methylated TWIST1 and NID2 genes through real-time methylation-specific polymerase chain reaction assays for the noninvasive detection of primary bladder cancer in urine samples. *Eur. Urol.* 58, 96–104. doi: 10.1016/j.eururo.2009.07.041

Ringuette Goulet, C., Bernard, G., Tremblay, S., Chabaud, S., Bolduc, S., and Pouliot, F. (2018). Exosomes induce fibroblast differentiation into cancer-associated fibroblasts through TGFβ signaling. *Mol. Cancer Res.* 16, 1196–1204. doi: 10.1158/1541-7786.mcr-17-0784

Robertson, A. G., Kim, J., Al-Ahmadie, H., Bellmunt, J., Guo, G., Cherniack, A. D., et al. (2018). Comprehensive molecular characterization of muscle-invasive bladder cancer. *Cell* 174, 1033. doi: 10.1016/j.cell.2018.07.036

Roger, T., Lugrin, J., Le Roy, D., Goy, G., Mombelli, M., Koessler, T., et al. (2011). Histone deacetylase inhibitors impair innate immune responses to Toll-like receptor agonists and to infection. *Blood* 117, 1205–1217. doi: 10.1182/blood-2010-05-284711

Romero-Cordoba, S. L., Salido-Guadarrama, I., Rodriguez-Dorantes, M., and Hidalgo-Miranda, A. (2014). miRNA biogenesis: biological impact in the development of cancer. *Cancer Biol. Ther.* 15, 1444–1455. doi: 10.4161/15384047.2014.955442

Roperch, J. P., Grandchamp, B., Desgrandchamps, F., Mongiat-Artus, P., Ravery, V., Ouzaid, I., et al. (2016). Promoter hypermethylation of HS3ST2, SEPTIN9 and SLIT2 combined with FGFR3 mutations as a sensitive/specific urinary assay for diagnosis and surveillance in patients with low or high-risk non-muscle-invasive bladder cancer. *BMC Cancer* 16, 1–9. doi: 10.1186/s12885-016-2748-5

Rosenberg, J. E., Hoffman-Censits, J., Powles, T., van der Heijden, M. S., Balar, A. V., Necchi, A., et al. (2016). Atezolizumab in patients with locally advanced and metastatic urothelial carcinoma who have progressed following treatment with platinum-based chemotherapy: a single-arm, multicentre, phase 2 trial. *Lancet* 387, 1909–1920. doi: 10.1016/S0140-6736(16)00561-4

Ross, J. S., Wang, K., Al-Rohil, R. N., Nazeer, T., Sheehan, C. E., Otto, G. A., et al (2014). Advanced urothelial carcinoma: next-generation sequencing reveals diverse genomic alterations and targets of therapy. *Mod. Pathol.* 27, 271–280. doi: 10.1038/modpathol.2013.135

Rothbart, S. B., and Strahl, B. D. (2014). Interpreting the language of histone and DNA modifications. *Biochim. Biophys. Acta - Gene Regul. Mech.* 1839, 627–643. doi: 10.1016/j.bbagrm.2014.03.001

Roudnicky, F., Dieterich, L. C., Poyet, C., Buser, L., Wild, P., Tang, D., et al. (2017). High expression of insulin receptor on tumour-associated blood vessels in invasive bladder cancer predicts poor overall and progression-free survival. *J. Pathol.* 242, 193–205. doi: 10.1002/path.4892

Roudnicky, F., Poyet, C., Wild, P., Krampitz, S., Negrini, F., Huggenberger, R., et al. (2013). Endocan Is Upregulated on Tumor Vessels in Invasive Bladder Cancer Where It Mediates VEGF-A-Induced Angiogenesis. *Cancer Res.* 73, 1097–1106. doi: 10.1158/0008-5472.CAN-12-1855

Roudnicky, F., Yoon, S. Y., Poghosyan, S., Schwager, S., Poyet, C., Vella, G., et al. (2018). Alternative transcription of a shorter, non-anti-angiogenic thrombospondin-2 variant in cancer-associated blood vessels. *Oncogene* 37, 2573–2585. doi: 10.1038/s41388-018-0129-z

Ruthenburg, A. J., Li, H., Patel, D. J., and David Allis, C. (2007). Multivalent engagement of chromatin modifications by linked binding modules. *Nat. Rev. Mol. Cell Biol.* 8, 983–994. doi: 10.1038/nrm2298

Sakaguchi, T., Yoshino, H., Sugita, S., Miyamoto, K., Yonemori, M., Osako, Y., et al. (2018). Bromodomain protein BRD4 inhibitor JQ1 regulates potential prognostic molecules in advanced renal cell carcinoma. *Oncotarget* 9, 23003. doi: 10.18632/ONCOTARGET.25190

Sánchez-Carbayo, M. (2012). Hypermethylation in bladder cancer: biological pathways and translational applications. *Tumor Biol.* 33, 347–361. doi: 10.1007/s13277-011-0310-2

Santos, M., Martínez-Fernández, M., Dueñas, M., García-Escudero, R., Alfaya, B., Villacampa, F., et al. (2014). In vivo disruption of an Rb-E2F-Ezh2 signaling loop causes bladder cancer. *Cancer Res.* 74, 6565–6577. doi: 10.1158/0008-5472.CAN-14-1218

Sasaki, H., Yoshiike, M., Nozawa, S., Usuba, W., Katsuoka, Y., Aida, K., et al. (2016). Expression Level of Urinary MicroRNA-146a-5p Is Increased in Patients With Bladder Cancer and Decreased in Those After Transurethral Resection. *Clin. Genitourin. Cancer* 14, e493–e499. doi: 10.1016/j.clgc.2016.04.002

Schenk, A., Bloch, W., and Zimmer, P. (2016). Natural Killer Cells–An Epigenetic Perspective of Development and Regulation. *Int. J. Mol. Sci.* 17, 326. doi: 10.3390/ijms17030326

Schlereth, K., Weichenhan, D., Bauer, T., Heumann, T., Giannakouri, E., Lipka, D., et al. (2018). The transcriptomic and epigenetic map of vascular quiescence in the continuous lung endothelium. *Elife* 7(e34423). doi: 10.7554/elife.34423

Schoepp, M., Ströse, A. J., and Haier, J. (2017). Dysregulation of miRNA Expression in Cancer Associated Fibroblasts (CAFs) and Its Consequences on the Tumor Microenvironment. *Cancers (Basel)* 9, 54. doi: 10.3390/cancers9060054

Schulte, J., Weidig, M., Balzer, P., Richter, P., Franz, M., Junker, K., et al. (2012). Expression of the E-cadherin repressors Snail, Slug and Zeb1 in urothelial carcinoma of the urinary bladder: relation to stromal fibroblast activation and invasive behaviour of carcinoma cells. *Histochem. Cell Biol.* 138, 847–860. doi: 10.1007/s00418-012-0998-0

Schulz, W. A. (2006). L1 retrotransposons in human cancers. *J. Biomed. Biotechnol.* 2006, 83672. doi: 10.1155/JBB/2006/83672

Schuyler, R. P., Merkel, A., Raineri, E., Altucci, L., Vellenga, E., Martens, J. H. A., et al. (2016). Distinct Trends of DNA Methylation Patterning in the Innate and Adaptive Immune Systems Europe PMC Funders Group. *Cell Rep.* 17, 2101–2111. doi: 10.1016/j.celrep.2016.10.054

Segovia, C., Martínez-Fernández, M., Dueñas, M., Rubio, C., López-Calderón, F. F., Costa, C., et al. (2017). Opposing roles of <i<PIK3CA</i< gene alterations to EZH2 signaling in non-muscle invasive bladder cancer. *Oncotarget* 8, 10531–10542. doi: 10.18632/oncotarget.14453

Segovia, C., and Paramio, J. M. (2017). Ezh2-dependent therapies in bladder cancer: Synthetic lethality. *Ann. Transl. Med.* 5, 3–6. doi: 10.21037/atm.2017.10.08

Segovia, C., San José-Enériz, E., Munera-Maravilla, E., Martínez-Fernández, M., Garate, L., Miranda, E., et al. (2019). Inhibition of a G9a/DNMT network triggers immune-mediated bladder cancer regression. *Nat. Med.* 25, 1073–1081. doi: 10.1038/s41591-019-0499-y

Serizawa, R. R., Ralfkiaer, U., Steven, K., Lam, G. W., Schmiedel, S., Schüz, J., et al. (2011). Integrated genetic and epigenetic analysis of bladder cancer reveals an additive diagnostic value of FGFR3 mutations and hypermethylation events. *Int. J. Cancer* 129, 78–87. doi: 10.1002/ijc.25651

Shah, M. Y., and Calin, G. A. (2014). MicroRNAs as therapeutic targets in human cancers. *Wiley Interdiscip. Rev. RNA* 5, 537–548. doi: 10.1002/wrna.1229

Shah, S. H., Miller, P., Garcia-Contreras, M., Ao, Z., Machlin, L., Issa, E., et al (2015). Hierarchical paracrine interaction of breast cancer associated fibroblasts with cancer cells *via* hMAPK-microRNAs to drive ER-negative breast cancer phenotype. *Cancer Biol. Ther.* 16, 1671–1681. doi: 10.1080/15384047.2015.1071742

Shang, D., Liu, Y., Matsui, Y., Ito, N., Nishiyama, H., Kamoto, T., et al. (2008). Demethylating Agent 5-Aza-2′-Deoxycytidine Enhances Susceptibility of Bladder Transitional Cell Carcinoma to Cisplatin. *Urology* 71, 1220–1225. doi: 10.1016/J.UROLOGY.2007.11.029

Shankar, S. R., Bahirvani, A. G., Rao, V. K., Bharathy, N., Ow, J. R., and Taneja, R. (2013). G9a, a multipotent regulator of gene expression. *Epigenetics* 8, 16–22. doi: 10.4161/epi.23331

Sharma, A., Jamil, M. A., Nuesgen, N., Dauksa, A., Gulbinas, A., Schulz, W. A., et al. (2019). Detailed methylation map of LINE-1 5′-promoter region reveals hypomethylated CpG hotspots associated with tumor tissue specificity. *Mol. Genet. Genomic Med.* 7, e601. doi: 10.1002/mgg3.601

Shi, H., Jiang, H., Wang, L., Cao, Y., Liu, P., Xu, X., et al. (2015). Overexpression of monocarboxylate anion transporter 1 and 4 in T24-induced cancer-associated fibroblasts regulates the progression of bladder cancer cells in a 3D microfluidic device. *Cell Cycle* 14, 3058–3065. doi: 10.1080/15384101.2015.1053666

Simm, C., Caridis, A., Di Maio, A., Knowles, P., Gorman, B., Jones, R., et al. (2018). Targeting of BRD4 with JQ1, combined with mitomycin C as a novel combination therapy for non-muscle invasive bladder cancer. *Eur. Urol. Suppl.* 17, e663. doi: 10.1016/S1569-9056(18)31300-9

Simon, J. M., Parker, J. S., Liu, F., Rothbart, S. B., Ait-Si-ali, S., Strahl, B. D., et al (2015). A role for widely interspaced zinc finger (WIZ) in retention of the G9a methyltransferase on chromatin. *J. Biol. Chem.* 290, 26088–26102. doi: 10.1074/jbc.M115.654459

Siomi, M. C., Sato, K., Pezic, D., and Aravin, A. A. (2011). PIWI-interacting small RNAs: the vanguard of genome defence. *Nat. Rev. Mol. Cell Biol.* 12, 246–258. doi: 10.1038/nrm3089

Smith, Z. D., and Meissner, A. (2013). DNA methylation: roles in mammalian development. *Nat. Rev. Genet.* 14, 204–220. doi: 10.1038/nrg3354

Sohel, M. H. (2016). Extracellular/Circulating MicroRNAs: Release Mechanisms, Functions and Challenges. *Achiev. Life Sci.* 10, 175–186. doi: 10.1016/j.als.2016.11.007

Sonpavde, G., and Bellmunt, J. (2016). Angiogenesis as a therapeutic target in urothelial carcinoma. *Nat. Rev. Urol.* 13, 306–307. doi: 10.1038/nrurol.2016.69

Stenzl, A., Cowan, N. C., De Santis, M., Kuczyk, M. A., Merseburger, A. S., Ribal, M. J., et al. (2011). Treatment of Muscle-invasive and Metastatic Bladder Cancer: Update of the EAU Guidelines. *Eur. Urol.* 59, 1009–1018. doi: 10.1016/j.eururo.2011.03.023

Stone, O. A., El-Brolosy, M., Wilhelm, K., Liu, X., Romão, A. M., Grillo, E., et al (2018). Loss of pyruvate kinase M2 limits growth and triggers innate immune signaling in endothelial cells. *Nat. Commun.* 9, 4077. doi: 10.1038/s41467-018-06406-8

Stubendorff, B., Wilhelm, K., Posselt, K., Catto, J., Hartmann, A., Bertz, S., et al. (2019). A three-gene methylation marker panel for the nodal metastatic risk assessment of muscle-invasive bladder cancer Keywords Muscle-invasive bladder cancer · Methylation · Biomarker · Metastasis. *J. Cancer Res. Clin. Oncol.* 145, 811–820. doi: 10.1007/s00432-018-02829-4

Su, H., Tao, T., Yang, Z., Kang, X., Zhang, X., Kang, D., et al. (2019). Circular RNA cTFRC acts as the sponge of MicroRNA-107 to promote bladder carcinoma progression. *Mol. Cancer* 18, 27. doi: 10.1186/s12943-019-0951-0

Su, S.-F., de Castro Abreu, A. L., Chihara, Y., Tsai, Y., Andreu-Vieyra, C., Daneshmand, S., et al. (2014). A panel of three markers hyper- and hypomethylated in urine sediments accurately predicts bladder cancer recurrence. *Clin. Cancer Res.* 20, 1978–1989. doi: 10.1158/1078-0432.CCR-13-2637

Sukari, A., Nagasaka, M., Al-Hadidi, A., and Lum, L. G. (2016). Cancer immunology and immunotherapy. *Anticancer Res.* 36, 5593–5606. doi: 10.21873/anticanres.11144

Sun, H., Tian, J., Xian, W., Xie, T., and Yang, X. (2015). miR-34a inhibits proliferation and invasion of bladder cancer cells by targeting orphan nuclear receptor HNF4G. *Dis. Markers* 2015, 1–8. doi: 10.1155/2015/879254

Sundar Rajan, V., Laurent, V. M., Verdier, C., and Duperray, A. (2017). Unraveling the receptor-ligand interactions between bladder cancer cells and the endothelium using AFM. *Biophys. J.* 112, 1246–1257. doi: 10.1016/j.bpj.2017.01.033

Tada, Y., Wada, M., Kuroiwa, K., Kinugawa, N., Harada, T., Nagayama, J., et al. (2000). MRD1 gene overexpression and altered degree of methylation at the promoter region in bladder cancer during chemotherapeutic treatment. *Clin. Cancer Res.* 6, 4618–4627.

Taheri, M., Omrani, M. D., and Ghafouri-Fard, S. (2018). Long non-coding RNA expression in bladder cancer. *Biophys. Rev.* 10, 1205–1213. doi: 10.1007/s12551-017-0379-y

Takeuchi, A., Shiota, M., Tatsugami, K., Yokomizo, A., Tanaka, S., Kuroiwa, K., et al. (2012). P300 Mediates cellular resistance to doxorubicin in bladder cancer. *Mol. Med. Rep.* 5, 173–176. doi: 10.3892/mmr.2011.593

Tan, Y., Wang, L., Du, Y., Liu, X., Chen, Z., Weng, X., et al. (2018). Inhibition of BRD4 suppresses tumor growth in prostate cancer *via the* enhancement of FOXO1 expression. *Int. J. Oncol.* 53, 2503–2517. doi: 10.3892/ijo.2018.4577

Tao, L., Huang, G., Song, H., Chen, Y., and Chen, L. (2017). Cancer associated fibroblasts: an essential role in the tumor microenvironment. *Oncol. Lett.* 14, 2611–2620. doi: 10.3892/ol.2017.6497

Taubert, H., Wach, S., Jung, R., Pugia, M., and Keck, B. (2015). Piwil 2 expression is correlated with disease-specific and progression-free survival of chemotherapy-treated bladder cancer patients. *Mol. Med.* 21, 371–380. doi: 10.2119/molmed.2014.00250

Taverna, S. D., Li, H., Ruthenburg, A. J., Allis, C. D., and Patel, D. J. (2007). How chromatin-binding modules interpret histone modifications: lessons from professional pocket pickers. *Nat. Struct. Mol. Biol.* 14, 1025–1040. doi: 10.1038/nsmb1338

Tian, Z., Cao, S., Li, C., Xu, M., Wei, H., Yang, H., et al. (2019). LncRNA PVT1 regulates growth, migration, and invasion of bladder cancer by miR-31/*CDK1*. *J. Cell. Physiol.* 234, 4799–4811. doi: 10.1002/jcp.27279

Tolkach, Y., Stahl, A. F., Niehoff, E. M., Zhao, C., Kristiansen, G., Müller, S. C., et al. (2017). YRNA expression predicts survival in bladder cancer patients. *BMC Cancer* 17, 1–7. doi: 10.1186/s12885-017-3746-y

Tsai, H.-C., and Baylin, S. B. (2011). Cancer epigenetics: linking basic biology to clinical medicine. *Cell Res.* 21, 502–517. doi: 10.1038/cr.2011.24

Vafaee, F., Colvin, E. K., Mok, S. C., Howell, V. M., and Samimi, G. (2017). Functional prediction of long non-coding RNAs in ovarian cancer-Associated fibroblasts indicate a potential role in metastasis. *Sci. Rep.* 7, 10374. doi: 10.1038/s41598-017-10869-y

Valenzuela, M. T., Galisteo, R., Zuluaga, A., Villalobos, M., Núñez, M. I., Oliver, F. J., et al. (2002). Assessing the use of p16(INK4a) promoter gene methylation in serum for detection of bladder cancer. *Eur. Urol.* 42, 622–628. discussion 628-30.

van der Heijden, A. G., Mengual, L., Ingelmo-Torres, M., Lozano, J. J., van Rijt-van de Westerlo, C. C. M., Baixauli, M., et al. (2018). Urine cell-based DNA methylation classifier for monitoring bladder cancer. *Clin. Epigenet.* 10, 1–10. doi: 10.1186/s13148-018-0496-x

van Kessel, K. E. M., Beukers, W., Lurkin, I., Ziel-van der Made, A., van der Keur, K. A., Boormans, J. L., et al. (2017). Validation of a DNA Methylation-Mutation Urine Assay to Select Patients with Hematuria for Cystoscopy. *J. Urol.* 197, 590–595. doi: 10.1016/j.juro.2016.09.118

van Rhijn, B. W. G., Burger, M., Lotan, Y., Solsona, E., Stief, C. G., Sylvester, R. J., et al. (2009). Recurrence and progression of disease in non-muscle-invasive bladder cancer: from epidemiology to treatment strategy. *Eur. Urol.* 56, 430–442. doi: 10.1016/j.eururo.2009.06.028

Van Rhijn, B. W. G., Van Der Kwast, T. H., Liu, L., Fleshner, N. E., Bostrom, P. J., Vis, A. N., et al. (2012). The FGFR3 mutation is related to favorable pT1 bladder cancer. *J. Urol.* 187, 310–314. doi: 10.1016/j.juro.2011.09.008

Vedadi, M., Barsyte-lovejoy, D., Liu, F., Rival-gervier, S., Allali-hassani, A., Labrie, V., et al. (2012). A chemical probe selectively inhibits G9a and GLP methyltransferase and genanylgeranyltransferase I with antitumor activity against brest cancer *in vivo*. *Nat. Chem. Biol.* 7, 566–574. doi: 10.1038/nchembio.599.A

Villar-garea, A., Fraga, M. F., Espada, J., and Esteller, M. (2003). Procaine Is a DNA-demethylating Agent with Growth-inhibitory Effects in Human. *Cancer Res.* 63, 4984–4989.

Viré, E., Brenner, C., Deplus, R., Blanchon, L., Fraga, M., Didelot, C., et al. (2006). The Polycomb group protein EZH2 directly controls DNA methylation. *Nature* 439, 871–874. doi: 10.1038/nature04431

Vivier, E., Tomasello, E., Baratin, M., Walzer, T., and Ugolini, S. (2008). Functions of natural killer cells. *Nat. Immunol.* 9, 503–510. doi: 10.1038/ni1582

Vo, J. N., Cieslik, M., Zhang, Y., Shukla, S., Xiao, L., Zhang, Y., et al. (2019). The landscape of circular RNA in cancer. *Cell* 176, 869–881.e13. doi: 10.1016/j.cell.2018.12.021

Wagner, E. K., Nath, N., Flemming, R., Feltenberger, J. B., and Denu, J. M. (2012). Identification and characterization of small molecule inhibitors of a plant homeodomain finger. *Biochemistry* 51, 8293–8306. doi: 10.1021/bi3009278

Wang, D., Quiros, J., Mahuron, K., Pai, C.-C., Ranzani, V., Young, A., et al. (2018a). Targeting EZH2 reprograms intratumoral regulatory T cells to enhance cancer immunity. *Cell Rep.* 23, 3262–3274. doi: 10.1016/j.celrep.2018.05.050

Wang, K. C., and Chang, H. Y. (2011). Molecular mechanisms of long noncoding RNAs. *Mol. Cell* 43, 904–914. doi: 10.1016/j.molcel.2011.08.018

Wang, M., Guo, C., Wang, L., Luo, G., Huang, C., Li, Y., et al. (2018b). Long noncoding RNA GAS5 promotes bladder cancer cells apoptosis through inhibiting EZH2 transcription. *Cell Death Dis.* 9, 238. doi: 10.1038/s41419-018-0264-z

Wang, P., Nishitani, M.-A., Tanimoto, S., Kishimoto, T., Fukumori, T., Takahashi, M., et al. (2007). Bladder cancer cell invasion is enhanced by cross-talk with fibroblasts through hepatocyte growth factor. *Urology* 69, 780–784. doi: 10.1016/j.urology.2007.01.063

Wang, S., Chen, J., Garcia, S. P., Liang, X., Zhang, F., Yan, P., et al. (2019). A dynamic and integrated epigenetic program at distal regions orchestrates transcriptional responses to VEGFA. *Genome Res.* 29, 193–207. doi: 10.1101/gr.239053.118

Wang, X.-S., Zhang, Z., Wang, H.-C., Cai, J.-L., Xu, Q.-W., Li, M.-Q., et al. (2006). Rapid Identification of UCA1 as a very sensitive and specific unique marker for human bladder carcinoma. *Clin. Cancer Res.* 12, 4851–4858. doi: 10.1158/1078-0432.CCR-06-0134

Wang, Y. M., Gu, M. L., Meng, F. S., Jiao, W. R., Zhou, X. X., Yao, H. P., et al. (2017). Histone acetyltransferase p300/CBP inhibitor C646 blocks the survival and invasion pathways of gastric cancer cell lines. *Int. J. Oncol.* 51 (6), 1860–1868. doi: 10.3892/ijo.2017.4176

Wang, Y., Xiang, W., Wang, M., Huang, T., Xiao, X., Wang, L., et al. (2014). Methyl jasmonate sensitizes human bladder cancer cells to gambogic acid-induced apoptosis through down-regulation of EZH2 expression by miR-101. *Br. J. Pharmacol.* 171, 618–635. doi: 10.1111/bph.12501

Weber, J. A., Baxter, D. H., Zhang, S., Huang, D. Y., How Huang, K., Jen Lee, M., et al. (2010). The MicroRNA Spectrum in 12 Body Fluids. *Clin. Chem.* 56, 1733–1741. doi: 10.1373/clinchem.2010.147405

Weinstein, J. N., Akbani, R., Broom, B. M., Wang, W., Verhaak, R. G. W., McConkey, D., et al. (2014). Comprehensive molecular characterization of urothelial bladder carcinoma. *Nature* 507, 315–322. doi: 10.1038/nature12965

Wiklund, E. D., Bramsen, J. B., Hulf, T., Dyrskjøt, L., Ramanathan, R., Hansen, T. B., et al. (2011). Coordinated epigenetic repression of the miR-200 family and miR-205 in invasive bladder cancer. *Int. J. Cancer* 128, 1327–1334. doi: 10.1002/ijc.25461

Winquist, E., Knox, J., Wood, L., Wainman, N., Reid, G. K., Pearce, L., et al., (2006). "Phase II trial of DNA methyltransferase 1 inhibition with the antisense oligonucleotide MG98 in patients with metastatic renal carcinoma," in *A National Cancer Institute of Canada Clinical Trials Group investigational new drug study. Invest. New Drugs* 24, 159–160. doi: 10.1007/s10637-006-5938-1

Witjes, J. A., Compérat, E., Cowan, N. C., De Santis, M., Gakis, G., Lebret, T., et al. (2014a). EAU guidelines on muscle-invasive and metastatic bladder cancer: summary of the 2013 guidelines. *Eur. Urol.* 65, 778–792. doi: 10.1016/j.eururo.2013.11.046

Witjes, J. A., Compérat, E., Cowan, N. C., De Santis, M., Gakis, G., Lebret, T., et al. (2014b). EAU guidelines on muscle-invasive and metastatic bladder cancer: summary of the 2013 guidelines. *Eur. Urol.* 65, 778–792. doi: 10.1016/j.eururo.2013.11.046

Wolff, E. M., Chihara, Y., Pan, F., Weisenberger, D. J., Siegmund, K. D., Sugano, K., et al. (2010). Unique DNA methylation patterns distinguish noninvasive and invasive urothelial cancers and establish an epigenetic field defect in premalignant tissue. *Cancer Res.* 70, 8169–8178. doi: 10.1158/0008-5472.CAN-10-1335

Wu, J., Li, W., Ning, J., Yu, W., Rao, T., and Cheng, F. (2019a). Long noncoding RNA UCA1 targets miR-582-5p and contributes to the progression and drug resistance of bladder cancer cells through ATG7-mediated autophagy inhibition. *Oncol. Targets Ther.* 12, 495–508. doi: 10.2147/OTT.S183940

Wu, J., Yu, C., Cai, L., Lu, Y., Jiang, L., Liu, C., et al. (2017). Effects of increased Kindlin-2 expression in bladder cancer stromal fibroblasts. *Oncotarget* 8, 50692–50703. doi: 10.18632/oncotarget.17021

Wu, M., Sheng, L., Cheng, M., Zhang, H., Jiang, Y., Lin, S., et al. (2019b). Low doses of decitabine improve the chemotherapy efficacy against basal-like bladder cancer by targeting cancer stem cells. *Oncogene* 38, 5425–5439. doi: 10.1038/s41388-019-0799-1

Wu, S., Yang, Z., Ye, R., An, D., Li, C., Wang, Y., et al. (2016a). Novel variants in MLL confer to bladder cancer recurrence identified by whole-exome sequencing. *Oncotarget* 7, 2629–2645. doi: 10.18632/oncotarget.6380

Wu, X., Liu, D., Tao, D., Xiang, W., Xiao, X., Wang, M., et al. (2016b). BRD4 Regulates EZH2 transcription through upregulation of C-MYC and represents a novel therapeutic target in bladder cancer. *Mol. Cancer Ther.* 15, 1029–1042. doi: 10.1158/1535-7163.MCT-15-0750

Wu, Z., Huang, W., Wang, X., Wang, T., Chen, Y., Chen, B., et al. (2018). Circular RNA CEP128 acts as a sponge of miR-145-5p in promoting the bladder cancer progression *via* regulating SOX11. *Mol. Med.* 24, 40. doi: 10.1186/s10020-018-0039-0

Xie, F., Li, Y., Wang, M., Huang, C., Tao, D., Zheng, F., et al. (2018). Circular RNA BCRC-3 suppresses bladder cancer proliferation through miR-182-5p/p27 axis. *Mol. Cancer* 17, 144. doi: 10.1186/s12943-018-0892-z

Xie, H., Liao, X., Chen, Z., Fang, Y., He, A., Zhong, Y., et al. (2017a). LncRNA MALAT1 inhibits apoptosis and promotes invasion by antagonizing miR-125b in bladder cancer cells. *J. Cancer* 8, 3803–3811. doi: 10.7150/jca.21228

Xie, Y., Ma, X., Chen, L., Li, H., Gu, L., Gao, Y., et al. (2017b). MicroRNAs with prognostic significance in bladder cancer: A systematic review and meta-analysis. *Sci. Rep.* 7, 5619. doi: 10.1038/s41598-017-05801-3

Xue, M., Pang, H., Li, X., Li, H., Pan, J., and Chen, W. (2016). Long non-coding RNA urothelial cancer-associated 1 promotes bladder cancer cell migration and invasion by way of the hsa-miR-145-ZEB1/2-FSCN1 pathway. *Cancer Sci.* 107, 18–27. doi: 10.1111/cas.12844

Xylinas, E., Hassler, M. R., Zhuang, D., Krzywinski, M., Erdem, Z., Robinson, B. D., et al. (2016). An epigenomic approach to improving response to neoadjuvant cisplatin chemotherapy in bladder cancer. *Biomolecules* 6, 37. doi: 10.3390/biom6030037

Yamaguchi, H., and Hung, M.-C. (2014). Regulation and Role of EZH2 in Cancer. *Cancer Res. Treat.* 46, 209–222. doi: 10.4143/crt.2014.46.3.209

Yamamoto, K., Tateishi, K., Kudo, Y., Hoshikawa, M., Tanaka, M., Nakatsuka, T., et al. (2016). Stromal remodeling by the BET bromodomain inhibitor JQ1 suppresses the progression of human pancreatic cancer. *Oncotarget* 7, 61469–61484. doi: 10.18632/oncotarget.11129

Yang, C., Yuan, W., Yang, X., Li, P., Wang, J., Han, J., et al. (2018a). Circular RNA circ-ITCH inhibits bladder cancer progression by sponging miR-17/miR-224 and regulating p21, PTEN expression. *Mol. Cancer* 17, 19. doi: 10.1186/s12943-018-0771-7

Yang, G.-J., Lei, P.-M., Wong, S., Ma, D.-L., and Leung, C.-H. (2018b). Pharmacological inhibition of LSD1 for cancer treatment. *Molecules* 23 (12), 3194. doi: 10.3390/molecules23123194

Yang, X., Han, H., De Carvalho, D. D., Lay, F. D., Jones, P. A., and Liang, G. (2014). Gene body methylation can alter gene expression and is a therapeutic target in cancer. *Cancer Cell* 26, 577–590. doi: 10.1016/j.ccr.2014.07.028

Yang, X., Yuan, W., Tao, J., Li, P., Yang, C., Deng, X., et al. (2017). Identification of circular RNA signature in bladder cancer. *J. Cancer* 8, 3456–3463. doi: 10.7150/jca.19345

Yang, Y., Qu, A., Liu, J., Wang, R., Liu, Y., Li, G., et al. (2015). Serum miR-210 contributes to tumor detection, stage prediction and dynamic surveillance in patients with bladder cancer. *PloS One* 10, e0135168. doi: 10.1371/journal.pone.0135168

Yang, Z., Liu, A., Xiong, Q., Xue, Y., Liu, F., Zeng, S., et al. (2019). Prognostic value of differentially methylated gene profiles in bladder cancer. *J. Cell. Physiol.*, 28515. doi: 10.1002/jcp.28515

Yates, D. R., Rehman, I., Abbod, M. F., Meuth, M., Cross, S. S., Linkens, D. A., et al. (2007). Promoter hypermethylation identifies progression risk in bladder cancer. *Clin. Cancer Res.* 13, 2046–2053. doi: 10.1158/1078-0432.CCR-06-2476

Yeh, C. R., Hsu, I., Song, W., Chang, H., Miyamoto, H., Xiao, G. Q., et al. (2015). Fibroblast ERalpha promotes bladder cancer invasion *via* increasing the CCL1 and IL-6 signals in the tumor microenvironment. *Am. J. Cancer Res.* 5, 1146–1157.

Yoon, C. Y., Park, M. J., Lee, J. S., Lee, S. C., Oh, J. J., Park, H., et al. (2011). The histone deacetylase inhibitor trichostatin a synergistically resensitizes a cisplatin resistant human bladder cancer cell line. *J. Urol.* 185, 1102–1111. doi: 10.1016/j.juro.2010.10.034

Yu, C., Longfei, L., Long, W., Feng, Z., Chen, J., Chao, L., et al. (2019). LncRNA PVT1 regulates VEGFC through inhibiting miR-128 in bladder cancer cells. *J. Cell. Physiol.* 234, 1346–1353. doi: 10.1002/jcp.26929

Yu, G., Yao, W., Xiao, W., Li, H., Xu, H., and Lang, B. (2014). MicroRNA-34a functions as an anti-metastatic microRNA and suppresses angiogenesis in bladder cancer by directly targeting CD44. *J. Exp. Clin. Cancer Res.* 33, 779. doi: 10.1186/s13046-014-0115-4

Yu, J., Walter, K., Omura, N., Hong, S.-M., Young, A., Li, A., et al. (2012). Unlike pancreatic cancer cells pancreatic cancer associated fibroblasts display minimal gene induction after 5-Aza-2′-Deoxycytidine. *PloS One* 7, e43456. doi: 10.1371/journal.pone.0043456

Yu, T., Wang, Y., Hu, Q., Wu, W., Wu, Y., and Wei, W., (2017). The EZH2 inhibitor GSK343 suppresses cancer stem-like phenotypes and reverses mesenchymal transition in glioma cells. *Oncotarget* 8 (58), 98348–98359. doi: 10.18632/oncotarget.21311

Yuan, T., Huang, X., Woodcock, M., Du, M., Dittmar, R., Wang, Y., et al. (2016). Plasma extracellular RNA profiles in healthy and cancer patients. *Sci. Rep.* 6, 19413. doi: 10.1038/srep19413

Yuan, Y., Wang, Q., Paulk, J., Kubicek, S., Kemp, M. M., Adams, D. J., et al. (2012). A small-molecule probe of the histone methyltransferase G9a induces cellular senescence in pancreatic adenocarcinoma. *ACS Chem. Biol.* 7, 1152–1157. doi: 10.1021/cb300139y

Yun, S. J., Jeong, P., Kim, W.-T., Kim, T. H., Lee, Y.-S., Song, P. H., et al. (2012). Cell-free microRNAs in urine as diagnostic and prognostic biomarkers of bladder cancer. *Int. J. Oncol.* 41, 1871–1878. doi: 10.3892/ijo.2012.1622

Zeisberg, E. M., Potenta, S., Xie, L., Zeisberg, M., and Kalluri, R. (2007). discovery of endothelial to mesenchymal transition as a source for carcinoma-associated fibroblasts. *Cancer Res.* 67, 10123–10128. doi: 10.1158/0008-5472.CAN-07-3127

Zeisberg, E. M., and Zeisberg, M. (2013). The role of promoter hypermethylation in fibroblast activation and fibrogenesis. *J. Pathol.* 229, 264–273. doi: 10.1002/path.4120

Zeng, Z., Zhou, W., Duan, L., Zhang, J., Lu, X., Jin, L., et al. (2019). Circular RNA circ-VANGL1 as a competing endogenous RNA contributes to bladder cancer progression by regulating miR-605-3p/VANGL1 pathway. *J. Cell. Physiol.* 234, 3887–3896. doi: 10.1002/jcp.27162

Zhang, C., Yao, Z., Zhu, M., Ma, X., Shi, T., Li, H., et al. (2012). Inhibitory effects of MicroRNA-34a on cell migration and invasion of invasive urothelial bladder carcinoma by targeting Notch1. *J. Huazhong Univ. Sci. Technol. Med. Sci.* 32, 375–382. doi: 10.1007/s11596-012-0065-z

Zhang, M., and Xin, Y. (2018). Circular RNAs: a new frontier for cancer diagnosis and therapy. *J. Hematol. Oncol.* 11, 21. doi: 10.1186/s13045-018-0569-5

Zhang, Q., Miao, S., Han, X., Li, C., Zhang, M., Cui, K., et al. (2018a). MicroRNA-3619-5p suppresses bladder carcinoma progression by directly targeting β-catenin and CDK2 and activating p21. *Cell Death Dis.* 9, 960. doi: 10.1038/s41419-018-0986-y

Zhang, Q., Zhao, W., Ye, C., Zhuang, J., Chang, C., Li, Y., et al. (2015). Honokiol inhibits bladder tumor growth by suppressing EZH2/miR-143 axis. *Oncotarget* 6, 37335–37348. doi: 10.18632/oncotarget.6135

Zhang, X., Zhang, Y., Liu, X., Fang, A., Wang, J., Yang, Y., et al. (2016). Direct quantitative detection for cell-free miR-155 in urine: a potential role in diagnosis and prognosis for non-muscle invasive bladder cancer. *Oncotarget* 7, 3255–3266. doi: 10.18632/oncotarget.6487

Zhang, Y., Huang, Z., Zhu, Z., Zheng, X., Liu, J., Han, Z., et al. (2014). Upregulated UHRF1 promotes bladder cancer cell invasion by epigenetic silencing of KiSS1. *PloS One* 9(10), e104252. doi: 10.1371/journal.pone.0104252

Zhang, Y., Liang, W., Zhang, P., Chen, J., Qian, H., Zhang, X., et al. (2017). Circular RNAs: emerging cancer biomarkers and targets. *J. Exp. Clin. Cancer Res.* 36, 152. doi: 10.1186/s13046-017-0624-z

Zhang, Y., Tian, S., Xiong, J., Zhou, Y., Song, H., and Liu, C. (2018b). JQ-1 Inhibits colon cancer proliferation *via* suppressing Wnt/β-catenin signaling and miR-21. *Chem. Res. Toxicol.* 31, 302–307. doi: 10.1021/acs.chemrestox.7b00346

Zhao, L., Duan, Y.-T., Lu, P., Zhang, Z.-J., Zheng, X.-K., Wang, J.-L., et al. (2019). Epigenetic targets and their inhibitors in cancer therapy. *Curr. Top. Med. Chem.* 18, 2395–2419. doi: 10.2174/1568026619666181224095449

Zhao, L., Ji, G., Le, X., Wang, C., Xu, L., Feng, M., et al. (2017). Long noncoding rna linc00092 acts in cancer-associated fibroblasts to drive glycolysis and progression of ovarian cancer. *Cancer Res.* 77, 1369–1382. doi: 10.1158/0008-5472.CAN-16-1615

Zhong, Z., Huang, M., Lv, M., He, Y., Duan, C., Zhang, L., et al. (2017). Circular RNA MYLK as a competing endogenous RNA promotes bladder cancer progression through modulating VEGFA/VEGFR2 signaling pathway. *Cancer Lett.* 403, 305–317. doi: 10.1016/j.canlet.2017.06.027

Zhong, Z., Lv, M., and Chen, J. (2016). Screening differential circular RNA expression profiles reveals the regulatory role of circTCF25-miR-103a-3p/miR-107-CDK6 pathway in bladder carcinoma. *Sci. Rep.* 6, 30919. doi: 10.1038/srep30919

Zhou, X., Zhang, X., Yang, Y., Li, Z., Du, L., Dong, Z., et al. (2014). Urinary cell-free microRNA-106b as a novel biomarker for detection of bladder cancer. *Med. Oncol.* 31, 1–7. doi: 10.1007/s12032-014-0197-z

Zhu, J., Jiang, Z., Gao, F., Hu, X., Zhou, L., Chen, J., et al. (2011). A systematic analysis on DNA methylation and the expression of both mRNA and microRNA in bladder cancer. *PloS One* 6, e28223. doi: 10.1371/journal.pone.0028223

Zhu, S., Denman, C. J., Cobanoglu, Z. S., Kiany, S., Lau, C. C., Gottschalk, S. M., et al. (2015). The narrow-spectrum HDAC inhibitor entinostat enhances NKG2D expression without NK cell toxicity, leading to enhanced recognition of cancer cells. *Pharm. Res.* 32, 779–792. doi: 10.1007/s11095-013-1231-0

Zhu, Y., Spitz, M. R., Zhang, H., Grossman, H. B., Frazier, M. L., and Wu, X. (2004). Methyl-CpG-binding domain 2: a protective role in Bladder Carcinoma. *Cancer* 100, 1853–1858. doi: 10.1002/cncr.20199

Zhuang, J., Lu, Q., Shen, B., Huang, X., Shen, L., Zheng, X., et al. (2015). TGFβ1 secreted by cancer-associated fibroblasts induces epithelial-mesenchymal transition of bladder cancer cells through lncRNA-ZEB2NAT. *Sci. Rep.* 11924. doi: 10.1038/srep11924

Ziani, L., Chouaib, S., and Thiery, J. (2018). alteration of the antitumor immune response by cancer-associated fibroblasts. *Front. Immunol.* 9, 414. doi: 10.3389/FIMMU.2018.00414

Zong, Y., Huang, J., Sankarasharma, D., Morikawa, T., Fukayama, M., Epstein, J. I., et al. (2012). Stromal epigenetic dysregulation is sufficient to initiate mouse prostate cancer *via* paracrine Wnt signaling. *Proc. Natl. Acad. Sci.* 109, E3395–E3404. doi: 10.1073/pnas.1217982109

Permissions

All chapters in this book were first published by Frontiers; hereby published with permission under the Creative Commons Attribution License or equivalent. Every chapter published in this book has been scrutinized by our experts. Their significance has been extensively debated. The topics covered herein carry significant findings which will fuel the growth of the discipline. They may even be implemented as practical applications or may be referred to as a beginning point for another development.

The contributors of this book come from diverse backgrounds, making this book a truly international effort. This book will bring forth new frontiers with its revolutionizing research information and detailed analysis of the nascent developments around the world.

We would like to thank all the contributing authors for lending their expertise to make the book truly unique. They have played a crucial role in the development of this book. Without their invaluable contributions this book wouldn't have been possible. They have made vital efforts to compile up to date information on the varied aspects of this subject to make this book a valuable addition to the collection of many professionals and students.

This book was conceptualized with the vision of imparting up-to-date information and advanced data in this field. To ensure the same, a matchless editorial board was set up. Every individual on the board went through rigorous rounds of assessment to prove their worth. After which they invested a large part of their time researching and compiling the most relevant data for our readers.

The editorial board has been involved in producing this book since its inception. They have spent rigorous hours researching and exploring the diverse topics which have resulted in the successful publishing of this book. They have passed on their knowledge of decades through this book. To expedite this challenging task, the publisher supported the team at every step. A small team of assistant editors was also appointed to further simplify the editing procedure and attain best results for the readers.

Apart from the editorial board, the designing team has also invested a significant amount of their time in understanding the subject and creating the most relevant covers. They scrutinized every image to scout for the most suitable representation of the subject and create an appropriate cover for the book.

The publishing team has been an ardent support to the editorial, designing and production team. Their endless efforts to recruit the best for this project, has resulted in the accomplishment of this book. They are a veteran in the field of academics and their pool of knowledge is as vast as their experience in printing. Their expertise and guidance has proved useful at every step. Their uncompromising quality standards have made this book an exceptional effort. Their encouragement from time to time has been an inspiration for everyone.

The publisher and the editorial board hope that this book will prove to be a valuable piece of knowledge for researchers, students, practitioners and scholars across the globe.

List of Contributors

Alka Singh and Manisha Sachan
Department of Biotechnology, Motilal Nehru National Institute of Technology, Allahabad, India

Sameer Gupta
Department of Surgical Oncology, King George Medical University, Lucknow, India

Tong Wang and Hui Gao
State Key Laboratory of Stem Cell and Reproductive Biology, Institute of Zoology, Chinese Academy of Sciences, Beijing, China

Wei Li and Chao Liu
State Key Laboratory of Stem Cell and Reproductive Biology, Institute of Zoology, Chinese Academy of Sciences, Beijing, China
College of Life Sciences, University of Chinese Academy of Sciences, Beijing, China

Xichun Wang, Sergio Branciamore, Grigoriy Gogoshin, Shuyu Ding and Andrei S. Rodin
Department of Computational and Quantitative Medicine, Beckman Research Institute and Diabetes and Metabolism Research Institute of the City of Hope, Duarte, CA, United States

Xin Feng
Department of Epidemiology and Biostatistics, School of Public Health, Jilin University, Changchun, China
Jilin Institute of Chemical Technology, Jilin, China
BioKnow Health Informatics Lab, College of Computer Science and Technology, and Key Laboratory of Symbolic Computation and Knowledge Engineering of Ministry of Education, Jilin University, Changchun, China

Xubing Hao
BioKnow Health Informatics Lab, College of Software, and Key Laboratory of Symbolic Computation and Knowledge Engineering of Ministry of Education, Jilin University, Changchun, China

Ruoyao Shi
BioKnow Health Informatics Lab, College of Life Sciences, Jilin University, Changchun, China

Zhiqiang Xia and Fengfeng Zhou
BioKnow Health Informatics Lab, College of Computer Science and Technology, and Key Laboratory of Symbolic Computation and Knowledge Engineering of Ministry of Education, Jilin University, Changchun, China

Lan Huang
College of Computer Science and Technology, and Key Laboratory of Symbolic Computation and Knowledge Engineering of Ministry of Education, Jilin University, Changchun, China

Qiong Yu
Department of Epidemiology and Biostatistics, School of Public Health, Jilin University, Changchun, China

Wenjing Zhang
NHC Key Laboratory of Reproduction Regulation (Shanghai Institute of Planned Parenthood Research), Fudan University, Shanghai, China
Reproductive Medical Center, Changhai Hospital of Shanghai, Shanghai, China

Min Li, Zhaofeng Zhang, Junwei Liu, Xiaowei Sun, Yupei Shen, Jianhua Xu, Maohua Miao, Bin Wu, Yao Yuan, Huijuan Shi and Jing Du
NHC Key Laboratory of Reproduction Regulation (Shanghai Institute of Planned Parenthood Research), Fudan University, Shanghai, China

Feng Sun
Department of Obstetrics and Gynecology, International Peace Maternity and Child Health Hospital, Shanghai Jiao Tong University, Shanghai, China

Xuting Xu
Huzhou Key Laboratory of Molecular Medicine, Huzhou Central Hospital, Zhejiang, China

Aiping Zhang
Bio-X Institutes, Key Laboratory for the Genetics of Developmental and Neuropsychiatric Disorders, Ministry of Education, Shanghai Jiao Tong University, Shanghai, China

Xianliang Huang
Shanghai Institute of Planned Parenthood Research Hospital, Shanghai, China

Michela Bottani
IRCCS Istituto Ortopedico Galeazzi, Laboratory of Experimental Biochemistry & Moelcular Biology, Milano, Italy

Giuseppe Banfi
IRCCS Istituto Ortopedico Galeazzi, Laboratory of Experimental Biochemistry & Moelcular Biology, Milano, Italy
Vita-Salute San Raffaele University, Milano, Italy

Giovanni Lombardi
IRCCS Istituto Ortopedico Galeazzi, Laboratory of Experimental Biochemistry & Molecular Biology, Milano, Italy
Department of Physiology & Pharmacology, Gdańsk University of Physical Education & Sport, Gdańsk, Poland

Zhiwei Qiao, Ying Jiang, Ling Wang, Lei Wang, Jing Jiang and Jingru Zhang
The Department of Gynaecology, Liaoning Cancer Hospital & Institute, Cancer Hospital of China Medical University, Shengyang, China

Marcelo L. Ribeiro
Laboratory of Experimental Hematology, Department of Hematology, Vall d'Hebron Institute of Oncology (VHIO), Vall d'Hebron University Hospital, Autonomous University of Barcelona, Barcelona, Spain
Laboratory of Immunopharmacology and Molecular Biology, Sao Francisco University Medical School, Braganca Paulista, São Paulo, Brazil

Diana Reyes-Garau, Marc Armengol, Miranda Fernández-Serrano and Gaël Roué
Laboratory of Experimental Hematology, Department of Hematology, Vall d'Hebron Institute of Oncology (VHIO), Vall d'Hebron University Hospital, Autonomous University of Barcelona, Barcelona, Spain

Carlos Eduardo Fonseca-Alves
Institute of Health Sciences, Paulista University—UNIP, Bauru, Brazil
Department of Veterinary Surgery and Anesthesiology, School of Veterinary Medicine and Animal Science, Sao Paulo State University—UNESP, Botucatu, Brazil

Priscila Emiko Kobayashi and Antonio Fernando Leis-Filho
Department of Veterinary Clinic, School of Veterinary Medicine and Animal Science, Sao Paulo State University—UNESP, Botucatu, Brazil

Patricia de Faria Lainetti and Renee Laufer-Amorim
Department of Veterinary Surgery and Anesthesiology, School of Veterinary Medicine and Animal Science, Sao Paulo State University—UNESP, Botucatu, Brazil

Valeria Grieco
Department of Veterinary Medicine, Università degli studi di Milano, Milan, Italy

Hellen Kuasne
International Center for Research (CIPE), AC Camargo Cancer Center, Sao Paulo, Brazil

Silvia Regina Rogatto
Department of Clinical Genetics, University Hospital of Southern Denmark, Institute of Regional Health Research, University of Southern Denmark, Vejle, Denmark

Nelson Varela
Laboratory of Chemical Carcinogenesis and Pharmacogenetics, Department of Basic-Clinical Oncology, Faculty of Medicine, Universidad de Chile, Santiago, Chile

Fernando Lanas
Department of Internal Medicine, Faculty of Medicine, Universidad de La Frontera, Temuco, Chile
Center of Molecular Biology and Pharmacogenetics, Scientific and Technological Bioresource Nucleus, Universidad de La Frontera, Temuco, Chile

Luis A. Salazar
Center of Molecular Biology and Pharmacogenetics, Scientific and Technological Bioresource Nucleus, Universidad de La Frontera, Temuco, Chile

Tomás Zambrano
Department of Medical Technology, Faculty of Medicine, Universidad de Chile, Santiago, Chile

Carolina Soler-Botija and Carolina Gálvez-Montón
Heart Failure and Cardiac Regeneration (ICREC) Research Program, Health Science Research Institute Germans Trias i Pujol (IGTP), Badalona, Spain
CIBERCV, Instituto de Salud Carlos III, Madrid, Spain

Antoni Bayés-Genís
Heart Failure and Cardiac Regeneration (ICREC) Research Program, Health Science Research Institute Germans Trias i Pujol (IGTP), Badalona, Spain
CIBERCV, Instituto de Salud Carlos III, Madrid, Spain
Cardiology Service, HUGTiP, Badalona, Spain
Department of Medicine, Barcelona Autonomous University (UAB), Badalona, Spain

Clara Snijders, Barbie Machiels, Gunter Kenis, Daniel van den Hove, Bart P. F. Rutten and Laurence de Nijs
Department of Psychiatry and Neuropsychology, School for Mental Health and Neuroscience, Maastricht University, Maastricht, Netherlands

Julian Krauskopf and Jos Kleinjans
Department of Toxicogenomics, Maastricht University, Maastricht, Netherlands

Marco P. M. Boks
UMC Utrecht Brain Center, Department of Psychiatry, Utrecht, Netherlands

Ehsan Pishva
Department of Psychiatry and Neuropsychology, School for Mental Health and Neuroscience, Maastricht University, Maastricht, Netherlands
College of Medicine and Health, University of Exeter Medical School, Exeter, United Kingdom
Department of Psychiatry, New York University School of Medicine, New York, United States

Lars Eijssen
Department of Psychiatry and Neuropsychology, School for Mental Health and Neuroscience, Maastricht University, Maastricht, Netherlands
Department of Bioinformatics (BiGCaT), NUTRIM School of Nutrition and Translational Research in Metabolism, Maastricht University, Maastricht, Netherlands

Myeong Ok Kim
Division of Applied Life Science (BK 21), College of Natural Sciences, Gyeongsang National University, Jinju, South Korea

Christiaan H. Vinkers
Amsterdam UMC (location VUmc), Department of Anatomy and Neurosciences, Amsterdam, Netherlands
Amsterdam UMC (location VUmc), Department of Psychiatry, Amsterdam, Netherlands

Eric Vermetten
Arq, Psychotrauma Research Expert Group, Diemen, Netherlands
Department of Psychiatry, Leiden University Medical Center, Leiden, Netherlands
Military Mental Healthcare, Netherlands Ministry of Defense, Utrecht, Netherlands

Elbert Geuze
UMC Utrecht Brain Center, Department of Psychiatry, Utrecht, Netherlands

Mónica Martínez-Fernández
Genomes & Disease Lab, CiMUS (Center for Research in Molecular Medicine and Chronic Diseases), Universidade de Santiago de Compostela, Santiago de Compostela, Spain

Victor G. Martinez, Cristian Suarez-Cabrera, Cristina Segovia and Iris Lodewijk
Biomedical Research Institute I + 12, University Hospital 12 de Octubre, Madrid, Spain
Molecular Oncology Unit, CIEMAT (Centro de Investigaciones Energéticas, Medioambientales y Tecnológicas), Madrid, Spain

Ester Munera-Maravilla, Alejandra Bernardini, Carolina Rubio, Marta Dueñas and Jesus Maria Paramio
Biomedical Research Institute I + 12, University Hospital 12 de Octubre, Madrid, Spain
Molecular Oncology Unit, CIEMAT (Centro de Investigaciones Energéticas, Medioambientales y Tecnológicas), Madrid, Spain
Centro de Investigación Biomédica en Red de Cáncer (CIBERONC), Madrid, Spain

Index

www.ingramcontent.com/pod-product-compliance
Lightning Source LLC
LaVergne TN
LVHW082154200926
848484LV00008B/2157

* 9 7 9 8 8 8 7 4 0 3 7 1 7 *